Radiology in
Medical Diagnostics

Evolution of
X-Ray Applications 1895–1995

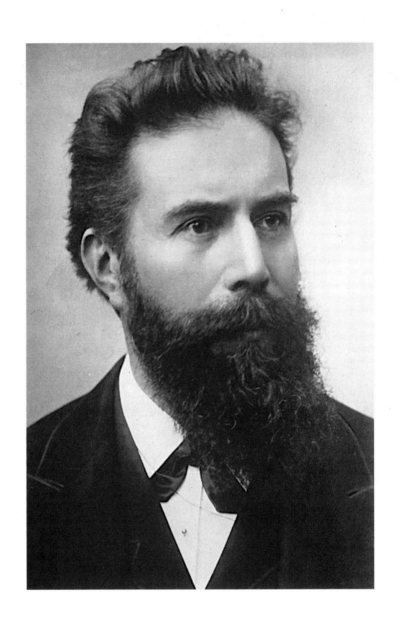

Radiology in Medical Diagnostics

Evolution of
X-Ray Applications 1895–1995

GERD ROSENBUSCH MD
Professor of Abdominal Radiology
Department of Radiology University Hospital St. Radboud
Nijmegen, The Netherlands

MATTHIJS OUDKERK MD, PhD, FACA
Department of Radiology Dr. Daniel den Hoed Cancer Center
University Hospital Rotterdam, The Netherlands

ERNST AMMANN Dr-Ing., Dipl-Ing
Siemens Medical Engineering Group
Erlangen, Germany

WITH CONTRIBUTIONS BY

H. Becker · L. Beltz · E. Boijsen · H. Heintzen · F. Heuck · W. Hoeffken
W.A. Kalender · E. Löhr · J.W. Ludwig · J.-W. Oestmann · P.E. Peters
J.H.J. Ruijs · Th. Schmidt · J.L. Sellink · U. Speck · H.-S. Stender · F.E. Stieve
E. Zeitler · B.G. Ziedses des Plantes (†)

ENGLISH LANGUAGE EDITION

PETER F. WINTER MD
Clinical Assistant Professor of Radiology
University of Illinois
College of Medicine at Peoria

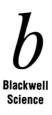

**Blackwell
Science**

© 1994 by
Blackwell Wissenschafts-Verlag
English language edition
© 1995 by
Blackwell Science Ltd
Editorial Offices:
Osney Mead, Oxford OX2 0EL
25 John Street, London WC1N 2BL
23 Ainslie Place, Edinburgh EH3 6AJ
238 Main Street, Cambridge
 Massachusetts 02142, USA
54 University Street, Carlton
 Victoria 3053, Australia

Other Editorial Offices:
Arnette Blackwell SA
1, rue de Lille, 75007 Paris
France

Blackwell Wissenschafts-Verlag GmbH
Kurfürstendamm 57, 10707 Berlin,
Germany
Feldgasse 13, 1238 Vienna, Austria

First published 1994
 (*Radiologie in der medizinischen
 Diagnostik*)
English translation 1995

Printed and bound in Germany

DISTRIBUTORS
Marston Book Services Ltd
PO Box 87
Oxford OX2 0DT
(*Orders:* Tel: 01865 791155
    Fax: 01865 791927
    Telex: 837515)

North America
Blackwell Science, Inc.
238 Main Street
Cambridge, MA 02142
(*Orders:* Tel: 800 215-1000
    617 876-7000
    Fax: 617 492-5263

Australia
Blackwell Science Pty Ltd
54 University Street
Carlton, Victoria 3053
(*Orders:* Tel: 03 347-5552)

A catalogue record for this title is
available from the British Library

ISBN 0-86542-899-9

Preface

'History is the umbilical cord to the present'
ANONYMOUS

The physician's actions are governed by the diagnostic process since it is the diagnosis that determines the therapy. Radiology, together with endoscopy, plays a central role in revealing the morphologic manifestation of a disease process. The morphologic abnormalities have to be correlated with the patient's history, clinical findings and laboratory results. Only the sensible integration of all findings can provide the right guidance for the therapeutic strategy.

The beginning of only a few medical specialities can be dated as precisely as that of radiology: November 1895. In honor of Wilhelm Conrad Roentgen, the discoverer of the new rays that made this speciality possible, it was first called roentgenology but today it is generally referred to as radiology though the original term is still in use. A centennial invites retrospection, which provides the opportunity of reviewing the origin and growth of such a fascinating and influential discipline. Neither the contributing authors nor the editors are historians, but developed an inclination for history through their work on this book, which was initiated by a general interest in the origin and growth of their specialties. Acknowledged specialists from Germany, The Netherlands and Sweden have written about their work and their impact, past and present, often relating their personal involvement and providing a lively account of the events.

The personal approach selected by some contributors to present their subject should enhance the readability. Similarly, the unique style of each presentation and any emphasis on an issue in a particular article should not be seen as detrimental but rather beneficial as to the book's objective. Some contributions are primarily historic reviews, others more scientific treatises and again others presentations of current developments. Repetitions and overlapping of topics were unavoidable. Though not intended, they should be seen positively since they allow selective reading of individual articles.

Recollections of the intellectual background at the time of the discovery of X-rays are followed by descriptions of the emergence of radiology as a diagnostic device within the context of the development of medicine. In the beginning, radiology was only applied for the evaluation of the skeleton, lungs and soft tissues, but its application soon spread to other organs and organ systems, in part advanced through the introduction of appropriate contrast media and in part through the development of tomographic techniques, with the cross-sectional method representing the latest and relatively new addition. The advances in radiographic equipment are described in detail and their effects on image interpretation and diagnostic information are emphasized. The radiologist's world encompasses physics, chemistry, and medicine, with physics and chemistry providing the means to produce images from which medically relevant information can be deduced. Imaging studies not based on X-rays, such as sonography, scintigraphy and magnetic resonance imaging, are not included, and interventional radiology is only briefly mentioned.

The history of radiology cannot be exhausted in one book, and the interested reader, perhaps enticed by one of the contributions, may wish to read more about certain topics. We gratefully consulted the following books: E.R.N. Grigg, The trail of the invisible light, C.C. Thomas, Springfield 1965; A.J. Bruwer (ed.), Classic descriptions in diagnostic roentgenology, 2 volumes, C.C. Thomas, Springfield 1964; R.L. Eisenberg, Radiology, an ilustrated history, Mosby Year Book, St. Louis 1992; and R.F. Mould, A century of X-rays and radioactivity in medicine (with emphasis on photographic records of the early years), Institute of Physics Publishing, Bristol, Philadelphia 1993.

The few historic accounts written in German are Otto Glaser's biography of Roentgen, 2nd edition, Berlin 1959, which includes the early development of roentgenology, R. Schinz's book

60 Jahre Radiologie (60 Years of Radiology), Stuttgart 1959 and Heinz Goerke's book 75 Jahre Deutsche Roentgengesellschaft (75 Years German Roentgen Society), Stuttgart 1980. A few doctoral theses, most of which written under the auspices of Heinz Goerke, deal with specific aspects or pioneers of radiology. Kurt M. Walther, Leer, has written commentaries for anniversaries and several biographic texts on eminent radiologists. It seems that the chronicle of radiology is far from being complete and is in need of further historic studies.

This book presents a journey into the past, but it is not a sentimental journey. The history revealed through this journey illuminates the present state of radiology, which should not only be of interest to those directly working with X-rays but also to general practitioners and specialists who are confronted with radiologic studies in their practice. Furthermore, this text will also be informative for the interested nonmedical reader, despite the unavoidable medical and technical terminology.

We are indebted to many people who have contributed to this book. Dr. Daniel de Moulin, professor of medical history at Nijmegen University, The Netherlands, awakened our interest in the history of radiology at the right time through an exhibition on medical history. Dr. Rudolf Schittenhelm, Kurt Steiner and Kurt Dietz provided valuable input from their many years of working in radiologic engineering.

We thank Barbara Ludwig, Irmgard Otto, Gerlinde Sippel, Charlotte Mikx-Suripatty and Tim Grainacher. Our appreciation belongs to the many translators Penny Klann, Eric Bach, Larry and Susan Ware, A.S. Hay, D.C. Lohrmann, J. McMinn, M.A. Schillhorn, E. Beese and especially to Dr. Peter Winter for revising and editing the English text. Photographic material was contributed by Ursula Buchholz of Siemens Medical Archives, and by Ulrich Hennig and Uwe Busch of the German Roentgen Museum. We thank Guenther Trapp for patent research.

We would like to express our gratitude to Dr. Peter Grassmann, Siemens AG, who supported this project from the very beginning. We are obliged to Rainer Kusche for faithfully shaping our ideas into a book. Last but not least, we thank Dr. Axel Beduerftig, Blackwell Wissenschaft, for taking the risk of publishing this book.

Again we have tried our spouses' understanding and are most grateful for their patience.

Gerd Rosenbusch – Matthijs Oudkerk – Ernst Ammann

Summer 1995

Table of Contents

Preface V

List of Contributors IX

Chapter 1   The invisible light
History

Roentgen in historical perspective
M. Oudkerk, G. Rosenbusch, E. Ammann .   1

A new kind of rays
G. Rosenbusch, M. Oudkerk, E. Ammann .   6

Medical science before 1895
G. Rosenbusch, M. Oudkerk, E. Ammann . 22

The pioneering age of radiology
G. Rosenbusch, M. Oudkerk, E. Ammann . 25

Chapter 2   The invisible light applied
The advancing diagnostic evaluation of the skeleton and thorax following Roentgen's discovery

Introduction
G. Rosenbusch, M. Oudkerk, E. Ammann . 37

Skeleton
F. Heuck 39

Thorax
H. S. Stender, J. Oestmann 67

Soft tissues - mammography
W. Hoeffken 98

Chapter 3   The invisible light captured
Diagnostics of organs by means of artificial absorption changes

Introduction
G. Rosenbusch, M. Oudkerk, E. Ammann . 115

Development of intravascular contrast media
U. Speck 121

Digestive tract
J. L. Sellink 131

Gallbladder and biliary tract
J. H. J. Ruijs 157

Urinary tract
E. Löhr 163

Heart and blood vessels –
evolution of angiography
E. Boijsen 176

Abdominal vessels
E. Boijsen 200

Heart and coronaries – the pioneering age
J.W. Ludwig 213

Heart and coronaries –
evolution of digital angiocardiography
P. H. Heintzen 225

Peripheral vessels
E. Zeitler 236

Lymphatic system
L. Beltz 248

Chapter 4   Invisible light sliced

Improved diagnostics by new representation of anatomy

Introduction
G. Rosenbusch, M. Oudkerk, E. Ammann . 261

Conventional tomography
F. E. Stieve 265

Computer tomography –
technical development
W. A. Kalender 281

Brain and spinal cord – before CT
B. G. A. Ziedses des Plantes, G. Rosenbusch 293

Brain and spinal cord – with CT
H. Becker 305

Torso
P. E. Peters 314

Chapter 5   The invisible light manipulated

Evolution of X-ray technology by interaction of physicians and engineers

Introduction
E. Ammann, M. Oudkerk, G. Rosenbusch . 335

X-ray tubes
E. Ammann, G. Rosenbusch, M. Oudkerk . 338

Generators
E. Ammann, G. Rosenbusch, M. Oudkerk . 357

Tables and stands, patient positioning and systems
E. Ammann, G. Rosenbusch, M. Oudkerk . 397

Fluoroscopy and recording of digital and image intensifier images
E. Ammann, G. Rosenbusch, M. Oudkerk . 440

Roentgen photography
G. Rosenbusch, E. Ammann, M. Oudkerk . 458

Radiation exposure:
changing risk and benefit over time
Th. Schmidt 471

Epilogue

G. Rosenbusch, M. Oudkerk, E. Ammann . 477

List of sources for the illustrations 487

Chronological index 497

Index of Names 501

Subject index 513

List of Contributors

Ernst Ammann, PhD
Siemens Medical
Engineering Group
Henkestraße 127
D-91052 Erlangen

Hartmut Becker, MD
Professor of Neuroradiology
Head of the Neuroradiology
Dept.
University Hospital
Konstanty-Gutschow Straße 8
D-30625 Hannover

Ludwig Beltz, MD
Professor of Radiology
Head of the Radiology Dept.
Maltese Hospital
Von Hompesch Straße 1
D-53123 Bonn

Erik Boijsen, MD PhD
Emeritus Professor of Radiology
Former Chairman of the
Diagnostic Radiology Dept.,
University Lund
Present address:
Thulehem 62
S-22467 Lund

Paul H. Heintzen, MD
Emeritus Professor of Radiology
and Pediatrics
Former Head of the Pediatric
Cardiology Dept. and
Biomedical Technics Dept.
Present address:
Birkenweg 112
D-24211 Preetz

Friedrich Heuck, MD
Emeritus Professor of Radiology
Former Head of the Diagnostic
Radiology Dept.
Katharinen Hospital Stuttgart
Present address:
Hermann Kurz Straße 5
D-70192 Stuttgart

Walther Hoeffken, MD
Professor of Radiology
Machabäerstraße 19-27
D-50668 Köln

Willi Kalender, PhD
Professor of Medical Physics
University of Erlangen-Nürn-
berg
Krankenhausstraße 12
D-91054 Erlangen

Eberhard Löhr, MD
Emeritus Professor of Radiology
Former Chairman of the
Diagnostic Radiology Dept.
University Hospital of Essen
Present address:
Hans Niemeyerstraße 1
D-4147 Essen

Jan W. Ludwig, MD PhD
Radiologist, former Consultant
of the Diagnostic Radiology
Dept.
Anthonius Hospital Utrecht
Present address:
De Holle Wierde
Baarnseweg 41c
NL-3735 ML Bosch en Duin

Jörg-Wilhelm Oestmann, MD
Professor of Radiology
Diagnostic Radiology Dept.
Robert Koch Straße 40
D-37075 Göttingen

Matthijs Oudkerk, MD PhD
FACA
Head of Radiology Dept.
Dr. Daniel den Hoed Cancer
Center
University Hospital Rotterdam
Groene Hilledijk 301
NL-3075 EA Rotterdam

Peter E. Peters, MD
Professor of Radiology and
Chairman of Clinical Radiology
University Hospital
Albert Schweitzer Straße 33
D-48129 Münster

Gerd Rosenbusch, MD
Professor of Abdominal
Radiology
Diagnostic Radiology Dept.
University Hospital St. Radboud
Geert Grooteplein 18
NL-6525 GA Nijmegen

Josephus H.J. Ruijs, MD PhD
Professor of Radiology and
Chairman of Diagnostic
Radiology Dept.
University Hospital St. Radboud
Geert Grooteplein 18
NL-6525 GA Nijmegen

Theodor Schmidt, PhD
Professor of Physics
Head of Medical Physics Dept.
Hospital of Nürnberg
Flurstraße 17
D-90419 Nürnberg

Johan L. Sellink, MD PhD
Emeritus Professor of Radiology
Former Chairman of the
Diagnostic Radiology Dept.
Open University of Amsterdam
Present address:
Groenloseweg 49
NL-7101 AC Winterswijk

Ulrich Speck, PhD
Professor of Chemistry
Research and Development of
Contrast Agents
Schering AG
Müllerstraße 170-178
D-13342 Berlin

Hans-S. Stender, MD
Emeritus Professor of Radiology
Former Chairman of the
Diagnostic Radiology Dept.
University Hospital Hannover
Present address:
Pregelweg 5
D-30916 Isernhagen NB/2

Friedrich E. Stieve, MD
Professor of Radiology
Institute of the Federal Govern-
ment for Radiation Protection,
Neuherberg
Ingelstädter Landstraße
D-85758 Oberschleißheim

Eberhard Zeitler, MD
Professor of Radiology
Head of the Diagnostic
Radiology Dept.
Hospital of Nürnberg
Flurstraße 17
D-90419 Nürnberg

Bernard G. Ziedses des Plantes,
MD PhD †
Professor of Radiology

Chapter 1

The invisible light

History

Roentgen in historical perspective of medicine

M. Oudkerk, G. Rosenbusch, E. Ammann

The twentieth century, which almost exactly coincides with the X-ray era, has seen a great change in medicine, particularly in the field of morphologic and functional diagnosis of the human body.

W.C. Roentgen's discovery of the 'invisible light' opened the living body noninvasively, making it accessible for the study of anatomy and function. At the same time, it launched the use of modern techniques for the examination of the human body.

Seen from the historic point of view, much ground had to be covered before the human body could be subjected to these modern techniques. Roentgen's discovery of 'invisible light' and its use on the human body meant the beginning of an era in which, one might say, the human body could be opened without a scalpel.

Less than four centuries ago, the anatomist Andreas Vesalius (1514–1564) shocked the world with his radical anatomical views that he had gained from examining human cadavers. Then, less than 300 years ago, the English physician William Harvey (1578–1657) broke with conventional, Galenic views of the function of the heart and other organ systems with his description of the blood circulation. In this century, within a few decades following Roentgen's discovery, the new knowledge as to morphology and function could be verified in living bodies or, where necessary, corrected and expanded.

The 'closed' body

For a long time, dissecting the human body was forbidden in most cultures as being sacrilegious. The Egyptians considered anatomical exploration of human body to be a crime. Embalming was a meticulous ritual. The person who made the first incision in the dead body was regarded as a lawbreaker, symbolically prosecuted with expressions of disdain and even stoned by the crowd.

Similarly, the Jews were ignorant of anatomy. The Torah prohibited contact with a corpse, as by touching it, one became unclean. The Arabs regarded the human body as unclean and were therefore not inclined to investigate inside the corpse. Despite their immense contribution to medicine, they added nothing of importance to the knowledge of human anatomy.

In India, the use of a knife on human beings was forbidden. Before burying the body, it lay in flowing water for seven days so that the parts most susceptible to decomposition were washed away. In China, even physical contact with a dead body was forbidden and knowledge of anatomy has developed only in modern times.

The only period in which systematic investigation of dead bodies was performed was in the third century BC, by Greek physicians in Alexandria, such as Herophilos (320–250 BC) and Erasistratos (d.280 BC), under the arts and sciences patronizing Ptolemy I, who ruled from 305 to 285 BC.

Galen (129–199 AD), a Greek physician from Pergamum, Asia Minor, tried to synthesize all that was known in antiquity about anatomy. After studying in Alexandria and Rome, he practised as a doctor and acquired his knowledge by dissecting animals, particularly monkeys. Galen did not, however, investigate the anatomy of the human body. His views, passed on in many of his books on anatomy and function of the human body, were the prevailing source of instruction until the seventeenth century, that is, over a period of nearly 15 centuries.

Galen's theories can be summarized as follows: blood is produced by the liver, the largest organ in the body, from nutrients carried through a large vessel from the intestines to the liver. Substances, such as air, heat and life (spirit) have to be added to the blood. This takes place in the heart where all things come together: the blood from the liver, the air from the lungs, the heat from the heart itself and the spirit, which arrives from the lungs together with the air. The new, liquid, living blood leaves the heart via the main arteries to reach the various organs in waves where it dissipates. The blood flushes through the organs like tidal waves. According to Galen, breathing serves three different purposes: for air to enter the body and to get to the heart via the air vessels where it is mixed, for air to cool the heart and the body, and, finally, to expel smoke and soot that are formed by the burning furnace in the heart.

These functional interpretations had anatomical correlates. It was impossible to distinguish between a right and left side of the heart since all substances were mixed in the heart. Consequently, the intraventricular septum of the Galenic anatomy had pores and holes for the flow of blood from one side of the heart to the other.

A second strange concept, which remained unchallenged over 1500 years, was that of the function of the vessels between the lungs and the heart. According to this concept, air went from the outside to the inside while blood went from the inside to the outside to remove smoke and soot. It is difficult to understand today the implications that these perceptions had for a doctor. Nevertheless, for 1500 years everyone adopted and learned these concepts. Although Leonardo da Vinci (1452–1519) wondered about the fact that such a large amount of blood was supposed to flow through the heart, he sketched a heart with pores in the septum that, of course, he could not have seen. Ultimately, we have the Arabs to thank for resolving Galenic misconceptions.

Opening the human body

Until the twelfth century, science was dormant in the Western Civilization, just as in the preceding Roman Empire, and did not introduce any advances. A notable exception was theology since the centers of learning were invariably in monasteries.

In the eighth century, Arabian culture flourished through the Moors, who had conquered an area stretching from India to Spain. Arab scientists had made considerable gains in scientific knowledge. Scientific centers in Bagdad (now in Iraq), Damascus (Syria) and Cordoba (Spain) combined Babylonian, Egyptian, Indian, Persian and, later, Chinese teachings with the teachings of the Greco-Roman world. Large hospitals staffed with licensed physicians were found in the major cities, which were population centers and had water mains and sewage canals. The libraries and universities contained tens of thousands of books, written on paper that was manufactured in local paper mills. Arab scientists defined the various sciences and developed the basis for systematic scientific methods. In Spain, the Arabs founded universities in several cities where scientific laboratories and observatories were available for scientific experiments and learning. In contrast, the largest library in the Western Civilization, located in a monastery in Bobbio (Italy), contained no more than 100 titles by the year 1000.

This development in scientific thought that had begun around the eighth century culminated in the works of the Arabian philosopher Averroes (medieval Latin name for Ibn Rushd) (1126–1198). According to Averroes, the only way to true knowledge was through logic, and by systematically applying it to physics, the human mind could arrive at a true understanding of reality. The complete work of Averroes, who had also translated and commented the works of Aristotle, was the source of European intellectual life. By advocating reason over religion, it helped to reject theological dogma for an experimental approach to physics and medicine. Already at the beginning of the eleventh century, Western scientists were in close contact with Arabic culture. They travelled to northern Spain and southern Italy to become acquainted with the many Arabic books on mathematics, astronomy, geometry and medicine.

The respected medical school in Salerno was established under the leadership of the great Arab physician Constantine of Africa (c.1010–1087, born at Carthage) at the place where the famous Monte Cassino monastery had been founded in 529. Salerno is generally considered the oldest medical school in the West. In the Middle ages, science achieved its growth in Europe through by translated Arabic works. The schools founded in Toledo (Spain) and Salerno were dedicated to the translations of Arabic texts, and all new knowledge was catalogued and discussed there. Constantine of Africa, as a mediator between Islam and Christianity, made the Arabic science and philosophy accessible to the Europeans through his translations of medical works from Arabic into Latin.

This new knowledge that swept through Europe came into conflict with the prevailing theological dogma, particularly in Paris. Between 1270 and 1277, Averroes' doctrines were condemned by 219 theses in Paris (Edict of Tempier). These theses primarily criticized the logical foundation of science and represented a confrontation of fundamental importance as all scientific centres were in monasteries. In Paris, the sciences exclusively served theology.

Only in northern Italy, free universities were established under the supervision of city councils. They were not under the influence of the church and did not have theological faculties. Erasmus of Rotterdam (1466–1536) called Padua 'the Athens of the West'. It had the oldest university that taught the complete quadrivium (the course of music, arithmetic, geometry and astronomy) and a sanctuary for studying modern science. Since the thirteenth century, even the city's clergy had been under the supervision of the city council. Theology was barely studied at the University of Padua, and the scientific curriculum concentrated on natural sciences, medicine and mathematics instead. The influence of the Arabic philosopher Averroes was so overwhelming that it was called averroistic. Towards the end of the Middle Ages, the scientific progress in Padua lead to a scientific revolution under averroistic colors, heralding a new era.

The astronomer Nicolas Copernicus (1473–1543) and the physicist Galileo Galilei (1564–1642), the founders of the modern world view, worked as professors in Padua. The Flemish anatomist Andreas Vesalius (1514–1564) and the English anatomist William Harvey (1578–1657), founders of modern anatomy, also worked in Padua and published their significant discoveries there.

Not far from Padua, in Bologna, which had the oldest law school (founded in 1158) and was together with the universities of Padua and Salerno under the patronage of Fredrick II of Sicily (1194–1250), scientists opened the human body to examine the anatomy of internal organs for the first time in a thousand years. It took place in 1305, when the Bolognese physician and anatomist Mondino de Liucci (1270–1326), also called Mundinus, investigated the 'contents' of the body.

It should be noted that Mundinus did not observe the anatomy accurately since he still viewed it through the prevailing Galenic anatomy. He mentioned five lobes of the liver, two uterine horns, a lower jaw consisting of two parts, a heart with a bone and a middle heart between right and left halves of the heart. Although Mundinus cut open the body, he left Galen's theories completely undisturbed.

For 250 years, anatomy was practised without thorough observation and without a challenge of the inaccuracy of the Galenic anatomy. This continued until Vesalius began his studies. He had to leave Paris because opening the human corpse was a crime, for which the penalty was death, and in 1538, he went to Padua where the bodies of executed convicts were given to the university.

Vesalius' voluminous work 'De Humani Corporis Fabrica' caused a tremendous sensation immediately after its publication in 1543. Vesalius refuted the Galenic views with new findings from his own observations. He stated to have seen with his own eyes that a woman had only a single uterus and that the heart did not have a bone. He described two lobes of the liver, not five as had been assumed for 1500 years. In the second edition of his work published in 1555, he also questioned the passage blood through pores from the right side of the heart to the left, one of the main theses in Galen's work. It was clear that, eventually and under severe opposition, Galen's morphology would be rejected, though not yet his views on the function of the organs. In this, Vesalius remained a disciple of Galen.

Drawn by the reputation of the University of Padua in the field of anatomy, the Englishman William Harvey arrived in Padua in 1600 to study medicine. He became a student of Fabricius of Aquapendente (1537–1619), who in turn was a student of the famous Gabriele Fallopio (Fallopius) (1523–1562). Fabricius had discovered the valves in the veins and concluded that blood could only flow in one direction, namely, towards the heart. This did not agree with the Galenic viewpoint of tidal movements in blood vessel. Vesalius' successor in Padua, Realdo Colombo (died 1599), had already discovered the lesser or pulmonary circulation based on his anatomical observations and had been teaching this at the university for many years.

In 1628, Harvey finally published his hypotheses on the function of several organs and thus broke with Galen's views. It was the first time that the complete blood circulation had been described. Nevertheless, even he still seemed to hold on to Galen's views, in that he was convinced that breathing was necessary to cool the heart which was 'hot' by nature. He suspected the existence of a capillary system which, immediately after his death, was described by the Dutchman Antonie van Leeuwenhoek (1632–1723) who had used the microscope, as well as by Marcello Malpighi (1628–1694).

Opening the living human body

The newly acquired knowledge in the fields of anatomy and physiology slowly spread from Padua throughout Europe and gradually broke the theological dominance at the universities.

Since the sixteenth century, numerous universities were founded and hospices evolved into hospitals and, at the beginning of the nineteenth century, the ground was laid to apply to the living body the theoretical knowledge derived from the dead body.

A person of note is the physiologist Johannes Mueller (1801–1858). He worked mainly in Berlin and had several famous students, including Rudolf Virchow (1821–1902), founder of the cellular pathology, the anatomist Rudolf A. von Koelliker (1817–1905), who was very influential in the development of the medical use of X-rays, and Hermann Ludwig von Helmholtz (1821–1894), physiologist and physicist.

Whereas before, tissue specimens had to be taken to study the pathological anatomy, the radiation discovered in 1895 could 'open' the living body for the first time without an incision. Although Roentgen described the fundamental possibilities of his discovery in detail, he would not and could not contribute to the development of its medical application. This can be ascribed mainly to the repetition of x-ray experiments by others immediately after the discovery of X-rays, which was initiated by the publication of the radiograph of a hand.

By current standard, it is a crude radiograph, but it revolutionized the thinking at the time. It was the dawning of a new era that could see into the interior of the living body without the use of a knife.

In the first five years following the discovery of X-rays, the fluoroscopic findings were exactly recorded and correlated with various pulmonary abnormalities and their corresponding clinical findings, providing an insight into disease processes that had remained obscure for thousands of years. For instance, pneumothorax, pleural effusion, pneumonia, pleural thickening, atelectasis etc. could now be differentiated. Using radiographs, fractures could be reset, the healing process assessed by evaluating the callus formation up to and including its osseous consolidation, and the time to resume full weight bearing determined. The rate and time of appearance of the ossification centers could be charted in a table and used as indicator of skeletal maturation. The wide range of normal variants to the early pathological skeletal changes were also described.

Following the introduction of contrast media, contractions of the oesophagus and stomach were observed, as well as intestinal peristalsis. Until then, clinical findings could not be related to defects of the diaphragm, congenital anomalies of the oesophagus, tumours or foreign bodies in the stomach etc. Injecting a contrast medium directly into the venous blood stream provided completely new knowledge as to the function of the kidneys and collecting system including ureters and bladder, and for the first time provided a physiopathological explanation for many clinical problems. Injecting contrast medium rapidly within seconds directly into the arterial blood stream contributed to the diagnosis of congenital heart diseases. The capillary system and the venous return of the blood to the heart could also be investigated.

Of equal importance was the injection of contrast medium straight into the coronary artery of the heart to diagnose coronary arteriosclerosis, the commonest disease of modern civilization. Surgical treatment or dilatation with balloon catheter would be unthinkable without the help of 'invisible light'.

The development of radiology reached its pinnacle when it became possible to measure the absorption coefficient of X-rays at every point in the body with exact precision, as achieved with computed tomography. This enabled the visualization of soft tissues that were only partly visible before. Obviating the need to dissect the corpse, it was possible to prove, within minutes, that the heart does not contain a bone, the human liver consists of two lobes, the airways are not connected to the heart, and the uterus normally does not have two horns.

In the hundred years following Roentgen's discovery, the morphologic knowledge of the human anatomy has been reexamined, improved and amended a thousand times, and the physiologic knowledge of the organ function markedly increased, by means of a variety of radiological examinations. Roentgen's discovery heralds the imaging without ionizing radiation, which was achieved with sonography and magnetic resonance imaging. Diagnostic radiology will increasingly employ these new technologies. This past century truly should be considered as 'the X-ray era'.

Roentgen's discovery coincided with the first publications on psychoanalysis. In 1895, 'Studien über Hysterie' (Studies on Hysteria) by Sigmund Freud (1856–1939) and Josef Breuer (1842– 1925), and in 1900, 'Die Traumdeutung' (The Interpretation of Dreams) by Sigmund Freud were published. While Freud's theory introduced the concept of 'shining light through the soul', Roentgen's discovery can be seen as 'shining light through the living body'.

'A new kind of rays'

G. Rosenbusch, M. Oudkerk, E. Ammann

W.C. Roentgen in Würzburg at the turn of the century

As early as 1894, the 49-year-old professor in physics in Würzburg, Wilhelm Conrad Roentgen (Fig. I, 1), ordered an *'approved discharge apparatus and discharge tubes'* from Mueller-Unkel. On 5 May 1894, he sent a postcard to his younger colleague, the German physicist Philipp Lenard (1862–1947), asking from which reliable source he could obtain the window plate. Cathode rays would be emitted from the discharge chamber and so become accessible for investigation through the 'Lenard window'. Lenard replied that he did not have any reliable source of reference at the moment, but he took the liberty of

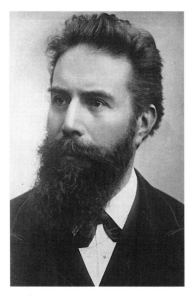

Fig. I, 1.
W.C. Roentgen
(1845–1923)

'sending two plates from my small stock. Their thickness is approximately 0.005 mm' (A. Hermann, 1981).

Under Heinrich Hertz (1857–1894), the great physicist in electrodynamics, the young Lenard had already carried out important investigations on cathode rays. Like so many other physicists of his time, Roentgen also wanted to be engaged in these strange luminous phenomena of discharge tubes and cathode rays. After all, much remained obscure and needed investigation. Initially he was only able to undertake a few experiments since he had already assumed the responsibilities and duties as dean of the respected University of Würzburg for the academic year 1894/95.

Würzburg, situated on both sides of the Main River and dominated by the Marienberg Castle, has maintained the character of a city that was built at the end of the Middle Ages and during the Baroque era. For a long time it was an episcopal see and finally fell under the rule of the Kingdom of Bavaria in 1814. In the second half of the nineteenth century and at the onset of the twentieth century, it had approximately 80 000 inhabitants.

A university was founded in Würzburg in 1402, but it existed for only a few years. The present university was founded in 1582. It had become a scientific centre for medicine, biology and chemistry. It was here that Rudolf Virchow (1821–1902) formulated his theory of cellular pathology in the 1850s, before returning to Berlin to announce this publicly. The physiologist Adolf Fick (1829–1901), the anatomists Rudolf von Koelliker (1817–1905) and Philip Stoehr (1849–1912), and the biologist Theodor Boveri (1862–1915) contributed through their research and knowledge to the fame of the city and its university. Emil Fischer (1852–1919), the distinguished organic chemist, attracted students from all over the world during his tenure at the University of Würzburg. The reputation of the city and its university attracted a growing number of students. In the year 1866, their number amounted to 603, with 261 attending medical school, and had increased by 1904 to 1289, with 401 attending medical school.

Although automobiles were already fabricated around 1895, the railways remained the main means of transport. Electricity was not yet generally available. Gas or kerosene were used as light source. The telephone had already been invented. The intellectual life was prospering. Im-

pressionism flourished in France. Many authors aroused debates: Arthur Schnitzler and Hugo von Hofmannsthal in Vienna, Emile Zola in Paris, Gottfried Keller in Switzerland, and Gerhard Hauptmann, with his sociocritical dramas, in Germany. In music, Guiseppe Verdi, Claude Debussy, Gustav Mahler and Richard Strauss introduced new tonal patterns. Richard Wagner had died in 1883, followed by Anton Bruckner in 1896 and Johannes Brahms in 1897.

In the autumn of 1895, Roentgen could finally dedicate himself completely to cathode rays (Figs I, 2 and 3). To carry out his experiments, he needed a discharge tube, an induction coil, a

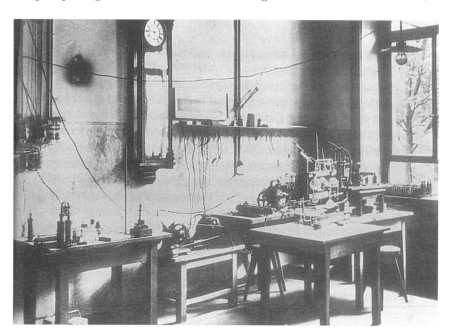

Fig. I, 2. Roentgen's laboratory in Wuerzburg.

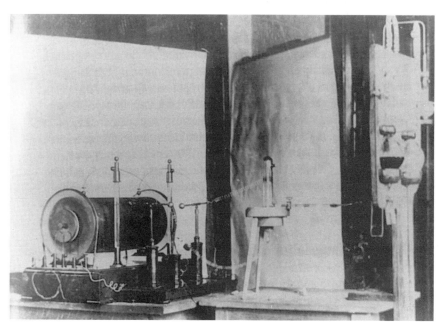

Fig. I, 3. Set-up of apparatuses used by Roentgen.

contact interrupter, a lead battery and a vacuum pump.

The following investigation protocol was used:

- In a vacuum glass tube, a high-voltage field was generated between the anode and cathode. As soon as the electric field was high enough, the electrons released in the cathode moved through the vacuum towards the anode and discharged the electrodes.
- The electric field was generated using an induction coil. The secondary winding of the Ruhmkorff induction coil had 200 000 turns of thin wire and the primary coil a few hundred turns of thick wire. The induction coil was adjusted in such a way that a tube voltage of 40 000–60 000 V was generated between the anode and cathode of the discharge tube.
- The induction coil was powered by a lead battery, which supplied 32 V.
- The primary current (approximately 20 A) from the lead battery was interrupted 15–20 times per second using a platinum contact breaker devised by Depréz. The spark gap was approximately 3 cm.
- Prior to these tests, the glass tube, usually a Hittorf or Geissler tube, had to be evacuated using a mercury vacuum pump which was connected to the laboratory water mains. A vacuum of 0.01 Torr (= mercury column) could be produced with this pump, developed by A. Raps only a few years earlier. This could take many hours or even days (U. Hennig, 1989).

8 November 1895: the overnight revelation (F. Dessauer)

In the late evening of 8 November 1895, in a darkened room, while experimenting with this equipment, Roentgen noticed a weak spot of light near the discharge tube. The light came from a piece of fluorescent paper next to the tube. It was coated with a layer of barium platinocyanide. In those days, such fluorescent screens were used to detect ultraviolet light. At first, he suspected that the phenomenon was generated from inside the tube itself, but the fluorescence was also present when he covered the glass tube with black paper. This observation could not be explained by the then prevailing knowledge of physics. The phenomenon aroused Roentgen's experimental and analytical talents.

To investigate this phenomenon further, Roentgen placed various objects between the fluorescent screen and the discharge tube: playing cards, a book, a piece of wood, several metal objects and also his own hand. He told his wife Bertha and his friend, the biologist Theodor Boveri, that he thought he had discovered something very exciting.

Later, in Davos in the winter of 1911/12, during lunch with the Roentgens and the physicist Friedrich Dorn, Bertha Roentgen was asked by Heinrich Franke how her husband was able to accomplish a comprehensive overview of the nature and significance of his discovery in such a short time. She answered that she could not tell, because in those first days she had hardly seen her husband at all. He had been completely absorbed in his experiments and his scientific imagination had taken over. He had therefore retreated in strict seclusion: *'He not only took his meals to his study, he even had his bed installed there for a longer period of time to be left undisturbed by any trivialities of life or such like interferences, so that during waking moments he could put his thought immediately to the test'* (H. Franke, 1926).

Due to the fact that he needed absolute darkness to observe the weak fluorescent light, Roentgen switched his working hours to nighttime. The Roentgen family, however, lived on the top floor of the institute's two-story building, immediately above the laboratory.

Ludwig Zehnder (1854–1949), a colleague and friend of Roentgen, reported that Roentgen asked the physiologist Adolf Fick, in the adjacent building, to observe his experiments with him. Adolf Fick told his son Rudolf, who later became famous for his research on the mechanism of joints, about these experiments. Rudolf Fick immediately recognized the importance of this new radiation for medicine, particularly in the field of surgery and anatomy. When Roentgen discovered the effect of the new radiation – the X-rays as he called them – on photographic plates, he took photographs of several objects, including his own hand.

On 28 December 1895, approximately seven weeks after the discovery, Roentgen, absolutely convinced of his observation, submitted his manuscript to the Secretary of the Physical Medical Society at Würzburg. The manuscript was printed without further discussion, because of its significance. This sensational article 'Ueber eine neue Art von Strahlen. Vorläufige Mitteilung' (On a new kind of rays. Preliminary report) was printed in 1895 (Figs I, 4 and 7).

On 1 January 1896, Roentgen sent a reprint of his 11-page paper, with copies of the radiographs of his wife's hand and several other objects, to his colleagues at home and abroad (Figs I, 5 and 6).

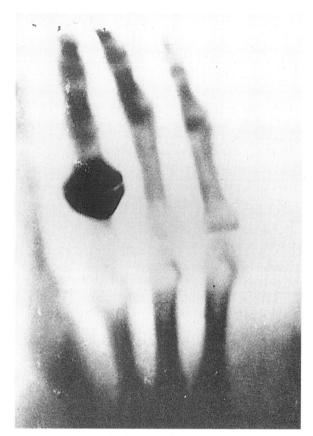

Ueber eine neue Art von Strahlen

von W. C. Röntgen.

(Vorläufige Mittheilung).

1. Lässt man durch eine Hittorf'sche Vacuum-röhre, oder einen genügend evacuirten Lenard'schen, Crookes'schen oder ähnlichen Apparat die Entladungen eines grösseren Ruhmkorff's gehen, und bedeckt die Röhre...

Fig. I, 4. First page of his manuscript Ueber eine neue Art von Strahlen (On a new kind of rays). The rest of the manuscript was destroyed after the death of Roentgen according to his will.

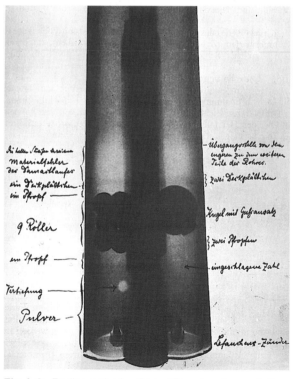

Fig. I, 5. Radiograph of the hand of Roentgen's wife 1895.

In his preliminary report, Roentgen listed 18 characteristics of X-rays, of which the following are the most important:
- The transmission of X-rays through various materials of the same thickness, fundamentally depends on the material's density.
- When the thickness is increased, all materials transmit fewer X-rays.
- In addition to barium platinocyanide, other substances also fluoresce, for example, the phosphorescent calcium compounds.
- Photographic dry plates are sensitive to X-rays.
- X-rays are not diffracted by a magnet, unlike cathode rays.

Fig. I, 6. Radiograph of a rifle and Roentgen's annotation, 1896.

Sitzungs-Berichte
der
Physikalisch-medicinischen Gesellschaft
zu
WÜRZBURG.

| Jahrgang 1895. | Der Abonnementspreis pro Jahrgang beträgt *M* 4.—. Die Nummern werden einzeln nicht abgegeben. Grössere Beiträge erscheinen in Sonderdrucken. | No. 9. |

Verlag der Stahel'schen k. Hof- und Universitäts-Buch- und Kunsthandlung in Würzburg.

Inhalt. *Konrad Rieger*: Demonstration des sogenannten „Vogelkopfknaben" Dóbos Janos aus Battonya in Ungarn (Fortsetzung), pag. 129. — *W. C. Röntgen*: Ueber eine neue Art von Strahlen, pag. 132. — *Wilhelm Wislicenus*: 46. Jahresbericht der physikalisch-medizinischen Gesellschaft zu Würzburg, pag. 142. — Mitglieder-Verzeichniss, pag. 146.

Konrad Rieger: Demonstration des sogenannten „Vogelkopf-Knaben" Dóbos Janos aus Battonya in Ungarn.

(Fortsetzung.)

Die Mikrocephalin Wolf, deren Gesammt-Hirngewicht seinem muthmasslichen am Nächsten steht, hatte für das Grosshirn allein nur 520 gr Gewicht, weil sie ihre vollen 130 gr Kleinhirn-Gewicht hatte. Geben wir aber Dóbos ein muthmassliches Gesammthirn-Gewicht von 600 gr, so haben wir durchaus keinen Grund dafür, auch ihm soviel für das Kleinhirn abzuziehen, wobei ihm für das Grosshirn nur c. 450 gr blieben. Sondern, da wir allen Grund haben, bei ihm auch in dieser Richtung normalproportionirte Verhältnisse vorauszusetzen, so brauchen wir seinem Kleinhirn nur ein Achtel des Grosshirns oder höchstens 70 gr zuzuschreiben, wobei dann für das Grosshirn allein über 500 gr blieben.

Neben dem Quotienten zwischen Hirn- und Körpergewicht und dem zwischen Kopf- und Gesichts-Grösse halte ich diesen Quotienten zwischen Gross- und Kleinhirn für den am Meisten charakteristischen hinsichtlich der Kennzeichnung aller, hier in

9

---

132   Sitzungsberichte der physikal.-medicin. Gesellschaft. Jahrg. 1895.

frühere Mitglieder der Gesellschaft lediglich deshalb nicht mehr im Personalverzeichnisse geführt würden, weil sie bei ihrem Weggange aus Würzburg vergessen hatten, den entsprechenden Antrag zu stellen.
Herr von Kölliker stellt deshalb einen Antrag auf diesbezügliche Aenderung der Statuten. — Ueber denselben soll in der ersten Sitzung des nächsten Geschäftsjahres berathen werden.

Am 28. Dezember wurde als Beitrag eingereicht:

W. C. Röntgen: Ueber eine neue Art von Strahlen.

(Vorläufige Mittheilung.)

1. Lässt man durch eine *Hittorf*'sche Vacuumröhre, oder einen genügend evacuirten *Lenard*'schen, *Crookes*'schen oder ähnlichen Apparat die Entladungen eines grösseren *Ruhmkorff*'s gehen und bedeckt die Röhre mit einem ziemlich eng anliegenden Mantel aus dünnem, schwarzem Carton, so sieht man in dem vollständig verdunkelten Zimmer einen in die Nähe des Apparates gebrachten, mit Bariumplatincyanür angestrichenen Papierschirm bei jeder Entladung hell aufleuchten, fluoresciren, gleichgültig ob die angestrichene oder die andere Seite des Schirmes dem Entladungsapparat zugewendet ist. Die Fluorescenz ist noch in 2 m Entfernung vom Apparat bemerkbar.

Man überzeugt sich leicht, dass die Ursache der Fluorescenz vom Entladungsapparat und von keiner anderen Stelle der Leitung ausgeht.

2. Das an dieser Erscheinung zunächst Auffallende ist, dass durch die schwarze Cartonhülse, welche keine sichtbaren oder ultravioletten Strahlen des Sonnen- oder des elektrischen Bogenlichtes durchlässt, ein Agens hindurchgeht, das im Stande ist, lebhafte Fluorescenz zu erzeugen, und man wird deshalb wohl zuerst untersuchen, ob auch andere Körper diese Eigenschaft besitzen.

Man findet bald, dass alle Körper für dasselbe durchlässig sind, aber in sehr verschiedenem Grade. Einige Beispiele führe ich an. Papier ist sehr durchlässig:[1] hinter einem eingebun-

1) Mit „Durchlässigkeit" eines Körpers bezeichne ich das Verhältniss der Helligkeit eines dicht hinter dem Körper gehaltenen Fluorescenzschirmes zu derjenigen Helligkeit des Schirmes, welcher dieser unter denselben Verhältnissen aber ohne Zwischenschaltung des Körpers zeigt.

Fig. I, 7. First publication of Roentgen's report in the proceedings of the "Physikalisch-medizinische Gesellschaft" in Wuerzburg.

- X-rays originate from a spot where cathode rays hit the glass wall. The generation of X-rays not only takes place in glass but also in aluminium.
- The new rays could be longitudinal ether waves.

For Friedrich Dessauer, one of the pioneers in radiology, this concise preliminary report reflected clarity, simplicity and devotion.

Among the congratulations Roentgen received were letters from Thomas Edison, Lord Kelvin (Fig. I, 8), Albert Einstein, Madame Marie Curie and Hendrik Antoon Lorentz. Emperor Wilhelm II sent Roentgen a congratulatory telegram and invited him to demonstrate his rays at the Imperial Court in Berlin, which he did on 12 January 1896.

Unfortunately, Heinrich Hertz (1857–1894), the pioneer in electrodynamics, August Kundt (1839–1894), Roentgen's scientific patron and mentor, and Hermann von Helmholtz (1821–1894), the authority on physics in Germany, did not live to see the discovery. They all had died in 1894, Heinrich Hertz at the young age of only 37 years.

In contrast, when E. Warburg (1846–1931) presented X-ray photographs that he had received from Roentgen on at the fiftieth anniversary of the Institute of Physics in Berlin on 4 January 1896, they did not cause any excitement, hardly drawing any attention (Goerke, 1971).

On 23 January 1896, Roentgen gave his only public lecture on X-rays at the Physical Medical Society in Würzburg. In front of the audience, Roentgen also produced an X-ray photograph of the hand of the well-known anatomist Rudolf von Koelliker (Fig. I, 9). For von Koelliker, this meeting at the Institute was the most important one of his life and, deeply moved, he proposed

THE UNIVERSITY,
GLASGOW. *January 17. 1896.*

Dear Prof. Röntgen,

When I wrote to you thanking you for your kindness in sending me your paper and the photographs which accompanied it I had only seen the photographs and had not had time to read the paper. I need not tell you that when I read the paper I was very much astonished and delighted. I can say no more just now than to congratulate you warmly on the great discovery you have made and to renew my thanks to you for your kindness in so early sending me your paper and the photographs.

Believe me,
Yours very truly,

Kelvin

Fig. I, 8. Lord Kelvin congratulates Roentgen for his important discovery. Shortly before, Kelvin had only acknowledged the receipt of Roentgen's article.

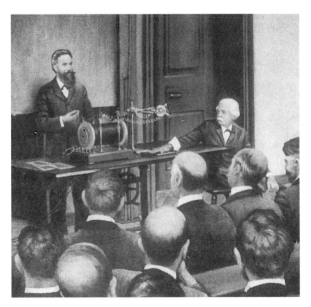

Fig. I, 9. The only public address Roentgen delivered on X-rays in Wuerzburg, 23 January 1896. Roentgen takes a photograph of the hand of the anatomist von Koelliker. Koelliker was profoundly impressed and proposed to name the new rays after Roentgen.

that the new rays be named after their discoverer, a suggestion received with a standing ovation. The enthusiasm here, compared with the almost reserved reception of the physicists in Berlin, showed that Roentgen's rays were immediately recognized as an important step forward in medicine and that they raised high expectations as to finding useful applications.

Roentgen published the results of further experiments on X-rays in two subsequent reports, in the spring of 1896 and in 1897, respectively.

In the second report, Roentgen was able to prove that air, irradiated with X-rays, discharged electric bodies with which it came into contact. If the electric bodies were in dry hydrogen instead of air, they were also discharged by X-rays but possibly at a slower rate. This result was the basis of dosimetry using an ionization chamber.

In the third report, Roentgen determined that, to evaluate the intensity of the X-rays, the best thing to use was spherical discharge apparatus with a flat polished platinum plate, which was struck by cathode rays at an angle of 45°.

From other experiments he concluded that the specific transperency of a substance increases with its thickness. This described the basis of the principle of 'hardening' X-rays.

Are X-rays waves?

Roentgen performed approximately 600 experiments. In spite of these, he had to admit that: *'I do not have a single experimental result, from which I could, to my own satisfaction, gain assurance of the existence of a diffraction of the X-rays.'* Could the absence of a diffraction be explained by the extremely short wavelengths?

In 1912, Max von Laue (1879–1960), Walter Friedrich (1883–1968) and Paul Knipping (1883–1935) finally succeeded in proving the diffraction of X-rays using crystals in the laboratory of the great physicist Arnold Sommerfeld (Figs I, 10–12). This proved that X-rays had a wavelike nature (Fig. I, 13). Their laboratory was next to Roentgen's in Munich. Roentgen followed these developments with keen interest and immense satisfaction. Studying crystals, which he resumed in Munich, had been his favorite subject in his early investigations.

In 1913, the English physicists William Henry Bragg (1862–1942) and William Lawrence Bragg (1890–1971) analyzed crystalline structures with X-rays, thus founding the science of X-ray spectroscopy.

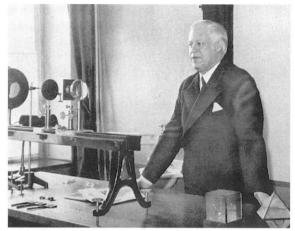

Fig. I, 10. Walter Friedrich (1883–1968) during a lecture at the University of Berlin in the thirties.
Already as a student from 1902–1904, Friedrich had made X-ray images in his own laboratory. Worked in Munich (assistant to A. Sommerfeld), Freiburg i. Br. (section-chief in the Gynecologic Clinic at the University) and since 1922 in Berlin as professor of medical physics. His thesis dealt with the interference of X-rays.

Fig. I, 12. Walter Friedrich's handwritten report on experimental evidence of the wavelike nature of Roentgen rays, 4 Mai 1912. Also signed by P. Knipping and M. von Laue.

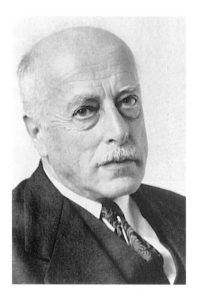

Fig. I, 11.
Max von Laue (1879–1960). Worked as physicist in Munich, Zurich, Frankfurt am Main and Berlin. Initiated the discovery of the interference of X-rays. Important contribution to the theory of relativity. Nobel prize for physics in 1914.

Accidental or rediscovered?

Given the importance of X-rays, it is not surprising that other people claimed to be the first in their discovery. Nevertheless, they had ignored their observations or misinterpreted them, as Arthur Willis Goodspeed (1860–1943) in Philadelphia and the Englishman William Crookes (1832–1919) had done. Similarly, J. J. Thomson (1856–1940), the famous teacher of physics in England, had seen phosphorescence on tubes

Fig. I, 13. Albert Einstein's congratulatory letter to M. von Laue: "Your experiments belong to the best achievements physics has ever seen".

of ordinary *'German glasses ... that were placed at a distance of several feet from a discharge tube.'* Other researchers complained that their photographic plates showed fogging when stored near a discharge tube. As we know today, these effects were the result of unrecognized X-rays (K. Simonyi, 1990).

While an assistant to Roentgen in Würzburg between 1888 and 1890, L. Zehnder had been interested in the ultraviolet spectrum and the processes in the Geissler tube. In his tests, he had observed the luminescence of a fluorescent screen. When, later, people wanted to acclaim him as the 'real' discoverer of the X-rays, he answered: *'To watch a mysteriously luminescent fluorescence screen is a long way from discovering a new physical phenomenon.'*

Kasper Marstaller, Roentgen's technical assistant at the Institute, is often mentioned as the discoverer of X-rays. Even if he had been the first to see the screen showing fluorescence, which is doubtful and even unlikely, the value of Roentgen's discovery is not lessened, because Roentgen did not leave it at a simple description of a light effect but, admirably, investigated it in greater depth. Because Roentgen usually performed his tests alone, he could well have been alone that particular night.

According to another version, it is alleged that Roentgen accused Marstaller of negligent treatment of the plates which were therefore useless for his investigations, although Marstaller had not exposed the plates. Marstaller protested his innocence whereupon Roentgen began to wonder. It had been said that this was the real reason to begin his investigation, finally leading up to the discovery of X-rays (situation similar to Zehnder). It is rumored that, half-seriously, the Würzburg students called the rays *'Marstaller rays'*, which hurt Roentgen deeply!

In 1893, following a proposal by Heinrich Hertz, Philipp Lenard (Fig. I, 14) succeeded in allowing cathode rays to pass through a small aluminum window for further investigation outside the glass tube. The characteristics of these rays were unknown and were therefore called Lenard rays. Lenard, in particular, could not get over the fact that Roentgen beat him to the discovery of X-rays. Hertz and Lenard were very close to the discovery, but Hertz died in 1894 and Lenard used a fluorescent substance unfit for X-rays (pentadecylparatylketone). To darken the tube, he did not use cardboard as Roentgen did, but a zinc sheet-metal, which at least partly absorbed the rays. In addition, Lenard was fully occupied with the publication of Hertz's scientific work.

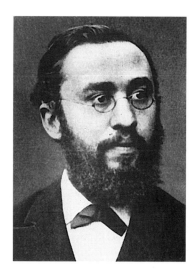

Fig. I, 14. Philipp Lenard (1862–1947). Born in Preßburg (Bratislava), university training in Budapest and Vienna, then in Germany. Worked, among other places, in Breslau, Bonn (under H. Hertz), Kiel, Heidelberg. Important experimental physicist. Investigations on cathode rays, phosphorescence, attenuation of radiation. Nobel prize for Physics in 1905.

Later, after the First World War, Lenard tried to belittle Roentgen's achievements. He did not refrain from slander and always called X-rays, even in later years, *'high-frequency rays'* rather than roentgen rays, as they are referred to in German. This was contrary to his statements made at a young age, when he wholeheartedly recognized Roentgen's discovery. In his work 'Grosse Naturforscher', which went into several editions, Roentgen's name is absent.

Why Roentgen should choose to investigate the discharge phenomena of cathode rays is not known. Was it intuition? Was it foresight? Was it that *'sacred curiosity, which distinguishes the true scientist and discoverer, capable of wonder and bent on discovery ...'*? (Schroedinger)

It may be true that Lenard's experiments with cathode rays encouraged Roentgen to explore this field further. *'I would very much like to see your important investigations on cathode rays in the free atmosphere, etc.'*, Roentgen stated in a letter to Lenard asking for the aluminum foil.

What was known about cathode rays?

Cathode rays were known to be emitted by the cathode, to be propagated in straight line, to be deflected by a magnet, have a discharging effect on charged bodies, to initiate chemical reactions and therefore expose photographic films, and to heat the anode and therefore transfer energy.

Occasionally, a particle structure of the cathode rays was unconvincingly talked about but a wavelike property was more probable, which was, at least, the prevailing opinion of the physicists in Germany, while the physicists in England favored the particle theory. It was not until two years after Roentgen's discovery that J.J. Thomson finally clarified the nature of cathode rays as negatively charged particles, which he called electrons.

Lenard related that von Helmholtz had the gift, *'to assess the possibility of unknown natural phenomena from known phenomena'* and that *'his proof that light beams of short enough wave length would penetrate everything in a straight line, three years prior to the discovery of rays that fitted this description and 20 years before the rays that became so important in medicine, was indeed identified as extremely short wavelength ether radiation (high-frequency radiation)'* (Ph. Lenard, 1930). This is the reason why von Helmholtz was called the mathematical discoverer of X-rays (A.W. Crane, 1934).

Roentgen, when he observed the new phenomenon that first night, was aware that he was dealing with something entirely new. His experiments, observations and conclusions were so explicit, unmistakable and thorough, that it took until 1912 before a new physical property, the discovery of the wave-nature of X-rays, could be added, supplementing and expanding Roentgen's work.

Although F. Dessauer (1882–1963) spoke about 8 November as the night of the revelation, T.S. Kuhn would not pinpoint the discovery to one particular date, but placed it in the period between 8 November and 28 December, as the phenomenon observed on 8 November had to be explained and defined. Only after the new explanation was ascertained, could the discovery be regarded as complete.

In his will, Roentgen stipulated that all his scientific papers should be destroyed, and this was carried out. A retrospective analysis of his investigations on the discovery of X-rays is therefore impossible. Only the first handwritten page of his manuscript 'Über eine neue Art von Strahlen. Vorläufige Mitteilung' was saved. This page is now in the proud possession of the Roentgen Museum in Lennep, Germany.

Roentgen's scientific integrity

On Roentgen's seventieth birthday, Arnold Sommerfeld (1868–1951) emphasized Roentgen's strong personality, his serious attitude towards scientific thoroughness. Time and again, Roentgen produced arguments against observations, had experiments repeated and proposed verifications to prevent false conclusions.

This brilliant, conscientious experimentalist, who knew how important his discovery was, refrained from taking part in the development of X-ray technology. He did not want to benefit financially from his investigations and discoveries, and renounced all patent applications. His discovery was intended to be for the good of mankind.

In 1901, Roentgen was the first to be awarded the Nobel Prize for outstanding achievments in the field of physics. The ceremonial address reads: *'The Academy has awarded Professor W.C. Roentgen from Munich the Nobel Prize for Physics on the grounds of the discovery, the name of which will always remain linked with him as 'roentgen rays', or as he calls them himself, X-rays ... . From the properties associated with roentgen rays, only those are considered that contribute to the far-reaching application these rays have found in medical practice.'*

The last wish of Alfred Bernard Nobel (1833–1896), in his will signed on 27 November 1895, a year before he died, was fulfilled with this award: *'The prize is to be awarded to those individuals who have contributed most towards mankind in the course of that year'*. Roentgen had received numerous other prizes and honors. Incidentally, Lenard received the Nobel Prize for Physics for his investigations on cathode rays in 1905.

Discoveries often stand on many shoulders

In 1897, S.P. Thompson wrote *'In the history of science, nothing holds more truth than the statement that the discoverer, even the most eminent, is but the descendant of his ancestors; in fact, he is the product of the times in which he was born'*.

Wilhelm Conrad Roentgen's discovery of X-rays on 8 November 1895, would not have been possible without the distinguished achievements of his predecessors, as well as the many smaller steps in the various fields of physics and engineering, in particular, photography, vacuum engineering, luminescence and electricity, where the ideas were still very ambiguous. Numerous scientists and experimenters prepared the way for the discovery of X-rays. Many names were soon forgotten. Tables I, 1a-e are time charts that list the dates relevant for the development in the various fields that contributed to the discovery of X-rays was based.

Roentgen: 'only' the discoverer of roentgen rays?

Roentgen's work did not only include the discovery of X-rays. He was renowned as one of the eminent experimentalists of his time for his investigations before 1895. Altogether, Roentgen published 58 papers on various fields of physics, such as light, heat, acoustics, electricity, crystallography, and elasticity.

P.P. Koch, a former student and, later, Roentgen's colleague, catalogued Roentgen's scientific activities chronologically:

- Topics of early works (1870–1879):
  - determinations of specific gas–heat ratios;
  - soldering platinized glass;
  - electrical discharges;
  - heat transmission in crystals;
  - intensity of sun rays;
  - capillarity;
  - design of instruments, e.g. aneroid barometer with mirror reading;
  - proof of electromagnetic rotation of polarization plane of light in gases (with Kundt).
- Topics investigated in Giessen, Germany (1879–1888):
  - Kerr's effect (magneto-optic effect);
  - pyro- and piezoelectricity;
  - heat absorption by steam;
  - construction of an apparatus to demonstrate Poiseuille's law;
  - inner friction of elements;
  - compressibility
  - refraction experiments;
  - dielectric constant;
  - galvanic conductivity;
  - discovery of displacement current (see 'Roentgen current' below).
- Topics investigated in Würzburg, Germany (1888–1900):
  - investigations of thick, coherent oil films on water surfaces;
  - water and ice molecules of water;
  - discovery of X-rays (three papers).
  From 1898 until 1907, Roentgen remained silent!
- Topics investigated in Munich, Germany (1901–1921):
  - thermal coefficient of expansion, particularly in diamonds at low temperatures;
  - electric conductivity in crystals after irradiation;
  - up-to-date determinations of the Curie piezoelectric constant of quartz.
  - At the time Roentgen was in Munich, 25 physicists, including W. Friedrich and R. Glocker, received their doctoral degrees on various subjects, some on the interpretation and clarification of the properties of X-rays.

Apart from his work on X-rays, two of Roentgen's investigations were of special interest and great importance: the photoacoustic effect and the displacement current.

Photoacoustic effect

When gas is periodically irradiated with light, the temperature changes and with it the pressure. These pressure changes can be recorded as sound with the use of a microphone. The absorption of light depends on the type of gas and on the wavelength of the light.

The publication, in 1881, of 'Über Töne, welche durch intermittierende Bestrahlung eines Gases entstehen' (On sounds produced by intermittent irradiation of gases) formed the basis of photoacoustic spectroscopy and is still used for gas analysis in medicine, biology and meteorology.

Displacement current (roentgen current)

According to Maxwell, not only conduction current but also each temporarily changing field is surrounded by closed magnetic boundaries. As a result, the displacement current joins, with equal status, the conduction current. The starting point of the investigation was the question of whether a non-conductor or insulator, moved in an electric field, exerted a magnetic effect. It could be concluded that a dielectric could be polarized using electricity.

Using a sophisticated experimental design, Roentgen could actually prove the existence of this displacement current indirectly. He published his findings in a five-page paper entitled 'Durch Bewegung eines im homogenen elektrischen Feld befindlichen Dielektrikums hervorgerufene elektrodynamische Kraft' (On the electromotoric force produced by moving a dielectric in a homogeneous electric field). Because of its significance, Hendrik Antoon Lorentz called this displacement current 'roentgen current'.

A few decades later, the work became very important in the formulation of the theories of relativity and electrons. A. Sommerfeld emphasized that only a few could appreciate this discovery. Even Roentgen himself thought that this dis-

Physical prolegomena of the discovery of X-rays

Table I, 1a. Evacuation

1643	Evangelista Torricelli (1608–1647): creates vacuum by turning an open glass tube filled with mercury upside down into a dish of mercury.
1654	Otto von Guericke (1602–1686): designs the first mechanical air pump.
1660	Robert Hooke (1635–1703) and Robert Boyle (1627–1691): improve the air pump.
1855	Heinrich Geissler (1814–1879): introduces a practical mercury air pump that can lower the gas pressure to 2 Torr.
1869	Johann Wilhelm Hittorf (1824–1914): increases the vacuum.
1874	R. Gill: develops the oil pump.
	August Raps (1865–1920): automatic mercury air pump.

Table I, 1b. Fluorescence examination

1602	Vincentius Casciarolus (1571–1624): shoemaker in Bologna discovers the Bolognese fluorescent stone during alchemic studies.
1675	Jean Picard (1620–1682): observes luminescence in the barometer tube when mercury is moved.
1838	Michael Faraday (1791–1867): discovers phosphorescence that originates from electrical charges in gases under low pressure.
1852	George Gabriel Stokes (1819–1903): discovers that certain materials and artificial compounds fluoresce when radiated with UV light (hydrofluoric, fluorspar/calcium, barium and strontium salts, particularly platinum cyanuric barium.
1859	Julius Pfluecker (1801–1868): observes greenish fluorescence on the walls of vacuum tubes during his research on cathode rays.
1866	Sidot: investigates zinc collimators.
1867	Alexander Edmund Becquerel (1820–1891) and Antoine Henri Becquerel (1852–1908): works on phosphorescence: 'La lumière, ses causes et ses effects'.

Table I, 1c. Manufacture of discharge tubes

1855	Heinrich Geissler (1814–1879) and
1859	Julius Pfluecker (1801–1868): melted platinum electrodes; expanded experiments.
1869	Johann Wilhelm Hittorf (1824–1914): develops tubes for high-pressure gas research.
1875	Friedrich W. Georg Kohlrausch (1840–1910): works on electrolysis, elasticity, electrochemistry – independent ion movements.
1879	William Crookes (1832–1919): develops concave cathode and the 45° anode.
1894	Otto Schott (1851–1935): improves resistance of industrial glass.

Table I, 1d. Photography

1553	Giovanni Battista della Porta (1535–1615): invents camera obscura.
1727	Johann H. Schulze (1687–1744) and
1802	Thomas Wedgewood (1730–1795): use light sensitivity of silver salts to reproduce letter stencils by means of sunlight.
	Carl Wilhelm Scheele (1742–1786): uses silver-chloride-covered paper to demonstrate the spectrum of the sun light.
1819	John Herschel (1792–1871): proves that sodium thiosulphate dissolves solid silver chloride; concept of 'photography'.
1826	Josephe Nicéphore Niepce (1765–1833): demonstrates first photography: uses light sensitive matter (protein emulsion containing silver iodide) in the camera obscura.
1839	Louis J.M. Daguerre (1789–1851): uses iodized silver plates and mercury silver development.
1839	William Fox Talbot (1800–1877): copies images on paper; invents negative-positive method achieving positive print on light-sensitive paper.
1851	Frederick Scott Archer (1813–1857): uses colloid instead of protein to bind silver iodide (must be moist on exposure and during development).
1871	Richard L. Maddox : uses gelatin silver bromide solution on glass plates (= dry plates), being more light sensitive.
1879	George Eastman (1854–1932): invents machine to coat plates
1889	George Eastman (1854–1932): invents paper roll-film using cellulose nitrate (transparent film).

Table I, 1e. Electricity and Magnetism

1600	William Gilbert (1544–1603): shows electrical phenomena by rubbing; 'electricity' is his concept.
1713	Francis Hauksbee (1670–1713): observes electrical discharge in vacuum.
1729	Stephen Gay (1666–1736): difference between conductor and insulator.
1733	Charles F. Dufay (1698–1739): discovers electric charge.
1755	Benjamin Franklin (1706–1790): there is no electric charge within a confined, charged container.
1757	Johann Carl Wilcke (1732–1796): interprets electrostatic induction.
1758	Benjamin Franklin (1706–1790): demonstrates that electricity and lightning are the same.
1775	Alessandro Volta (1745–1827): electrostatic induction device with 30 kV to 100kV.
1778	Georg Ch. Lichtenberg (1742–1799): separates the electric charge into positive and negative.
1800	Alessandro Volta (1745–1827): develops the first battery.

Table I, 1e. Electricity and Magnetism (continuted)

1820	Hans Christian Oersted (1777–1851): discovers the magnetic effect of an electric current and founded the theory of electromagnetism.
1821	André Marie Ampère (1775–1836): deflection of a coil in a magnetic field; outlines elementary electrodynamic research and its laws.
1822	Humphrey Davy (1778–1829): generates electrical arcs with Volta's batteries.
1827	Georg Ohm (1789–1854): finds quantitative correlation of voltage, resistance and current.
1831 –1834	Michael Faraday (1791–1867): discovers electromagnetic induction and self-induction; laws of electrolysis.
1848	Franz Ernst Neumann (1798–1895): proposes theory of magnetic induction. Heinrich Daniel Rühmkorff (1803–1877): designs the spark inductor.
1857	Julius Pfluecker (1801–1868): is first to observe cathode rays and (without identification) their deflection under the influence of magnetism.
1859	Gaston Planté (1834–1899): concept of lead battery.
1865	Holz (1836–1912) and Toepler: electrostatic – induction machine.
1866	Werner von Siemens (1816–1892): dynamo electric principle.
1871	James Clerk Maxwell (1831–1879): proposes electromagnetic light theory.
1876	Eugen Goldstein (1850–1930): introduces concepts of cathode light and cathode rays.
1879	Thomas Alva Edison (1847–1931): invents incandescent lamp.
1881	Johnstone Stoney (1826–1911): introduces concept of electrons.
1882	Hendrik Antoon Lorentz (1853–1928): proposes electron theory.
1883	Lucien Goulard (1850–1888) and Gaulard J.W. Gibbs (1839–1903): develop voltage transformer.
1885	Colley: first recording of a curve of alternating current.
1886	Hermann L.F. von Helmholtz (1821–1894): works on electromagnetic theory.
1888 –1892	Heinrich R. Hertz (1857–1894): discovers that cathode rays can penetrate through thin metal sheets. Proposes analogy between optic and electromagnetic waves.
1889	Henry Rowland (1848–1901): moving charges show magnetic effect.
1891	Nikola Tesla (1856–1943): performs tests with high-frequency current.
1893	Joseph John Thomson (1856–1940): measures velocity of cathode rays with a rotating mirror (lower than velocity of light).
1894	Philipp Lenard (1862–1947): is able to transmit cathode rays through thin aluminum window into the atmosphere ('Lenard rays').
1895	Jean Baptiste Pervin (1870–1942): provides experimental evidence that cathode rays consist of negative electric particles.

covery would prove to be more important than the discovery of X-rays, possibly because of the greater problems encountered in the experiments, and of the concept behind it (Sommerfeld, 1915).

Roentgen was nominated for admission to the Berlin Academy, the proposal signed by E. Warburg and other members of the Academy, on 4 February 1896. This nomination was a general acknowledgement of Roentgen's entire work up to 1896:

'Roentgen's first investigation dealt with the experimental determination of the ratio of both specific heats of gases. It came about at the instigation of Kundt and was a first rate precision job. By using large containers, they succeeded in reducing the interfering influence of heat exchange with the glass walls to a minimum, as had been seen by Kundt and others. Further extraordinary precision tasks that had been performed from 1884 to 1894 were on the compressibility of liquid and also on the influence of pressure on capillarity, viscosity and refraction of light of these elements. These investigations were carried out together with Schneider and Zehnder.

While the works mentioned above dealt with fields governed by well-known laws, the experiments investigating the electrical properties of quartz had to find general features that can explain subordinate phenomena of less clarity. Roentgen deduced from his investigations that the electric excitation of quartz by changes of temperature and radiation could be related to the electrical excitation pressure. He also discovered the peculiar result that a cylindric quartz rod, whose axis lay parallel to the main axis, became electric after torsion.

Roentgen proved his great constructive talent in his investigation of the electromagnetic effect of dielectric polarization and his skillfulness in finding new methods, among others, in his investigation of the absorption of heat in gases and vapors. He had the genial idea to measure directly the temperature rise of the gas caused by the heat remaining in the gas instead of measuring the rays after transmission through the gas. Through this method, he succeeded in solving the old controversy on water vapour absorption.

All of Roentgen's works mentioned as well as those omitted are distinguished by their reliability and diligence in detecting and eliminating sources of error. Remarkable new relationships between properties of con-

stituents are not derived from these works and they were not much noticed. They were also not comparable to the importance of Roentgen's new discovery which engaged the world at the time. While the initial observation leading to this outstanding discovery was a stroke of luck, the same skillfulness that had made his previous experiments successful enabled Roentgen to determine the properties of the newly discovered rays with great precision and expediency. He hardly touched upon the important and evidently practical meaning of the discovery. He only discussed the scientific questions, which is admirable.'

This proposal was put forward and signed by Warburg, Kohlrausch, Planck, Fischer and Bezold.

Roentgen - a German or a Dutchman?

Roentgen was influenced by three countries: Germany, The Netherlands and Switzerland. His formative years were spent in The Netherlands, his scientific education took place in Switzerland and his professional life was spent in Germany.

Wilhelm Conrad Roentgen was born on 27 March 1845 in Lennep, a small, pretty village with slate-roofed houses, 35 km west of Duesseldorf. It is now part of Remscheid. The house where Roentgen was born, now houses the Library of the German Roentgen Museum.

Wilhelm Conrad was an only child. In 1848, the Roentgen family left Lennep and moved to the city of Apeldoorn in The Netherlands, possibly to find better economic conditions or to escape the political circumstances in the Rhineland which were uncertain because of the revolution. Apeldoorn, at the border of the Veluwe Nature Reserve, had, in 1850, about 3000 inhabitants, mostly belonging to the Dutch Reformed Church, as did father and son. His mother, however, was a member of the Walloon Reformed Church.

Both parents had ties with Holland. Roentgen's mother was born in Amsterdam. Roentgen's father and grandfather were linen merchants. His parents were prosperous, exemplified by the securities invested in railways in various countries, which were found in Roentgen's estate.

When Wilhelm Conrad Roentgen was 17 years old, he attended the technical school in Utrecht, one of the oldest cities in The Netherlands, with its many canals and dominated by its cathedral. He got good reports. However, when he refused to divulge the name of a classmate, who had drawn a caricature of a teacher, he was expelled from the school. He took the entrance examination at the University of Utrecht but did not pass. After preparing for only 8 months, he attempted to pass the examination in classical languages but the time was obviously too short. He was allowed to attend lectures on zoology, Latin, Greek, physics, botany, stereometry, analytic geometry and logic at Utrecht University for two terms from 1864 until 1865, but only as a guest student.

In Utrecht, he stayed with Dr J.W. Gunning (1827–1900), a chemist, who was later appointed to a professorship in Amsterdam. In 1896, Roentgen wrote a moving letter to Gunning saying that: *'You will always have a place in my heart and I have never forgotten how much I have to thank you both'* (W.A.H. van Wylick, 1975). In 1865, Roentgen compiled a 58-page brochure with questions pertaining to the chemistry book written by Dr J.W. Gunning. This brochure was Roentgen's first publication.

Later, Roentgen remembered Holland as a country that: *'I owe so much and where I had a happy childhood.'* (Roentgen to Lorentz, 12 April 1915, in W.A.H. van Wylick, 1975).

When Roentgen learned that it was possible to attend the Polytechnical Institute in Zurich without a school-leaving certificate, he went there in 1865. Because of his good school records and the preparatory studies in Utrecht, he was allowed to study without an entrance examination. After three years, he received a diploma in mechanical engineering. One of his teachers was Rudolf Clausius, the physicist who extended the kinetic theory of gases.

In 1869, Roentgen submitted his doctoral thesis on 'Studien über Gase' (studies on gases) to the University of Zurich, which shared several facilities with the Polytechnical Institute. He had lost interest in his initial plan to work in industry. Then he met August Kundt, a young Professor in Physics at the University of Zurich, who asked him about his future plans, and when he replied that he did not have any, Kundt advised him *'to try physics'*. Roentgen then began *'to study and pursue'* physics.

During his stay in Switzerland, he became fascinated by the mountains. From all his subsequent homes, he went on mountain hikes during the autumn holidays, usually in Pontresina or Cadenábbia, while in spring he spent his holidays in Italy. Roentgen knew about the positive and negative aspects of travelling and wrote later: *'Travelling belongs to the best educational means. I admit that this mean can turn to "poison" and it already has in many of today's travellers'* (S. Woelfflin, 1955).

He met Anna Bertha Ludwig in Zurich. She was the daughter of an innkeeper, who, as a student of classical languages, had left Germany on political grounds and settled in Switzerland in 1830. In the first half of the nineteenth century, Zurich was an asylum for many German intellectuals who as liberals and fighters for democracy were persecuted in their homeland. In Zurich, Roentgen became interested in the debates of these intellectuals and loved to participate.

In 1872, Wilhelm Conrad Roentgen and Anna Bertha Ludwig were married in Apeldoorn. The marriage remained childless. Later they adopted the daughter of Anna Bertha Roentgen's brother.

Roentgen went as Professor Kundt's assistance to Würzburg in 1871 and, in 1872, to Strasbourg. Kundt valued Roentgen for his accurate investigations. They also published some papers jointly. Roentgen was subsequently offered a position as Professor of Physics in Hohenheim (1875), Strasbourg (1876), Giessen (1879) and Würzburg (1888). In Würzburg, the Institute of Physics had moved into a new building only a few years earlier. It was, perhaps, satisfying for him to work at the very university that, a few years previously, had refused his admission because of lacking the appropriate certificate. He declined an invitation to come to Utrecht in 1888. The correspondence between Roentgen and the Utrecht University reveals that, even at that time, he was already famous in Europe. The series of articles he had published from 1870 to 1888 proved Roentgen's versatility. They were on subjects dealing with elasticity, acoustics, crystallography and electricity. He also declined invitations to come to the universities in Jena and Freiburg, even before his discovery of the X-rays.

For Roentgen, the periods spent in Giessen and Würzburg were the most productive. In both cities, he had made friends for life, the ophthalmologist von Hippel, the surgeons Kroenlein and Schoenborn, the classical scholar Hitzig, the anatomist Stoehr, the ophthalmologist Woelfflin, his younger colleague Zehnder and, especially, Boveri, with whom he had extensive discussions, went hunting and undertook mountain tours. He later said that the time spent in Würzburg was the happiest time of his life.

In 1900, he accepted the professorship of physics offered by the University of Munich. In 1915, Roentgen lost his best friend Boveri, and in 1919, his wife after 47 years of happy marriage. He became lonely, and retired in 1920. The attacks by his colleagues had left their marks on him. However, he regarded most of the honors he had re-ceived as formalities. He wholeheartedly disliked everything that was artificial, pretentious and pompous. He was deaf to flattery and he did not know what prejudice was. G. Forssell, the great Swedish radiologist, was impressed by his natural simplicity, cautious circumspection and farsightedness. On 10 February 1923, he died of an ileus caused by cancer of the colon. He was buried in a shared tomb, alongside his parents and wife, in Giessen.

The importance of the discovery of roentgen rays

Physics before 1895: was it 'complete'?

In the second half of the nineteenth century, physics was characterized by theories that found technical applications. The electromagnetic theories (Michael Faraday, 1837; James Clerk Maxwell, 1864; Heinrich Hertz, 1890) resulted in electric light and radio transmission, and the theory of thermodynamics (Rudolf Clausius, 1850; Josiah Gibbs, 1876) resulted in the development of the steam engine and combustion motor. The mechanical world pictured by Galilei and Newton was considered to be definitive. According to this world, space and time are absolute, and the processes and movements continual, with ether playing an important role as a universal medium. It is therefore not surprising that, in 1875, a professor of physics said to Max Planck, who wanted to study physics: *'Young man, why should you want to destroy your future? Theoretical physics has been completed. The differential equations are formulated, the methods to solve them have been worked out. A few special cases are left to be calculated. But is it worthwhile to devote one's entire life to such a case?'* This is how the well-known Russian physicist A.F. Joffé, who had been Roentgen's assistant for many years in Munich, quoted Max Planck.

Even H. von Helmholtz declared in 1894 that the task of physics was *'the mere general presentation of facts and their laws, as given to physics by the systems of differential equations'* (Gerlach, 1980).

The importance of the year 1895

The start of the heroic period of physics

The place of Roentgen in a historic perspective was clearly described in his nomination for corresponding membership of the Berlin Academy on 18 November 1920:

'The importance of Mr. Roentgen's scientific accomplishments is so vast and so widely known, and has been appropriately acknowledged in the records of the Academy in conjunction with his nomination for membership and on the occasion of the fiftieth anniversary of receiving his doctorate, that it is superfluous to recite it again. Roentgen is generally considered to be the father of German experimental physics, and it seems quite appropriate to honor him by nominating him for corresponding membership. The obvious reason to submit this proposal at this particular time is the fact that exactly 25 years have passed this December since the discovery of X-rays, which heralded a new era in the history of physics.'

This nomination was proposed by H. Rubens and signed by Rubens, Laue, Liebisch, Nernst, Schwanz, Mueller, Hellmann, Erhard, Schmidt, Einstein, Haber, Warburg and Planck.

The years between 1895 and 1916 have been called 'the heroic period of physics' by J.D. Barnal. It began with the discovery of X-rays in 1895 by Roentgen, and continued with the discovery of natural radiation by Henry Becquerel only a few months later (1896). In 1898, Marie Curie's investigations with 'Becquerel rays' resulted in the discovery of radium. For the phenomenon of spontaneous radiation of elements, Marie and Pierre Curie invented the term 'radioactivity'.

Although, over a period of 100 years, the existence of atoms had been debated in chemistry and physics, the boundaries of imagination were soon reached. For example, the structure of the atom was unknown. The new fundamental investigations on X-rays, radioactivity and others (such as the discovery of the electron by J. J. Thomson in 1897, with subsequent measurements of the electron's charge) formed the experimental basis on which the great theories of modern physics could be developed: the quantum theory (Max Planck, 1900); the theory of special and general relativity (Albert Einstein, 1905 and 1916; important pioneers Ernst Mach and Hendrik Antoon Lorentz, 1892); and the proposed model of the atom (Ernest Rutherford, 1910; Niels Bohr, 1913; Arnold Sommerfeld, 1916). It almost seemed as if physics had to be written all over again. However, because of new information, the classical laws gained a new foothold, expressed by W. Gerlach (1980) when he stated that: *'The basic laws of classical physics are still true, but the atomic phenomena have additional unique laws.'*

The beginning of the reign of technology in medicine

'When the hand is held between the discharge apparatus and the screen, one can see the dark shadows of the bones of the hand and within the less dark shadows of the hand itself,' Roentgen wrote in his preliminary report. The reign of technology in medicine began with this observation.

Of all principles and methods of visual diagnosis in medicine, X-rays have affected the most significant changes. The evolving technology has become of great importance for diagnosis but also for therapy (S.J. Reiser, 1991).

X-rays in non-medical disciplines

Other disciplines, not related to medicine, were heavily influenced by the discovery of X-rays, including crystallography, structural analysis, material testing, biology, archaeology and art.

'Medical deeds rest on two pillars' (Karl Jaspers)

The constantly expanding scientific approach, and the technically perfectionistic way of thinking and acting in medicine brought about a counter-movement of which psychoanalysis is the most important (R. Winau, 1973). It is not by chance that 1895, the year X-rays were discovered, also saw the birth of psychoananlysis with the publication of 'Studien ueber Hystery' (Studies on Hysteria) by Sigmund Freud and Josef Breuer.

References

Barnal, J.D.: Wissenschaft Bd. 3. Rororo Hamburg 1970

Clark, G.L.: The contribution of a quarter century of electron physics to Roentgen-ray science. Am. J. Roentgenol. 26 (1931) 528–539

Crane, A.W.: The research trail of the x-ray. Radiology 23 (1934) 131

Dessauer, F.: Wilhelm C. Röntgen. Die Offenbarung einer Nacht. Walter, Olten 1945

Forssell, G.: Wilhelm Conrad Röntgen. Acta Radiol 19 (1923) 101–109

Franke, H.: Zur Geschichte der Röntgenschen Entdeckung. Fortschr Röntgenstr 34 (1926) 441

Gerlach, W.: Physik und Chemie. In: Propyläen-Weltgeschichte Bd. IX S. 477. Hrsgg. von G. Mann, Prisma-Verlag Gütersloh 1980

Glasser, O.: The genealogy of the Roentgen rays. Am J Roentgenol 30 (1933) 180

Glasser, O.: Scientific forefathers of Röntgen. Am J Roentgenol 54 (1945) 545–546

Glasser, O.: Wilhelm Conrad Röntgen. 2. Auflage. Springer-Verlag, Berlin-Göttingen-Heidelberg 1959

Goerke, H.: Röntgen und die Ärzte. Berichte d. Physik.-Med. Gesellsch. zu Würzburg 79 (1971) 55–68

Hennig, U.: Deutsches Röntgen-Museum Remscheid-Lennep. Westermann, Braunschweig 1989

Hermann, A.: Weltreich der Physik. Bechtle, Esslingen 1981

Joffe, A.F.: Begegnungen mit Physikern. Teubner, Leipzig 1967

Koch, P.P.: Wilhelm Conrad Röntgen als Forscher und Mensch. Z techn Phys 4 (1923) 273–279

Kuhn, Th.S.: Die Entstehung des Neuen. Suhrkamp, Frankfort a.M. 1978

Lenard, Ph.: Grosse Naturforscher. J.F. Lehmanns Verlag, München 1930

Patton, D.D.: Insights on the radiological centennial - a historical perspective. Roentgen and the "new light". I. Roentgen and Lenard. Invest Radiol 27 (1992) 408–414

Physiker über Physiker. Wahlvorschläge zur Aufnahme von Physikern in die Berliner Akademie 1870-1929 von Hermann v. Helmholtz bis Erwin Schrödinger. Bearb. von C. Kirsten u. H.-G. Körber Akademie-Verlag Berlin 1975

Reiser, S.J.: Medicine and the reign of technology. Cambridge Univ. Press 1991

Röntgen, W.C.: Über eine neue Art von Strahlen. (Vorläufige Mitteilung). Sitzungsber. Physik.-med. Ges. Würzburg (1895) 132–141

Röntgen, W.C.: Über eine neue Art von Strahlen. (Fortsetzung). II. Mitteilung. Sitzungsber. Physik.-med. Ges. Würzburg (1896) 11–17

Röntgen, W.C.: Weitere Beobachtungen über die Eigenschaften der X-Strahlen. III. Mitteilung. Sitzungsber. Kgl. preuss. Akad. Wissensch. Berlin (1897) 576

Schrödinger, E.: Die Natur und die Griechen. Rowohlts Deutsche Enzyklopädie 1956

Simonyi, K.: Kulturgeschichte der Physik. Deutsch, Frankfurt 1990.

Sommerfeld, A.: Zu Röntgens siebzigstem Geburtstag. Physik Zeitschr 16 (1915) 89–93

Thomson, J.J.: zit. nach Simonyi.

Thompson, S.P.: zit. nach Glasser (1933)

Winau, R.: Röntgens Entdeckung und die Medizin. Inter Nationes, Bonn-Bad Godesberg, I 1973

Wölfflin, S.: Meine persönlichen Erinnerungen an W.C. Röntgen. 1955

Van Wylick, W.A.H.: Röntgen und die Niederlande. Remscheid-Lennep 1975

Zakovsky, J.: Die zwei ersten Veröffentlichungen zu Röntgens Entdeckung der neuen Strahlen. Röntgenstrahlen, Sommer 1959

Zehnder, L.: W.C. Röntgen. Briefe an L. Zehnder. Rascher, Zürich 1935

Medical science before 1895

G. Rosenbusch, M. Oudkerk, E. Ammann

At the beginning of the nineteenth century, romanticism prevailed in Germany and natural philosophy (Naturphilosophie) was taught by Friedrich Wilhelm Schelling (1775–1845) and, from a medical viewpoint, by Carl Gustav Carus (1779–1868). Natural philosophy believes in the unity of nature and that spirit and matter are one. Since it was a belief in a universal order of metaphysical validity, natural phenomena were interpreted to conform with this pattern. There was no need to perform experimental studies and speculative thinking prevailed. Analogies were made that are incomprehensible today, such as between blood cells and the earth or tophaceous deposits of gout and onions, and the physician was empowered by divine grace and exercised his art through authority. Science and medicine were seen as servants of philosophy (Shryock, The development of modern medicine, 1979).

A radical change got under way in the mid-nineteenth century, beginning in France where the situation was quite different than in Germany. The French Revolution (1789) encouraged the concept of progress and raised intelligence to an eminent status. It is therefore not surprising that the natural scientific method was first developed in France and spread from there.

The rural exodus as a result of the Industrial Revolution caused the cities to grow enormously. Malnutrition, lack of hygiene, lack of sunlight in the narrow streets and alleys led to diseases and epidemics. There was an urgent need for health care. Many physicists and chemists, such as Jean le Rond d'Alembert (1717–1783), Antoine-Laurent Lavoisier (1743–1794) and Pierre Simon Laplace (1749–1827), had good relations with physicians in Paris who extended and inspired their scientific ideas.

The physicians wanted to apply the principles of physics and medicine to their examinations and treatments. This approach concurred with the ideas of John Locke (1632–1704), the founder of empiricism, the doctrine that our knowledge is derived from experience and that there are no innate ideas or principles.

Around 1800, Paris was the fourth medical centre of Europe, in addition to Vienna, Dublin and London. In the early nineteenth century, there were as many as 30 hospitals in Paris with 10 000 beds: the Hôtel Dieu alone had 1000 beds. The Parisian medical school housed many eminent specialists, such as the pathologist Xavier Bichat (1771–1802), the internists Jean-Nicolas Corvisart (1755–1821), René Théophile Laënnec (1781–1826) and Victor Broussais (1772–1838), the bacteriologist Louis Pasteur (1822–1895), Ferdinand Widal (1862–1929), the surgeons Jean Dominique Larrey (1766–1842) and Guillaume Dupuytren (1777–1835). Corvisart and Laënnec, in particular, deserve credit for the introduction of the stethoscope and the technique of percussion.

Foreign physicians and people with an interest in science came to Paris to become familiar with the development and ideas of true science. Precise, independent research was important for the scientific approach, necessary to observe and explain the healthy and diseased organism. It brought about new and important results, which contributed considerably to the body of medical knowledge. In Germany, natural philosophical views were first suppressed but later expanded through science. At the end, both science and natural philosophy complemented each other. Nevertheless, the teachers of the new scientific approach characterized natural philosophy as the plague or Black death of the century (Justus von Liebig 1803–1873).

Johannes Mueller (1801–1858), the founder of modern scientific physiology, accused the philosophic natural healers, of which he was once a member, in his inaugural lecture in Bonn 1824: *'The virtues of the naturalists are very simplistic, but the real essence of observation, the real power of observation and its application have become rare among scientists who occupied themselves with living organisms.'*

Mueller characterized the progress of medicine from a philosophically orientated discipline to a scientific discipline in the following words: *'Medicine can only then make true progress when physics, chemistry and all the natural sciences are applied in their entirety, thus raising medicine also to their current elevated levels and in step with their marvelous advances.'* Observation is of central importance and it must only be explained scientifically.

In the first half of the nineteenth century, anatomical observations were primarily descriptive, although fundamental investigations on histology had been performed. Later, there were attempts to classify the human anatomy in an historical context: was humankind a creation in its own right or an extraordinary development of nature?

Comparative anatomy looked for similarities and differences between living creatures, while developmental biology (embryology) looked at the development of an organism from conception to adulthood and the concomitant differentiation. Significant similarities were found in the construction and development of the various groups of organisms. The study of heredity became the next subject of interest. Darwin's (1809–1882) theory on the evolution of living species was epoch-making. On the basis of his observations of the geographic distribution of animals on the South American coast, he became *'fully convinced that species are not immutable'*. Here, basic religious beliefs were indeed questioned.

The use of newly developed recording equipment and measuring techniques in physics and chemistry helped physiology to flourish under Johannes Mueller and his students Hermann von Helmholtz (1821–1894), Carl Ludwig (1816–1895) and Emil Du Bois-Reymond (1818–1896). Likewise, pathology prospered under Rudolf Virchow (1821–1902) and his students Edwin Klebs (1834–1913), Julius Cohnheim (1838–1884) and Friedrich von Recklinghausen (1833–1910). While Mueller made considerable contributions towards reviving logical research in

physiology, Ludwig laid the foundation of modern physiology that employs experiments, causal reasoning, and physicochemical quantitative analysis. Ludwig was of the opinion that the role of physiology was to ascertain the basic functions of the living animal and to deduce these as a necessity from its elementary conditions.

The topics covered in Ludwig's institute comprised a broad spectrum of subjects, from the movements of organs through diffusion and secretion on to circulation. The kymograph, the mercury pump and the flow meters were developed in this institute, instruments that were indispensable for physiologic investigations for many years.

In Vienna, Karl von Rokitansky (1804–1878) had already contributed important fundamental work to pathology through systematic comparison of autopsy findings and clinical observations. Simultaneously, Virchow considered the cell to be the basic morphologic element, encompassing life, disease and death. It is for this reason that he ascribed a particular role to the examination under the microscope. His seminal work 'Cellular Pathology' was published in 1858, only a few years after he had left Wuerzburg and had accepted an appointment in Berlin. The wide range of his extraordinary intellectual power – his specialities were pathology, epidemiology, anthropology and, ultimately, politics – made him the greatest personality in German medicine and one of the world's most eminent medical scientists. For him, medicine was *'a social science and politics is nothing but medicine on a large scale.'*

The chemist Emil Fischer (1852–1919), in cooperation with his students, analyzed animal proteins and expanded knowledge of organic chemistry considerably. His studies on carbohydrates, amino acids and peptides were the foundation for much research in the fields of blood, nutrition and metabolism.

The Dutch chemist, Jacobus Hendricus van't Hoff (1852–1911) created the basis for physical chemistry. His theory on electrolytic dissociation was important in explaining osmotic pressure, seen in blood, lymphogenesis, secretion and resorption.

Arising from studies about heat balance in the human body under tropical conditions, Julius Robert Mayer (1814–1878) formulated the law of the conservation of energy, which played an important role in scientific debates.

Broadening the medical foundations of physiology, pharmacology, chemistry and pathology had in turn an effect on the clinical practice. Johann Lukas Schoenlein (1791–1864) extended laboratory research so that blood and urine were not only judged by appearance alone but also by the results of chemical analysis and microscopic examinations. Schoenlein, just as Skoda and Rokitansky, stressed the necessity for a close relationship between internal medicine and pathological anatomy and encouraged clinicopathological conferences. He perfected the physical examination, percussion and auscultation, and documented the course of the diseases for correlation of the obtained results.

Pathologic conditions were artificially induced and analyzed, primarily by Ludwig Traube (1818–1876) and Julius Cohnheim (1839–1884), whereby Traube's investigations concerned breathing, circulation and the related pharmacology, and Cohnheim's investigations inflammatory processes and vascular pathology including thrombosis and embolism. Claude Bernard (1813–1878) in France and Ivan Pavlov (1849–1936) in Russia were the masters of experimental physiology. Claude Bernard was famous for his basic approach to experimental medicine and for his new insight into the carbohydrate metabolism, the sympathetic nervous system and the role of the pancreas in digestion. Pavlov was known for his studies on gastric secretion, especially under the influence of psychological factors. Applied physiology and pathophysiology, founded at that time, formed the basis for research in diseases and finally in clinical medicine. Virchow already considered *pathological physiology the crown of scientific medicine to which the pathological anatomy and clinical studies are only attached.*

Even though in the meantime travelers reported their experience from remote countries, the medical yield was limited. In 1836, Christoph Wilhelm Hufeland (1762-1836), an influential physician and professor at the University of Berlin, as well as the personal physician of the King of Prussia, mentioned bloodletting, opium and emetics as the *'three capital remedies of medicine'*: *'They equally represent the three fundamental methods of medicine, the antiphlogistic, the gastric, the excising method; and at the same time the three fundamental systems, bloodletting for the irritable, the vomitive for the reproductive and opium for the sensitive … . They immediately intervene. …; they can give life but also death; they decide the battle in the critical moment; on its use depend the fortune and good name of the physician … . Whosoever knows how to use these three correctly, is a master and can be recognized as such.'* These statements concur with the natural philosophical tradition of medicine. As early as 1816, the French physician François Magendie

(1783–1855) stated that the entire knowledge of medicine had been of no value until that date.

In the second half of the nineteenth century, established remedies, which were usually extracted from plants, were analyzed, to identify their potent components and their composition and how they could be manufactured or altered to increase their potency. Dosages and routes of application had so far been vaguely stated and were experimentally unsubstantiated. Nothing was known about actions, side-effects and elimination of drugs. A lot was ahead for pharmacology and pharmacy. At the end, research did not remain confined to the universities but was taken over to a large extent by the newly developing pharmaceutical industry.

It was important for pharmacology that chemistry could deliver relevant results that lead to new methods for analysis and synthesis. Using physical methods in chemistry, physical chemistry, which deals with the kinetics of chemical reactions and their determining factors, was founded, in addition to organic and inorganic chemistry. Wilhelm Ostwald (1853–1932), Jacobus Hendricus van't Hoff (1852–1911) and Svante August Arrhenius (1859–1927) have earned their place in this field.

The chemical industry boomed at the turn of the century. During this time, many now well-known companies were founded. In 1869, alizarin was synthesized, representing the beginning of industrial manufacturing of synthetic dyes, and in 1873, salicylic acid, serving as the basis for acetylsalicylic acids, aspirin. Phenacetin followed in 1882 and sulfonal in 1886. Natural products were broken down into their components which, in turn, formed the basis of new drugs or household products.

Furthermore, other methods of treatment came into existence, such as hydrotherapy (according to Kneipp) and heliotherapy. Climatic resorts and spas were built. Tuberculosis, in particular, was subjected to this kind of treatment. In low altitude mountains and the high altitude alpine mountains, sanatoria were built where a variety of nonspecific treatments were offered, such as rest, fresh air, sunbathing and nutritional food.

The introductions to the following chapters will present the developments in serology, bacteriology, hygiene, and surgery with anesthetics and asepsis that took place in the second half of the nineteenth century .

Within the framework of these major changes in medicine, the diagnosis underwent an unprecedented growth through the application of X-rays since 1896.

The pioneering age of radiology

G. Rosenbusch, M. Oudkerk, E. Ammann

The news travels around the world

At the turn of the year 1895/96, Roentgen sent a reprint with copies of his first 'radiographs' to, among others, the professor of physics Franz Exner in Vienna, who was a former fellow student in Zurich. At the very next evening meeting of physicists, Exner demonstrated the radiographs. The physicist Ernst Lecher, who saw them, told his father, an editor of the Vienna newspaper 'Presse', about the demonstration. Ernst Lecher wrote a brief summary which was published the next day, 5 January 1896, on the front page of the *Presse* under the heading *'a sensational discovery'*. The article also described future perspectives and ideas, probably not written by Lecher.

A representative of Reuter's news agency was informed about the article in the 'Presse' by colleagues. He immediately passed the news on by cable, so that word got around the world within a few days.

The editorial in the 'Presse' had misspelled 'Roentgen' as 'Routgen', this mistake was printed in all newspapers for several days. The 'Presse' had already recognized and rectified the mistake the very next day, but the damage had already been done. Other countries got to know the name of the discoverer as Routgen.

Roentgen himself was greatly disturbed by the uproar brought about by the press. Forebodingly, he told his wife after his discovery that *'all hell might brake loose now'*.

The press talked about an epoch-making discovery: *'in which the pathfinders in the specialized field of photography would shortly come to grips with the discovery and would experiment how to improve it and put it to practical use. As to its practical use, biologists and physicians and especially surgeons will be interested, because it seems that they are being offered a new, and very valuable, diagnostic means. Concerning such a sensational discovery, it is difficult to avoid fantastic futuristic speculations in the style of Jules Verne'* ('Frankfurter Zeitung', Tuesday, 7 January 1896).

On 10 January 1896, the physiologist Sigmund Exner demonstrated before the Royal Association of Physicians in Vienna: 'Photographs produced using newly discovered rays by the Professor in Physics in Wuerzburg, Roentgen'. He also lectured about Roentgen's results [1].

E. Haschek, an assistant in physicist Franz Exner's laboratory, succeeded in taking radiographs of various objects, and had his friend G. Kaiser, a young doctor with an interest in physical problems, present during the experiments. Franz Exner's brother Sigmund, the physiologist, heard of the successful experiments and asked the Privy Councillor E. von Neussner, director of the II. Medical Clinic in Vienna, for permission to try the new rays on living human beings.

The first medical radiographs

Von Neussner visited the Physics Society with a few colleagues the next day. He ordered his assistant Kaiser to take radiographs. Kaiser took the first for ever medically indicated radiographs: a gunshot wound of a hand; a badly set forearm fracture; and a double toe. This occurred between 10 and 17 January 1896, about one to two weeks before the memorable meeting of Physikalisch-medizinische Gesellschaft (Physical Medical Society) in Wuerzburg on 23 January 1896 (Glasser, 1959; Thurnher, 1964; Maurer and Weber, 1977).

On 23 January 1896, the article 'A contribution to the practical application of Roentgen photography' was published in the clinical journal 'Wiener klinische Wochenschrift' by E. Haschek and O.Th. Lindenthal from Professor Franz Exner's Society of Physical Chemistry [2]. In the paper, there was a picture of a hand taken from a cadaver, in which Teichmann's substance, a solution of chalk, cinnabar and petroleum, had been injected into the brachial artery. The radiograph, with an exposure time of 57 minutes, showed not only the skeleton but also the arterial blood vessels (s. Fig. III, 96). An illustration of a little finger of the left hand was also published, which, as the result of a bullet injury, showed a *callus replacing a bone defect in angular position'*.

Furthermore, they made mention of the successful fluoroscopy of the upper arm and forearm of a child, as well as a foot, and of an attempt 'to radiograph the head or torso according to Roentgen's method', which failed due to lack of means. They concluded: *'Should it be possible to succeed with the necessary improvements to picture the other types of tissue of which the organism is composed, a new field would be opened for the well-being of suffering mankind.'*

These same radiographs were already shown by Sigmund Exner at the meeting of the Association of Physicians in Vienna on 17 January 1896. At the meeting of the same society on 24 January 1896, Mosetig-Moorhof demonstrated two radiographs of a hand and a foot. As a result of the radiographs, a 6 mm lead projectile could be located. It had penetrated the palm, due to careless handling of a revolver and could not be located by palpation. The second radiograph showed a malformation of the left big toe, consisting of a duplication [3]. The radiographs were taken in the Exner brothers' laboratory. A few months later, new radiographs were published in the 'Wiener klinische Wochenschrift', this time by R. Poech, who located a foreign body in the lungs using two different projections [4]. In the paper 'Threatened fatal haemorrhage after ingesting a foreign body' by J. Hochenegg, experiments were performed to establish: *'to what extend fluoroscopy with X-rays was appropriate to diagnose a foreign body that got stuck in the throat or oesophagus'*. These experiments were performed at the pathologic institute in cooperation with Poech. Foreign bodies, such as chicken bones, a denture and pieces of metal, were introduced into a cadaver. The radiographs were of remarkable quality. Unfortunately, their Ruehmkorff coil got damaged and the authors had to terminate their investigations.

Birth of radiology in Vienna

At the beginning of 1896, G. Kaiser had a small laboratory, whose staff at first only worked for the II. Medical Clinic but who soon started working for many of the clinics in the General Hospital.

The hospital management promised him an efficient unit on condition that he would perform: *'fluoroscopies and where possible radiographs of patients'* for all the departments. This 'Roentgen department' at the General Hospital in Vienna, under the supervision of Kaiser and his collaborators, Dr Poech and Dr Stoeckl, was the nucleus of the later rather famous Central Roentgen Institute. Kaiser retired from his work in the hospital because of severe radiation injuries and only worked in a private practice. In 1902, the young G. Holzknecht took over the supervision of the institute from A. Stoeckl, and was able to make it independent as early as 1914 (Fig. I, 15). Holzknecht knew how to attract capable collaborators, and founded, together with R. Kienboeck, the famous Viennese Roentgenologic School, which produced such well-known names as Schwarz, Mayer, Hitzenberger, Haudek, Schueller, Fleischner, Paluqyay, Lenk, Freund, Czepa, Eisler, Weiss and Zdansky (Freund, 1937). This school, which excelled in diagnostic, therapeutic and fundamentally scientific areas, collapsed in the forties as many of its best people were forced to leave during the Third Reich.

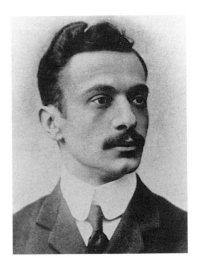

Fig. I, 15. Guido Holzknecht (1872–1931). He founded the once world famous Viennese school of radiology. Worked in many areas of diagnostic and therapeutic radiology. Classic contributions to the diagnosis of gastric tumors, roentgenologic examinations of the Lung parenchyma (1901), and dosimetry. Great organizational talent.

Reactions to the discovery of X-rays in Berlin

While the radiographs taken with roentgen rays did not overly impress the members attending the convention of Society of Physics in Berlin on 4 January 1896, the neurologist and psychiatrist from Berlin, Moritz Jastrowitz, who had seen a reprint with Roentgen's radiograph of his wife's hand, immediately understood the significance of the discovery.

Already on 6 January 1896, he talked about X-rays before the Society of Internal Medicine in Berlin. By 13 January 1896, a 36-line review article had appeared in the section 'Medical Society Proceedings' in the 'Berliner klinische Wochenschrift' [6].

The report stated that the discovery of X-rays was one of the most important of its time. Initially, it was solely a physical phenomenon but could *also be of importance for both internal and external medicine. As proof, the speaker included the radiograph of the human hand, which looked 'exactly as if it had been a photographed skeleton, but was actually taken from a living human being'*. The report concludes with the parenthetic remark: *'The new discovery will undoubtedly be of the utmost importance for medicine'*.

At the meeting of the Society of Internal Medicine on 13 January 1896, under the chairmanship of the well-known internist von Leyden, M. Jastrowitz performed a demonstration with a few pieces of lead, put together to make up the form of the letter 'A'. *'These were put inside a wooden box and radiographed with the new X-rays.'* Because the light passed through the wooden box but not through the lead, the shadow was clearly visible on the negative [7]. According to Goerke, this radiograph was taken by the physicist Spies of the 'Urania'. The 'Urania' was a popular scientific association in Berlin that, in the rooms of their meeting place, had many scientific instruments to be used for simple experiments. The medical journal 'Deutsche medizinische Wochenschrift' (German Medical Weekly) of 30 January 1896 printed two lectures by M. Jastrowitz, given on 6 and 20 January 1896, on 'Roentgen experiments with cathode rays and their diagnostic usefulness', with a reproduced radiograph of a hand with a glass splinter near the joint of the middle finger. This radiograph was probably taken on 12 January 1896.

At the meeting of the Berlin Medical Society on 15 January 1896, under the chairmanship of R. Virchow, R. Neuhauss, apparently a practising physician, was allowed *to submit photographs taken by the Roentgen technique. These were produced by Professor Karger, Dr Mendelssohn and S. Joffé in Posen'* [8]. There was no mention of which objects were radiographed, but it was emphasized that the technique *'therefore has a special significance for us practising physicians, and using this technique, we will be able to determine the position of projectiles which have entered the body'*. The technique would also be of use in diagnosing comminuted fractures. Neuhauss stated that *'radiographs of thigh bones are not yet available'*, but that they would undoubtedly get positive results: *'It may only need a tenfold longer exposure time than with the hand'*. With an exposure time of half an hour for a hand, an hour and a half for a forearm, this would mean several hours for a thigh!

On 3 February 1896, a radiograph of a normal foot was published in a one-page article 'On Roentgen's rays' by E. Goldstein, a physicist at the Berlin Observatory. This radiograph was probably taken at the club 'Urania'. It was the first publication of a radiograph in the 'Berliner klinische Wochenschrift' (Berlin Clinical Weekly) [9].

During the meeting of the Berlin Medical Society on 29 January 1896, Wohlgemut showed a *'radiograph taken of a plucked chicken'* [10]. It was stated: *'The long bones in the radiograph are clearly visible and the brighter bone marrow cavity can be clearly distinguished by its sharp contours. The sacrum is also distinctly outlined. A longitudinal fracture of the lower leg is clearly visible. However, head and vertebrae are blurred. The speaker therefore expressed his hope that a wider range be found for medical applications of Roentgen's discovery.'*

At the next meeting of 5 February 1896, Koenig reported on 'Fluoroscopy by means of Roentgen's methods' [11]. He reported that he was: *'in the position to see and treat a patient with a neoplasm in the tibia. I further had the opportunity, not in vivo, because the patient had died, to obtain a radiograph as a postmortem picture of the disease.'* He compared the operative specimen with the 'photograms' (used here synonymously with 'fluoroscopy') and concluded: *'To read from the shadows, the tibia was destroyed, not by a festering infection, but through a neoplasm'*.

On 17 February 1896, Huber demonstrated *'a number of photographs, which also proved the usefulness of Roentgen's rays for internal medicine. These radiographs of patients of the first medical clinic were taken at the Imperial Physical Technical Institute in Berlin.'* These were radiographs of four hands with acute rheumatoid arthritis, chronic rheumatic arthritis, gout, and residual stiffening after blood poisoning. In addition, there was a *'radiograph of an arteriosclerotic aorta'*.

In the discussion following Huber's lecture, Thorner spoke about the substantial progress in radiographic techniques. He commented on the prices of equipment and advised waiting a little longer before buying an X-ray apparatus, because shortly rather cheap units would be marketed.

In the discussion, Ewald referred to a report in the latest 'British Medical Journal' which stated that: *'One could also work with electric light bulbs with broken filaments, to produce X-rays. The matter has thus become so much easier'*. Today, this statement appears absurd considering the further technical development of radiology!

On 22 June 1896, following a few demonstrations, E. Grunmach wrote, in a three-column article 'X-rays in the diagnosis of internal disorders' [12], that *'thanks to technical advancements it has become possible, by means of X-ray tubes and the fluorescent screen, to see important internal organs, to determine their position and size, and to follow their motion'*. In collaboration with the physiologist René Du Bois-Reymond and the engineer Levy, Grunmach examined both healthy and sick individuals in the A.E.G. laboratory. Fluoroscopy of the neck, thorax and abdomen were described. The movements of different organs were investigated. *'If the X-ray tube and the fluorescent screen are moved further down to observe the region of the stomach, from back to front, the diaphragm can be clearly distinguished from the gastric fundus, and when the stomach is filled with a barium mixture, its full expansion can be seen.'*

For the first time, gas was used as a negative contrast medium, a medium that absorbs X-rays to a lesser degree than, for instance, water or soft tissues. Furthermore, several pathologies were discussed, such as arteriosclerosis, pulmonary tuberculosis, and hypertrophy of the left ventricle. The article concluded that: *'The use of X-rays not only confirms the results of our current methods used to examine patients, but already enables the recognition of all anomalies, that were up to now undetectable with the available methods. With the help of X-ray tube and the fluorescent screen, it has even become possible to see changes in organs that were impossible to diagnose with other methods.'*

After publication of 'removal of foreign bodies with the help of X-rays' [13] and the demonstration of radiographs, 'On the current state of roentgenological technique' was published by W. Cowl on 27 July 1896, [14], in which he wrote: *'As a result of considerable improvements, the shadow image of internal organs of living human beings may assume fundamental meaning for internal medicine'*. In this impressive article, he stated that: *'The use of the photographic plate … forms an indispensable confirmation and completion of the immediate observation using the fluorescent screen'*. After a discussion on the transmission of X-rays through different tissues, he continued: *'From this follows the possibility of performing a thorough examination of the chest wall as well as the chest's contents by means of X-ray penetration. Applying the same to the abdomen, particularly to the pelvis, is more difficult as the increasingly thicker muscles of the trunk are very much in the way, especially in healthy, muscular individuals.'* Cowl had already spoken of: *'the composite nature of Roentgen's shadow images.'* General comments upon the analysis of the thorax followed.

Individual demonstration of radiographs took place thereafter and, on 7 September 1896, a case report on a congenital anomaly of the right hemithorax and corresponding hand was published by Joachimsthal [15].

On 23 November 1896, Max Levy-Dorn (Fig. I, 16) [16] described the radiological appearance of an asthmatic attack and, on 2 December 1896, he gave an address called 'Contribution to the method of examination with X-rays' [17] at the meeting of the Berlin Medical Society. He stated that they have still been unsuccessful *'in brightening the darkness of most of the internal organs using X-rays, despite improved technique. The fault, as may well be known, lies in the impossibility of avoiding the superimposition of the many shadows, which become more or less obscured and thus blur the image.'* Levy-Dorn considered the use of intracavitary X-rays tubes, e.g. in the rectum, vagina and mouth but the hazards of working with the tubes were too great in those days. He also contemplated using X-ray sensitive substances, such as fluorescent plates that are inserted into body cavities.

A comparison of both leading journals of the two German-speaking radiological centres – Vienna and Berlin – reveals that in the first months after the discovery of X-rays the articles with radiographic content were more foresighted and comprehensive in the journal from

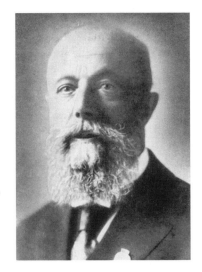

Fig. I, 16. Max Levy-Dorn (1863–1929). Opened in October 1896 a roentgenologic laboratory in Berlin, was in 1906 appointed physician-in-charge of the roentgenologic ward of the Rudolf-Virchow-Hospital. Immediately used all new methods. Liked to organize popular seminars.

Berlin. Reviewing journals in such a way worldwide can provide information that is representative of the different views and investigations. Each country keeps in memory its pioneers who contributed to the development of this new specialty, whether through science or organizations.

Radiographs as evidence

It is remarkable that radiographs as evidence in court were used in a case of malpractice as early as November 1896 in Denver, Colorado, USA. It concerned a boy who had been injured falling from a ladder. A famous surgeon, who had been consulted, did not immobilize the thigh, but instead ordered exercises as appropriate for contusion. The boy's attorney sought the advice of a person who became an expert in photography and radiography by taking radiographs, for the last eight months, for his own enjoyment and the entertainment of his friends. He accepted the invitation to take a radiograph of the boy's hip.'

'The electric apparatus, batteries, Crookes' tubes, etc. were all in the court room.' The photographer first introduced the basic principles of radiographic imaging. By shining the light of a candle through a small opening in a box onto a screen, he demonstrated to the judges a shadow image cast by a hand. Then he showed images of a hand and a watch, produced by X-rays on a fluoroscopic screen. The sight of the bones of the judge's hand caused quite a commotion, as it was reported by the press the following day. Finally, the shadow image of a femur cast by a candlelight and the radiographic images of the boy's femur were demonstrated. The exposure time was 80 minutes!

The radiograph showed that the femoral head was not in normal position in relation to the major trochanter and femoral shaft. The radiograph was presented to the judge as evidence of an impacted fracture.

In a remarkable comment it was documented that 'Courts of Justice had opened their doors wide for all well-studied scientific discoveries. Modern science had made it possible to see beneath the tissues of the human body and helped surgery to reveal the hidden mysteries' (Withers, 1931). With the possibility of documentation, radiology would play an important role in judging medical activities in the future (Collins, 1964).

Who took the radiographs and how can the new trade be learned?

Wherever equipment similar to that used by Roentgen was installed, attempts were made to take radiographs. Primarily, this applied to university institutes of physics but also to high schools. Photographers interested in the new radiographic technique purchased equipment and advertised in newspapers (Figs I, 17–20). In addition, institutes of physical medicine, e.g. the popular Zander Institutes, which were dedicated to gymnastics and physical therapy, got involved in the application of the new radiation.

Mainly the younger physicians took an immediate interest in the new X-rays and dedicated their lives to them but, unfortunately, also became their victims. Other young physicians with an aptitude for technique and physics were often appointed to investigate the new rays. They had a background in surgery, orthopaedics and internal medicine, and visited many laboratories and institutes of radiography to learn the method, often subjecting themselves to extensive traveling.

In Britain, only four months after Roentgen's discovery, the 'Archives of Clinical Skiagraphy' was founded by Sidney Rowland, the first radiologic journal, which later (in 1924) became the 'British Journal of Radiology'.

In 1897, 'The American X-ray Journal' followed as the first American periodical and as the predecessor of the 'American Journal of Roentgenology', and in the same year in Germany, 'Fortschritte auf dem Gebiete der Roentgenstrahlen' (Advances in the Field of Roentgen Rays), which has been continuously published for 98 years in the year of the 100th anniversary of the discovery of X-rays, except for a few months after the Second World War. Radiographic journals were founded in nearly all countries. There was a surprisingly good exchange of experience and knowledge between the USA and Europe.

To keep up with the rapid development of technique and speciality and to exchange experience, associations were founded shortly after the discovery of the X-rays. The Roentgen Society was founded in England on 3 June 1897, and locally in Berlin, on 18 March 1898, the 'Roentgen Vereinigung' (Roentgen Association), which on 2 May 1905 during their first convention helped to form the 'Deutsche Roentgengesellschaft' (German Roentgen Society) (Fig. I, 21). The

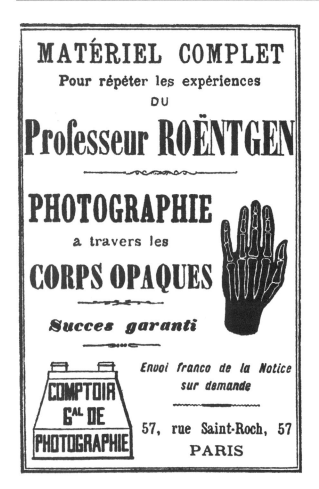

Fig. I, 17. Advertisement for Roentgen photographs.

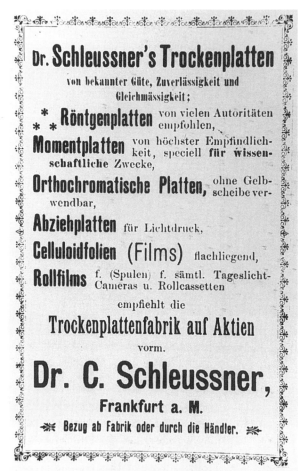

Fig. I, 18. Advertisement by Dr. Schleussner, 1899.

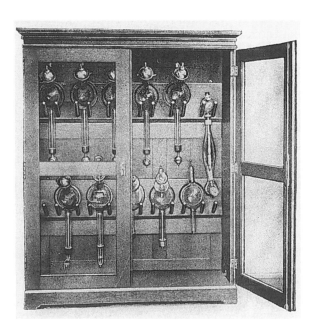

Fig. 1.19. Roentgen tubes for different applications

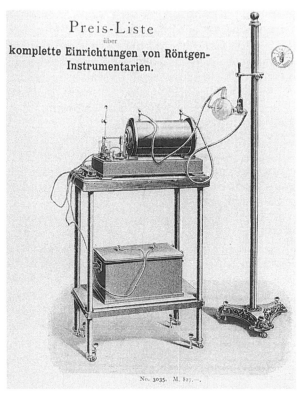

Fig. I, 20. Price of a complete roentgenologic equipment (RGS 1897, Elektromed. Apparate).

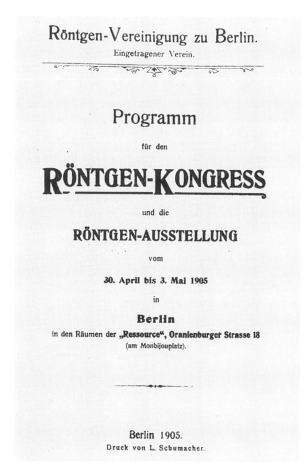

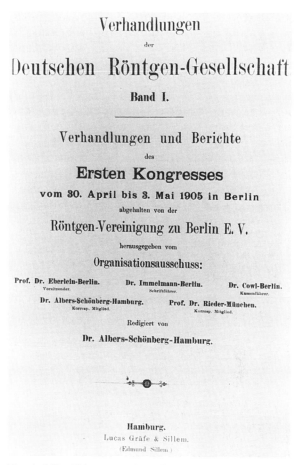

Fig. I, 21a. Program of the first German Roentgen Kongress (Convention of Roentgenology) in 1905.

Fig. I, 21b. Title-page of the German Roentgen Society Conference, Volume I.

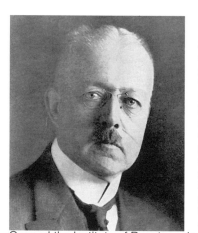

Fig. I, 22. Heinrich Ernst Albers-Schoenberg (1865–1921). Opened a private institute with Georg Deycke in Hamburg in 1897. First physician in Germany certified in roentgenology. Cofounder of the Fortschritte auf dem Gebiete der Röntgenstrahlen (Advances in the Field of X-rays) in 1897. Opened the Institute of Roentgenology at the General Hospital St. Georg in Hamburg. Contributions to technology and areas of diagnostic radiology.

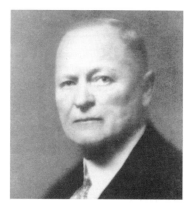

Fig. I, 23. Hermann Gocht (1869–1938). As assistant in the surgical department of General Hospital Hamburg-Eppendorf, he established an institute of roentgenology (first x-ray image on 20 March 1896!). Contribution to diagnostic and therapeutic radiology. Lehrbuch der Röntgenuntersuchung (Textbook of Roentgenologic Examination) 1898. Röntgenliteratur (Roentgenologic Literature), a multivolume work with references from the pioneering age to 1934. Eventually, worked as orthopedic specialist.

founders of the German Roentgen Society were: H.E. Albers-Schoenberg (Fig. I, 22), Hamburg; W. Cowl, Berlin; R. Eberlein, Berlin; H. Gocht (Fig. I, 23), Halle; R. Grashey, Munich; M. Immelmann, Berlin; A. Koehler, Wiesbaden; H. Rieder, Munich; and B. Walter, Hamburg. As early as

1900, the first International Congress of Radiology was held in Paris under A. Béclère (Fig. I, 24) (Walther, 1955).

The interest in the new diagnostic possibilities was also reflected in the number of rapidly appearing monographs, textbooks, manuals and atlases during the first few years following the discovery of X-rays. Hermann Gocht, an unrelenting collector of roentgenological literature from the outset and an orthopaedist by profession, wrote in 1898/1899 his 'Das Lehrbuch der Roentgen-Untersuchung zum Gebrauche fuer Mediziner' (Textbook of Roentgen Examination in its Application to Medicine). His book was considered to be the first textbook on diagnostic radiology; it had 232 pages and went through several revisions and additions.

Of great importance in German speaking countries were 'Die Roentgentechnik' (Roentgen Technique) by Albers-Schoenberg (1903), 'Lehrbuch der Röntgenkunde' (Textbook of Roentgen Studies) by Rieder and Rosenthal (1913), and, 1928, 'Lehrbuch der Roentgendiagnostik' (Textbook of Roentgen Diagnostics) by Baensch and Friedl, later known under the name 'Schinz' (H.R. Schinz, Fig. I, 25). In other countries, similarly important and influential books were published, e.g. in the USA, 'Roentgen Rays in Medicine and Surgery' by F. Williams (1901) and, in France, 'Les Rayons de Roentgen et le Diagnostic des Maladies Internes' (Roentgen Rays and the Diagnosis of Internal Diseases) by A. Béclère (1904).

It was only slowly recognized that this rapidly expanding field required special training. As early as 1933, the American radiologist Case quoted the roentgenologist Feodor Haenisch, in Hamburg, as saying: *'Incompetent and dishonest elements are occupying the field of radiology. Only a few were not led by anticipated financial motives.'*

The Swede G. Forssell (Fig. I, 26) and the Austrian G. Holzknecht were among the most influential lecturers in radiology. In 1899, J.K.A.

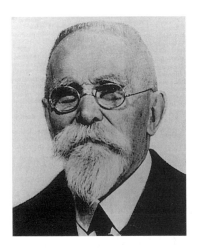

Fig. I, 24. Antoine Béclère (1856–1939). After immunologic studies, dedicated himself to examinations with x-rays. Considered the founding father of the French roentgenology. Worked in the areas of diagnosis, therapy and technology. Cultivated international connections. President of the 3. International Roentgen Congress in Paris in 1931.

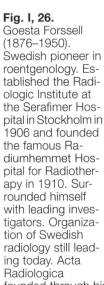

Fig. I, 26. Goesta Forssell (1876–1950). Swedish pioneer in roentgenology. Established the Radiologic Institute at the Serafimer Hospital in Stockholm in 1906 and founded the famous Radiumhemmet Hospital for Radiotherapy in 1910. Surrounded himself with leading investigators. Organization of Swedish radiology still leading today. Acta Radiologica founded through his initiative.

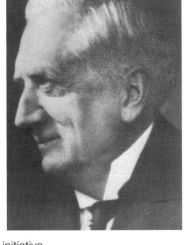

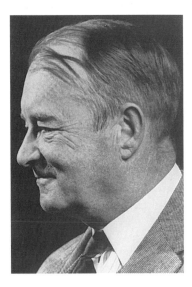

Fig. I, 25. Hans Rudolf Schinz (1891–1966). Radiologist in Zurich. Great influence on the organization and education in radiology in Europe. Editor of famous textbook of diagnostic roentgenology (1. edition 1928). President of the 4. International Roentgen Congress in Zurich.

Fig. I, 27. Johannes Karl August Wertheim Salomonson (1864–1922). Pioneer of the Dutch roentgenology. Founded the Dutch Association of Radiologists. First professor of roentgenology in The Netherlands (Amsterdam).

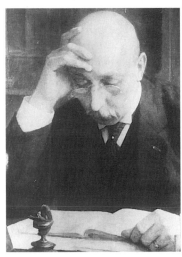

Wertheim Salomonson (Fig. I, 27) became the first professor in roentgenology in Amsterdam.

In 1934, the Board of Radiology was introduced in the USA. Five nationwide radiological organizations followed the example of other speciality boards, delegated three members to the Board, which laid down the conditions for board certification in radiology. The standards improved in the course of time. In addition to moral and ethical qualification, basic medical training and training in radiology were required.

Candidates had to limit their practice to the field of radiology and finally had to pass a comprehensive examination, which at first covered the entire field of radiology, including diagnosis and therapy, and later was confined to diagnostic radiology or radiotherapy. Not only physicians practising radiology need special training but also nurses and technologists working in this field must be trained, as illustrated in the following example.

In 1924, Max Levy-Dorn reported *'the death of a doctor and his nurse by an electric current while performing an X-ray examination.'* Shocked by the report in the newspaper of these deaths in a Finnish village, the engineer Dr Grossmann travelled to Finland to investigate the exact circumstances of the accident. The owner of the X-ray apparatus had no training in roentgenologic technique and had only been informed of the basics of the new equipment by the mechanic who had installed it. At their very first attempt to *'radiograph'* the right leg of a young sailor, the physician and his nurse were killed. *'Because he thought that the X-ray tube was not properly centered, he wanted to improve its position. In doing so, he took the cathode, which was already switched-on with a high-voltage of a 40,000 volt, in his right hand, while the nurse took the anode in her left hand. The two must have touched each other with their free hands and, therefore, induced some sort of short circuit. The burns on both bodies proved this beyond any doubt.'*

Max Levy-Dorn now demanded that, in the future, only specially trained personnel should be allowed to work with roentgen rays.

The other side of the coin

That the new radiation had not only positive characteristics, namely the ability to penetrate organs and create images of previously unknown structures, but also negative attributes became soon apparent.

As early as 23 March 1896, a letter was published in 'Science', stating that 21 days after the image of a boy's skull was taken, his hair fell out where the tube had been nearest the head. The exposure time was one hour at a distance of approximately 1.3 cm. The skin, however, looked normal. The authors stated that they *'were interested to observe the late effects.'*

Other instances were reported in which patients had been subjected to X-rays for several hours to locate projectiles. The next day and subsequent days, the patients noticed skin changes, such as redness resembling a sunburn (dermatitis), and noticed the beginning of hair loss (alopecia).

It was not without consequence that during early years of roentgenology the practicing physicians used their own hands to adjust *'the brightness of the light'* (A. Koehler, 1937). Within days of intensive exposure to X-rays, hair loss, redness, swelling and blisters were found. These changes appeared later with shorter and more frequent radiation. Even as late as 1948, a study showed that 48% of radiologists had radiation-induced skin lesions on the hands. In the early years, it was not uncommon for such skin lesions to lead to amputation of the hand.

Another notable change was the occurrence of azoospermia, i.e. the lack of living spermatozoa in the semen, found in men who had worked with X-rays over an extended period of time. Other parts of the body were also inadvertently exposed to X-rays. Acute effects of whole body irradiation were reported, such as high fever, diarrhoea and vomiting, representing systemic symptoms similar to those occurring with a severe sunburn.

Leukaemia and other neoplastic diseases occurred more frequently in practising radiologists (Henshaw and Hawkins, 1944; Schuettmann, 1988). The list of people who lost their lives through X-rays is long.

In the first few years of its use, it was questioned whether the accompanying ultraviolet light could cause the side effects or perhaps the radiation-incuded ozone on the skin. Furthermore, platinum particles from the anode, the fluoroscopic screen and the induction apparatus were implicated, as well as, an individual idiosyncrasy.

It was obvious that efforts were required to measure the radiation exposure and to understand the biologic effects of X-rays, to protect patient as well as examiner from the radiation.

The application of the negative effects of X-rays: radiotherapy

The Viennese physician Leopold Freund had a pediatric patient with a large hairy naevus on the back. He had heard of an American engineer, who had suffered hair loss after working intensely with X-rays. This report gave him the idea of depilating the hairy naevus with X-rays.

Freund discussed this possibility with the child's mother, who immediately agreed to the experiment with X-rays. He also succeeded in convincing the Privy Councillor Eder of the Graphic Learning and Experiment Institute to be given the institute's apparatus at his disposal. Between December 1896 and January 1897, Freund radiated the naevus daily in the neck region for two hours. After ten treatments, hair loss began to show in the treated area. After another 4 days, the child's neck was hairless, but the skin looked normal. He then radiated the naevus in the lumbar region. In this instance, he used a thin aluminum plate between skin and X-ray tube, and skin necrosis later developed in the irradiated area, which later had to be excised. On 15 January 1897, Freund reported his observations and experiences. They caused him to reflect on the exposure time, tube distance, hardness of tube and radiation intensity (Freund, 1937).

The treatment of this naevus using the side-effects of X-rays can be considered the birth of radiotherapy, which went through a rapid development paralleling that of diagnostic radiology. Today, radiotherapy has become an important part of oncology.

First steps to quality control: birth of dosimetry, radiation biology and radiation protection

The first and rather simple step was to adjust the *'brightness of the light'* with the help of a skeleton rather than with one's own hand. Of course, the subjective nature of this evaluation was not eliminated. Next, it was recommended to wear lead aprons, jackets, and gloves as well as spectacles with X-ray absorbing lead glass. Dressed in such a manner a radiologist could look like a knight in armor ('from head to toe in lead', 1907) (Fig. I, 28).

The lead-glass spectacles were necessary not only for fluoroscopy with a portable cryptoscope but also for the inspection of the X-ray tube before its use. The X-ray tube was no longer placed immediately on the area to be examined, but at a considerable distance from patient and examiner. It was shielded with a radiation-absorbing mantle and had an appropriate diaphragm, so that the X-ray exposure was confined to the region of the body under investigation. These recommendations were already made in 1901 by the American Rollins.

In 1899, the government of Lower Austria asked the City Council of Vienna to inspect Drs. Schroeder and Ehrenfeld's Institute of Roentgen Examinations. This request did not refer to the use of X-rays in general, but merely to their therapeutic applications. The committee was formed by physicians and a technical expert, Dr. Eder. The committee's report opens with a review of the side-effects of radiation as known from the literature. Two cases of acute radiation sickness were also exhaustively discussed. It was emphasized that careful dosage of the X-rays

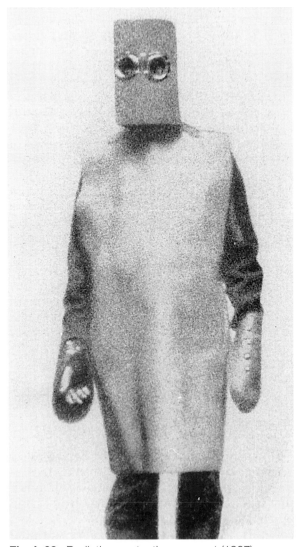

Fig. I, 28. Radiation-protection garment (1907).

could prevent such effects. One quoted article stated that only a few of the more than 2000 cases developed dermatitis.

The committee concluded that little progress in research had been accomplished so far, and that experimental work is desperately needed. In addition, they stated that theoretical foundation, special expertise, practical experience and carefully selected and well-tested equipment were necessary to avoid detrimental and harmful effects. The dependence of dose rate, exposure time and source to skin distance on the radiation effect was mentioned (Tschurlovits and Karacson, 1986). Dosimetry, radiation protection and radiation biology were already discussed.

It was not until 1925 that official protection standards were introduced; radiation was considered to be at a safe level if it did not exceed 1/100 of the erythema dose every 30 days (in today's terms 2 mSv). Regulations and laws were drawn up regarding radiation protection, which included diagnostic applications. Emphasis was on proper indication, optimization of the procedure, and lowest possible dose.

In the course of time, regulations for the installation and operation of institutes working with ionizing radiation were introduced as well as regulations to protect the general population and professionals against radiation. These radiation safety regulations included maximum permissible dose, restricted areas, protective barriers, medical supervision, dosimeters.

Of particular importance was the appropriate training of the personnel, from radiologist to technologist.

Roentgen technique and medicine

In the early years, the radiographic equipment, including the one used by W.C. Roentgen, was simple compared to present-day standards. Roentgen's apparatus consisted of a Rühmkorff coil with contact breakers, a gas-discharge tube and a battery (24–30 V). These parts stood in the room separately and were connected by wires. Those interested in performing radiographic studies had to invest time and energy to operate and to maintain the machines and tubes, requiring the skill of a physician and an engineer.

On the one hand, the operational life of the tubes was short, and on the other hand, the vacuum in the tube increased with use, which changed the radiation quality. Since tubes with different levels of 'hardness' were necessary, the tubes

had to be exchanged depending on the objects to be examined, and a supply of tubes with different grades of hardness was essential in every radiographic institute or laboratory. The increase in the tube's vacuum with use was caused by entrapment of the remaining gas in the metal parts (Koehler, 1937; Dessauer, 1945). For a longer operational life, 'hardened' tubes could be connected to a small palladium tube, which was heated until enough gas had been released for the required hardness and vacuum, respectively.

The dawn of the X-ray era brought with it the beginning of a new industry, which immediately began to implement technical improvements. The exposure times had to be reduced to eliminate motion unsharpness. The resolution of the radiographs had to be improved for better detail recognition. Finally, a decrease in dosage was desirable.

The equipment had to meet the different demands of the various examinations. The industry was required to build equipment that was more reliable, safer, easier to operate, and more durable. In addition, the radiographic data had to be reproducible, and the radiographic plates more sensitive and better suitable for filing. The search for a different carrier, other than glass, for the photosensitive layer became essential. The glass plates took good radiographs but were breakable and used up a lot of storage space. Radiation safety measures had to be implemented for patients and personnel, and the necessary accessories designed. These developments brought into existence completely new branches of industry. By continually communicating and exchanging ideas with the radiologic community, the industry significantly contributed to the development and success of radiology.

The pioneer Friedrich Dessauer (Fig. I, 29) stated in his article, 'Reminiscences on the develop-

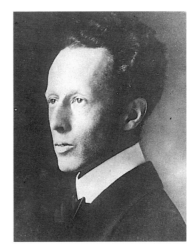

Fig. I, 29. Friedrich Dessauer (1882–1963). Initially trained as engineer. He had his own roentgen factory Veifa in Aschaffenburg for manufacturing important new equipment. Later biophysicist in Frankfurt/Main, with fundamental contributions to radiation effects and therapy. Emigration. Also known as writer.

ment of roentgen technique' (1945), that, after the discovery of X-rays, physicists and engineers remained uncertain about the nature of the cathode rays and the new rays, since both were still interpreted as longitudinal ether waves.

As late as 1912, Max von Laue, W. Friedrich and P. Knipping discovered the interference of X-rays and deduced their wavelike property. Dessauer continued: *'The interrelationship between voltage, current, beam hardness and brightness of the rays (intensity was the term then used and not as accurate) was a topic of hot dispute throughout the years. One had to experiment and construct without reliable foundations, often even with hypotheses that later turned out to be wrong.'*

List of Sources

1.	Wiener klin. Wschr. 9 (1896),	48
2.	ibid.	63
3.	ibid.	83
4.	ibid.	1065–1067
5.	ibid.	1207–1214
6.	Berl. klin. Wschr.33 (1896),	47
7.	ibid.	66
8.	ibid.	85
9.	ibid.	106
10.	ibid.	133
11.	ibid.	150
12.	ibid.	574
13.	ibid.	586
14.	ibid.	682
15.	ibid.	804
16.	ibid.	1046
17.	ibid.	1142

References

Collins, V.P.: Origins of medico-legal and forensic roentgenology. In: Bruwer, A.J. (ed.): Classic descriptions in diagnostic roentgenology, vol. 2: 1578. Thomas, Springfield 1964

Dessauer, F.: Erinnerungen aus der Entwicklung der Röntgentechnik. Experientia 1 (1945) 307–316

Freund, L.: 40 Jahre Röntgentherapie. Wien. Klin. Wschr. 147 (1937) 147–153

Glasser, O.: Wilhelm Conrad Röntgen. 2. Aufl. Springer, Berlin-Göttingen-Heidelberg 1959

Goerke, H.: Frühe röntgendiagnostische Arbeiten in Berlin 1896–1902. Röntgenstrahlen, Heft 15 (1966) 3–16

Henshaw, P.S., J.W. Hawkins: Incidence of leukemia in physicians. Cancer 4 (1944) 339–346

Jastrowitz, M.: Die Roentgen'schen Experimente mit Kathodenstrahlen und ihre diagnostische Verwertung. Dtsch. Med. Wschr. 22 (1896) 65–67

Köhler, A.: Ärztlicher Röntgenbetrieb um die Jahrhundertwende. Strahlentherapie 60 (1937) 283–289

Levy-Dorn, M.: Die Tötung eines Ärztes und seiner Gehilfin durch den elektrischen Strom bei Vornahme einer Röntgenuntersuchung. Med. Klinik 22 (1924) 1762–1763

Maurer, H.-J., W. Weber: Die Entdeckung der Röntgenstrahlen in der Trivialliteratur und der Fachpresse von 1896–1901. Technikgeschichte 44 (1977) 324–339

Schüttmann, W.: Zur Geschichte der Kenntnisse von den Strahlenschäden. Z. gesamte Hyg. 34 (1988) 674–680

Thurnher, B.: Die II. Medizinische Universitätsklinik, Geburtsstätte des Zentral-Röntgeninstituts der Universität Wien. Wiener. Z. inn. Med. 45 (1964) 213–219

Tschurlovits, M., P. Karacson: Licencing of medical X-ray equipment in 1899: background and procedure. Appl. Radiat. Isot. 37 (1986) 373–381

Walther, K.: Die Gründer der Deutschen Röntgengesellschaft. Röntgenblätter 8 (1955) 290–352

Withers, S.: The story of the first roentgen evidence. Radiology 17 (1931) 99–103

Chapter 2

The invisible light applied

The advancing diagnostic evaluation of the skeleton and thorax following Roentgen's discovery

Introduction

G. Rosenbusch, M. Oudkerk, E. Ammann

Bacteriology and serology contributed greatly to the understanding of inflammatory diseases in the second half of the nineteenth century. Louis Pasteur (1822–95) and Robert Koch (1843–1910) made outstanding contributions. Even at the beginning of the nineteenth century, little was known about infection. Despite evidence of widespread infections, many physicians were of the opinion that such a thing did not exist and only a few (the contagionists) thought otherwise.

Koch's publication in 1876 on *Bacillus anthracis* was important in that it was the first publication dealing with a detailed description of the aetiology of an inflammatory disease. The discovery of *B. tuberculosis* and *B. cholerae* followed. Until then many physicians firmly believed that tuberculosis was a hereditary disease.

Koch stated that: *'In the future it will not be difficult to identify what is tuberculous and what is not. Not the characteristic structure of the tubercle, not its lack of vessels and the presence of giant cells will be decisive, but the proof of the presence of tuberculous bacilli. . . . I have performed my investigations in the interest of public health care and I hope for its widespread use as a result of this. In the future, the battle against this horrible plague of mankind will no longer be against an unidentifiable something, but against a fathomable parasite, its conditions for living known to a large extent and open for further investigation.'*

Koch's wish for a quick and effective treatment for tuberculosis unfortunately remained unfulfilled. The cholera epidemic, which caused more than 9000 deaths in Hamburg in 1892, still showed how significant the consequences of infection were.

Based on bacteriological findings, serological tests were developed to discover clinical symptoms at a relatively early stage and a corresponding therapy administered, by injecting attenuated bacteria or viruses, or drugs. In particular, Louis Pasteur, Emil von Behring (1854–1917), Paul Ehrlich (1854–1915) and Fernand Widal (1862–1929) had made a mark in this field. The diphtheria serum had been a blessing for children: many had previously died from the disease. Von Behring was awarded the Nobel Prize in 1901 for the development of this serum, at the same time as Roentgen received his.

It was not until the discovery of the various pathogenic organisms that prophylactic measures could be taken. Hygiene had found an advocate in Max von Pettenkofer (1818–1901) who was concerned with the improvement of drinking water and the construction of sewage systems. In the fields of bacteriology, serology and hygiene, particularly, progress was proven by the fact that, since the Hamburg cholera epidemic of 1892, no major epidemics of dysentery, plague, smallpox, typhoid or cholera have occurred in Western countries.

Today, these diseases only occur in isolated cases and are immediately and aggressively treated. Coordinated government or communal health care has certainly contributed to the retreat of these epidemics. Using registry, statistics and geographical classification, significant epidemiological conclusions can be drawn and applied to newly discovered cases. In Germany, the sociomedical measures taken by the state under Bismarck were decisive in improving and maintaining the national health and in creating a compulsory sickness insurance.

In 1900, tuberculosis was the principal cause of death in the USA. Early and rapid diagnosis of this disease was essential for implementing therapeutic measures, such as pneumothorax or light therapy. Chest radiography evolved as the most important diagnostic method in the initial evaluation of the disease and in following its course.

As a result of hygienic and sociomedical measures, pulmonary tuberculosis has become a relatively rare disease in recent times. The main indications for radiographs of the lungs therefore shifted towards neoplasms of the bronchial system, nonspecified pulmonary disease and parenchymal changes. Pulmonary radiographs still constitute a major part of routine radiological examinations. The technical demand to obtain high-quality radiographs with the lowest possible radiation exposure increased in the course of time.

In the skeletal system, radiographs can reveal fractures, inflammatory and degenerative changes, and tumours. In soft tissues, radiography was used to locate metallic foreign bodies caused by industrial accidents or war injuries. Mammography, at first performed hesitantly, achieved its current role only after technical improvements.

Because W.C. Roentgen had given significance to the use of X-rays for bones with the publication of the photograph of his wife's and Professor R. Koelliker's hand, it was only natural that the X-rays were first used to diagnose skeletal diseases. Friedrich Heuck, whose main interest are skeletal diseases, including density measurements, illustrated the progress of skeletal radiology. The history of the interpretation of chest radiographs – easier for some than others – is written by Stender and Oestmann. Stender has primarily distinguished himself in the diagnosis of parenchymal diseases of the lungs.

Hoeffken, the senior master and pioneer of mammography, illustrates the slow and gradual, but finally successful development of mammography.

The radiologist's demand on the technology was shortening of the exposure times, to avoid or, at least, to minimize motion blurring. This had to be achieved without loss of detail and with a concomitant decrease in radiation exposure. Great efforts were required to improve generators, tubes and imaging systems. Obtaining radiographs of the various organs often demanded a modification or even entirely new design for specific organs. The simple equipment of the early days became more complex and differentiated through continuous integration of new technologies. Today, numerous technical disciplines contribute to the manufacturing of radiographic equipment: mechanical engineering, oscillation theory, statics and dynamics, material science, low and high voltage electrical engineering, high voltage capacitor, actuator devices, control engineering, data processing, communication techniques, optics, air conditioning techniques, vacuum techniques, production techniques, software programs, quality control, communication techniques, test protocols, tool making, and installation engineering.

Organizations are also required for design, transport, installation, service, control, standardization, cost-effect analysis, basic research, etc.

Important work emerges not only from university institutes but also from industry institutes dedicated to research without the immediate goal of new product development. Without active basic research, the known techniques are utilized inefficiently and new technologies cannot be conceived. This also relates to the history of the application of X-rays. The industries that produced electrical devices, such as light bulbs, electric motors or generators, recognized early the value and benefit of X-rays in medicine and, jointly with the medical community, developed the needed applications, mutually stimulated by clinical necessity and technical potential. This "Give and Take" still applies today, even after incorporating other industries, such as producers of glass, contrast agents and films. In this way, radiology could achieve its important role it has in medicine today.

Skeleton

F. Heuck

Radiographic evaluation of the skeleton: the beginning

While experimenting with cathode rays on the 8. November 1895, W.C. Roentgen unexpectedly created an image of the bones of his hand on a photographic plate. This encouraged him to investigate the properties of this 'new type of rays'. In his first presentation on X-rays before the Wuerzburg Physical Medical Society, Roentgen made a radiographic image of the hand of the anatomist von Koelliker and thus laid the cornerstone for the development of Roentgenologie und Strahlenheilkunde or radiology. The use of X-rays in medicine opened the door to study, in vivo, size, topography, morphology and structure of individual bones that are part of the skeleton and to visualize the teeth and their osseous sockets. All osseous structures or mineral-containing connective tissues are rendered visible by using X-rays, providing information down to microscopic levels. A new scientific era had commenced in medicine, pertaining the diagnosis and therapy.

Beginning in 1896, X-rays used for diagnostic purpose discovered a large number of previously unknown anatomical changes in the skeleton during growth and maturity as well as normal variants and pathologic osseous processes. The rapid increase in profound knowledge primarily benefited orthopaedics and surgery. Comparing morphological changes of bones and joints visible in radiographic images with the relevant pathoanatomical findings of surgical and pathologic specimens have increased the knowledge of numerous diseases of the skeleton, hitherto often even unknown to pathologists. With this increase in knowledge, surgical interventions and conservative treatments could be markedly improved.

The names of several pioneers of radiology are still remembered today. First and foremost, Alban Koehler (Fig. II, 1) [129] who, in 1910, published the first edition of a book on the current knowledge of the skeleton in roentgenographic diagnosis, entitled 'Lexikon der Grenzen des Normalen im Röntgenbild' *[Encyclopedia of Normal Limits in Roentgen Images]* (Fig. II, 2), which became renowned worldwide. The second edition was published only five years later. This standard work, now known as Koehler/Zimmer: 'Grenzen des Normalen und Anfänge des Pathologischen im Röntgenbild des Skelets' *[Borderlands of the Normal and Early Pathologic in Skeletal Roentgenology]* has been revised many times, and the current thirteenth edition, translated as the fourth English edition, remains of enormous value in the daily work of radiologists, orthopaedists, surgeons and paediatricians.

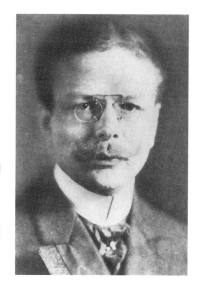

Fig. II, 1. Alban Koehler (1874–1947), one of the pioneers in radiology, was widely recognized for his "Lexikon der Grenzen des Normalen im Röntgenbild" published in 1910. He worked as roentgenologist at St. Joseph Hospital in Wiesbaden and since 1903 in private praxis. In addition to publications about skeletal radiology also publications about technique.

LEXIKON

DER

GRENZEN DES NORMALEN

UND DER

ANFÄNGE DES PATHOLOGISCHEN

IM

RÖNTGENBILDE

VON

DR. ALBAN KÖHLER

SPEZIALARZT FÜR RÖNTGENOLOGIE IN WIESBADEN.

MIT 73 ABBILDUNGEN IM TEXT.

HAMBURG

LUCAS GRÆFE & SILLEM (EDMUND SILLEM)

1910.

Fig. II, 2. The first edition of this well-known standard work by Alban Koehler was published in 1910 bound as a single volume with Jugendstil cover: "Lexikon der Grenzen des Normalen im Röntgenbilde", in the second edition of 1915 entitled: "Grenzen des Normalen und Anfänge des Pathologischen im Röntgenbild" published by Lucas Graefe and Sillem, Hamburg, Germany. After G. Thieme-Verlag had published Alban Koehler's work up to the eighth edition, Emil Alfred Zimmer had continued this up to the twelfth edition and restricted its contents to the skeleton. It was written in German and translated into English, French, Italian and Spanish.

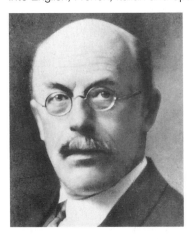

Fig. II, 3. Rudolf Grashey (1876–1950). As assistant in the surgical clinic at the University of Munich in charge of the roentgenologic laboratory since 1902. Worked primarily on localization of foreign bodies. "Atlas typischer Röntgenbilder vom normalen Menschen" published in 1905. In Cologne since 1912. Became chairman of the Department of Roentgenology at the University of Cologne in 1929. Succeeded Karl Frik at the Charité in 1944.

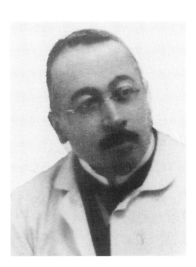

Fig. II, 4. Robert Kienboeck (1871–1954). Austrian pioneer in roentgenology. Director, Department of Roentgenology, General Outpatient Clinic in Vienna since 1904. Works on skeletal diseases and on radiation therapy of sarcomas. Multivolume textbook on bone and joint diseases. Cooperation with G. Holzknecht.

In addition, H.E. Albers-Schoenberg [2], E. Bircher [17], H. Fischer [54], E. Fraenkel [58, 59], R. Grashey (Fig. II, 3) [71, 72, 73], F. Haenisch [80], A. Hasselwander [88] and R. Kienboeck (Fig. II, 4) [120, 121, 122] should be mentioned as pioneers and researchers in the field of skeletal radiology. In the field of orthopaedics, not only Max Immelmann [102], who also was Permanent Secretary of the German Roentgen Society from the outset, deserves recognition in investigating bone and joint diseases using X-rays but also A. Hoffa [98, 99], G. Joachimsthal [106, 107], Jüngling [111], W. Kuemmel [135], A. Lorenz [159] and J. Wolff [261, 262]. It is not surprising to encounter numerous names of German-speaking European countries among the first physicians working in the field of skeletal radiology.

Adding radiology to the examination of the skeleton has greatly benefited the diagnosis and treatment of fractures and dislocations. The obvious value of X-rays to demonstrate foreign bodies in soft tissue was first recognized in military medicine [7, 201]. A British expeditionary corps in the Egyptian Sudan was equipped with two X-ray units as early as 1896 [78]. In the Greek–Turkish War of 1897, and in the Spanish–American War of 1898, X-ray equipment was used successfully [7, 13, 24, 47, 74, 78, 103, 113, 162]. The Army Medical Corps in World Wars I and II had much more advanced equipment at their disposal but often lacked qualified physicians in the field hospitals to assure adequate treatment of the wounded soldiers.

In traumatology, the outcome of the treatment of fractures could be improved by serial radiographic studies to check the position of the bony fragments. Kuentscher and colleagues [136, 137] developed 'marrow nailing', a treatment for fractures in which a metal rod is inserted into the bone marrow cavity after the fracture fragments have been anatomically aligned under radiological guidance. This paved the way for an ideal fracture therapy, later known as 'stable osteosynthesis'.

Further improvements and modifications of the X-ray equipment, particularly the development of the 'C-arm' [19] for use in the operating room, allowed considerable progress of the treatment of fractures by means of osteosynthesis [25, 172, 178]. To quote from Max Immelmann [102], in his first report on 'Ten Years of Orthopaedics and Roentgenology': *Surely orthopaedics could not have developed to this extent, if it had not received major support from radiology'.*

Genetic bone diseases could be classified through pathoanatomic and histologic analysis [30, 182, 202] revealing that a variety of deformities and abnormal structures are not a disease in its true sense.

With newly developed examination methods, such as computed tomography and magnetic resonance imaging, it is now possible to diagnose congenital deformities and defects at the fetal stage [33, 139, 213]. Congenital dislocation of the hip – its etiology had long been in dispute – cannot only be recognized earlier and understood better but can also be treated more effectively. It had become possible to divide pathomorphological changes of the skeleton into those that need urgent therapy and those that change to a normal finding during growth if left alone [54, 71, 88, 128, 129, 188, 207].

Generalized skeletal diseases, systemic diseases or osteopathies could be analyzed and classified with the increasing knowledge of mineral metabolism and hormonal regulation. Comparative pathoanatomic and histomicroscopic radiological studies have led to a better understanding of the pathogenesis of bone diseases. Using quantitative bone radiology, osteopathies could be diagnosed early and its course after therapeutic procedures objectively followed [96].

Using radiomorphological criteria, infectious bone diseases of different aetiologies could be detected and their response following surgery or conservative treatment monitored, leading to unprecedented progress in the control of these diseases, which previously were serious, if not fatal.

The early radiological diagnosis of bone tumours, the radiomorphologic investigation of their various types and their radiological moni-toring after surgical intervention have resulted in a considerably improved treatment of these diseases, previously considered to be incurable.

The breathtaking increase in medical knowledge at the beginning of this century has continued to the present through incessant improvement of equipment and examination methods, and today clinical radiology plays an important role in the delivery of health care in all countries throughout the world.

Findings of skeletal ossification during growth

Using X-rays, the development of the bony skeleton could be easily analyzed *in vivo* from the third embryonic month onwards without any intervention [33, 139]. Before the third month, the mineral content of the bones is too low for radiographic detection and intrauterine assessment was therefore not feasible. The first ossification centres can be detected in the clavicles in the seventh embryonic week. At the end of the third embryonic month, ossification centres are distinguishable in many bones. When the diaphyses become visible, the epiphyses of the long bones are not yet detectable since they remain cartilaginous for a long time. The onset of the endochondral ossification can be recorded, and an ossification centre is known to be distinguished in the distal femur epiphysis from the thirtieth week onwards, a fact which is important in forensic medicine [225].

Careful monitoring of the ossification in cartilaginous bone after birth by various groups of radiologists resulted in a solid basic knowledge that can be applied to separate normal ossification and healthy growth of the skeleton from disorders due to a variety of causes. Hormonal disorders of the growing child are in the forefront [88, 97, 214, 258]. Fundamental results from these studies helped to explain accessory ossification and the origin and development of sesamoid bones. In addition, the diagnosis and differential diagnosis of persistent epiphyses and apophyses, which frequently occur, could be advanced. In this context the works by M. Wilms and C. Sick [257], R. Grashey [72], W.W. Greulich and S.I. Pyle [75], A. Koehler [129] and F. Schmid and H. Moll [215] deserve special attention. The time and sequence of the appearance of all important ossification centres of the skeleton have been recorded (Fig. II, 5). With this knowledge, persistent epiphyseal ossification centres and persistent apophyseal ossifications encoun-

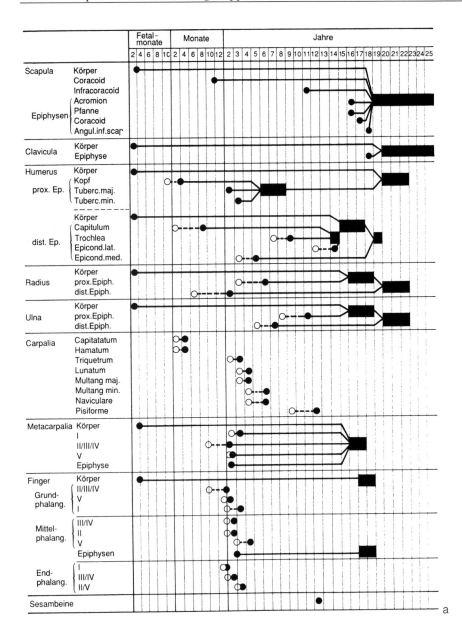

Fig. II, 5. Diagrams of the rate and time of appearance of the ossification centers of the bones of a) the upper and b) the lower extremity, to illustrate the contribution to the radiology of skeletal growth and maturation, connected with the names of R. Grashey, W.W. Greulich and S.J. Pyle. Similar diagrams were worked out for the ossification centers of the spine and skull.

tered in adulthood can be recognized, suggesting a hormonal disturbance. The ossification centres appear delayed in myxedema and irregular in mongolism. In hypothyroidism, the incidence of persistent growth plates and apophyses is increased.

Regional findings of ossification

Topographical peculiarities of the ossification of the skeleton of the hand had been investigated from the fetal period to the completion of skeletal maturation. As early as 1905, books and atlases on the normal anatomy of the hand were pre-

sented at the first German Roentgen Congress [14, 189]. The development of the finger and toe phalanges were of particular interest. The multifarious configuration of the ungual tuberosity of the distal phalanges and its gross morphological changes in pathological conditions such as acromegaly had already been described in the first two editions of Alban Koehler's [129] internationally renowned book, "Borderlands of the Normal and the Early Pathologic in Skeletal Roentgenology". The sesamoid bones and their great variety in form and location in the hand and foot skeleton had already been studied in detail at an early date [1, 54, 69, 88, 183, 195].

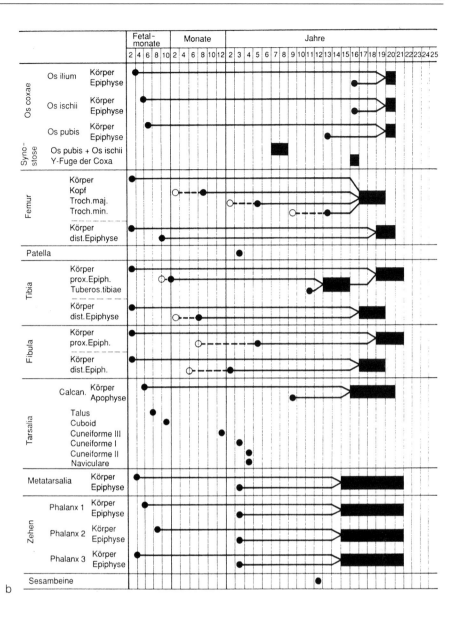

Fig. II, 5. (continued)   b

In the critical analysis of misinterpreted radiological images after osseous trauma, attention was drawn to small accessory bones, such as the trapezoid. Small, exostotic or thorn-shaped prominences on normal hand bones were described. Sclerotic densities in the spongiosa as manifestation of 'bone islands' were recognized as normal variants [72, 73].

The duplication of the navicular bone and the aplasia of navicular and lunar bones were also recognized [100, 129, 214].

Grashey's [7, 72, 73] roentgenographic atlases of normal anatomy already point out the difficult distinction between fractures and avulsions, particularly in injuries involving the epiphyseal and apophyseal centres of the elbow. Irregularities in the ossification of the olecranon apophysis were recognized early. An osseous apposition at the olecranon was described as 'olecranon spur' but its pathogenesis could not be explained. Malformations such as 'Madelung's deformity' [164] and the differential diagnosis of fractures of the processus styloideus of the ulna and radius have been discussed, as well as specific fractures such as parry fractures, longitudinal fissures and avulsions and their diagnostic problems.

Bernardeau [16] and von Lilienfeld [150] dealt with the problems of ossification of the os acromial. The variations of ossification of the scapula were recognized [72]. Fractures or dislocations of the clavicles were described. The implications of uncommon fractures, avulsions or fissures of the humerus were reported at an early date. A bony apposition on the flexor side was described as supracondylar process of the humerus.

The thickness of the articular cartilage, which should range between 2 and 4 mm, was especially mentioned in the discussion about the sequelae of fractures of the articulating bones of the shoulder joint. Pathological calcium deposits in the soft tissues and the bursae of the shoulder joint (bursa subacromialis and subdeltoidea) were described.

The ossification of the skeleton of the foot were described by Hasselwander [88], with mention of accessory ossicles analogue to those found in the skeleton of the wrist [54, 97]. Already Pfitzner (1891, 1895) [183] described the os tibiale externum and its variations as well as partial synostoses. It could be definitely proved that an os trigonum and the various manifestations of the posterior process of the talus are not pathological, but represent normal variants.

The ossification of the calcaneus, particularly of the calcaneal apophysis, was at first puzzling. It has now been ascertained that the appearance of more than one ossification centre in this apophysis can be considered a completely normal ossification process.

In the metatarsus, atypical accessory bones were detected and described. The effect of contemporary shoe design on the development of the skeleton of the foot was already discussed early. Much attention was given to the radiomorphological changes of gout and its differentiation from other disorders [129]. Luetic changes of the foot skeleton were recognized relatively early. For instance, abnormalities of the second metatarsal associated with ossifying periostitis was always suspicious for a gumma [83, 237].

In the proximal tibia, the often multiple ossification centres of the tibial tuberosity initially posed diagnostic problems before they were recognized as normal variants. C. Schlatter [216] reported a specific clinical entity related to pain during the ossification. Tuberculosis was also considered in the differential diagnosis when the irregularities of the ossification were first discovered [108, 128, 129, 141].

The diagnosis and differential diagnosis of the various types of bone injuries to the distal ends of the tibia and fibula often proved to be difficult. Accessory ossification centres in the region of the malleoli were discovered later and are now considered to be normal variants. The persistence of such ossifications as os subfibulare and os subtibiale could be established [188].

Early attention was given to the sesamoid bone in the quadriceps tendon: the patella. Duplica-tion or triplication of the patella as well as marginal appositions could be confirmed as normal findings [206].

A shell-like new bone formation in the region of the medial condyle of the femur initially caused considerable diagnostic difficulties until Stieda (1908) [236] could explain this peculiar bone density as an avulsion injury (inferior tear of the medial collateral ligament or periosteal avulsion of the adductor magnus tendon), representing a typical injury of the distal femur. Later, follow-up observations confirmed that this abnormality appeared approximately 3 weeks after trauma without prior visible pathologic radiographic changes, thus proving its traumatic aetiology.

Efforts of the radiologic assessment of the meniscus of the knee began very early, although direct delineation was not possible at first. After insufflating air into the knee joint capsule, the intra-articular soft tissues could be visualized [263, 264] and the diagnosis of meniscal injuries became feasible (Fig. II, 6). Only much later, the double-contrast method was introduced, refining the diagnosis of meniscal injuries [203].

In the pelvis, an initially described 'atypical and strange ossification zone' in the region of

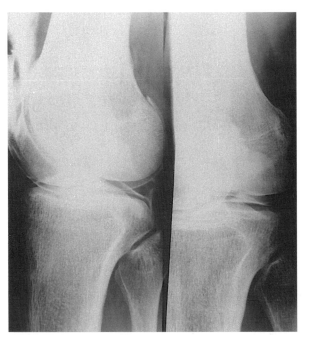

Fig. II, 6. The intra-articular structures of the knee joint with the menisci could be visualized and assessed radiologically by air insufflation [263] and later by double-contrast examination. Radiographs in oblique views could demonstrate the joint cavity with menisci (observation by Dr. Bosnjakovic-Buescher, Dept. of Radiology, Municipal Hospital, Sindelfingen, Germany).

the iliac crest was later found to be the apophysis. The hip joint was exhaustively studied with regard to various diagnostic questions. Congenital hip dislocations were diagnosed and correctly classified. In addition, deformities of the femoral neck, such as coxa vara or valga, and conditions after epiphyseolysis with a slipped epiphysis were correctly analyzed and classified [151, 202].

The phenomenon of the 'wandering acetabulum' was recognized and correctly diagnosed. Initially, the classification of the 'arthritis deformans infantilis' in terms of a pathogenetic interpretation dominated by a deformity of the epiphysis of the femur head was incorrect. Children, primarily boys, between the ages of 5 and 12 years developed a peculiar hip condition, in which the femoral head exhibited a cylindrical deformity. Only much later, this radiographic finding was correctly interpreted as Perthes disease in terms of an ossification disorder or an osteochondronecrosis [170, 179].

Bony ridges are present on the femur along the insertion of muscles and tendons and are visible radiographically.

Ample attention was given to form and contour of the lesser pelvis because of its obstetrical implication. Osteomalacia was not uncommon in women in the first half of this century, often leading to 'heart-shaped' deformities of the not always evenly developed pelvic skeleton. Consideration was also given to the pubic symphysis.

In the first decade of diagnostic application of X-rays, many calcifications in the pelvic region were correctly analyzed and classified, encompassing calcified myomas, dermoid cysts, mural calcification of the iliaca arteries, calcified uterine vessels, bismuth residues and calcifications after tuberculosis, particularly in the urinary bladder. Alban Koehler already cautioned that the fetus *in utero* should not be misinterpreted.

The growth-related ossification of the cartilaginous vertebral bodies could be studied. In parti-

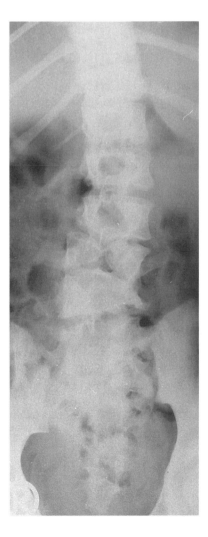 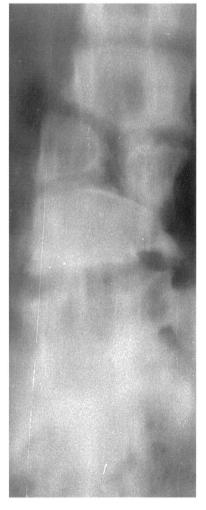

Fig. II, 7. Deformations of the vertebral bodies could be established as the cause of distortions of the spinal column, such as kyphoses and scolioses. This example shows complex vertebral anomalies in a 14-years-old girl resulting in slight bending of the spinal axis. The third lumbar vertebral body is a "butterfly vertebra". There is a compensating deformity of the adjacent vertebrae (plain radiograph and tomogram in a.p. projection).

cular, the ring apophyses of the vertebral bodies as seen in the lateral view had been misinterpreted in children between the ages of 10 and 13 years or even older, often incorrectly diagnosed or suspected as tuberculosis [8, 72, 82, 84]. The radiographic analysis of the vertebral bodies initially posed certain difficulties, though the intervertebral spaces were soon attributed to the anatomical substrate of the disk. The 'intervertebral disk spaces' vary in width, increasing from cranial to caudal. The radiographic presentation of the transverse, spinous and articular processes were analyzed early and the importance of correct positioning for radiographic exposure was soon recognized [128, 129].

Fractures of the odontoid process, the not infrequently bifurcated spinous processes of the cervical spine, the occurrence of cervical ribs, and the various forms of spinous processes of the thoracic and lumbar spine were described. Special views of the spine were introduced (the open mouth view of the odontoid process, oblique views of the spine and, later, tomography).

Congenital deformities of the vertebral bodies were analyzed and recognized as the cause of kyphosis or scoliosis (Fig. II, 7) [35, 116, 119, 173, 199, 221]. The lumbosacral vertebra was described as a 'transitional vertebra'. An occult spina bifida could be detected radiographically and was found to be a frequent defect. Often a fissure is not detectable, only a slight deformity of the spinous processes. It could be established that an occult spina bifida is present in one of ten patients. Fissures in the lower lumbar spine, and later also in the remaining spine, were correctly considered to be incidental and rare [125, 134, 194, 221, 244].

By studying the development of the cranial skeleton, disturbances of the ossification process were recognized. The sella was of particular interest from the beginning. Its pathological changes could be ascribed to underlying diseases, such as an enlarged sella to a tumour of the pituitary gland [171, 192, 222].

The cranial sutures were distinguished from fracture lines. It could be established that in elderly people the cranial sutures show partial osseous fusion [66, 129, 160]. In general, the skull is asymmetric, including orbits and nasal sinuses. To improve the visualization of the skull, special radiographic views of the base of the skull and nasal sinuses were introduced. Variations in the size of the sinuses were recognized. The development of the paranasal sinuses during childhood was studied. The ethmoidal cells were studied separately. In addition, the radiomorphology of the sphenoid sinuses attracted considerable attention [193, 232].

Diseases of the nasal sinuses, such as accumulation of pus, mucus and polyps, were identified radiographically.

In the orbital region, small foreign bodies, in particular metal splinters, were demonstrated and successfully removed. Fractures of the facial bones, including orbits, were correctly diagnosed. Malignant tumours of the paranasal sinuses were detected and analyzed radiographically.

The different radiographic manifestations of the petrous bone, particularly of its mastoid process, were the subject of intensive comparative studies [112, 129, 163, 192, 231]. A 'shadowing' of the pneumatization of the mastoid process was found in infective diseases of the internal ear. The radiographic changes of cholesteatomas were recognized. Already early, large abscess cavities were discovered in the cortex of compact bone. A comparison with the healthy contralateral petrous pyramid was found to be essential for the correct and reliable diagnosis of a pathological condition. The normal anatomical structures and diseases of the mandible and the dentition could be diagnosed and classified correctly without difficulty [34, 228].

'Osteochondronecroses' – ossification and growth disorders

A wide range of osteochondronecroses in adolescence were described during the first decade of skeletal radiology. Osteochondritis deformans coxa juvenilis (Fig. II, 8) was recognized early through studies by Calvé [29], Legg [142] and Perthes [179]. Additional early discoveries include Osgood–Schlatter's disease [175] of the tibial apophysis [216, 217], Koehler's disease of the navicular bone [130, 131] and Freiberg–Koehler's disease of the metatarsal II head [129, 132], as well as a few osteochondropathies of other epiphyses and apophyses of the skeleton [9, 67, 121, 122, 123, 140, 167, 188, 204, 205, 214, 242].

The comparative histomorphological and radiological analysis of the pathoanatomical findings led to several hypotheses as to the pathogenesis and pathomechanism of the so-called osteochondronecroses. After healing following completion of growth, they leave behind deformities of the affected epiphyseal or apophyseal regions. They are not a 'necrosis' of the bone in the true sense of the word since normal ossification re-

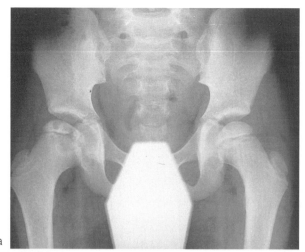

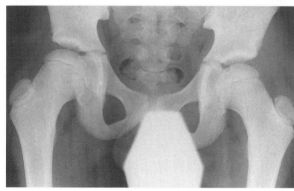

Fig. II, 8. Among the numerous disorders of enchondral ossification in children, "juvenile osteochondrosis deformans coxae" or "morbus Perthes" is the most frequent disease and can only be detected and analyzed by evaluation of subtle radiographic findings. This condition is attributed to osteochondronecrosis and heals completely with resultant flattening of the femoral head. This example shows the radiographic findings of active Perthes disease of the right hip in a 9-years-old boy **(a)**. The follow-up examination, two and a half years later, shows regeneration of the femoral head and a widened metaphysis of the femoral neck **(b)**. (Observation by Prof. Hauke, Dept. of Radiology, Olga Hospital, Stuttgart, Germany).

sumes after "revitalization" of what at first appears as a grossly pathologic process. Though many comprehensive papers and books have been devoted to their pathogenesis, the osteonecroses remain a controversial, enigmatic and problematic entity of the growing skeleton [81, 169, 188].

Discovery of genetically determined, congenital skeletal abnormalities

Many bone abnormalities previously only known pathoanatomically or even entirely unknown

were analyzed further or discovered by radiographic imaging [30, 76, 77]. The congenital skeletal abnormality of "multiple cartilaginous exostoses" produces rather impressive radiographic findings of unusual deformities of the bones [18, 168, 177]. Osteopetrosis is another, previously unknown disease discovered and described by Albers-Schoenberg (1904) [2]. Its various modes of inheritance (dominant or recessive monophenic or polyphenic) has since been ascertained. The radiographic appearance is characterized by spongiosclerosis with an extreme increase in epiphyseal and metaphyseal density (Fig. II, 9). In adolescence, periosteal appositions can also be found along the diaphyses. The morphological appearance gives the impression of an intermittently progressing pathoanatomical process. In addition to osteopetrosis, Albers-Schoenberg (1915) [3] has described the familial condition of osteopoikilosis that produces small bone islands in the spongiosa, predominantly found in the epiphyses and metaphyses.

Densities of this kind are not seen in the diploic space. The compact bone islands are mainly spindle-shaped, occasionally round and clearly related to the trabecular structure and architecture of the spongiosa (Fig. II, 10). A confluence of these sclerotic foci could be recognized [251]. On the basis of the pathohistology, the small enostomas can be assumed to develop during the growth phase of the bones. The sclerotic foci also participated in the transformations of the osseous structure. An nodular cutaneous thickening accompanying these osseous changes was already observed early and named lenticular dermatofibrosis [28].

The rare Léri's melorheostosis (1921) [144, 145] belongs to the group of hereditary bone changes of variable penetrance. The pathogenetic relationships are still completely obscure.

A disease recognized as hyperostosis generalisata, with and without pachydermia, may be considered to be a systemic connective tissue disorder, though its pathogenetic relationship at the cellular or molecular level remains unknown even today [39, 248].

The various forms of osteogenesis imperfecta [154] were already discovered in the early days of radiology, but their pathogenetic implication has become better understood only through research of the histology and biochemistry of connective tissues. The numerous hereditary defects of the skeleton are beyond the scope of this book [155, 230].

The opportunity to detect congenital skeletal abnormalities allowed, for the first time, a differ-

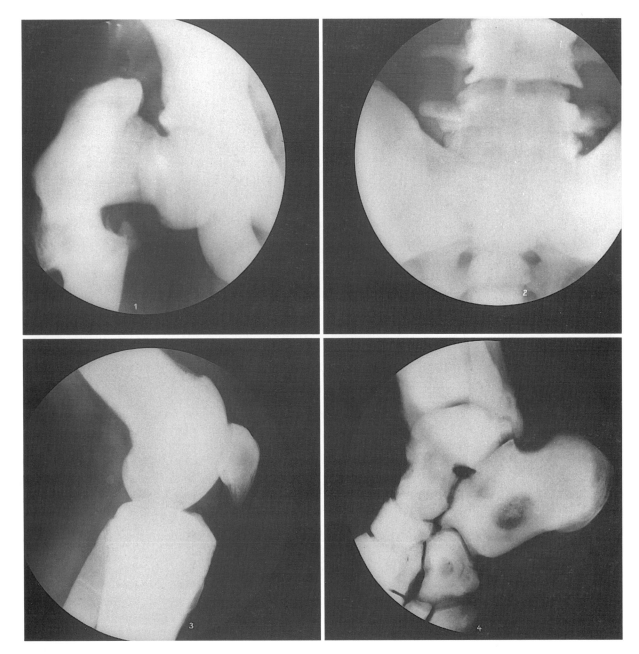

Fig. II, 9. Heinrich Ernst Albers-Schoenberg discovered the genetic congenital disorder of bone formation, "marble bones", at first by a roentgenologic examination in 1904 and later confirmed by pathoanatomic and histologic examination, characterized by an extreme increase in bone density. These radiographs were copied from the original publication and already show the findings clearly.

entiation between congenital and acquired deformities through the delineation of secondary skeletal changes according to diseases and their specific sequelae [49, 76, 77, 79, 100, 101, 129, 226, 229, 253, 255]. Congenital club foot was considered to be the result of a defect in the navicular bone or tibia. Defects of the hand were better understood and classified by subtle analysis of the radiographic images [12, 20, 40, 115, 213, 238].

A large number of theories on the origin of congenital hip dislocation could be replaced by objective knowledge gained through radiographic findings. It became apparent that the acetabulum did not deepen into a 'cavity', but is formed like a dish, while the femoral head corresponds in size to the child's age. The opinion that a congenital hip dislocation is an inherited disease was confirmed [159, 255]. Subtle analysis

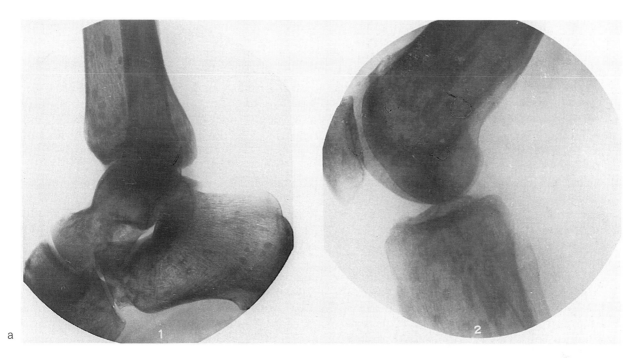

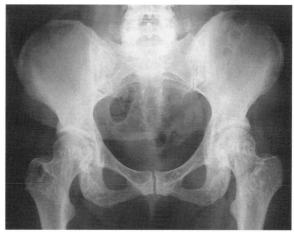

Fig. II, 10a, b. An additional condition with distinct oval densities in trabecular bone was discovered by H.E. Albers-Schoenberg in 1915 and called "osteopoikilosis". Later, nodular thickening of the skin (dermatofibrosis lenticularis) as manifestation of a systemic connective tissue disorder was found in patients with this rare, frequently familial condition. **(a)** These images are copies of the original publication and shown in comparison with **(b)** a recent radiograph of a quality that allows a subtle image analysis. The distribution pattern of compact islets and somewhat thickened trabecular structures can vary considerably.

b

of radiographic images could confirm the fact, emphasized by Hoffa (1905) [98], that in a large number of unilateral hip dislocations changes are also found in the contralateral hip. In addition, radiologic investigations could establish the differential diagnosis between congenital dislocation and acquired changes of the hip joint, e.g. tuberculous coxitis. The frequently debated theories and erroneous interpretations of hip-joint diseases were rectified with the help of radiographic analysis. According to Immelmann (1906) [102], it became impossible to overlook a dislocated hip.

Creating stereoscopic radiographic images provided additional information as to the relationship of depth of the acetabulum and the position of the femoral head in the hip joint.

The increased knowledge through radiographic and pathological findings of the hip joint contributed decisively to the improvement of therapeutic procedures. As a result, the indications for either conservative therapy or surgical correction increased. Even if it was not yet possible, at the beginning of the century, to reconstruct a normal joint, good functional results could be achieved.

Radiology had a considerable influence on the concepts of scoliotic curvatures of the spine and their treatment [21, 22, 129, 194, 210, 221]. Using fluoroscopy, it could be shown that, in severe scolioses, moveable portions of the spine could be realigned while the actual curvature did not really change. It was concluded that by means of 'redressment' slight corrections and thus improvements of the static function of the spine could be achieved. Not until later, the various types of vertebral deformities were recognized as the cause of scoliotic curvature of the entire spinal column (Fig. II, 7) [42, 82, 84, 211, 252].

The causative deformities of the lower extremities, such as bow legs and knock knees, were analyzed radiographically, influencing therapeutic measures. The outcome of careful studies and follow-up observations converted a large number of earlier theories on the curvatures of the legs into actual knowledge. When surgery seemed necessary, radiographs were essential to plan the operation and to achieve successful orthopaedic correction of numerous deformities of the foot skeleton [20, 202].

In the differential diagnosis, it was for the first time possible to quantify the impact of static forces on the morphology of the bones as components and structures of the skeleton. The importance of the internal structure and the architecture of the bones was increasingly understood [126, 138, 208, 261, 262].

It was established that increased pressure could induce thickening of the diaphyseal compact bone while marked decompression or rest would lead to a depletion of the osseous substance resulting in 'atrophy'. Skeletal changes caused by inappropriate weight bearing and other manipulations were recognized, such as extremely tightly laced corsets, inappropriate shoes (Chinese!) and long-standing unilateral faulty weight bearing. Deformities caused by static pressure as found in club foot or growth disturbances of the radius or tibia were understood for the first time.

Detection of fractures and their sequelae

Shortly after the first application of X-rays it was undisputed that fractures as the result of osseous trauma [266] were clearly recognizable. This advance allowed considerable improvements in fracture treatment and made it possible to develop the stable osteosynthesis [19, 136, 178, 256]. In contrast, fractures involving the growth plates could only be recognized and assessed through more subtle analysis of the radiographic images [123, 129].

A particular diagnostic problem that had been recognized early is the lack of or only partial understanding of the sequelae of heavy contusions and injuries caused by joint dislocations and their reduction, which often could not be identified by conventional radiographic studies. The experi-

ence gained from ligamentous or capsular tears as well as from periosteal injuries called for radiographic follow-up to look for the development of discrete ossifications after a several weeks or months. This was the beginning of an objective assessment of osseous findings following injuries to joints, connective tissue, soft tissues and muscle insertions. In addition, conspicuous atrophic changes of the bone structure after trauma, such as Sudeck's bone atrophy [240, 241], were identified early [90]. This porosity of the bones, later called 'acute bone atrophy', had to be differentiated from systemic changes found in bones, particularly the senile bone atrophy (Fig. II, 11).

The physical and geometrical requirements for an adequate radiographic examination of fractured bones and healing fractures were recognized. It was found that 'soft' X-rays (generated by low anode voltage) do not penetrate the bones and could produce changes simulating 'scleroses'. Only 'hard' X-rays delineate the sclerosis of a 'bony scar' and are feasible for evaluating the osseous bridging of a healing fracture. Impaired healing process of bones were recognized and analyzed further. The evolution of 'false joints' or 'pseudarthroses' and their causes became known [26, 110, 148, 161, 187, 191, 200, 218].

Radiographs of fractures of the growing skeleton show particularly profuse, often exuberant callus formation. The periosteal bone appositions, that is, the role of the fibrous membrane

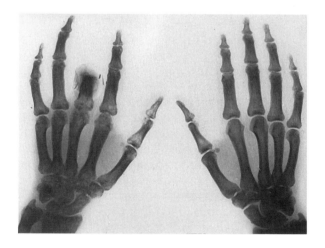

Fig. II, 11. In 1900/1901, Sudeck recognized "acute bone dystrophia", a hyperemia caused after injury and accompanied by pain and bone changes.
The original radiograph shows structural loss of trabeculations and cortex, visible as patchy radiolucencies and called "acute bone atrophy".

covering the surface of the bone or "periosteum" in the healing process, was recognized and documented [184, 187, 214, 265].

Joints affected by trauma could be analyzed with respect to secondary damage. It became apparent that the radiographically visualized 'articular space' corresponded to the articular cartilages covering both joint-forming bones. Atrophy of the cartilage was visible as a narrowing of the joint space. Conversely, an increase in the joint space in comparison with a previous examination or an established standard had to be interpreted as a joint effusion!

The role of radiology for expert testimony

Already the initial reports on the unimaginable diagnostic possibilities of X-rays stated that it was absolutely necessary to use this new tool for expert testimony of accidental injuries. Each case of osseous trauma at risk for financial compensation should be subjected to radiological objectivity of the findings. Appropriate radiographs of the injured bony region require at least two projections [89, 129, 214].

In this context, Immelmann (1906) [102] already emphasized that *evidence, on which so much depends should be made by a physician with postgraduate training in roentgenological techniques. The difficulty in taking a suitable radiograph resulted in establishing laboratories dedicated to this purpose. It is well known that different roentgen images of the same bone injury can turn out dissimilar. What applies to taking radiographs is also true for their interpretation*. Only experience gained over a long time can protect against diagnostic errors and misinterpretations. Furthermore, Immelmann pointed out that an appropriate radiographic image could unequivocally prove the sequelae of a bone injury even at a later date. It was emphasized that in all questionable cases the radiographic examination could objectively confirm the diagnosis and its sequelae. Already these expositions of the first decade of radiology pointed out that an examiner should be aware of all skeletal abnormalities to prevent misdiagnosis. The differential diagnosis between accessory bones and traumatic avulsions is often difficult. Pfitzner (1895) [183] deserves credit for the systematical compilation of all normal variants of the skeleton.

Radiology was of great benefit in assessing war injuries since rejected claims of war related disabilities could be corrected. Type and consequences of a bone injury and residual functional impairment could be substantiated by radiographic examinations [71, 143, 147, 148].

The importance of a meticulous radiological diagnosis was recognized early in forensic medicine. Foreign metal fragments in the body, such as the broken tip of a knife or a bullet, and the kind of gunshot wound could be assessed radiographically. It was possible to determine if the wound was inflicted by a pistol, shotgun or a rifle. While forensic physicians could previously assess a gunshot wound with a probe only, they can now answer all important questions by means of radiological examination [162].

Radiomorphology of inflammatory diseases

Inflammatory diseases were already differentiated around the turn of the century. In addition to osteomyelitis during childhood – its radiographic manifestation has changed due to considerable therapeutic improvements over the last two decades – tuberculosis of the joints and bones [133] was frequent at the beginning of this century. Elaborate studies of morphological changes found in the various skeletal regions led to a better understanding of the propagation of these serious, specific inflammatory diseases. Furthermore, the differential diagnosis was refined and today it is no longer a problem differentiating a tuberculous bone disease from other inflammatory or tumorous entities [11, 27, 85, 108, 111, 124, 128, 141, 227, 246, 250].

Tuberculous diseases of the hip played an important role, particularly in the growth period. The early findings of tuberculous coxitis as seen radiographically allowed its differentiation from a hip dislocation. It was emphasized that the contours of the joint-forming bones of the hip were blurred on the diseased side, while the healthy side always showed sharp contours. Radiographic follow-up of tuberculous coxitis allowed the assessment of increasing destruction of the joint-forming bones, resulting in spontaneous dislocations. Immobilization of the joint in extension was recommended, with very good results. If an ankylosis of the diseased joint developed, osteotomy could not only correct the deformity but also lengthen the limb. It became possible to diagnose and treat abscesses secondary to tuberculous coxitis. Follow-up examinations revealed that tuberculous hip infection has a protracted course over a period of several years.

In addition to tuberculosis of the hip, tuberculous spondylitis was recognized and analyzed radiographically. Of great concern was a tuberculous spondylitis accompanied by severe necroses and bone loss. Orthopaedic measures should prevent severe gibbus formation due to bone resorption [37, 153].

Using a compression aperture (after Albers-Schoenberg) in lateral fluoroscopy, the extent of the destruction of the vertebral body, which could lead to scoliosis, could be estimated. It was recognized early on that the unaffected spinous processes remain clearly visible in the lateral view. By counting the spinous processes, conclusions could be drawn about the number of fused vertebral bodies. This had therapeutic consequences.

Tuberculosis was a major cause of infectious arthritis. Tuberculous arthritis could lead to various types of contractures, and the recommended orthopaedic treatment consisted of immobilization with a plaster cast or splints before contractures have developed [133].

The objective was to let the joint ankylose in the best possible position. The radiographic analysis of the healing process of tuberculous arthritis revealed that occasionally reactive new bone formation produces osseous bridging and, at the same time, tuberculous granulation tissue in the middle of the joint prevents osseous fusion. The resulting ankylosis requires surgical intervention and correction.

In the first decade of radiology, rheumatic diseases also played a role in the differential diagnosis of inflammatory diseases of the bones and joints. Knowledge of the morphological and structural changes of bones, however, was limited. Only until radiologic techniques and spatial resolution had improved, the characteristic findings of rheumatic diseases could be established. Direct magnification techniques advanced the meticulous evaluation of the contours and structures of bones. Fine focus exposure and low kilovoltage immersion techniques for detailed analysis of the bones of the hand and soft tissues promoted further progress in the radiological diagnosis of rheumatic disease [53, 94, 95].

At the beginning of this century, a particular type of inflammatory disease was identified as syphilitic infection of the skeleton. Differences between infantile syphilis of the bones and joints and the luetic changes acquired in adulthood could be objectified [15, 58, 83, 129, 237]. Actinomycosis of the bones, often localized in the jaw, also deserves mention here as an inflammatory disease.

Lymphogranulomatosis of the bones is no longer classified as an inflammatory disease.

The eosinophilic granuloma and other histiocytomas have been diagnosed as an disease entity in their own right and classified as such [245].

Some rare inflammatory bone diseases were analyzed and correctly classified according to their pathogens. These conditions, which are primarily observed in African countries, include bone echinococcus [117, 198, 243], bone blastomycoses, sporotrichoses, Madura foot (mycetoma pedis), bone leprosy and bone malleomycoma.

Generalized bone diseases

The improvement in radiology coincided with an increasing knowledge of new and less well-known diseases through pathohistological and chemical investigations. This particularly applies to the generalized bone diseases or osteopathies. Whereas, previously, a porosity was merely defined as osteoporosis, which only had to be differentiated from an osteomalacia, three important types of systemic skeletal diseases evolved through the results of clinical research and biochemistry, laboratory medicine and radiology:

1 genetic disorders of bone formation and bone transformation;
2 disorders of mineral and vitamin metabolism with secondary involvement of the bones;
3 hormonal diseases with involvement of the bones [45, 65, 165, 174, 185].

The pattern of skeletal changes in deficiency rickets [186] became first known to pathologists. In the growth period, radiographic findings were primarily demonstrated in the epiphyses and metaphyses. The diaphyses are also involved in disturbances of bone formation and transformation, but the changes were less conspicuous radiographically, even though they were histologically recognizable. Bone distortions may occur as a result of decreased mineralization of the osseous matrix in rickets [60, 68, 156, 219, 260].

'Osteomalacia' was considered to be a disease of vitamin D deficiency in adulthood. The resulting disturbance of mineralization also leads to static insufficiency, which produces 'Looser zones' and pathological fractures of the bones, as well as bone deformities, such as *Kartenherzbecken* (pelvic deformity), indentations of the ribs and bowing of the long bone of the lower extremities [105, 109, 156, 166].

Before the diagnostic use of X-rays, little was known about skeletal changes due to vitamin C deficiency, which is sometimes still seen today (Moeller–Barlow syndrome in childhood or scurvy in adults). The radiographic appearance includes structural changes in the region of the growth plates of epiphyses and metaphyses, which also affect the diaphyses. Often, after separation of the periosteum due to bleeding and subsequent uncommon calcifications, bizarre deformities of the bones occur [59, 63, 259].

Bony changes after long periods of starvation or intestinal malabsorption (sprue) were described as gastrointestinal osteopathy. Increased porosity and substance loss of the osseous matrix are seen in these conditions. Similar changes can be seen after or with severe liver damage as manifestation of cholestatic diseases and hepatic cirrhosis as well as alcohol-induced hepatocellular disease. The 'hepatogenic osteopathy' shows changes of the bone structure similar to those found in gastrointestinal osteopathy. Secondary changes of the severe atrophy and demineralization of the osseous structure can lead to compression of the weight-bearing bones, such as vertebrae, femoral neck and calcaneus.

Of the hormonal bone diseases, disturbances mediated by the effect of the parathyroid hormone on bone turnover play a major role. Primary hyperparathyroidism is connected with the name of the pathologist J. Erdheim [43, 44]. He discovered a tumour growth of the glandula parathyroidea (epithelial bodies), first described by von Recklinghausen [196] as early as 1891. The 'osteodystrophia fibrosa generalisata cystica Recklinghausen' and its unusual changes of the bones were already known before the diagnostic use of X-rays. In an excellent contribution in the 'Handbuch der speziellen pathologischen Anatomie und Histologie' [Handbook of Special Pathological Anatomy and Histology] L. Haslhofer [86] acknowledged the contribution of skeletal radiography to medicine. In his opinion, it was the only method that provided information on the pathoanatomical changes of bony tissue far beyond the scope of the clinical examinations. In support of his position, every case he had observed so far confirmed this. Radiographic examinations are particularly valuable for regions of the skeleton that cannot be easily evaluated clinically, such as the bones of the hand and foot. The comparison skeletal radiographs of the diseased and healthy side brings out the radiographic manifestation of the disease to better advantage [105].

The bones were found to be considerably more radiolucent in cases of Recklinghausen's disease or in primary hyperparathyroidism. We are indebted to Looser [158] and Kienböck [120] for their elaborate descriptions of the radiomorphological findings of this disease. A decrease in calcified bone substance, i.e. less radiation absorption, was determined as the underlying cause. Already at the beginning of our understanding of this entity, the finding of the 'vanishing' cortex was described as replacement of bony tissue by connective tissue or by calcium-deficient bones. In severe cases, the bone exhibits a high-grade, honeycombed rarefaction and is only visualized as a delicate, irregular mesh. Despite the severe 'porosity' (as this condition was called in those days), the bones usually remain normal in shape.

In the tubular bones, cyst-like changes were found that were described as 'brown tumours'. These cystic, shell-like foci could be visualized and analyzed in detail with X-rays (Fig. II, 12) [62, 105, 158, 185, 186].

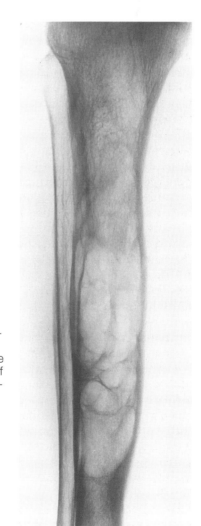

Fig. II, 12. The unusual, multilocular pseudocystic defect in the middle of the tibial shaft of a 64-years-old woman corresponds to a histologic "brown tumor" in primary hyperparathyroidism that had been initially called "osteodystrophia fibrosa generalisata cystica – Recklinghausen".

It was emphasized that the number of 'cysts' or 'brown tumours' did not indicate the seriousness of the disease. Based on a large number of radiomorphological findings, various forms of hyperparathyroidism (Recklinghausen's disease of the bone) were distinguished. A classification was developed by Albright, Aub and Bauer (1934) [5], which related the pathomorphological skeletal changes to diseases of the urinary system. As associated findings of this disease and its systemic disturbance of the bone metabolism, nephrocalcinosis and nephrolithiasis as well as involvement of other internal organs should also be mentioned.

Secondary hyperparathyroidism became well known through research performed on patients with chronic renal disease, The disease process, also known as 'renal osteopathy', led not only to an accelerated osseous turnover but also to the formation of pseudocysts in the bone, similar to the ones seen in primary hyperparathyroidism. During its later course, this secondary bone disease presents with pathological fractures, epiphyseolysis in the growing skeleton, and regional fine or coarse spongiosclerosis, which appears as sclerosis along the endplates of the vertebral bodies, producing the 'rugger jersey spine' [105].

Pituitary dysfunction leads to various bone changes. Hypofunction may lead to disturbances of the intercartilaginous ossification in adolescence, resulting in pituitary dwarfism. The acromegalic syndrome due to pituitary hyperfunction became better known by studying its radiographic skeletal findings. Not only an enlarged sella caused by tumour-like enlargement of the pituitary gland, but also osseous appositions in terms of acral growth in the hands and feet, along the ventral border of the vertebral bodies, and in the skull have long been known to characterize this hormonal osteopathy (Fig. II, 13). In addition, the bone turnover was found to be abnormal.

Characteristic skeletal changes in Cushing's disease include not only an abnormal turnover consisting of a hypomineralization of the osseous matrix, but also a distinct rarefaction in terms of an osteoporosis. Observed secondary findings include vertebral compression, impaired osseous turnover with osteonecroses affecting the large joints and changes in the skull.

Dwarfism or gigantism may result from a disorder of the sex hormones in adolescence. All bones may show a generalized osteoporosis [197, 207, 214].

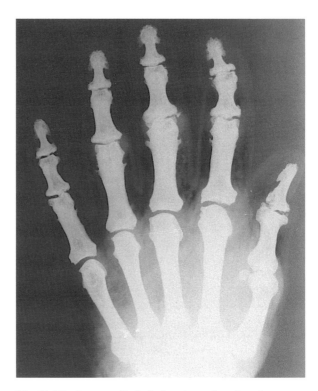

Fig. II, 13. As a result of pituitary hyperfunction, bone apposition occurs, particularly at the acral skeleton (bones of the hand and foot), and is called "acromegaly". This hormonal osteopathy can be reliably recognized by its typical findings in the hand skeleton, such as small, exostoses-like bone formations at the interphalangeal joints and ungulate processes and abnormally thick phalanges as well as thickening of the skin. (Low voltage immersion technique, left hand of a 75-years-old woman).

An often severe osteoporosis is commonly diagnosed in postmenopausal women and has been of considerable interest in the last few decades because its often debilitating course may lead to disability. The early diagnosis of this condition of severely increased bone turnover can be established by 'quantitative radiology' [92, 95, 96].

The effect of the thyroid gland on the skeleton has been thoroughly studied in the last few decades. Hyperthyroidism leads to an accelerated osseous turnover, often progressing to a loss of the osseous matrix with a resultant osteoporosis. In the growth period, the impaired thyroid function may lead to cretinism [17] or hypothyroidism, often associated with growth disturbances consisting of persistent ossification centers in the epiphyses and, even more, in the apophyses. After hormonal substitution, the persistent epiphyseal growth centers usually fuse with the main bone.

In long-standing diabetes mellitus, bone and joint changes of still unsatisfactorily explained etiology can be observed. Microangiopathy in diabetes has been thought to be the principal cause of this bone disease, but it should be kept in mind that a generalized abnormal bone turnover and rarefaction of the compacta and spongiosa could be detected as well. Moreover, a severe arthropathy may occur, possibly caused by a neuropathy.

In addition to these disturbances attributable to abnormal bone metabolism and turnover, not yet adequately analyzed forms of complex hormonal osteoporosis have been observed.

Unusual systemic bone diseases

Medullar osteopathies

The mutual effects of diseases of the bone marrow and osseous matrix can be seen in the manifestation of medullary osteopathies. In osteomyeloreticulosis, irregular spongiosclerotic changes appear in the final phase. The congenital diffuse generalized hyperostosis should be mentioned as an instance of unusual structural changes.

Toxic osteopathies

Applying a meticulous structural analysis of bone radiographs, changes could be found and were later classified in subsequent clinical and laboratory studies as skeletal damage secondary to exogenic toxic substances. These conditions includes bone damage from exposure to phosphorus or strontium. Bone changes were also seen with lead ingestion. Initially thought to be less important were spongiosclerosis and metaplastic calcifications in the tendons and ligaments induced by an increased fluorine intake. Only later could these findings be attributed to fluorine poisoning. The changes occur not only in humans but also in domestic animals, and has been observed in cattle that has grazed on fluorine-contaminated land. Through continual accumulation of knowledge, exhaustive and comprehensive classifications of all toxic osteopathies could be compiled [36].

Systemic osteoscleroses

A review of books on clinical radiology and even older textbooks on pathological anatomy and histology reveal that many of the skeletal changes of spongiosclerosis or hyperostosis were first recognized radiographically and then analyzed pathoanatomically and histologically.

Circulation disorders of the bones

At the beginning of the century, studies comparing radiomorphological and pathoanatomical findings could reveal the relationship and the great influence of the circulation on the turnover and mineralization of bone tissue [87]. P. Sudeck (1900) [239, 241] aroused particular attention with the first description of acute inflammatory bone atrophy, observed after injury of the extremities but also in connection with inflammation. Hyperaemia with rarefaction in terms of 'osteoporosis' was recognized and described by Pommer (1925) [186]. Venous hyperaemia, caused by circulatory disturbance from congestion in the venous system, was in the forefront of the considerations and discussions [90, 114, 118].

Quantitative analysis of the bones

In the last few decades, the accumulated knowledge of systemic skeletal diseases has stimulated the quantitative analysis of the osseous structures. In addition to measurements applied to the thickness of the diaphyseal compacta and cortex or electronic analysis applied to the structure of the spongiosa, X-ray densitometry was developed for the determination of the mineral concentration present in a circumscribed bone area [92, 95, 96, 233].

To eliminate incorrect measurements and methodical distortion, it was recommended to use a reference phantom measured together with the bone (Fig. II, 14). In addition to animal bones or aluminium, the bone-equivalent mineral alkaline hydroxylapatite was used as a reference substance. Quantitative computed tomography (QCT) was used to measure vertebral bodies, representing pure spongiosal bone. A large amount of data has already been accumulated regarding healthy test subjects and various skeletal diseases [96].

Microradiography of bone

The use of specific quality X-rays in the investigation of tissue or very thin bone sections has furthered scientific insight [41, 91, 93, 109]. The

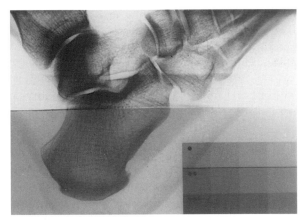

Fig. II, 14. A densitometric analysis of the general mineral content of a trabecular bone region in systemic skeletal diseases or osteopathies was at first investigated by means of reference substances of known compounds that were simultaneously imaged. As a practical bone-equivalent reference system, a step wedge of water-equivalent plastics containing various hydroxylapatite concentrations was used. Suitable measurement zones are found in the calcaneus (a generalized trabecular sclerosis is present in the shown case), the distal end of the radius and femoral neck. By using computed tomography, the trabecular bone in the vertebral bodies can be measured.

Fig. II, 15. The distribution and concentration of mineral components in the bone matrix can be demonstrated by means of a microradiograph.

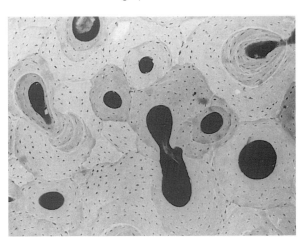

Fig. II, 15a. An undecalcified 50 µm slice of normal bone tissue from the proximal femur compacta.

bones were in the forefront of these investigations, but their preparation was difficult until now without prior decalcification. With the introduction of microtomes, bone sections of only 20 µm can be prepared without prior decalcification. Excellent studies of the microscopic distribution and concentration of the calcium salts in the osseous matrix areas can be performed using low energy X-rays with a maximum wave length in the region of the absorption edge of calcium (3.06 Å). Even discrete differences in mineral concentrations of the osseous matrix can be recorded. The resolution of the method extends down to the cellular level so that pericellular changes of the mineral concentration can be recognized and assessed (Fig. II, 15). Quantitative analysis of the mineral concentration of the osseous matrix is possible.

Comparative radiographic studies of the pathomorphological findings at the macroscopic level and down to the microscopic dimensions of tissue structures and cells contributed fundamentally to the understanding of many clinical entities.

Skeletal microradiography was used for investigating the pathological findings of hormonal or gastrointestinal systemic skeletal diseases, new

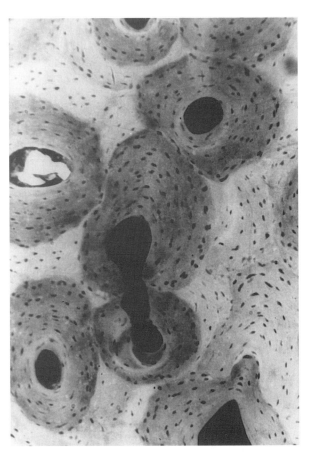

Fig. II, 15b. A 50 µm slice of bone of from the femoral cortex in renal osteopathy (secondary hyperthyroidism), revealing a very irregular mineralization of the osseous matrix.

bone formations, and metastatic bone tumours, and for studying interesting inherited structural changes, such as genetically altered bone formation. It can be hoped that the outcome will contribute to the understanding of the pathogenesis of currently obscure bone changes.

Discovery of bone dysplasia

A few bone diseases are classified as dysplasias. They are characterized by irregular bone transformations with associated replacement of the connective tissues and corresponding changes in shape and structure. The various types of hyperparathyroidism have already been mentioned under the systemic osteodystrophia. Fibrous dysplasia (Jaffe–Lichtenstein disease) and osteitis deformans (Paget's disease) are still aetiologically undefined bone diseases (recent findings suggest that Paget's disease is a viral infection).

Fibrous dysplasia of bone

After the discovery of this disease, which manifests itself in the first two decades of life, the pathohistological investigations revealed bone transformation with replacement of the spongiosa by connective tissue and formation of fibrous bone. Not only the spongiosa, but also the compact bone is replaced by fibrous bone interlaced with connective tissue. The lamella of the outer osseous contour remains, but the diaphyseal compacta is diminished throughout. Wherever fibrous bone with its low calcium content appears, bone deformities and distortions can be

expected. Several types are currently known. The combination of fibrous dysplasia with a pubertas praecox and café-au-lait spots was described by Albright [4, 6]. Monostotic and oligo-ostotic types of bone disease have been observed. The pathogenesis of this disease is still unknown [149, 247].

Osteitis deformans (Paget's disease)

This peculiar, still somewhat enigmatic disease had already been exhaustively and pathoanatomically described by Paget in 1877 [176], even before the discovery of X-rays. Radiography opened the way for a better understanding of the changes that are often confined to a single bone. Osteitis deformans was primarily considered to be a chronic infectious disease with a protracted course over several decades. The viral aetiology is currently under discussion again. The early diagnosis is characterized by demineralization of the osseous matrix, which usually is well delineated [220]. A characteristic early manifestation of Paget's disease of the skull is known as 'osteoporosis circumscripta cranii', first described by Schueller (1929) [223]. At this stage of the demineralized osseous matrix, the diseased bones become deformed, leading, for instance, to a heart-shaped compression of the pelvic inlet or bowing of the femur and tibia (Fig. II, 16). A diseased vertebra may be compressed despite its increasing size. The typical course of this condition will pass through different pathomorphological manifestations. The demineralization phase is followed by an exuberant osseous transformation that may vary in its appearance. Coarsing of the

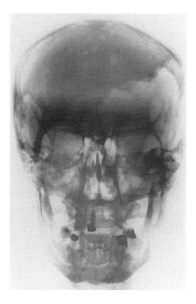 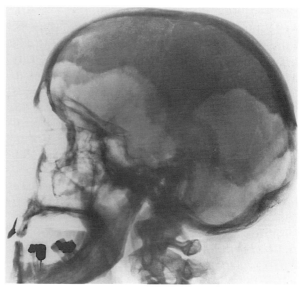

Fig. II, 16. The "osteoporosis circumscripta cranii" of the skull bones was described by Schueller in 1929 and has been established as an early phase of osteitis deformans or "Paget's disease". It corresponds to a reduced mineral content of the diplospongiosa. The different stages of Paget's disease were discovered by diagnostic radiology.

spongiosa develops as well as areas of localized consolidation, in addition to enlargements and deformities of the diseased bone, which may lead to Looser zones or increased fracture risk.

Pathologists have conducted elaborate studies of this disease. Erdheim (1935) [46] was the first to publish profound results of scientific research. Some authors have suggested a hereditary component.

It is a disease that is seen in elderly individuals and peaks between the ages of 60 and 70 years. The latter stages are characterised by a severe thickening and deformity of the bones. In addition, the tubular bones show an 'exfoliation' or funnelling of the diaphyseal compacta through coarsening and thickening of the spongiosa as manifestation of a spongiosclerosis [62]. Its course over years and even decades does not affect the patient's general condition, and often the patient merely complains of rheumatic pain of varying severity. Only the increasing thickness and distortion of an extremity and an obvious enlargement of the skull draws the patient's attention to Paget's disease. The static impairment of the strength of pagetic bones may lead to Looser zones or pathological fractures. Follow-up studies have shown that the dynamics of the Paget's disease subsides with advancing age [157].

In a late phase of the Paget's disease, sarcomatous degeneration of the bones can lead to osteogenic sarcomas [51, 224]. This is a truly interesting and unique skletal disease, which is suitable for studying transformation processes of the osseous matrix.

Radiomorphology of bone tumours

In addition to determining the most frequent localizations of various bone tumours, radiographic studies can evaluate size, shape, contour and structure of benign, semi-malignant and malignant bone tumours by morphologic analysis. The characteristic radiographic findings of benign bone tumours and those absolutely typical of malignant neoplasm of the bone have been established (Fig. II, 17) [70, 116, 120, 122, 152, 212, 214, 245, 249].

In addition to rare primary bone tumours, the more common secondary bone tumours or metastases could be recognized and often even related to their site of origin. Cognizance of the radiomorphology of metastatic bone tumours is important for surgery and radiotherapy. 'Pattern recognition' of tumours holds a prominent

place in the diagnostic process. Many books have been dedicated to both primary tumours and skeletal metastases [10, 31, 48, 55, 56, 57, 104, 120, 122, 128, 152, 209].

Comparative pathoanatomical and radiological studies have also been published [32, 80, 181, 249].

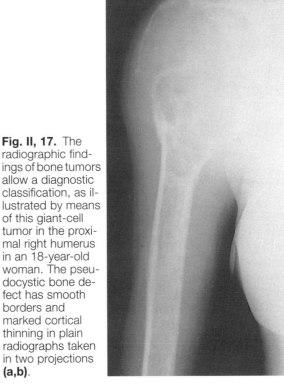

Fig. II, 17. The radiographic findings of bone tumors allow a diagnostic classification, as illustrated by means of this giant-cell tumor in the proximal right humerus in an 18-year-old woman. The pseudocystic bone defect has smooth borders and marked cortical thinning in plain radiographs taken in two projections **(a,b)**.

a

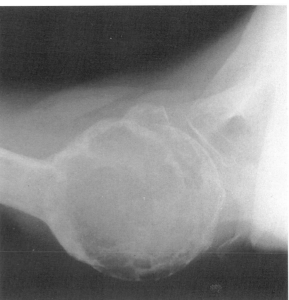

b

Tomography, and later computed tomography, of primary and secondary bone tumours have advanced the radiomorphological tumour diagnosis. The basic concept of diagnosing a particular tumour by analyzing its characteristic structure has not changed. Further investigations addressing the analysis of the primary tumour and its spread are important for therapy planning.

Assessment of osteoarticular diseases

In addition to correlating the radiomorphological findings with primary diseases of the joint-forming bones, meticulous analysis of the radiographic images was applied to study and understand subluxations, dislocations and dislocation-fractures [38, 71, 116, 121, 129, 146, 214, 255].

The characteristic radiographic findings of rheumatic joint diseases were recognized, with only limited contribution to clarify the pathogenesis. It has been recently stressed that, in addition to regional articular changes, a systemic disturbance of bone turnover may lead to secondary osteoporosis.

An unusual form of arthritis, known for hundreds of years, could be explained by its radiographic manifestation: Arthritis urica (gouty arthritis), caused by a disorder of the uric acid metabolism. Besides increasing the pathoanatomical knowledge of this osteoarticular disease, the radiomorphological findings [128] have improved the delineation of the extent, peripheral zones and osseous involvement of early gouty arthritis (Fig. II, 18).

Radiology made an important contribution to the detection and analysis of degenerative joint diseases [254], the so-called arthroses, particularly clarifying the neuropathic arthropathies. Furthermore, the arthrosis deformans that develops in various joints in the course of the ageing process could be recognized and evaluated [190]. Its underlying or precipitating disturbance has not yet been investigated adequately [9, 25, 113, 141].

With the introduction of contrast media in radiology, appropriate substances became available and were further developed for use in arthrography [52, 64, 99, 203, 264].

The soft tissue structures of the knee joint could now be evaluated. Severe lesions and tears of the menisci as well as ruptures of the ligaments and joint capsule could be diagnosed (Fig. II, 6), allowing planning of the surgical approach. As a result, the operations became more extensive and increasingly sophisticated. Finally, fluoroscopically guided arthroscopy, which followed the development of endoscopy, has become an invaluable addition, and even minute, subtle changes can be directly identified and treated arthroscopically.

Evaluation of the soft tissues

Radiology can also study the skeletal soft tissues. In addition to radiolucencies caused by air or gas-forming infections in the soft tissues (gas gangrene), increased densities within the soft tissues can be evaluated. Calcifications or ossifications in the muscles or subcutaneous tissues can be differentiated from ossifications or calcifications in the tendons and ligaments [129, 214, 236]). In addition, it was recognized that several soft tissue calcifications exhibit features characteristic of their primary diseases (trichinosis, cysticercosis) [234] (Fig. II, 19).

Foreign bodies in the soft tissues could now be detected and localized before surgical removal. In critical organs, such as the eye, the position of foreign bodies can be determined by measuring its depth.

Computed tomography greatly improved and expanded the diagnostic evaluation of the skeletal soft tissues. Its density resolution is considerably superior to that of conventional radiology. High-resolution computed tomography can delineate and analyze the most delicate soft tissue structures.

The different radiographic projections of the skeletal structures are summation images of the spatial absorption of X-rays and contain valuable information as to size, shape, contour and density

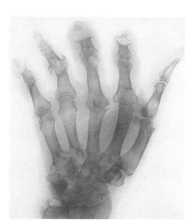

Fig. II, 18. In gout, deposits of uric acid in the bones lead to characteristic defects in the joint-forming bones that are referred to as tophi. They cause typical radiographic findings in the hand skeleton, as seen in this radiograph of a 58-year-old man obtained in 1917 (collection, E. Looser, Zurich, Switzerland).

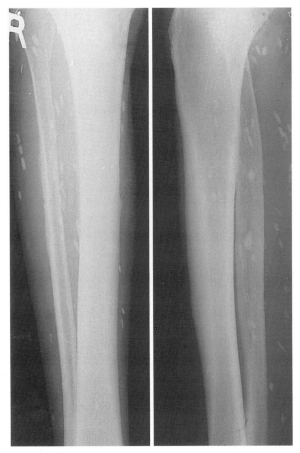

Fig. II, 19. The radiographic visualization of calcifications in the soft tissues often allows a classification as to their underlying disease. Cysticercosis can be recognized by numerous very dense, elliptic calcifications in the muscles.

(composition) of the bone in question and its surrounding soft tissues. The inherent superimposition of spongiosa, cortex and compacta, however, compromises the information content. The sectional display by means of conventional tomography, computed tomography and magnetic resonance imaging improves the spatial resolution and renders these macrostructures in great detail. This provides further pathomorphological evidence of diseases, obtained noninvasively with the patient fully awake. Moreover, the course of a disease can be monitored over a long period of time and the therapeutic results assessed. The following chapters will present the progress in diagnostic radiology and the continuing efforts of substantiating the value of its divers methods.

References

1. Åkerlund, A.: Entwicklungsteilen in Röntgenbildern von Hand, Fuß und Ellbogen im Mädchen- und Knabenalter. Fortschr. Röntgenstr. (1918) Erg.Bd. 33.
2. Albers-Schönberg, H.E.: Röntgenbilder einer seltenen Knochenerkrankung. (Arztverein Hamburg) Münch. med. Wschr. 51 (1904) 365
   Eine bisher nicht beschriebene Allgemeinerkrankung des Skelettes im Röntgenbild. Fortschr. Röntgenstr. 11 (1907) 261–263.
3. Albers-Schönberg, H.E.: Eine seltene, bisher nicht bekannte Strukturanomalie des Skelettes. Fortschr. Röntgenstr. 23 (1915/1916) 174–175.
4. Albright, F.: Syndrome characterized by osteitis fibrosa disseminata, areas of pigmentation and endocrine dysfunction, with precocious puberty in females. Report of five cases. New. Engl. J. Med. 216 (1937) 727–746.
5. Albright, F., J.C. Aub, W. Bauer: Hyperparathyreoidism: Common and polymorphic condition as illustrated by seventeen proved cases from one clinic. J. Amer. med. Ass. 102 (1934) 1276–1287.
6. Albright, F. E.G. Reifenstein: The parathyroid glands and metabolic bone disease. Selected studies. Williams and Wilkins Company, Baltimore 1948.
7. Allen, K.D.A.: Pioneer descriptions in military roentgenology. In: Bruwer A.J., ed.: Classic descriptions in diagnostic roentgenology, vol. 3: 1305–1405. Thomas, Springfield 1964.
8. Alexander, B.: Die Entwicklung der knöchernen Wirbelsäule. Fortschr. Röntgenstr. (1906) Erg.Bd. 13.
9. Axhausen, G.: Über den Abgrenzungsvorgang am epiphysären Knochen (Osteochondritis dissecans König). Virchows Arch. 252 (1924) 458.
10. Baetjer, F.H.: Differential diagnosis of bone tumors. Am. J. Roentgenol. 5 (1918) 260–264.
11. Baetjer, F.H.: Osteomyelitis. Am. J. Roentgenol. 6 (1919) 259–263.
12. Baisch, B.: Bau und Mechanik des normalen Fußes und des Plattfußes. Zschr. f. orthop. Chir. 31 (1913) 218.
13. Battersby, J.: The present position of the roentgen rays in military surgery. Arch. Roentgen Ray 3 (1899) 74–80.
14. Behrendsen: Studien über die Ossifikation der menschlichen Hand mittels des Röntgenverfahrens. Dtsch. med. Wschr. 27 (1897) 433.
15. Beitzke, H.: Syphilis der Gelenke. In Henke-Lubarsch, Hb. d. spez. Anat. u. Hist. (1934) Bd. 10.
16. Bernardeau: L'os acromial. These Bordeaux 1907.
17. Bircher, E.: Entwicklung und Bau des Kretinenskelettes. Verlag Gräfe und Sillem, Hamburg 1909.
18. Birkenfeld, W.: Zur Erblichkeit der multiplen kartilaginären Exostosen (Exostosen bei eineiigen Zwillingen). Dtsch. Z. Chir. 266 (1930) 397.
19. Bischoff, K. W. Gellinek: Geräte für die Anwendung ionisierender Strahlen. In: Diethelm, L., O. Olsson, F. Strnad, H. Vieten, A. Zuppinger (Hrsg.): Handbuch der med. Radiologie. Bd. I/2: 121–319. Springer Verlag 1965.
20. Blencke, A.: Über congenitale Femurdefekte. Zschr. orthop. Chir. 9 (1901) 584–656.
21. Böhm, M.: Beiträge zur Pathologie und Ätiologie der "Haltungstypen" der menschlichen Wirbelsäule. Ztsch. orthop. Chir. 13 (1909) 81–87.
22. Böhm, M.: Die Varietäten der Wirbelsäule. Röntgenpraxis 5 (1933) 81–84.

23. Böhm, M.: Die numerische Variation des menschlichen Rumpfskelettes. F. Enke Verlag Stuttgart 1907.

24. Borden, W.C.: The use of the roentgen ray by the medical department of the United States Army in the war with Spain (1898). Washington DC, U.S. Government Printing Office, 1900.

25. Brailsford, J.F.: The radiology of bones and joints. 3 Ed, Churchill, London 1945.

26. Brandt: Verzögerte Knochenheilung und Pseudarthrosenbildung. Thieme Leipzig 1937.

27. Bürgel, E., G. Bierling: Entzündliche Knochenerkrankungen. In: Diethelm, L., O. Olsson, F. Strnad, H. Vieten, A. Zuppinger (Hrsg.): Handbuch der med. Radiologie. Springer Verlag, Bd. V/2 (1973) 38–254.

28. Buschke A., H. Ollendorf. Ein Fall von Dermatofibrosis lenticularis disseminate und Osteopathia condensans disseminata. Derm.Wschr. 86 (1928) 257–262.

29. Calvé J.: Sur une forme particulière de pseudo-coxalgie greffée sur des déformations caractéristique de l'extremité supérieure du fémur. Rev. Chir. (Paris), 42 (1910) 54–84.

30. Cocchi, U.: Erbschäden mit Knochenveränderungen. In: Schinz, H.R., W.E. Baensch, E. Friedl, E. Uehlinger (Hrsg.): Lehrbuch der Röntgendiagnostik. G. Thieme Verlag Stuttgart, 5 Auflage, Bd. II/1 (1952) 621–636.

31. Codman, E.A.: Bone sarcoma, an interpretation of the nomenclature used by the Committee on the Registry of Bone Sarcoma of the American College of Surgeons. P.B. Hoeber, New York 1925.

32. Dahlin, D.C.: Bone Tumors. Charles C. Thomas, Springfield, Illinois, USA 1957.

33. Danelius, G.: Osteogenesis imperfecta intrauterin diagnostiziert. Arch. gynäk. 154 (1933) 160.

34. Dieck, W.: Anatomie und Pathologie der Zähne und Kiefer im Röntgenbilde. Verlag Gräfe und Sillem, Hamburg 1911.

35. Diethelm, L.: Fehlbildungen des Corpus vertebrae. In: Diethelm, L., F. Heuck, O. Olsson, K. Ranniger, F. Strnad, H. Vieten, A. Zuppinger (Hrsg.): Handbuch der med. Radiologie. Springer Verlag, Bd. VI/1 (1974) 190–264.

36. Diethelm, L. H. Fritz: Toxische Osteopathien. In: Diethelm, L., F. Heuck, O. Olsson, F. Strnad, H. Vieten, A. Zuppinger (Hrsg.): Handbuch der med. Radiologie. Springer Verlag, Bd. V/5 Osteopathien (1983) 649–815.

37. Diethelm, L., J. Kastert: Die entzündlichen Erkrankungen der Wirbelsäule. II Die spezifischen Entzündungen der Wirbelsäule. In: Diethelm, L., F. Heuck, O. Olsson, K. Ranniger, F. Strnad, H. Vieten, A. Zuppinger (Hrsg.): Handbuch der med. Radiologie. Springer Verlag, Bd. VI/2 (1974).

38. Dihlmann, W.: Gelenke-Wirbelverbindungen. G.Thieme-Verlag, Stuttgart-New York 1982.

39. Engelmann, G.: Ein Fall von Osteopathia hyperostotica (sclerotisans) multiplex infantilis. Fortschr. Röntgenstr. 39 (1929) 1101–1106.

40. Engels, W.: Über den normalen Fuß und den Plattfuß. Zschr. f. orthop. Chir. 12 (1904) 461.

41. Engström, A.: Microradiography of normal bone. In: Diethelm, L., O. Olsson, F. Strnad, H. Vieten, A. Zuppinger (Hrsg.): Handbuch der med. Radiologie. Springer Verlag, Bd. IV/1 (1970) 296–316.

42. Erdély, M.: Die komplexen Entwicklungsanomalien der Wirbelsäule. In: Diethelm, L., O. Olsson, F. Strnad, H. Vieten, A. Zuppinger (Hrsg.): Handbuch der med. Radiologie. Springer Verlag, Bd. VI/1 (1974) 583–620.

43. Erdheim, J.: Zur normalen und pathologischen Histologie der Glandula thyreoidea, Parathyreoidea und Hypophysis. II Epithelkörperchen (Glandula parathyreoidea). Beiträge zur pathologischen Anatomie und zur allgemeinen Pathologie. Jena-Fischer 33 (1903) 205–220.

44. Erdheim, J.: Über Epithelkörperchenbefunde bei Osteomalacie. S.-B. Akad. Wiss. Wien, math.-nat. Kl. 116 (1907) 311–370.

45. Erdheim, J.: Morphologische Studien über die Beziehungen der Epithelkörperchen zum Kalkstoffwechsel. Frankf. Z. Pathologie 7 (1911) 175–230.

46. Erdheim, J.: Über die Genese der Pagetschen Knochenerkrankung. Beitr. path. Anat. 96 (1935) 1.

47. Ernst, E.C.: Reminiscences of roentgenology during the last war, 1917–1919; Review of 17.000 examinations and x-ray equipment employed. Radiology 36 (1941) 421–438.

48. Evans, W.A.: Multiple myeloma of bone. Am. J. Roentgenol. 6 (1919) 646–649.

49. Ewald, P.: Über den Knick- und Plattfuß. Zschr. f. orthop. Chir. 24 (1909).

50. Fairbank, H.A.T.: An Atlas of general affections of the skeleton. E. and S. Livingstone, Edinburgh 1951.

51. Fedder, L.: Ostitis deformans mit sekundärer Rundzellensarkomatose. Fortschr. Röntgenstr. 31 (1923/1924) 391.

52. Fischedick, O.: Arthrographie des Kniegelenks. In: Diethelm, L., O. Olsson, F. Strnad, H. Vieten, A. Zuppinger (Hrsg.): Handbuch der med. Radiologie. Springer Verlag, Bd. V/2 (1973) 455–542.

53. Fischer, L.: Weichteildiagnostik an den peripheren Extremitäten mittels Weichstrahlentecknik. I. Indikationen und Bemerkungen zur Aufnahmetechnik. Radiologe 14 (1974) 454–456.

54. Fischer, H.: Beitrag zur Kenntnis der Skelettvarietäten (überzählige Karpalia und Tarsalia, Sesambeine, Kompaktaninseln. Fortschr. Röntgenstr. 19 (1912) 43.

55. Fraenkel, E.: Über Wirbelgeschwülste im Röntgenbilde. Fortschr. Röntgenstr. 16 (1910/1911) 245–257.

56. Fraenkel, E.: Über die sog. Hodgkin'sche Krankheit (Lymphomatosis granulomatosa). Dtsch. med. Wschr. (1912) 637.

57. Fraenkel, E.: Über multiple Enchondrome. Fortschr. Röntgenstr. 33 (1925) 775.

58. Fraenkel, E.: Die kongenitale Knochensyphilis im Röntgenbild. Fortschr. Röntgenstr. (1907) Erg. Bd. 26.

59. Fraenkel, E.: Die Möller-Barlowsche Krankheit. Fortschr. Röntgenstr. (1908) Erg. Bd. 18.

60. Fraenkel, E., U. Lorey: Die Rachitis im Röntgenbilde. Fortschr. Röntgenstr. (1910) Erg. Bd. 22.

61. Frangenheim, P.: Chondrodystrophische Zwerge. Fortschr. Röntgenstr. 12 (1911) 69.

62. Frangenheim, P.: Ostitis deformans Paget und Ostitis fibrosa v. Recklinghausen. Erg. d. Chir. u. Orthop. 14 (1921) 1.

63. Frank, H.: Röntgenologische Nachuntersuchungen bei klinisch geheilter Möller-Barlowscher Krankheit. Zschr. f. Kinderheilkd. 27 (1921) 127.

64. Freiberger, R.H., P.J. Killoran, G. Cardona: Arthrography of the knee by double contrast method. Am. J. Roentgenol. 97 (1966) 736–747.

65. Friedl, E., H.R. Schinz: Zur Frage der Knochenatrophie. In: Ergebnisse der medizinischen Strahlenforschung. G. Thieme Verlag Leipzig, Bd. I (1925) 95–130.

66. Friedmann, G.: Die Schädelnähte und ihre Pathologie. In: Olsson, O., F. Strnad, H. Vieten, A. Zuppinger (Hrsg.): Handbuch der med. Radiologie. Springer Verlag, bd. VII/1 (1963) 122–152.

67. Friedrich, H.: Über ein noch nicht beschriebenes, der Perthes'schen Erkrankung analoges Krankheitsbild des sternalen Klavikulaendes. Dtsch. Z. Chir. 187 (1924) 385.

68. Fromme, A.: Die Spätrachitis, die spätrachitische Genese sämtlicher Wachstumsdeformitäten und die Kriegsosteomalazie. Erg. Chir. u. Orthop. 15 (1922) 1.

69. Gebhardt, W.: Über die funktionelle Knochengestalt. Verh. Deutsch. orthop. Ges. 9/10 (1910/1911) 121.

70. Geschickter, C.F., M.M. Copeland: Tumors of bone. New York, Am. J. Cancer, 1931.

71. Grashey, R.: Atlas chirurgisch-pathologischer Röntgenbilder. Lehmann-Verlag München 1909.

72. Grashey, R.: Atlas typischer Röntgenbilder von normalen Menschen. Atlas I. 2. Aufl., Lehmann Verlag München 1912.

73. Grashey, R., R. Birkner: Atlas typischer Röntgenbilder von normalen Menschen. Urban und Schwarzenberg, München-Berlin 1964.

74. Grashey, R.: Röntgenologie. In: v. Schjerning: Handb. ärztl. Erfahrungen im Weltkriege, 9 (1922) 1914–1918.

75. Greulich, W.W., S.I. Pyle: Radiographic Atlas of Skeletal Development of the Hand and Wrist. Calif. University Press, Stanford 1959.

76. Gruber, G.B.: Hypoplasie, Mikromelie, Phokomelie, Amelie, Peromelie. In: Schwalbe: Die Morphologie der Mißbildungen III. Jena 1937.

77. Gruber, G.B.: Chondrodystrophia foetalis. In: Schwalbe: Morphologie der Mißbildungen III. Jena, 17 (1937) 333.

78. Guleke, N., H. Dietlen: Kriegs-Chirurgischer Röntgen-Atlas. Springer Verlag Berlin 1917.

79. Hackenbroch, M.: Der Hohlfuß. Erg. Chir. u. Orthop. 17 (1924) 457.

80. Haenisch, F.: Zur röntgenologischen Differentialdiagnose "zystischer" Knochentumoren. Fortschr. Röntgenstr. 30 (1922/1923) 84.

81. Häuptli, O.: Die aseptischen Chondro-Osteonekrosen. Walter de Gruyter-Verlag Berlin 1954.

82. Hahn, O.: Scheinbare Spaltbildung der Wirbelkörper in der Adoleszenz. Fortschr. Röntgenstr. 29 (1922) 211.

83. Hahn, O., U. Deycke-Pascha: Knochensyphilis im Röntgenbilde. Fortschr. Röntgenstr. Erg. Bd. 14 (1917).

84. Hanson, R.: On the development of spinal vertebrae, as seen on skiagrams, from late foetal life to the age of fourteen. Acta Radiol. 5 (1926) 112.

85. Hart, V.L.: Acute haematogenous osteomyelitis in children. J. Am. Med. Ass. 108 (1937) 524.

86. Haslhofer, L.: Die Engel-Recklinghausen'sche Knochenkrankheit (Ostitis bzw. Osteodystrophia fibrosa generalisata v. Recklinghausen). In: Lubarsch, O., F. Henke, R. Rössle (Hrsg.): Knochen und Gelenke. Handbuch der spez. pathologischen Anatomie und Histologie. Springer Verlag Berlin, Bd. IX/3 (1937) 342.

87. Haslhofer, L.: Kreislaufstörungen des Knochens. In: Lubarsch O., F. Henke, R. Rössle (Hrsg.): Knochen und Gelenke. Handbuch der spez. pathologischen Anatomie und Histologie. Springer Verlag Berlin, Bd. IX/3 (1937) 87–117.

88. Hasselwander, A.: Untersuchungen über die Ossifikation des menschlichen Fußskelettes. Z. Morph. u. Anthropol. 5 (1903) 438.

89. Hellner, H.: Knochenerkrankungen und -geschwülste in der Begutachtung. Heft 50 der "Hefte zur Unfallheilkunde". Hrsg. A. Hübner, Springer Verlag 1955.

90. Herfarth, H.: Beiträge zur Frage der Sudeckschen Knochenatrophie. Bruns Beitr. 132 (1924) 165.

91. Heuck, F.: Mikroradiographische Untersuchungen der Mineralisation des gesunden und kranken Knochengewebes. Radiologe 9 (1969) 142–154.

92. Heuck, F.: Die radiologische Erfassung des Mineralgehaltes des Knochens. In: Diethelm, L. (Hrsg.): Skelettanatomie. Handbuch der med. Radiologie. Springer Verlag, IV/1 (1970) 106–295.

93. Heuck, F.: Mikroradiographie. Verh. dtsch. Ges. Pathol. 58 (1974) 114–134.

94. Heuck, F., M. Schilling: Informationswert der Weichstrahl-Immersions-Radiographie (WIR) der Hand bei hormonalen und metabolischen Osteopathien. Radiologe 25 (1985) 573–581.

95. Heuck, F., E. Schmidt: Die quantitative Bestimmung des Mineralgehaltes des Knochen aus dem Röntgenbild. Fortschr. Röntgenstr. 93 (1960) 523–554.

96. Heuck, F., K. Vanselow: Radiologische Methoden. "Röntgenologie, Densitometri, Neutronen- und Protonenaktiverungsanalyse und Ultraschalluntersuchungen". In: Schwiegk, H. (Hrsg.): Handbuch der inneren Medizin, Bd. 6 Kuhlencordt, F., H. Bartel-Heimer (Hrsg.): Erkrankungen der Knochen, Gelenke und Muskeln. Springer Verlag, 1980.

97. Hickey, P.M.: The development of the skeleton. Trans Amer Roentgen Ray Soc. 4 (1903) 120–125.

98. Hoffa, A.: Die angeborene Coxa vara. Dtsch. med. Wschr. 31 (1905) 1257.

99. Hoffa, A.: Über Röntgenbilder nach Einblasung von Sauerstoff in das Kniegelenk. Berl. Klin. Wschr. 43 (1906) 28–30.

100. Hoffmann, L.: Mißbildungen der oberen Extremität. Fortschr. Röntgenstr. 17 (1911) 301.

101. Hurler, G.: über einen Typ multipler Abartungen vorwiegend am Skelettsystem. Z. Kinderheilkunde 24 (1919) 220–234.

102. Immelmann, W.: Zehn Jahre Orthopädie und Röntgenologie. 1896–1906. Otto und Emil Klett, Berlin 1906.

103. Israel, A.: Myositis ossificans neurotica nach Schußverletzung des Rückens. Fortschr. Röntgenstr. 27 (1910) 365.

104. Jaffe, H.L.: Tumors and Tumorous Conditions of the Bones and Joints. Lea and Febiger, Philadelphia 1958.

105. Jaffe, H.L.: Metabolic, Degenerative and Inflammatory Diseases of Bones and Joints. Urban und Schwarzenberg, München, Berlin, Wien 1972.

106. Joachimsthal, G.: Die angeborenen Verbildungen der oberen Extremitäten. Fortschr. Röntgenstr. Erg. Bd. 2 (1900).

107. Joachimsthal, G.: Über angeborene Verbildungen am Oberschenkel. Arch. Gebh. 65 (1902) 113.

108. Johansson, S.: Knochen- und Gelenktuberkulose im Kindesalter. G. Fischer, Jena 1926.

109. Jowsey, J.: Metabolic diseases of Bone. Saunders, Philadelphia 1977.

110. Jüngling, O.: Über Pseudarthrose im Kindesalter. Bruns Beitr. 90 (1914) 649.

111. Jüngling, O.: Ostitis tuberculosa multiplex cystica (eine eigenartige Form der Knochentuberkulose). Fortschr. Röntgenstr. 27 (1920) 375.

112. Jungherr: Die bisherigen Leistungen der Röntgenographie auf dem Gebiet der Rhinologie, Laryngologie und Otologie. Ztsch. med. Eletrol. Röntgenk. 4 (1908).

113. Kaiser, F.: Die spontane Regeneration Schußverletzter Gelenke im Röntgenbilde. Fortschr. Röntgenstr. 27 (191/1921) 119.

114. Kienböck, R.: Über akute Knochenatrophie bei Entzündungsprozessen an den Extremitäten (fälschlich sog. Inaktivitätsatrophie der Knochen) und ihre Diagnose nach dem Röntgenbild. Wien. med. Wschr. 51 (1901) 1346–1348.

115. Kienböck, R.: Zur radiographischen Anatomie und Klinik der enchondralen Dysplasie der Knochen mit multiplen kartilaginären Exostosen. Wien. med. Wschr. 47 (1903).

116. Kienböck, R.: Chirurgisch-radiologische Fehldiagnosen bei Knochenkrankheiten. Fortschr. Röntgenstr. 29 (1922) 81.

117. Kienböck, R., E. Klayer: Ein Fall von Echinococcose des Beckenknochens. Fortschr. Röntgenstr. 39 (1929) 1026–1034.

118. Kienböck, R.: Altersosteoporose. Wien. klin. Wschr. 432 (1931), 671 (1935).

119. Kienböck, R.: Angeborene Skelettanomalien der Lumbosacralgegend bei Kyphoskoliose. Fortschr. Röntgenschr. 60 (1939) 134–144.

120. Kienböck, R.: Differentialdiagnose der geschwulstigen Knochenkrankheiten. Urban und Schwarzenberg, Berlin-Wien 1933.

121. Kienböck, R.: Röntgendiagnostik der Knochen- und Gelenkkrankheiten. II Band: Gelenkkrankheiten, 1 und 2 Teil. Urban und Schwarzenberg, Berlin-Wien 1938.

122. Kienböck, R.: Röntgendiagnostik der Knochen- und Gelenkkrankheiten. I Band: Knochenkrankheiten. Urban und Schwarzenberg, Berlin-Wien 1941.

123. Kirchner, A.: Zur Frage der juvenilen Frakturen der Tuberositas tibiae, Tuberositas naviculare und des Tub.calc. Arch. klin. Chir. 84 (1907).

124. Kisch, E.: Fehldiagnosen bei Knochen- und Gelenktuberkulose. Langenb. Arch. 118 (1921) 481.

125. Klippel, M., A. Feil: Anomalie de la colonne vertébrale par absence des vertebres cervicales, cage thoracique remontant jusqu'á la base du crâne. Bull. mem. Soc. anat. (Paris) 87 (1912) 185–188.

126. Knese, K.H.: Knochenstruktur als Verbundbau. Heft 4 der "Zwanglosen Abhandlungen auf dem Gebiet der normalen und pathologischen Anatomie". G. Thieme Verlag, Stuttgart 1958.

127. Knese, K.H.: Mechanik und Festigkeit des Knochengewebes. In: Diethelm, L., O. Olsson, F. Strnad, H. Vieten. A. Zuppinger (Hrsg.): Handbuch der med. Radiologie. Springer Verlag, Bd. IV/1 (1970) 417–539.

128. Köhler, A.: Knochenerkrankungen im Röntgenbilde. Bergmann, Wiesbaden 1901.

129. Köhler, A.: Grenzen des Normalen und Anfänge des Pathologischen im Röntgenbilde, 2. Auflage. Verlag Gräfe und Sillem, Hamburg 1915.

130. Köhler, A.: Über eine häufige, bisher anscheinend unbekannte Erkrankung einzelner kindlicher Knochen. Münch. med. Wschr. 55 (1908) 1923–1925.

131. Köhler, A.: Das Köhler'sche Knochenbild des Os naviculare pedis – keine Fraktur. Langenb. Arch. 101 (1913) 560.

132. Köhler, A.: Eine typische Erkrankung des 2. Metatarsophalangealgelenkes. Münch. med. Wschr. 67 (1920) 1289–1290.

133. König, Fr.: Tuberkulose der Gelenke. In: Kirschner-Nordmann. Die Chirurgie, Bd. 2, Berlin 1928.

134. Kühne, K.: Die Zwillingeswirbelsäule (eine erbgenetische Forschung). Z. Morphol. und Anthropol. 35 (1936) 1–2.

135. Kümmel, H.: Die posttraumatischen Wirbelerkrankungen (Kümmell'sche Krankheit). Langenbecks Arch. 118 (1921) 876.

136. Küntscher, G.: Die Technik der Marknagelung des Oberschenkels. Zbl. Chir. (1940) 1145 und (1941) 1138.

137. Küntscher, G.: Die Technik der Marknagelung. Thieme Leipzig 1945.

138. Kummer, B.: Bauprinzipien des Säugerskelets. G. Thieme Verlag, Stuttgart 1959.

139. Lambertz,: Die Entwicklung des menschlichen Knochengerüstes während des föntalen Lebens. Fortschr. Röntgenstr. Erg. Bd. I, Verlag Gräfe und Sillem, Hamburg 1900.

140. Lang, F.: Über Art und Bedeutung der Kreislaufunterbrechung in der Ätiologie und Pathogenese der aseptischen Epiphyseonekrosen. Bruns Beitr. 171 (1941) 581.

141. Lange, M.: Knochen- und Gelenktuberkulose. II. Spezieller Teil erg. Tbk. -Forschg. Bd. 8 (1937) 319.

142. Legg. A.T.: An obscure affection of the hip-joint. Boston med. surg. J. 162 (1910) 202–204.

143. Lehmann, W.: Zur Frage der neurotischen Knochenatrophie, insbesondere nach Nervenschüssen. Bruns Beitr. 107 (1917) 605.

144. Léri, A.: Une maladie congénitale et héréditaire de l'ossification: la pléonostéose familiale. Bull. Mém. Soc. méd. Hop. Paris 3 (1921) 1228–1230.

145. Léri, A., Joanny: Une affection non décrite des os: Hyperostose en coulée sur toute la longueur d'un membre ou "Mélorhéostose". Bull. Soc. med. Höp. Paris 46 (1922) 1141–1145.

146. Lexer, E.: Gelenkchondrome. Dtsch. Z. Chir. 88 (1907) 311.

147. Lexer, E.: 20 Jahre Transplantationsforschung. Langenb. Arch. 138 (1925) 251.

148. Lexer, E.: Über die Entstehung von Pseudarthrosen nach Frakturen und Knochentransplantationen. Langenb. Arch. 119 (1922) 520.

149. Lichtenstein, L., H.C. Jaffe: Fibrous dysplasia of bone. Arch. Path. 33 (1942) 777–816.

150. Lilienfeld, A. von: Über das Os acromiale secundarium und seine Beziehungen zu den Affektionen der Schultergegend. Fortschr. Röntgenstr. 21 (1914) 198–204.

151. Lindemann, K.: Das erbliche Vorkommen der angeborenen Coxa vara. Z. Ortho. 72 (1941) 326.

152. Lodwick, G.S., C.L. Haun, W.E. Smith, R.F. Keller, E.D. Robertson: Computer diagnosis of primary bone tumors. A Preliminary report. Radiology 80 (1963) 273–275.

153. Löffler, F.: Die Pathogenese und Therapie der Spondylitis tuberculosa. Erg. Chir. u. Orthop. 15 (1922) 391.

154. Looser, E.: Über Osteogenesis imperfecta tarda. Verh. Dtsch. path. Ges. 1906 (1905) 239–242.

155. Looser, E.: Zur Kenntnis der Osteogenesis imperfecta congenita und tarda (sog. idiopathische Osteopsathyrosis). Mitt. Grenzgeb. Med. u. Chir. 15 (1906) 161.

156. Looser, E.: Über Spätrachitis und Osteomalacie. Klinische, röntgenologische und pathologisch-anatomische Untersuchungen. Dtsch. Z. Chir. 152 (1920) 210.

157. Looser, E.: Über Ostitis deformans und mit ihr angeblich und wirklich verwandte Knochenerkrankungen. Schweiz. med. Wschr. 1 (1926) 5.

158. Looser, E.: Über die Zysten und braunen Tumore der Knochen. Dtsch. Z. Chir. 189 (1924) 113.

159. Lorenz, A.: Die sog. angeborene Hüftverrenkung. F. Enke Verlag, Stuttgart 1920.

160. Lorenz, R.: Röntgendiagnostik des Schädeldaches. In: Olsson, O., F. Strnad, H. Vieten, A. Zuppinger (Hrsg.): Handbuch der med. Radiologie. Springer Verlag, Bd. VII/1 (1963) 340–429.

161. Maatz, R. K. Haasch: Vorgänge bei der Bruchheilung und Pseudarthrosenentstehung. In: Diethelm, L., O. Olsson, F. Strnad, H. Vieten, A. Zuppinger (Hrsg.): Handbuch der med. Radiologie. Springer Verlag, Bd. IV/1 (1970) 540–616.

162. Marwedel, G.: Das steckengebliebene Geschoss. In: Borchard und Schmieden "Die deutsche Chirurgie im Weltkrieg 1914–1918". 2, 1920.

163. Mayer, E.G.: Ergebnisse der röntgenologischen Untersuchungen des Schläfenbeines bei Erkrankungen des Ohres. Fortschr. Röntgenstr. 32 (1924) 39.

164. Melchior, E.: Die Madelungsche Deformität des Handgelenkes. Erg. Chir. 6 (1913) 324.

165. Michaelis, L.: Systemerkrankungen des Skelettes. Fortschr. Röntgenstr. 45 (1932) 187.

166. Milkman, L.A.: Pseudofractures (hunger osteopathy, late rickets, osteomalacia): report of a case. Am. J. Roentgenol. 24 (1930) 29–37.

167. Möller, F.P.: The clinical observation after Heating of Calvé-Perthes disease compared with the final Deformities left by that disease and the bearing of those final Deformities on the ultimate prognosis. Acta Radiol. 5 (1926) 1.

168. Müller, F.: Über hereditäre multipele kartilaginäre Exostosen und Enchondrome. Zieglers Beitr. 57 (1914) 232.

169. Müller, W.: Die erbliche multipele Störung der Epiphysenverknöcherung als typisches Krankheitsbild. Fortschr. Röntgenstr. 59 (1939) 65.

170. Müller, W.: Die Perthessche Krankheit als Erscheinungsform der Ermüdungs- und Abnutzungsreaktionen des Skelettes und ihre Abgrenzung gegenüber den verschiedenen Epiphysenstörungen. Fortschr. Röntgenstr. 63 (1941) 247.

171. Muntean, E.: Die Rö.-diagn. der Schädelbasis. In: Olsson, O., F. Strnad, H. Vieten, A. Zuppinger (Hrsg.): Handbuch der med. Radiologie. Springer Verlag, Bd. VII/1 (1963) 430–500.

172. Nägeli, Th.: Einführung in die chirurgische Röntgendiagnostik. Band IV "Bonner Röntgenbücher". Hrsg. A. Grebe und H. Martius. Friedrich Cohen Verlag, Bonn 1923.

173. Nau, P.: Les scolioses congénitales. Paris, Thèse No 446 (1904).

174. Nonne: Über radiographisch nachweisbare akute und chron. Knochenatrophie (Sudeck) bei Nervenkrankheiten. Fortschr. Röntgenstr. 5 (1901/1902) 293.

175. Osgood, R.B.: Lesions of the tibial tubercle occurring during adolescense. Boston med. surg. J. 148 (1903) 114–117.

176. Paget, J.: On a form of chronic inflammation of bones (Osteitis deformans). Med. chir. Trans. Lond. 60 (1877) 37.

177. Pels-Leusden: KLinische, pathologisch-anatomische und radiologische Studien über Exostosis cartilaginea multiplex. Dtsch. Z. Chir. 86 (1907) 434.

178. Peltier, L.F.: The impact of Röntgen's discovery upon the treatment of fractures. Surgery 33 (1953) 579–586.

179. Perthes, G.C.: Über Arthritis deformans juvenilis. Dtsch. Z. Chir. 107 (1910) 111–159.

180. Perthes, G.C., G. Welsch: Über Entwicklung und Endausgänge der Osteochondritis deformans des Hüftgelenkes (Calvé-Legg-Perthes) sowie über das Verhältnis der Krankheit zur Arthritis deformans. Bruns Beitr. 127 (1922) 477.

181. Pfahler, G.E.: The roentgen diagnosis of metastatic malignant disease of bone with special reference to the spinal column. Am. J. Roentgenol., 4 (1917) 114–122.

182. Pfaundler, M.V.: Demonstrationen über einen Typus kindlicher dysostose. Jb. Kinderheilkd. 92 (1920) 420–421.

183. Pfitzner, W.: Beiträge zur Kenntnis des menschlichen Extremitätenskelettes. In: Morphol. Arbeiten von Schwalbe. Bd. 1, 1891–1892. Bd. 4, 1895.

184. Pochhammer, K.: Über die Entstehung periostaler Kallusbildungen und künstliche Kalluserzeugung an Tieren und Menschen. Langenb. Arch. 94 (1911) 352.

185. Pommer, G.: Bemerkungen zu den Lehren vom Knochenschwunde. Arch. mikr. Anat. 102 (1924) 324.

186. Pommer, G.: Über Osteoporose, ihren Ursprung und ihre differentialdiagnostische Bedeutung. Langenb. Dtsch. Arch. Klin. Chir. 136 (1925) 1–35.

187. Pommer, G.: Zur Kenntnis der mikroskopischen Befunde bei Pseudarthrose. Wien. klin. Wschr. (1917) 328.

188. Pöschl, M.: Juvenile Osteo-Chondro-Nekrosen. In: Diethelm, L., O. Olsson, F. Strnad, H. Vieten, A. Zuppinger (Hrsg.): Handbuch der med. Radiologie. Springer Verlag, Bd. 5/4 (1971)

189. Poland, J.: Skiagraphic atlas showing the development of the bones of the wrist and hand. Smith, Elder and Co., London 1898.

190. Preiser, G.: Statische Gelenkerkrankungen. F. Enke Verlag, Stuttgart 1911.

191. Preiser, G.: Zur Frage der typischen traumatischen Ernährungsstörungen der kurzen Hand- und Fußwurzelknochen. Fortschr. Röntgenstr. 17 (1911) 360–362.

192. Psenner, L.: Die Röntgendiagnostik des Schläfenbeins. In: Olsson, O., F. Strnad, H. Vieten, A. Zuppinger (Hrsg.): Handbuch der med. Radiologie. Springer Verlag Bd. VII/2 (1963) 365–672.

193. Psenner, L.: Die Röntgendiagnostik der Nase, der Nasennebenhöhlen und des Epipharynx. In: Olsson, O., F. Strnad, H. Vieten, A. Zuppinger (Hrsg.): Handbuch der med. Radiologie. Springer Verlag, Bd. VII/2 (1963) 130–364.

194. Putti, V.: Die angeborenen Deformitäten der Wirbelsäule. Fortschr. Röntgenstr. 14 (1909) 285–313 und 15 (1910) 65–92, 243–292.

195. Ranke, H. von: Die Ossifikation der Hand unter Röntgenbeleuchtung. Münch. med. Wschr. 43 (1898) 1365–1369.

196. Recklinghausen, F. von: Die fibröse oder deformierende Ostitis, die Osteomalacie und die osteoplastische Carcinose in ihren gegenseitigen Beziehungen. Festschr. Rudolf Virchow, Reimer-Berlin 1891.

197. Redlich, E.: Ein Fall von Gigantismus infantilis. Wien. klin. Rdsch. 26 (1906).

198. Reich, A.: Über Echinokokken der langen Röhrenknochen. Bruns Beitr. Klin. Chir. 59 (1908) 1–39.

199. Reinhardt, K.: Krankhafte Haltungsänderungen, Skoliosen und Kyphosen. In: Diethelm, L., F. Heuck, O. Olsson, K. Ranniger, F.Strnad, H. Vieten, A. Zuppinger (Hrsg.): Handbuch der med. Radiologie. Bd VI/3 Röntgendiagnostik der Wirbelsäule. Springer Verlag 1976.

200. Rentsch: Der Verlauf der Frakturheilung im Röntgenbild. Arch. orthop. Chir. 36 (1936) 557.

201. Reynolds, L.: The history of the use of the roentgen ray in warfare. Carman-Caldwell Lecture, 1945. Am. J. Roentgenol. 54 (1945) 649–672.

202. Ribbing, S.: Studien über hereditäre multipele Epiphysenstörungen. Acta Radiol. Suppl. 34, Stockholm 1937.

203. Ricklin, P., A. Rüttiman, M.S. Del Buono: Die Meniskuslaesion. G. Thieme Verlag, Stuttgart 1964.

204. Riedel, G.: Zur pathologischen Anatomie und Ätiologie der Osteochondritis deformans coxae juvenilis. Virchows Arch. 244 (1923) 335.

205. Rieder, W.: Zur Ätiologie der Schlatter'schen Krankheit. Langenb. Arch. 120 (1922) 588.

206. Rieder, H., J. Rosenthal: Lehrbuch der Röntgenkunde. J.A. Barth, Leipzig 1913.

207. Rössle, R.: Wachstum und Altern. Zur Physiologie und Pathologie der postfötalen Entwicklung. J.F. Bergmann, München 1923.

208. Roux, W.: Anpassung, Histomechanik, Histochemie. Virchows Arch. 209 (1912) 168.

209. Rumpel: Über Geschwülste und entzündliche Erkrankungen der Knochen. Fortschr. Röntgenstr. (1908) Erg. Bd. 16.

210. Scheuermann, H.W.: Kyphosis dorsalis juvenilis. Z. Orthop. Chir. 41 (1921) 305–317.

211. Scheuermann, H.W.: Kyphosis dorsalis. Acta Chir. 54 (1922) 29.

212. Schinz, H.R., E. Uehlinger: Zur Diagnose, Differentialdiagnose, Prognose und Therapie der primären Geschwülste und Zysten des Knochensystems. In: Ergebnisse der medizinischen Strahlenforschung. G. Thieme Verlag, Bd. V (1931) 387–506.

213. Schinz, H.R.: Ergebnisse der physiologischen Genetik und ihre Bedeutung für die menschliche Erbforschung. Arch. Julius-Klaus-Stiftung für Vererbungslehre 16 (1941) 645.

214. Schinz, H.R., W. Baensch, F. Friedl: Lehrbuch der Röntgendiagnostik – mit besonderer Berücksichtigung der Chirurgie. G. Thieme Verlag, Leipzig 1928.

215. Schmid, F., H. Moll: Atlas der normalen und pathologischen Handskelettentwicklung. Springer Verlag, Berlin 1960.

216. Schlatter, C.: Verletzungen des schnabelförmigen Fortsatzes der oberen Tibia-epiphyse. Beitr. klin. Chir. 38 (1903) 874–887.

217. Schlatter, C.: Unvollständige Abrißfrakturen der Tuberositas tibiae oder Wachstumsanomalien. Bruns Beitr. 59 (1908) 518.

218. Schlotheim, A.: Über Kallusbildung aufgrund systematischer Röntgenaufnahmen bei heilenden Knochenbrüchen. Dtsch. Z. Chir. 144 (1918) 289.

219. Schmorl, G.: Die pathologische Anatomie der rachitischen Knochenerkrankung mit besonderer Berücksichtigung ihrer Histologie und Pathogenese. Erg. Inn. Med. 4 (1909) 403.

220. Schmorl, G.: Über Ostitis deformans Paget. Virchows Arch. 283 (1932) 694.

221. Schmorl, G., H. Junghanns: Die gesunde und die kranke Wirbelsäule im Röntgenbild und Klinik. 5 Auflage. G. Thieme Verlag, Stuttgart 1968.

222. Schüller, A.: Die Schädelbasis im Röntgenbilde. Verlag Gräfe und Sillem, Hamburg 1905.

223. Schüller, A.: Über zirkumskripte Osteoporose des Schädels. Med. Klin. I (1929) 615.

224. Schürch, O., E. Uehlinger: Sarkomatöse Entartung bei Ostitis deformans Paget. Schweiz. med. Wschr. 68 (1938) 631.

225. Schumacher P.H.: Röntgenuntersuchung des Neugeborenen. Kapitel IX, Die Röntgendiagnostik in der Geburtshilfe. In: Ergebnisse der medizinischen Strahlenforschug. G. Thieme Verlag, Bd. VI (1933) 305–310.

226. Siegert, F.: Der chondrodystrophische Zwergwuchs (Mikromelie). Erg. inn. Med. 8 (1912) 64.

227. Simon, S.: Zur Diagnose der frühkindlichen Extremitätentuberkulose im Röntgenbild. Fortschr. Röntgenstr. 40 (1929) 448.

228. Sonesson, A.: Die Röntgendiagnostik der Kiefer und Zähne. In: Olsson, O., F. Strnad, H. Vieten, A. Zuppinger (Hrsg.): Handbuch der med. Radiologie. Springer Verlag, Bd. VII/2 (1963) 886–988.

229. Speiser, F.: Ein Fall von systematisierter Enchondromatose des Skeletts. Virchows Arch. 258 (1925) 126.

230. Spranger, J.W., L.O. Langer, H.R. Wiedemann: Bone Dysplasias. G. Fischer Verlag, Stuttgart 1974.

231. Steurer, O.: Die Röntgendianostik des Ohres. In: Ergebnisse der medizinischen Strahlenforschung. G. Thieme Verlag, Bd. III (1928) 45–88.

232. Steurer, O.: Die Röntgendiagnostik der Nase und der Nasenebenhöhlen. In: Ergebnisse der medizinischen Strahlenforschung. G. Thieme Verlag, Bd. III (1928) 1–44.

233. Steven, G.D.: "Standard bone". A description of radiographic technique. Ann. rheum. Dis. 6 (1947) 184–185.

234. Stieda, A.: Verkalkte Parasiten (cysticerous cellulose) im Röntgenbilde. Bruns Beitr. Klin. Chir. 42 (1904) 245–250.

235. Stieda, A.: Über umschriebene Knochenverdichtungen im Bereich der Substantia spongiosa im Röntgenbilde. Bruns Beitr. Klin. Chir. 45 (1905) 700–703.

236. Stieda, A.: Über eine typische Verletzung am unteren Femurende. Langenb. Arch. Klin. Chir. 85 (1908) 815–826.

237. Stolper, P.: Über die Beziehungen zwischen Syphilis und Trauma, insbesondere in gerichtlich und versicherungsrechtlich medizinischer Hinsicht. Dtsch. Z. Chir. 65 (1902) 117.

238. Ströer, F.H.: Familiäres Auftreten von Hand- und Fußabweichungen in fünf Generationen. Genetica 17 (1935) 299.

239. Sudeck, P.: Zur Altersatrophie und Inaktivitätsatrophie der Knochen. Fortschr. Röntgenstr. 3 (1899/1900) 201.

240. Sudeck, P.: Über die akute (reflektorische) Knochenatrophie und Entzündungen und Verletzungen an

den Extremitäten und ihre klinischen Erscheidungen. Fortschr. Röntgenstr. 5 (1901/1902) 277.

241. Sudeck, P.: Die Akute entzündliche Knochenatrophie. Langenb. Arch. Klin. Chir. 62 (1900) 147.

242. Thiemann, H.: Juvenile Epiphysenstörungen. Fortschr. Röntgenstr. 14 (1909/1910) 79.

243. Titow, L.: Über Knochenechinokokkus. Langenb. Arch. 94 (1910) 186.

244. Töndury, G.: Embryonale und postnatale Entwicklung der Wirbelsäule. In: Diethelm, L., O. Olsson, F. Strnad, H. Vieten, A. Zuppinger (Hrsg.): Handbuch der med. Radiologie. Springer Verlag, Bd. VI/1 (1974) 15–64.

245. Uehlinger, E.: Über Knochen-Lymphogranulomatose. Virchows Arch. 288 (1933) 36.

246. Uehlinger, E.: Die Hämatogene Tuberkulose der extrapulmonalen Organe. Schweiz. med. Wschr. (1933) 1150.

247. Uehlinger, E.: Osteofibrosis deformans juvenilis. (Polyostische fibröse Dysplasie Jaffé-Lichtensten). Virchows Arch. Path. Anat. 306 (1940) 255–299. Fortschr. Röntgenstr. 64 (1941) 41–46.

248. Uehlinger, E.: Hyperostosis generalisata mit Pachydermie. (Idiopathische familiäre, generalisierte Osteophytose Friedreich-Erb-Arnold). Virchow Arch. Path. Anat. 308 (1941) 396.

249. Uehlinger, E.: Die pathologische Anatomie der Knochengeschwülste. Helv. chir. Acta 26 (1959) 597–620.

250. Uehlinger, E., M. Künsch: Über Zwillingstuberkulose. Untersuchungen an 46 Paaren. Beitr. Klin. Tbk. 92 (1938) 275.

251. Voorhoeve, N.: L'image radiologique non encore décrite d'une anomalia du squelette: ses rapports sont la Dyschondroplasie et l'Osteopathie condensans disseminata. Acta radiol. 3 (1924) 407–416.

252. Wackenheim, A.: Fehlbildungen am Schädel-Halsübergang. In: Diethelm, L., F. Heuck, O. Olsson, K. Ranniger, F. Strnad, H. Vieten, A. Zuppinger (Hrsg.): Handbuch der med. Radiologie. Springer Verlag, Bd. VI/1 (1974) 391–436.

253. Weiss, K.: Über den Halbseitentyphus des multiplen Chondroms. Fortschr. Röntgenstr. 31 (1923/1924) 615.

254. Weiss, K.: Degenerative Gelekerkrankungen. In: Diethelm, L., O, Olsson, F. Strnad, H. Vieten, A. Zuppinger (Hrsg.): Handbuch der med. Radiologie. Springer Verlag, Bd. V/3 (1968) 543–602.

255. Weyers, H.: Erbliche Gelenkleiden. In: Diethelm, L., O. Olsson, F. Strnad, H. Vieten. A. Zuppinger (Hrsg.): Handbuch der med. Radiologie. Springer Verlag, Bd. V/3 (1968) 407–511.

256. Wilbert, M.I.: A comparative study of fractures of the extremities. Trans. Am. Roentgen Ray Soc. (1904) 195–204.

257. Wilms, M., C. Sick: Die Entwicklung der Knochen der Extremitäten von der Geburt bis zum vollendeten Wachstum. Fortschr. Röntgenstr. 9 Erg. Bd. (1902).

258. Wimberger, H.: Röntgenometrische Wachstumsstudien am gesunden und kranken Säugling. Z. Kinderheilkd. 35 (1923) 182.

259. Wimberger, H.: Die Spätdiagnose des Säuglingsskorbuts. Fortschr. Röntgenstr. 32 (1924) 17.

260. Wimberger, H.: Klinisch-radiologische Diagnostik von Rachitis, Skorbut und Lues congenita im Kindesalter. Erg. Inn. Med. u. Kinderheilkd. 28 (1925) 264.

261. Wolff, J.: Die Lehre von der funktionellen Knochengestalt. Virchows Arch. Path. Anat. n. Physiol. 155 (1899) 256–315.

262. Wolff, J.: Das Gesetz der Transformation der Knochen. Hirschwald, Berlin 1892.

263. Wollenberg, G.A.: Apparat zur Einblasung chemisch reinen Sauerstoffes in die Körpergewebe und in die Körperhöhlen. Med. Klin. 2 (1906) 20.

264. Wollenberg, G.A.: Die normale Anatomie des Kniegelenks im Röntgenbild nach Aufblasung der Gelenkkapsel. Ztschr. orthop. Chir. 19 (1908) 245.

265. Zuppinger, H.: Die Dislokation der Knochenbrüche. Bruns Beitr. 49 (1906).

266. Zuppinger, H.: Über die mechanischen Vorgänge beim Brechen der Diaphysen der Röhrenknochen. Bruns Beitr. 52 (1907) 301.

Thorax

H.S. Stender, J. Oestmann

The 'new rays' were used for chest examinations immediately after their discovery by W.C. Roentgen. Only limited information could be extracted from these first images on photographic plates or fluorescence screens. The poor performance of the initial equipment with inductors, contact breakers, ionic tubes and photographic plates of low sensitivity led to long exposure times of up to 60 minutes for a chest radiograph. The resulting images showed severe blurring due to movement, low contrast and little detail. The images on the fluorescent screen gave some insight into organ motion and large structures of the chest; subtle changes of low contrast, however, could not be detected on these grainy screens. In addition, the short distance between the photographic plate and focus led to considerable magnification and distortion.

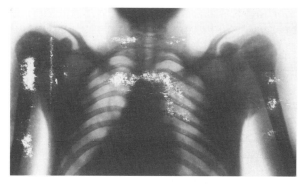

Fig. II, 20. Roentgen photograph of the torso of a living 16-year-old individual, taken in 1896 with a tube manufactured by Reiniger, Gebbert and Schall and operated with an induction coil with a 15 cm spark gap. Exposure time: 12 minutes (Siemens Archiv Erlangen, the original was damaged by water). – Side-reversed picture

The early years

The first blurred radiographs (Fig. II, 20) primarily showed the configuration and position of the diaphragm, large opacities due to pleural effusions or adhesions, extensive pulmonary infiltrations, transparencies due to pneumothorax, changes in size and configuration of the heart, dilatations of the aorta and widening of the mediastinum (Grunmach, 1896; Levy, 1896; Thomson, 1896; Rosenfeld, 1897; Rumpf, 1897). The thoracic skeleton close to the photographic plate was also recognized in these images (Williams, 1897). Oudin and Barthélemy (1896), Bouchard (1896), Marragliano (1897) and Béclère (1899) all published early descriptions of tuberculous changes in the lung with and without pleural effusion. Bergonié (1896) reported on the radiological characteristics of pulmonary echinococcus

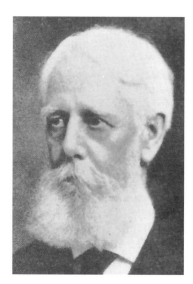

Fig. II, 21. Francis Henry Williams (1852–1936). American pioneer in radiology. After radiographic studies at MIT in Boston, became the director of the Department of Radiology at Boston City Hospital in 1913. Fundamental investigations of fluoroscopy of the heart and lungs. Important textbook Roentgen Rays in Medicine and Surgery, published in 1901. Also involved in technical developments, such as fluorometer.

and enlarged hilar lymph nodes. Williams (1897) (Fig. II, 21) was the first to point to the decreased motility of the diaphragm on the side of an apical tuberculous process. Grunmach (1898) outlined the findings in pulmonary tumours. Bouchard (1897) and Wassermann (1897) diagnosed cavernous lesions in the infiltrated lung. Levy-Dorn (1896) discovered that the low diaphragmatic position in bronchial asthma was due to hyperinflation of the lung. Levy (1896) and MacIntyre (1898) assigned segments of the cardiac contour to the separate heart chambers.

Fluoroscopy of the chest

Fluoroscopy allowed the radiologist to observe thoroughly particular segments of the lungs, heart and mediastinum by looking at oblique or craniocaudally angled projections (Benedikt, 1897; Holzknecht, 1901), supplemented by spot films of specific regions (Albers-Schoenberg, 1903). The quality of the fluoroscopic images was soon improved through lead encasement of the tube (Easton, 1896), lead box collimators (Albers-Schoenberg, 1903) (Fig. II, 22) or the use of a lead shield between tube and patient, for containing the primary radiation and decreasing the scattered radiation (Levy, 1898; Holzknecht and Kienboeck, 1901; Rieder, 1902; Dessauer, 1903; Rollins, 1904).

Levy (1896), Gocht (1898) and Albers-Schoenberg (1903) emphasized the importance of centering, i.e. the proper alignment of the focal point of the anticathode (focus) with the centre of the collimator and the object to be examined along a straight line, to achieve a true representation of the object for fluoroscopy and film exposure.

Despite the steadily improving quality of fluoroscopic and radiographic images, Dumstrey and Metzner (1898) as well as Schjerning and Kranzfelder (1896) questioned the diagnostic value of fluoroscopy in comparison with percussion and auscultation. They pointed out that the examination with X-rays only confirmed the diagnosis already established by physical examination. They considered it inconceivable that X-rays could find very subtle pathological changes that evaded detection by auscultation and percussion and were of the opinion that an uncertain diagnosis of early tuberculosis could not be substantiated by fluoroscopy or radiographic films. The improvements through technical advancements and increasing interpretative experience soon refuted this critical and skeptical view.

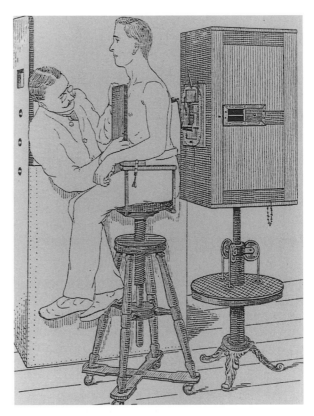

Fig. II, 22. Thorax fluoroscopy with lead-box collimator (Albers-Schoenberg 1909).

Béclère (1901), Holzknecht (1901), Rieder (1902), Williams (1901) and many others could show that the fluoroscopic results were more reliable than those of percussion and auscultation.

Improvements of the exposure technique

Long exposure times were soon identified as the main reason for poor image quality. Efficient ionic tubes, more sensitive plates and, eventually, intensifying screens were developed to obtain chest radiographs with less unsharpness and more detail. In his analysis of 8000 different chemical compounds, Edison (1896) found calcium tungstate ($CaWO_4$) to be especially suitable as a fluorescent agent. The first intensifying screens with $CaWO_4$ were manufactured by Pupin and Kahlbaum in 1897. A considerable decrease in exposure dose and time was achieved with these screens.

Levy (1897) primarily investigated the technical aspects. By analyzing radiographic images of the thorax as to their diagnostic information, he investigated the effect of the high-voltage generator, the required spark gap (30-60 cm), the performance of the tubes (in particular, the influence of the degree of evacuation), the efficiency of intensifying screens, and the sensitivity of the photographic plates coated on one side or on both sides with light sensitive emulsion. The use of a glass plate with a double-sided emulsion or a celluloid film placed between two intensifying screens reduced the exposure time to a tenth or even a fifteenth of the usual time, thus achieving exposure times of less than a minute.

The use of intensifying screens was initially limited by the high granularity and the often nonuniform density of the photographic image obtained with film-screen combinations, potentially masking diagnostic relevant structures (Levy-Dorn, 1897). Good thoracic images visualizing finer structures could be realized with improved tubes and highly sensitive photographic plates ('Schleussner plates'). With this technique, the exposure time could be reduced to about 45 s.

After 1897, Cowl as well as Stechow and Guilleminot tried to take photographs of the chest using respiratory gating of the exposure through mechanically control of the aperture. The exposure time was between 10 and 15 minutes. However, the diagnostic improvement of this technique, the 'rheotomy method', proved to be negligible.

In 1899, Rieder and Rosenthal in Munich reported instantaneous photographs of the chest with suspended breathing with an exposure time of only fractions of a second. The technical parameters were: an inductor with a 60 cm spark gap, an electrostatic contact breaker, a single-emulsion Schleussner plate and two intensifying screens. The resulting chest images showed relatively sharp contours of the diaphragm, the heart and of the ribs near the plate. Additional smaller tuberculous lesions, not usually detected by percussion or auscultation, could now be seen in the thoracic image. Rieder and Rosenthal pointed out that the reduced dose of these instantaneous photographs eliminated the dermatitis (caused by skin dosages higher than 4 Sv) that had been previously observed in a few cases. Using highly sensitive 'Lumière-Sigma-Films' with two intensifying screens, the exposure time could be reduced to less than one second and the image detail improved.

Many authors such as Holzknecht (1901) and Gocht (1903) renounced the use of intensifying screens because of disturbing image noise. Albers-Schoenberg (1903) wrote:

'Better images can be achieved by working with extraordinarily short exposure times, that is, to use three to ten seconds of exposure. The patient is well capable of holding his breath during this period. The lungs and the contours of the diaphragm, the bronchi as well as the arteries and veins of the lungs will, as a result, be more conspicuous. An intensifying screen is not necessary in these photographs, which has the advantage that we get nice, clear plates.

Particularly in photographs of tuberculous lungs or calcified processes in the apices, it is important to have a plate that is produced without the intensifying screen since the graininess does not allow an accurate diagnosis of apical lesions, etc. in many cases.'

Chest fluoroscopy as primary examination

Despite increased efficiency of the X-ray apparatus, adequately evacuated X-ray tubes with 'correct beam hardness', increased sensitivity of the photographic plates and films, and the use of intensifying screens, the photographic images of the chest obtained in suspended respiration were only adequate under the best of circumstances, and fluoroscopy with variable lead collimators between X-ray tube and patient was used as the primary examination method for quite some time. Fluoroscopy especially allowed the observation and assessment of the movements of thoracic organs, such as diaphragm, heart and mediastinum, in various respiratory phases, projections and tube positions (Bouchard, 1896; Thomson, 1896; Benedikt, 1897; Williams, 1897; Kienboeck, 1898; Immelmann, 1899; Holzknecht, 1901).

The documentation of radiological findings initially consisted of marking the patient's skin or by copying the screen image onto paper. Fluoroscopy was increasingly used to select the regions of interest for further documentation

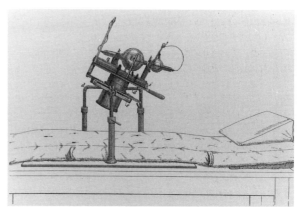

Fig. II, 23. Spot-film device with compression collimator (Albers-Schoenberg, 1903).

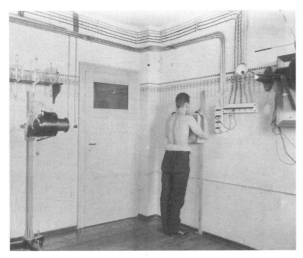

Fig. II, 24. X-ray apparatus manufactured by VEIFA in 1907 (Siemens Archiv, Erlangen).

by spot-films (Bergonié and Carrière, 1897; Béclère, 1899; Williams, 1897; Garrigou, 1897; Holzknecht, 1901). Albers-Schoenberg recommended taking spot-films with a compression collimator (Fig. II, 23). If the close-ups turned out to be satisfactory, complete photographs of the chest were taken only in selected cases (Fig. II, 24).

Because of these technical developments, it became repeatedly evident during clinical use that fluoroscopy was generally more reliable than percussion and auscultation (Walsh, 1897; Béclère, 1899; Immelmann, 1899; Rieder, 1899; Tuffier, 1899; Bade, 1900; Holzknecht, 1901). Films taken with suspended respiration under favourable conditions also showed small abnormalities in the lung as seen in the early phase of pulmonary tuberculosis (Rieder and Rosenthal, 1899; Williams, 1899; Levy-Dorn, 1900; Béclère, 1901; Albers-Schoenberg, 1903).

Initial conclusions (ca. 1900–1910)

Improvements in X-ray generating equipment, photographic plates and fluorescent screens allowed a closer look at the thorax and produced images of physiological and pathological processes. The experiences of physicians who used X-rays around the turn of the century were reflected in the essays and books published in the first decade. Pointing the way ahead, Holzknecht (1901) described in depth the technical aspects of diagnostic radiology, the normal thor-

acic image, the pathological processes of lung and pleura as well as the appearance of the normal and pathological heart, thoracic aorta, mediastinum and diaphragm. Further informative surveys were published by Béclère (1901), Williams (1901), Weinberger (1900), Cabot (1901), Rieder (1902), Gocht in Hamburg (1903), Albers-Schoenberg (1903), Pfahler (1905), Walsham and Orton (1906), Koehler (1906), Otten (1906) and Groedel (1909).

The experiences of the first 5 to 15 years of X-rays in the diagnosis of thoracic diseases illustrated the usefulness, limitations and still unfulfilled expectations of diagnostic radiology, and, at the same time, disclosed the need for improvements.

Anteroposterior or posteroanterior sagittal views of the chest were usually taken, depending on the location of the suspected pathology. In addition, the height and the angle of the tube was altered in the craniocaudal direction to improve the visualization of the various thoracic components. Some chest films were taken with the patient sitting on a special chair intended to minimize patient movement and to facilitate suspended respiration, thus avoiding blurring. On good, short-exposure films, hazelnut- or walnut-sized consolidations and translucencies due to pneumothorax, cavities or emphysema could be seen.

The slow rotation of the erect patient in front of a flat, inflexible screen produced an almost three-dimensional image of the lungs, heart and diaphragm. Changes in the shape and size of thoracic organs were interpreted anatomically, and movements of the diaphragm, heart, chest wall and mediastinum were analyzed. Fluoroscopy often failed to visualize small nodular, linear and low-contrast densities. By using lead collimators with an opening of 2–5 cm placed between the X-ray tube and the patient, the fluoroscopic image could be improved and the patient's radiation burden due to scattered radiation markedly reduced.

A thorough fluoroscopy ("radioscopy"), lasting 5–45 minutes, was typically the first step of a regular roentgen examination of the chest. Depending on the result, the diagnostic questions and the necessity of documentation, radiographs were subsequently taken as spot film or survey film.

To extract the entire information contained in a radiographic image, Albers-Schoenberg (1903) recommended that the negative is studied in front of an otherwise covered window. Holzknecht (1901) used a special viewing device,

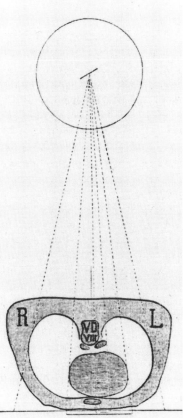
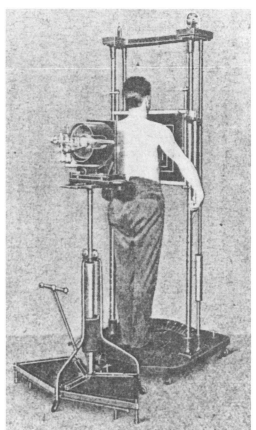
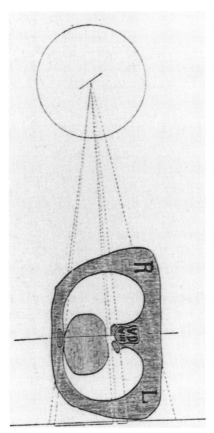
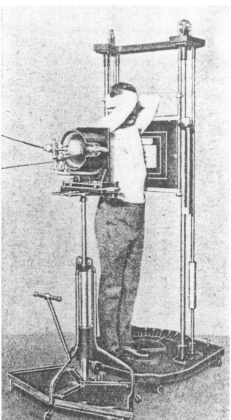

Fig. II, 25a,b. Chest radiographs in dorsoventral and lateral dextrosinistral projection (Groedel, 1921).

the "negative stand", which consisted of a view box that illuminated the plate with a diffuse, unfocused light of adjustable intensity. This was felt to be the only way to avoid interfering visual effects, such as glare, disturbing shadows or suboptimal illumination.

Anatomy of the chest in various projections

The radiographic anatomy of the chest was investigated and documented in several projections. In the sagittal path (anteroposterior or posteroanterior view) (Fig. II, 25), the lungs, which absorb few rays, could be recognized as two bright fields (lung fields). The darker shadow in the middle of the mediastinal organs, the heart and the spine as well as the basal border of the lungs and the lateral boundary of the chest wall and ribs (Weinberger, 1900; Holzknecht, 1901) were also identified. The midline shadow showed the spine and trachea and, in some cases, the main stem bronchi. The right margin of the midline shadow was found to be formed by the superior vena cava and its branches cranially, and by the right atrium caudally. On the left, the upper bulge was identified as the aortic arch, the intermediate pulmonary branch or the left auricle, the middle bulge as the pulmonary trunk or the left atrium with its appendage, and the lower bulge as the wall of the left ventricle.

In the transverse path (lateral view), the thoracic image was described as an 'irregular rectangle of uneven translucency' (Holzknecht, 1901). The retrosternal and retrocardiac region became more translucent during inspiration, outlining the frontal and dorsal borders of the heart. The ascending aorta was seen to demarcate the retrosternal space dorsally, and the descending aorta to form the dorsal border of the retrocardiac space below the seventh vertebral body, where it projects in front of the thoracic spine.

The outline of the mediastinum and lungs was clearly observed in oblique projections (von Criegern , 1899; Holzknecht, 1901; Rieder, 1902). It also became clear that the height of the pulmonary fields, the size of the lung apex and the way the heart rested on the diaphragm depended not only on the respiratory phase and the position of the diaphragm, but also on the height of the X-ray tube and the direction of the central ray.

In many radiographs, the surroundings of the pulmonary hilus showed only irregular, patchy shadows. Von Criegern described radiating structures in the lungs, which extend caudally and parallel to the heart border, as 'companion shadows

of the heart'. The majority of authors assumed that these structures were pulmonary vessels. Because of the limited quality of the radiograph, these prominent arteries and veins were not clearly delineated, and it was assumed that centrally located pathological changes of corresponding size were undetectable (Holzknecht, 1901). The hilar structures and their peripheral extensions could be better visualized on radiographs obtained with short exposure times during breath holding.

Density changes in lung field

The elasticity of the lungs was reflected by the changing pulmonary translucency and by the diaphragmatic movements with inspiration and expiration. Pulmonary emphysema and interstitial fibrosis (sclerosis) reduce the excursions of the diaphragm and the respiratory changes of the pulmonary translucency. The pulmonary translucency was found to be increased in emphysema and decreased in fibrosis (Béclère, 1901; Holzknecht, 1901; Rieder, 1902). A diffusely increased density in both lungs and indistinctness of the pulmonary structures were described in acute or chronic pulmonary congestion. Similar patterns were found in diffusely disseminated pulmonary foci and in pneumoconioses.

Large consolidations seen in survey views were assigned to specific pulmonary lobes, and were generally ascribed to pneumonia or tumours (Levy-Dorn, 1899; Holzknecht, 1901; von Jaksch and Rotky, 1908).

The detectability of individual pulmonary opacities depends on their minimum size. Opacities have to be sufficiently different to the background of normal pulmonary structures and not too far away from the recording plane. It is for this reason that radiographs are recommended in both anteroposterior and posteroanterior directions if specific questions are to be addressed (Holzknecht, 1901; Rieder, 1902; Albers-Schoenberg, 1903; Pfahler, 1905).

The radiography of small pulmonary opacities and interstitial markings requires adequate hardness of the X-ray beam, reduced scattered radiation by using collimators, a favourable projection, a sensitive photographic plate and a short exposure time during breath holding (Holzknecht, 1901; Albers-Schoenberg, 1903; Gocht, 1903; Pfahler, 1905). In fluoroscopy, the brightness of the fluorescent screen should be kept low for the detection of delicate pulmonary densities (Béclère, 1899; Holzknecht, 1901).

Specific chest diseases

Radiologic examinations gradually allowed better differentiation of the various manifestations of diseases. Bacterial pneumonias show regional, sometimes lobar densities, frequently assuming a typical radiographic pattern (von Jaksch and Rotky, 1908). They exhibit an irregular margin towards the parenchyma, but are sharply outlined along the lobar fissure. The intensity of the density depends on the extent of the pneumonia in the direction of the X-ray path. In the evolving phase as well as in the resolving phase, the affected pulmonary regions could appear to be 'brighter'. Extensive opacification throughout an entire lobe is rare (de la Camp, 1904; Pfahler, 1907). Adjacent parts of other lobes could be involved. Abnormal percussion and auscultation found with pneumonia can always be confirmed by radiographically demonstrated findings. In contrast, centrally located processes often are only recognized on radiographic images (Rieder 1906). During resolution, the pathologic findings persist longer radiographically than clinically. Conversion into chronic pneumonia, fibrosis and bronchiectasis can be monitored by serial radiographic examinations. Pleural effusion as well as diaphragmatic, pericardiac, interlobar and costal pleural thickening show characteristic manifestations, which can be particularly well appreciated with fluoroscopy. Evaluating the course of pneumonic processes by serial examinations can be difficult because of inconstant technical factors of the X-ray tubes. It has been repeatedly stated in the medical literature that the radiographic evaluation should be seen as only one, though important, of many parameter in the diagnostic process.

Opacities caused by gangrenous processes and abscesses do not differ from other parenchymal densities. A 'cavity' as manifestation of a centrally necrotic lesion has to be diagnosed with caution since increased translucency could also represent atypically localized air within a pulmonary opacity (Holzknecht, 1901). Clinical symptoms and corresponding sputum usually lead to the correct diagnosis. Thin-walled lung cysts were described by Pfahler (1907).

Holzknecht (1901) and Rieder (1902) described the peripherally located opacification of pulmonary infarction. These localized densities can be detected by scrutinizing the periphery of the lungs during fluoroscopy.

Lobular pneumonia (bronchopneumonia) with small focal opacities is often poorly recognized. These opacities are ill-defined and low in contrast. Larger confluent opacities form pulmonary densities that are more conspicuous (Béclère, 1901; Holzknecht, 1901).

Diaphragmatic, costal and interlobar pleural effusions and the respiratory fluid movements in the pleural space can be well studied fluoroscopically. If a seropneumothorax is present, the changing air-fluid level can be shown (Bergonié and Carrière, 1897; Williams, 1901). The displacement and distortions of the heart and mediastinum caused by pleural effusion, pleural scars and interlobar effusions were fluoroscopically analysed by Paget (1897), Holzknecht (1901), Walsham (1901) and Gerhardt (1907).

Tumours

Centrally and peripherally located lung tumours were described by Pfahler (1907), Krause (1921), Tuffier and Aubourg (1904) and Otten (1910). The number of observations, however, remain relatively small at first. Radiographic findings of massive densities extending from the hilus, finger-shaped shadows or small opacities are described. Ill-defined densities suggest atelectases.

Peripheral tumours appear as dense shadows that can be separated from the central lung by a 'bright stripe' in oblique projections (Holzknecht, 1901). They show respiratory motion and are to be differentiated from pleural scars and pleural tumours.

Tumour metastases in the lungs form large round lesion that can be seen as pea-sized or hazelnut-sized shadows on radiographs taken during suspended respiration, but can escape radiographic detection if the image quality is inadequate. In 1909, Heinecke described ossifying sarcoma metastases.

The pulmonary echinococcal lesions are described as smooth, round, homogeneous or cavity-like shadows by Levy-Dorn and Zadek in 1899 as well as by Arnsperger in 1909 and Berenroth in 1913.

Mediastinal tumours project as well-demarcated soft tissue structure into the adjacent lung fields and can be shallow, lobulated or massively bulging. They can shift or compress the trachea, and have to be differentiated from retrosternal and intrathoracic goitre (Kienboeck, 1908; Hochsinger, 1910). By means of the fluoroscopically observed location and configuration, mediastinal tumours should be distinguished from vascular pathologies, particularly those of the aorta and the heart (Finny and Watson, 1902).

Displacement of the mediastinum during breathing indicates respiratory disorders, such as unilateral bronchostenosis (Holzknecht, 1901; Jacobsen, 1903), pulmonary fibrosis or emphysema, pleura fibrosis (Béclère, 1901) and paralysis of the diaphragm (Holzknecht, 1901).

Pulmonary tuberculosis

The pulmonary manifestations of tuberculosis were investigated by Béclère (1901), Holzknecht (1901), Immelmann (1899), Williams (1899) and Pfahler (1905). In 1903, Rieder pointed out that diagnostic radiology was still in its early stage, but had already advanced the early diagnosis of phthisis. According to Holzknecht, radiology complements and clarifies the clinical findings, contributes to the discovery of early or chronic processes, and provides information as to location, extent and course of the tuberculous process.

The delineation of the individual foci depends heavily on the previously described technical factors, such as hardness of the X-ray beam, distance of the imaging plane and projection of the central ray. Radiological detection of localized apical foci is rarely successful (Rieder, 1903; Pfahler, 1905; Albers-Schoenberg, 1908; Groedel, 1908). Often only diffuse opacities caused by superimposed multiple small adjacent foci are detected. The inspiratory increase in radiolucency is absent. A unilateral apical lesion is frequently accompanied by reduced diaphragmatic mobility (Williams' sign). In larger tuberculous lesions, low density and indistinct borders indicate active progressive foci, while high density and well-demarcated borders favor chronic changes (Béclère, 1901; Holzknecht, 1901; Rieder, 1903; Cohn, 1910). According to de la Camp (1903) and Rieder (1903), cavities appear as mostly sharply demarcated radiolucency within a pulmonary opacification.

Round opacities in the hilus represent tuberculous enlargements of the peribronchial lymph nodes (Rieder, 1903; Koehler, 1906; Allbutt and Rolleston, 1909). Swelling of the peribronchial tissues primarily develops centrally as manifestation of tuberculous lymphangitis.

Shrinking tuberculous processes lead to irregular opacifications which can be associated with compensatory ipsilateral or contralateral pulmonary emphysema (Béclère, 1901; Holzknecht, 1901; Rieder, 1903; Pfahler 1905).

In general, the course of the pulmonary tuberculosis can be followed radiographically, but the evaluation must consider the technical conditions and projections and requires a critical assessment of the radiographic and fluoroscopic findings. The faithful delineation of delicate changes was not always reproducible in the early years (Albers-Schoenberg, 1903).

Heart and aorta

The position and size of the heart as well as the border-forming components of the heart were investigated thoroughly (Benedikt, 1896; Thomson, 1896; Rosenfeld, 1897; Bouchard, 1898; Guilleminot, 1899; Levy-Dorn, 1899; Weinberger, 1900). Oblique projections of the heart were primarily studied by von Criegern (1899), Holzknecht (1901) and Rieder (1902).

Determining the size and configuration of the heart by percussion and by radiography led to different results (Moritz, 1901) (Fig. II, 26). The palpable pulsation of the cardiac apex does not correspond to the most lateral border of the radiographically visualized cardiac silhouette, but projects approximately 1.5 cm medial to it (Benedikt, 1896; Schwarz, 1911).

The configuration of the cardiac contour depends on the level of the diaphragm and the position of the heart. A change between the upright and supine position is accompanied by a characteristic change in the size, position and shape of the heart (Cowl, 1901; Moritz, 1905) (Fig. II, 27). In the lateral view, the retrocardiac radiolucency corresponds to the space between the dorsal heart border and the anterior border of the vertebral column. The rhythmic contractions of the ventricles and atria as well as extrasystoles can be observed fluoroscopically (Benedikt, 1896; Hoffmann, 1911). At the turn of the century, attempts were made to document these temporal changes of the heart by cinematography (MacIntyre, 1898; Guilleminot, 1899; Levy-Dorn, 1899; Kaestle, Rieder and Rosenthal, 1909).

The exact size of the heart could not be established on survey views of the chest because of the short distance between anticathode and photographic plate or, respectively, fluoroscopic screen and the resultant magnification and distortion. This projectional distortion (see above) can only be avoided by using a beam of parallel X-rays that are perpendicular to the recording device (orthodiagraphy). Levy-Dorn (1900), Moritz (1902), Guilleminot (1899), Holzknecht (1901) and others employed this method for exact measurements. In particular, Moritz built a workable fluoroscopic measuring device to record the

Fig. II, 26. Relationship between percussion and orthodiagraphic heart borders (schematic drawing after Moritz and Groedel).

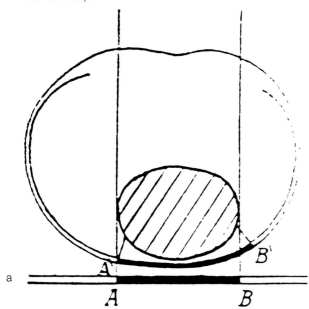

a

Fig. II, 26a. Healthy thorax and heart.

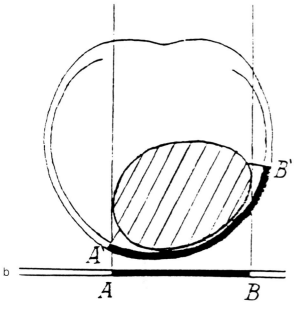

b

Fig. II, 26b. Predominantly cylindric thorax with enlargement of the heart to the left. The cardiac dullness on percussion A B exceeds the transversal projection of the heart A B in a) slightly, in b) considerably.

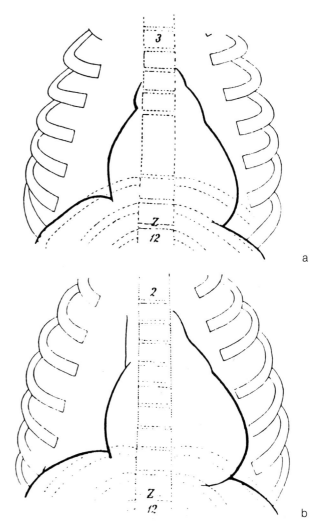

a

b

Fig. II, 27. Vertical **(a)** and horizontal **(b)** body orientation (H. Assmann, 1922).

heart contour with an orthogonal beam (Fig. II, 28). The focus of the roentgen tube, the center of the lead collimator, the central axis of the screen and the recording equipment were positioned in one straight line. Orthodiagraphy (Fig. II, 29) was performed with the patient supine, only rarely upright. The silhouette of the heart had to be charted in relation to thoracic landmarks, such as the median line, rib cage, diaphragm and lung bases. Special attention was given to comparable patient positioning and diaphragmatic level during the measurements. The size of the heart was determined by the following measurements (Fig. II, 30): distance of the right and left cardiac contours to the median line; largest longitudinal diameter; largest transverse diameter; and total surface in square centimetres. According to Albers-Schoenberg (1903), the radiological investigation of the heart with the orthograde beam was 'the greatest progress the roentgen method has achieved'. Teleradiography using an anticathode-plate distance of

Fig. II, 28. Groedel's orthodiagraphic diagram (H. Assmann, 1922).

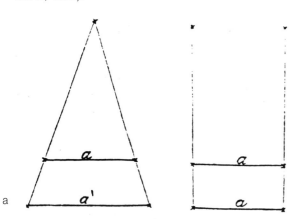

a

Fig. II, 28a. Diverging rays produce a magnified image of the object a and parallel rays an image of the same size.

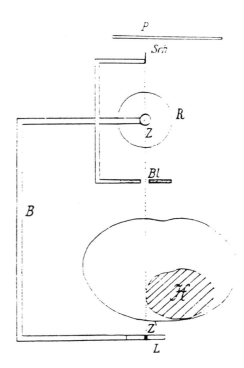

b

Fig. II, 28b. P paper, Sch pen, R tube, Bl collimator, L screen, B movable arc that connects tube, pen, collimator and screen, ZZ central beam, H heart of the patient.

1.5–2 m which can assess the cardiac size with similar reliability was recommended by Koehler in 1908.

Positional changes and dilatation of the thoracic aorta were described by Thomson (1896), Weinberger (1900), Holzknecht (1901), von Criegern (1902), Orton (1905) and Béclère (1910). Sac-like and fusiform dilatations of the aorta are seen with aneurysms. Dilatations over a long segment are observed in arteriosclerosis. Small aneurysms of the ascending aorta can be best seen in the left anterior oblique view. Detecting changes in the descending aorta is more dif-

ficult. Many aneurysms show pulsations. Similar though transmitted movements are also observed in mediastinal tumours (Levy-Dorn, 1897). Rapid aortic movements stand out in aortic valve insufficiency and with hyperthyroidism.

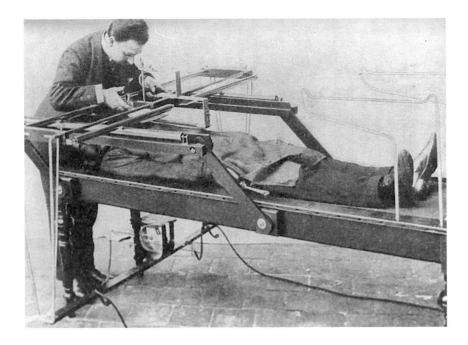

Fig. II, 29. Orthodiagraph according to Moritz, (from Albers-Schoenberg, 1903).

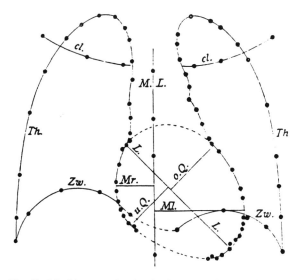

Fig. II, 30. Heart projection in the orthodiagram (from H. Assmann, 1922).
Mr. = maximum distance of the right side from the midline; Ml. = maximum distance of the left side of the heart from the midline; Mr.+Ml. = Tr. = transverse diameter; L = axial projection; O.Q. = upper cross-section distance; u.Q. = lower cross-section distance.

Expansion of radiographic observations (c. 1910–1920)

The efficiency of ionic tubes and spark inductors continued to improve. With increased experience, the regeneration of the X-ray tube could be improved and the appropriate beam hardness achieved for chest radiography and fluoroscopy. The tubes usually had a lead encasement and movable collimators that could limit the field of radiation to the object of interest. The thoracic exposures were preferably taken in inspiration and with suspended breathing. The exposure times were reduced to between 0.1 and 1 s for 'fast'-exposures and under 0.1 s for 'instantaneous' exposures (Rieder and Rosenthal, 1899; Dessauer and Wiesner, 1915; Groedel, 1921). Typical chest radiographs required an exposure time of several seconds. The newer intensifying screens, which operate without an afterglow effect, produce images with less graininess. Wooden cassettes are used to press the intensifying screen against the photographic plate (Gocht, 1903).

As a result of the general technical improvements, even smaller lung changes can now be vizualized on radiographs of the chest.

Fluoroscopy in sagittal and additional oblique projections remains the first step of the radio-graphic examination of the chest (Rieder, 1903; Dessauer and Wiesner, 1915; Groedel, 1921). In addition, a survey view consisting of a radiograph of the entire chest was felt to be state-of-the-art. Spot-films, particularly of the pulmonary apices in early tuberculosis, were specifically recommended by Albers-Schoenberg and Assmann (1914). Stereoscopic views assist in the spatial assignment of the pulmonary changes (Fraenkel and Lorey, 1909; Haenisch, 1912; Hasselwander, 1912; Groedel, 1921).

The normal radiographic image of the lung

The issue of the anatomical substrate of the pulmonary and hilar markings was settled only after very intense discussions. The observed passage of contrast medium in oesophagotracheal fistulas into the bronchi made this decision easier. According to Arnsperger (1909) and de la Camp (1904), the visualized structures are not the bronchi but the pulmonary vessels, as was proven by Albers-Schoenberg (1903), Holzknecht (1901), Rieder (1913) and Assmann (1914). The prominent main blood vessels form the hilus, which can appear rather irregular due to the superimposition of orthograde vessels and central bronchi (Koehler, 1906). Assmann measured the width of the hilar shadow and found a diameter of 13 mm in healthy men between 18 and 45 years of age. This width frequently increases in heart diseases (Groedel, 1912; Dietlen, 1913; Assmann, 1922).

The large central bronchi appear as radiolucency with double contours or as linear stripes along the arteries (de la Camp, 1904; Groedel, 1909; Krause, 1921). Perihilar bronchi seen in orthograde projection are depicted as small circular densities.

Only enlarged lymph nodes are visualized in the radiographic image (Koehler, 1906; Engel, 1913; Groedel, 1921). Calcified lymph nodes in the hilar region often show irregular opacification. Superimposed large vessels can be mistaken for enlarged lymph nodes.

The 'streaky and branched shadow tracings' emanating from the hilus and tapering peripherally (Assmann, 1914) correspond to the pulmonary vessels. The vessels seen in orthograde projection appear as round densities ('blood spots'). In increased pulmonary blood flow, pulmonary blood volume and congestion, the central vascular densities widen in diameter and the peripheral small vessels become visible as 'shadow spots' (Assmann, 1914).

Lymph vessels and interstitial tissues are only discernible after they have undergone pathological changes (lymph congestion, lymphangitis, malignant lymphangiosis) (Assmann, 1914).

Mediastinum and trachea

The mediastinum is evaluated with rotating fluoroscopy and radiographic views in sagittal and oblique projections. Enlarged mediastinal lymph nodes are particularly conspicuous in oblique views, which also delineates the course and width of the aorta to better advantage. The thymus can only be identified radiographically if it is enlarged (Hochsinger, 1910; Kienboeck, 1898, 1912). Displacement and narrowing of the trachea due to retrosternal and intrathoracic thyroid goitre, aortic dilatation, aortic aneurysms, mediastinal tumours, extensive pleural effusion, atelectases and pulmonary fibrosis can be recognized and its cause differentiated (Curschmann, 1905; Pfeiffer, 1906; Engel, 1913; Fraenkel, 1921). In 1921, Spieß and Pfeiffer published a complete overview on the radiographic evaluation of the upper respiratory tract.

Calcification of the trachea is primarily found in elderly patients. Only a few tracheal tumours have been mentioned in the literature (Pfeiffer, 1906; Kamnitz, 1912). The radiographic evaluation of the trachea and central bronchi is helpful in the search of aspirated foreign bodies. Determining the location of an atelectases in the lung can suggest the position of the aspirated material. An occluded main stem bronchus leads to an unilateral atelectasis. This is associated with abnormal respiratory movements of the thoracic organs, particularly of the mediastinum, which, on inspiration, shifts to the diseased hemithorax (Holzknecht, 1899; Jacobsen, 1903).

In 1914, Assmann described the pattern of mediastinal emphysema in a case of bronchiolitis with bright band-like streaks parallel to the cardiac and spinal contour. However, he could not recognize the interstitial pulmonary emphysema in the same patient.

Findings in pulmonary diseases

The X-ray attenuation of the diseased lung depends on the nature of the pathologic process, with increased radiolucency found if the air content is increased (emphysema, pneumothorax, cavity formation) and decreased radiolucency if the air content is decreased or if soft tissue densities are added (infections, tumours).

Diseases of the pulmonary parenchyma

In pneumonia with alveolar exudate, the radiographic density of the alveolar exudate does not only correlate with the extension of the process in the direction of the X-ray beam, but also with the position and angulation of the X-ray tube during fluoroscopy and radiographic exposure. The pneumonic infiltrate exhibits a sharp demarcation where it abuts the fissure. Frequently, the apex of the upper lobe remains uninvolved in upper lobe pneumonia (Rieder, 1913; Assmann, 1914). The resolution of the radiographic densities clearly lags behind the improvement of the clinical findings.

Bronchial pneumonia (Hemophilus influenzae, Diplococcus pneumoniae) shows scattered 'focal shadows' in the lung fields, often associated with an accentuated hilar shadow and perihilar stripe-like densities. This finding is also observed in pulmonary infections in children (Gerhardt, 1907). Necrosis due to gangrene and abscesses (Fig. II, 31) can only be recognized radiographically after a large air-filled cavity is formed (Pfahler, 1907; Dietlen, 1908; Assmann, 1914; Chaoul and Stierlin, 1920). In aspiration and hypostatic pneumonia, basal confluent opacities, frequently located paravertebrally, are found and can be accompanied by atelectases and oedema (Dietlen, 1908). Following the inflammatory processes with subsequent chest radiographs add crucial information and might reveal evolving empyemas, abscesses and hilar lymph node enlar-

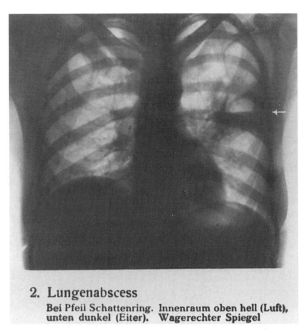

2. Lungenabscess
Bei Pfeil Schattenring. Innenraum oben hell (Luft), unten dunkel (Eiter). Wagerechter Spiegel

Fig. II, 31. Pulmonary abscess (from H. Assmann, 1922).

gements. The pulmonary densities of atelectases are more homogeneous in comparison with infiltration processes or oedema. A reliable differentiation between these processes on the basis of the radiographic manifestation is considered impossible. Parenchymal densities caused by lung infarcts were often obscured by pulmonary congestion (Rieder, 1913; Assmann, 1914).

Syphilitic lungs of the interstitial pneumonic type are described as showing sharply outlined opaque streaks, which emanate from an enlarged hilus and branch out into the lung periphery (Schroeder, 1919). The gummatous, coarsely nodular type shows massive round densities, partially perihilar in location. In case of necrosis, these densities develop a central radiolucency. Smaller nodular densities in the periphery of the lungs or in the vicinity of the hilus represent miliary gummas and are rarely observed (Groedel, 1909; Schroeder, 1919).

Bronchial asthma and lung emphysema

Increased radiolucency of the lungs due to an increased air content and a low position of the diaphragm are found in bronchial asthma. The diaphragmatic mobility is severely reduced. The inspiratory movement of the diaphragm appears to be jerky (Assmann, 1914; Krause, 1921).

The increased pulmonary radiolucency found in emphysema is attributed to increased air content as well as to loss of lung tissue. Additional findings of emphysema are widened intercostal spaces and a flattened diaphragm with restricted respiratory excursions. The heart usually is vertically oriented. Depending on the technique, the pulmonary vessels can appear more prominent on the chest radiograph.

Pulmonary tuberculosis

Improving the examination procedures and exposure techniques and the increasing number of pulmonary tuberculosis studied both pathoanatomically and radiologically in comparative series have definitely established the diagnostic value of the X-ray examination (Rieder, 1909; Cohn, 1910; Assmann, 1914; Krause, 1921; Lorey, 1914).

The diagnosis of early pulmonary tuberculosis relies on changes in the lung apices. The apical densities seen during fluoroscopy and on radiographs are exhaustively discussed in the literature. Improved radiographic image quality in-

creases the detectability of the small focal density of apical tuberculosis. In 1914, Assmann pointed out that the infraclavicular foci are of particular importance for the development of tuberculosis. A 'streaky shadow formation' running towards the hilus is felt to indicate an accompanying lymphatic reaction in the peribronchial tissues (Stuertz, 1907; Rieder, 1913).

Pulmonary tuberculosis can be accompanied by enlargement of the lymph nodes (Koehler, 1906; Engel, 1913; Assmann, 1914) (Fig. II, 32). Caution in assessing the hilar changes is recommended since many other pulmonary and nodal disease processes can involve the hilus. In children, a positive Pirquet's reaction favors the diagnosis of tuberculosis. The triangular shadow resting on the hilus, described by Sluka in 1912, has been attributed to many causes.

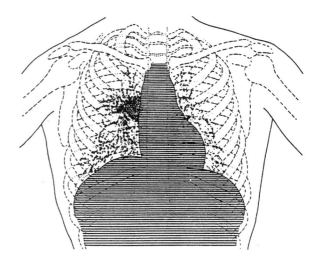

Fig. II, 32. Hilar tuberculosis, primarily on the right. Here, infiltration of the central pulmonary parenchyma. A few enlarged lymph nodes are in the right lower lung field as well as in the left hilus (Rieder, 1913).

Disseminated fine spots are diffusely spread throughout the lung fields in miliary tuberculosis (Fig. II, 33). Due to a summation effect, these focal densities appear as generalized opacification on fluoroscopy, but can be discerned as clusters of tiny spots on good radiographs. According to Lorey (1914), Matthes (1912), Vogl (1912) and Assmann (1914), the size of these spots correspond fairly well to the pathoanatomic lung lesions. Assmann believed that the miliary tubercles close to the image plane form the discrete spots on the radiographic image while those further away form the image plane are subjected to summation and produce the generalized opacification.

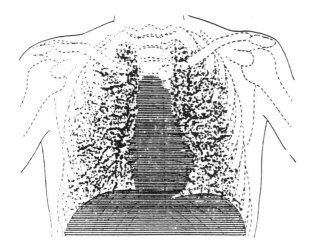

Fig. II, 33. Disseminated bilateral tuberculosis. Innumerable submiliary lesions, irregularly distributed throughout both lungs, producing a patchy image (Rieder 1913).

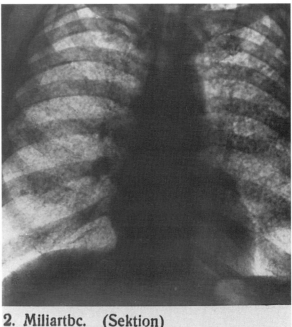

2. Miliartbc.   (Sektion)

Fig. II, 34. Miliary tuberculosis (H. Assmann, 1914).

Incorporating the observations of Béclère (1901), Holzknecht (1901), Marragliano (1897), Williams (1901), Rieder (1903), Hawes (1913), and Assmann (1914), localized pulmonary tuberculosis not detected by percussion and auscultation was radiographically observed with increasing frequency. According to Aschoff, the image of pulmonary tuberculosis is characterized by small densities of acinonodular foci (Fig. II, 34), 'peribronchitic tubercles' and 'bronchopneumonic densities' (Assmann, 1914). These are generally located in the upper lung fields, particularly below the clavicle. The development of phthisis can have a variable course in the various lung fields so that caseation, cavity formation, dissemination and regression can be observed alternately. Often dense streak-like densities representing lymphangitic and peribronchitic changes extend towards the hilus, (Rieder 1913; Krause, 1921).

Fibrotic processes lead to pronounced densities with volume loss, particularly in the upper lung, associated with the tissue cords that extend towards the hilus. The dense and streaky densities of the fibrotic and cirrhotic processes are radiographically more apparent than the densities of acute pulmonary processes. The activity of the tuberculous process cannot be inferred from the intensity of radiographic densities (Hawes, 1913; Rieder, 1913; Assmann, 1914; Krause, 1921). Krause proposed the following classification:
– pneumonic type
– cirrhotic-indurative type
– disseminated-nodular type.

The publications of the period illustrate how the improvement of the radiological chest examination benefited the early diagnosis and the assessment of the course of pulmonary tuberculosis.

Pneumoconioses

Chalicosis (stone-masons' lung) is one of the few diseases with a characteristic radiographic finding (Dietlen, 1921). After exposure to dust over a substantial period of time, the lungs become studded with tiny, irregular, dense spots, ranging 1 to 4 mm in diameter. This grainy infiltration is primarily observed in the middle and lower lung fields. In advanced cases, the small foci coalesce to form larger densities. In less affected parts of the lungs, a reticular pattern can develop (Staub-Oetiker, 1916). For the differential diagnosis, it is important to keep in mind that the minute nodules of dust disease are less clustered than those of miliary tuberculosis, and that their general appearance is more radiopaque (Dietlen, 1921). Diffusely disseminated mottled densities have also been described in bronchiolitis obliterans, septicemia, miliary carcinosis and syphilis.

Chest tumours

The radiographic visualization of lung tumours is of great importance since detection by clinical methods is limited to advanced stages owing to their central position. Through the large number of observed cases accumulated over the years, a wide range of manifestations could be documented. The central bronchial carcinoma, which develops in the main stem bronchi in the vicinity of the hilus, leads to 'frayed' fine or coarse peribronchial and perihilar streak-like densities (Otten, 1906, 1910).

With further growth, large masses form in the hilar region (hilus carcinoma) (Chaoul and Stierlin, 1920). Regionally increased density in the lung adjacent to the hilar carcinoma and the 'contraction signs of the diaphragm and ribs' indicate a bronchial stenosis with atelectasis. Carcinomatous infiltrations, atelectases and obstructive pneumonitis of a lung lobe lead to the dense opacification of the 'lobar carcinoma', which has a preference for the upper lobes.

The lobar lung carcinomas can extend to the hilus or pleura via lymphatic vessels (Chaoul and Stierlin, 1920).

Pulmonary metastases from carcinomas and sarcomas present as single nodule or multiple nodules with a diameter ranging from 0.5 to 10 cm, with renal carcinoma, thyroid carcinoma, chorionepithelioma, bone sarcoma, mammary carcinoma and gastric carcinoma comprising the most often described primary sites (Holzknecht, 1901; Dietlen, 1921; Krause, 1921; Munk, 1914).

Only a few benign pulmonary masses, such as a pulmonary angioma reported by Tuffier and Aubourg (1909), have been described in the early years.

Tumours of the pleura or chest wall can mimick lung tumours. Rotating fluoroscopy is helpful in assigning these tumours (Assmann, 1914; Dietlen, 1921; Krause, 1921). Mediastinal tumours lead to compression and displacement of neighbouring organs.

Fluoroscopy facilitates recognition, classification and assessment of the effects of mediastinal tumours (Kienboeck, 1912; Koehler, 1914). In particular, it can differentiate aortic pathology, such as aortic aneurysm. Mediastinal widening can be caused by tumours of the lymph nodes (lymphogranulomatosis, leukaemia, metastases, tuberculosis), cystic tumours (dermoid cysts, teratomas, bronchial cysts, echinococcosis), substernal and intrathoracic strumata as well as thymic tumours (Krause, 1921; Rieder, 1913; Dietlen, 1921). The observed upward gliding found in strumata during swallowing and coughing assists in the assignment (Fraenkel, 1921).

The importance of diagnostic radiology in evaluating tumours in the thoracic cavity was increasingly acknowledged by physicians outside the field of radiology such as the pathologist Fraenkel (1921).

Diseases of the pleura

The changes of the pleura and the costal, diaphragmatic and interlobar pleural space were elaborately described, particularly their fluoroscopic findings. Diaphragm and chest wall show restricted motion in pleuritis sicca. The distribution of the effusion at the pleural base and along the costal pleural space produces a characteristic radiographic image. In large exudates, the displacement of the heart is not only attributed to pressure but also to changed elastic tension in either lung (Gerhardt, 1907; Brauer, 1914, 1921). Pleural adhesions modify the appearance of pleural fluid. Dependent or encapsulated pleural effusion usually shows a sharp margin. Residual fluid in pleural scars is identified through radiographically guided pleural punctures (Holzknecht, 1901; Brauer, 1921). Radiographic examinations made a great contribution to the recognition and differential diagnoses of interlobar effusion and thickening (Bouchard, 1897; Dietlen, 1913; Brauer, 1914, 1921; Da Costa, 1914).

Interlobar effusion and fibrosis change greatly in appearance with the projection, and the manifold patterns can best be clarified by fluoroscopy performed in different degrees of obliquity.

Pleural effusion in pneumothorax (seropneumothorax) is characterized by horizontal air-fluid interfaces as long as the fluid does not completely fill the pleural cavity. Retraction of the collapsed lungs towards the hilus is restricted by pleural adhesions. An increase in intrapleural pressure (tension pneumothorax) can lead to displacement of the mediastinum, including trachea and heart. More pronounced mediastinal shifts (mediastinal hernias) occur in the two more mobile segments of the mediastinum: retrosternally about the level of the first to third rib, and retrocardially between descending aorta and oesophagus. In cases of severe tension pneumothorax, the transmitted respiratory movements of the collapsed lung become negligible (Holzknecht, 1901; Williams, 1901; Brauer, 1921). Brauer (1910), Haenisch and Lorey

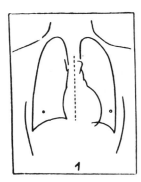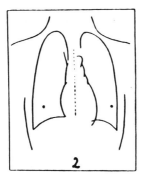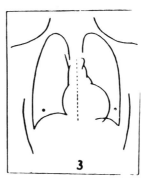

Fig. II, 35. 1) Normal heart. 2) Vertically oriented and median positioned heart in an elongated thorax. 3) Recumbent heart in a transverse thorax (obesity, old age, etc.) (from H.R. Schinz et al, 1928).

(1914) emphasized the crucial role of radiology in general and radiologic stereoscopy in particular, for the indication of thoracic surgery and for postoperative care.

Diaphragm and respiration

The fluoroscopic investigations by Bouchard and Guilleminot (1899), Williams (1897), Cowl (1898), Levy-Dorn (1908), Hasselwander (1912), Hofbauer and Holzknecht (1907) showed the basic spectrum of physiological and pathological findings of the diaphragm. Koehler and Groedel tried to document the respiratory excursions with cinematographic studies. The changes in shape and position of the diaphragm in upright or supine position, lying on the left or right side, during inhalation and exhalation as found in posteroanterior and frontal projections were investigated exhaustively by means of radiography, teleradiography or thoracic orthodiagrams. Diseases of the abdomen were found to influence the position and movement of the diaphragm (Jamin, 1906, 1921; Hofbauer and Holzknecht, 1907; Foerster, 1920). Paralysis of the diaphragm, phrenicotomy (Sauerbruch, 1913), tonus disorders (Eppinger, 1911), congenital elevation of the diaphragm (Glaessner, 1917) and diaphragmatic hernia (Koehler, 1907) show a relatively distinct fluoroscopic and radiographic behaviour.

Heart and large vessels

The knowledge of the shape, position and size of the heart in the radiographic image could be advanced through extensive investigations. Many observations contributed to the increasing experience in recognizing changes in shape and size of the various cardiac components found in specific heart diseases.

Fluoroscopy, orthodiagraphy, teleradiography and survey radiographs of the chest were used in the diagnosis of heart diseases.

According to Groedel (1912, 1921), the heart was a 'long egg-shaped structure' which varied largely in shape and position during breathing (upright, oblique and transverse positions, Fig. II, 35).

Fluoroscopy in the first oblique projection (the left anterior oblique, LAO) primarily provides information about enlargement of the left atrium and distention of the pulmonary outflow tract. The radiolucent retrocardiac space (Holzknecht's space) is encroached by the enlarged atrium. Course and width of the aorta are also easily appreciated in this oblique view. Orthodiagraphic measurements of the heart are applied to determine the cardiac size and any change on comparison studies (Moritz, 1908; Groedel, 1912; Dietlen, 1913; von Romberg, 1915). The extensive investigations provided, within certain limits, a constant ratio between the size of the heart, as determined in the orthodiagram, and the height, weight, age and gender of the individual. Normal values in themselves were reported to be of little value (Groedel, 1912). The physiological variations in the size of the heart generally did not exceed 1.5 cm (Groedel, 1921).

Including width and mass of the lung adds further reference parameters (Groedel and Groedel, 1912). The ratio between the transverse diameter of the heart and the transverse diameter of the lung is found to be highly constant (1:1.9–1.99) (Fig. II, 36).

Gradually, teleroentgenography replaced the time-consuming orthodiagraphy in daily practice. Teleroentgenography, which uses a focal spot and an increased focus-film distance, provides adequate data on the size of the heart (Koehler, 1908; Munk, 1914; Hammer, 1918), but a comparison between both methods has to take into account the position of the patient and the level of respiration (degree of inspiration).

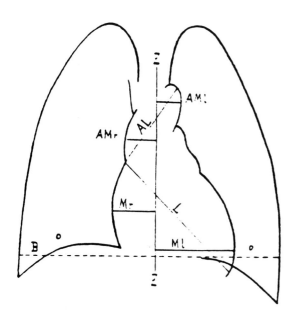

Fig. II, 36. Measurements of the heart, vessels and thorax. Heart measurements: Mr. = distance to the right from the midline; Ml. = distance to the left from the midline line; L = axial length.
Vascular measurements: AMr. = distance to the right from the midline; AMl. = distance to the left from the midline; AL. = length of the aorta; B (dotted line) = thorax width; Z-Z = midline. (from H.R. Schinz et al, 1928)

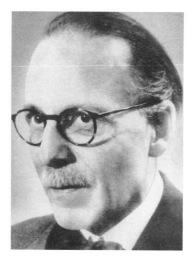

Fig. II, 37. Franz Maximilian Groedel (1881–1951). Since 1910 in charge of the Department of Radiology at the Hospital of the Holy Spirit in Frankfurt am Main and since 1926 associate professor at the University of Frankfurt. At the end of the twenties, founder and director of the William-G.-Kerckhoff-Institute in Bad Nauheim. Forced to emigrate in 1933. Worked on the radiologic diagnosis of lung and heart as well as stomach. Several important books about diagnostic radiology. Popular lecturer at conventions. Respected teacher.

After acute physical stress, a decrease in the size of the heart could be observed (Dietlen, 1908; Kienboeck, 1912). According to de La Camp (1903), an increase in size can be attributed to a diseased heart muscle. Heavy physical stress over a long period of time can lead to a slight increase in heart size (Schieffer, 1906; Dietlen and Moritz, 1908).

Serial radiographs and electrocardiograms revealed additional pendular movements of the entire heart during cardiac contractions (Groedel and Groedel, 1912). Diagnostically significant deviation of the cardiac movements are described in defects of the ventricular septum, heart block and extrasystoles. Abnormal pulsations of the pulmonary artery are in a patent ductus arteriosus (ductus of Botalli) and of the aorta in aortic insufficiency.

The enlargement of individual cardiac sections can be suspected from changes in the shape and contraction of the heart. The fluoroscopy in various oblique projections is very informative. Hypertrophy and early dilatation of the left ventricle have been critically investigated (Schwarz, 1911; Groedel, 1912; Vaquez and Bordet, 1913; Grangérard, 1920; Palmieri, 1920).

According to Groedel (1912) (Fig. II, 37), the acquired valvular diseases of the heart can be divided into two types: 'The vertical, usually spherical mitral type heart and the horizontal aortic heart'. In aortic insufficiency, the enlargement of the left ventricle leads to a left-sided enlargement of the heart. The aorta elongates, primarily its ascending segment, and shows swinging pulsations. In aortic stenosis, the left lower cardiac contour increases its curvature and the ascending aorta becomes moderately dilated. Combined aortic valve defects and cardiac decompensation can produce multifarious radiographic findings.

In mitral stenosis, the heart forms a vertically oriented egg-like configuration. The enlarged left atrium and the dilatated outflow tract of the right ventricle accentuate the left second and third cardiac bulge (Fig. II, 38). Mitral insufficiency leads to a moderate bilateral enlargement of the heart. The left ventricle contour is elongated, the pulmonary contour pronounced, the right heart border more curved and the left atrium moderately extended dorsally. Combined mitral–aortic defects often show an oblique position of the heart and a prominently segmented left heart border. Tricuspidal and pulmonary defects have only been described infrequently at this time. The changes of the various cardiac components in cardiac defects were passionately debated (Ebertz and Stuertz, 1912; Groedel, 1912; Dietlen, 1913; Zehbe, 1916).

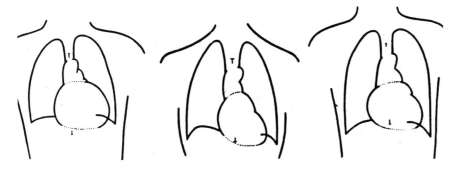

Fig. II, 38. Diagrams of radiographic findings of the heart with mitral valve disease: left, mitral insufficiency; middle, mitral stenosis; right, mitral insufficiency and stenosis (F.M. Groedel, 1921).

The pulmonary vessels become dilated and the lung fields blurred in cardiac decompensation due to cardiac defects and diseases of the myocardium. In fluoroscopy, the lung structure appear indistinct and the hilar structures enlarged (Schwarz, 1911; Groedel, 1912; Assmann, 1914; Vaquez and Bordet, 1913; Chaoul, 1920). After treatment with digitalis, pulmonary congestion can be observed to resolve within a few days (Groedel, 1921).

The number of observed congenital defects was still limited. The patterns found with a patent ductus arteriosus (ductus of Botalli), defects of the ventricular septum, congenital pulmonary stenosis and aortic stenosis as well as with transposition of the large vessels, dextrocardia and situs inversus were described (Burghardt, 1898; Groedel and Groedel, 1912; Miller and Orton, 1913; Weinberger, 1919; Vaquez and Donzelot, 1920). Positional anomalies of the heart due to pulmonary and pleural changes, elevation of the diaphragm and diaphragmatic hernia or thorax deformities could be readily explained radiologically.

According to Lorey, pericardial effusion leads to pouch-like enlargements of the cardiac silhouette, which frequently shows shallow movements of its border. It can be difficult to differentiate an exudative pericarditis from an enlarged heart with relative tricuspid insufficiency (Dietlen, 1921). Pneumopericardium presents a characteristic radiolucent halo around the heart, possibly with air-fluid levels (Brauer, 1921). Localized fibrotic plaques of either pericardial membranes cannot be detected radiologically, but pleuropericardial thickening can be easily recognized. Pericardial calcifications can encase the heart (armoured heart) and change the haemodynamics, primarily causing inflow congestion (Groedel, 1912; Rieder, 1913; Vaquez and Bordet, 1913; Mueller, 1917; Brauer, 1921).

Aorta

The thoracic aorta shows age-related dilatations and calcifications. The aortic dimensions were determined by Groedel (1912), Vaquez and Bordet (1913) and von Teubern (1916). Groedel measured the distance between the aortic arch and the median line in dorsoventral projection, the transverse diameter of the aortic arch and the length of the aortic shadow (Fig. II, 36). The differential diagnosis of the aortic aneurysms, which have a multifarious appearance, was discussed in detail (Thomson, 1896; Holzknecht, 1901; Williams, 1901; Walsham and Orton, 1906; Béclère, 1910). The influence of the aorta on the adjacent organs (trachea, main stem bronchi, lung atelectasis, oesophagus) was described by Krause in 1921.

Further expansion between 1920 and 1950

During the first 25 years, the radiology succeeded in visualizing the gross anatomical and pathological structures of the thoracic organs by means of fluoroscopy and radiographic films. Extensive clinical observations were systematically gathered and the most significant diseases described according to their radiological patterns. Except for extremely favourable circumstances, the technique could not visualize finer structures. In 1922, Assmann emphasized that a satisfactory chest radiograph requires a sharp demarcation of diaphragm, heart, ribs and lung markings.

These requirements could be increasingly met in subsequent years through technical improvements. The contribution of radiology to enrich the clinical diagnosis and to recognize otherwise undetectable pathological changes is increasingly acknowledged (Struempell, 1914; Sauerbruch, 1920; Assmann, 1922; Lichtheim, 1922; Engel, 1924; Brunner, 1926; Sante, 1925; Volhard, 1930; Brauning, 1938).

Technical developments

In the twenties, the introduction of the thermionic tube in conjunction with efficient generators (transformer and rectifier tubes) (Coolidge, 1913, 1917) allowed an independent selection of exposure voltage and milliampere per second (mAs). With this technique, beam hardness, exposure rate and exposure time can be controlled and adapted to the needs. The 'line focus' of the anode of the X-ray tube (Goetze, 1918) reduces the effective focal spot size and improves the geometric sharpness as well as increases the tube capacity. The introduction of the rotating anode (Bouwers, 1928) further increased the heat capacity of the X-ray tubes considerably and allowed shorter exposure times. As a result, the chest radiographs contain more detail and the interpretation of chest film findings improves. Stereoscopic views serve the spatial assignment of intrathoracic changes (Hasselwander, 1914; Durham, 1911; Lewis and Morgan, 1946).

The steady improvement of intensifying screens and the use of radiographic films with an emulsion on both sides (double-emulsion films) contributed decisively to a better image quality.

In the early thirties, the more high performance three-phase generators are being installed. First attempts with phototimers to standardize the optical density were made by Franke in 1929, Pape in 1936 and Morgan in 1940, but the routine application of phototimers was only introduced after 1945.

Applied examination techniques

Fluoroscopy remains at the beginning of the radiographic examination of the chest. To visualize the entire chest, including its subtle structures, for diagnostic evaluation, chest radiographs are taken in deep inspiration and during breath holding, using a focus-film distance of 1.5–2 m, a tube voltage of 60-80 kV and the shortest possible exposure time. Schinz et al. (1928) wrote: *'Indeed, the physical examination of the thoracic organs is only complete if the roentgen method is also included.'*

The newly developed X-ray tomography achieves a better separation of generalized and focal pulmonary densities. This enables the demonstration of caseation, cavities and abscesses, enlargements of hilar and mediastinal lymph nodes, changes of the trachea and main stem bronchi, stenoses and obstructions of the major bronchi, and bronchiectases (Vallebona, 1937; Ziedses des Plantes, 1932; Chaoul, 1935; Greineder, 1935; Grossmann, 1935; Kremer, 1936; Gebauer et al.., 1940, 1959).

For the examination of the heart, especially for better visualization of an enlarged left atrium, a barium swallow outlining the oesophagus and a right anterior oblique (RAO) projection were added (Frik, 1922). With barium in the esophagus, the extent of mediastinal tumours, intrathoracic goitres, impressions caused by right-sided aorta, aortic dilatations, and aortic aneurysms can also be visualized, as well as pseudo-widenening of the mediastinum caused by a dilated oesophagus or mediastinal pleural effusion.

Kymography can assess the movements of the heart, aorta and main pulmonary arteries (Cignolini, 1934; Sabat, 1934). The area kymography (Stumpf, 1937) provides a general overview of the motion of the heart borders as a reflection of volume changes due to cardiac contractions, but also shows rotation, pendular motion and deviation of the cardiac axis. The topography of the border-forming cardiac segments, myo- and pericardial changes and pulsation patterns of the aorta and pulmonary artery can be studied in depth (Delherm and Fischgold, 1936; Carvalho, 1934; Zdansky and Ellinger, 1933; Heckmann, 1935; Stumpf, 1937). Using a vertical slit position and a horizontal grid movement (Stumpf, Weber and Weltz, 1936), the area kymography can also be applied for the analysis of diaphragmatic, costal and mediastinal motion. Electrokymography can record the amplitude of moving segments of the heart border and, through phase analysis, can reconstruct the kinetic activities of the entire heart (Heckmann, 1959; Luisada et al.., 1948; Haubrich, 1955).

Bronchography, which was first performed with oily contrast media, gave new insights into changes of the bronchi (Lynah and Stewart, 1921; Sicard and Forestier, 1922; Lorey, 1927). Since iodized oil led to complications, bronchography could only be used successfully after the introduction of viscous, iodine-containing, water-soluble contrast media (Fischer, 1948; Morales and Heiwinkel, 1948; di Rienzo, 1949; Stutz and Vieten, 1955).

The radiopaque bronchogram can visualize changes that are only infrequently recognized on the chest film, such as inflammatory, stenotic, destructive and ectatic changes of the bronchi, and congenital bronchopulmonary defects. The bronchographic findings provide important information before and after surgery.

Additional diagnostic methods are fistulography, pleural punctures and diagnostic pneumothorax.

The experience from observing lung tuberculosis has revealed that the disease has to be recognized in the clinically silent early stage, that is, at a stage when it can only be discovered radiologically (Redeker, 1927; Brauning and Redeker 1931). The first radiographic survey for early tuberculosis in 'healthy' pupils, recruits, officials and students showed a considerable number of cases of active and quiescent lung tuberculosis (Wiewiorowski, 1931; Kattentidt, 1932). The number of cases that escaped detection in mass screening programs was relatively high (20%) in the experience of Redeker and Walter (1929). The need for greater reliability, better imaging and longer film storage stimulated the introduction of more appropriate, possibly mobile, photographic systems. Two photographic methods were used in mass screening: the roll-film-paper method (Heisig, 1938) and the photofluorographic method (de Abreu, 1938; Holfelder and Berner, 1938; Janker, 1938). Photofluorography prevailed (size 24/24 mm), although a high-quality, normal chest film was needed to confirm the diagnosis in cases with suspected pathologic findings (Griesbach and Wieda, 1938; Holfelder and Berner, 1938). Holfelder 1939 in Germany, Holm et al 1948 in Denmark, Cauley 1950 in the USA, Fischer and Schinz 1948 in Switzerland, and Wegelius and Noschis 1948 in Sweden reported positive experiences with mass chest screening.

Radiographic findings

Pulmonary diseases

The different patterns of pulmonary diseases were repeatedly studied with increasingly refined methods. Acute pulmonary oedema shows confluent patchy densities (Zdansky, 1924, 1933; Barden and Cooper, 1948). In the chronic stage of pulmonary congestion (congestive fibrosis), tiny nodules appear and the vasculature in the upper lung fields become dilated, while the basal are narrowed (Sylla, 1935; Zdansky, 1939).

For the localization and spreading of pneumonic processes and atelectases, the lung segments play an important role (Herrnheiser, 1936; Huizinga and Behr, 1940; Warembourg and Graux, 1947; Esser, 1949; Cocchi, 1951). According to Engel in 1924, the pneumonic processes in children primarily involve paravertebral subsegments. In the frequent absence of clinical findings, only the radiographic image can reveal the pulmonary findings (Engel, 1924). The manifold patterns of pneumonia caused by a vast number of organisms, bacteria, viruses, rickettsiae and mycoplasma, have been described, but patterns characteristic of specific infectious agents could not be found. Only the fleeting pulmonary infiltrates with eosinophilia reported by Loeffler in 1932 might represent a notable exception.

Most pneumomycoses show localized, progressive opacities or disseminated small foci (Schinz and Blangley, 1934; Carter, 1936; Doub, 1940).

The radiological analysis of the tuberculosis has continued. Its early stage, various manifestations and course have been related to their clin-

Fig. II, 39. Chest radiographs – partial views.

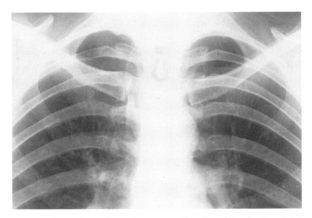

Fig. II, 39a. In 1937, minute patchy densities in the right pulmonary apex caused by apical tuberculosis. Dystelectatic azygos lobe.

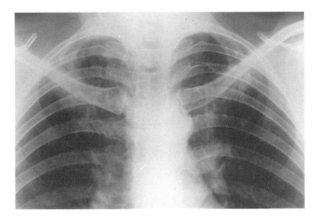

Fig. II, 39b. In 1942, indistinct large density in the right pulmonary apex with peribronchial opacities towards the right hilus. Patchy densities in the left apex and bean-sized opacity in the infraclavicular region. Accentuated linear densities towards the left hilus. Active pulmonary tuberculosis, spreading from apical lesions.

ical and pathological findings. The radiographic findings are found to be decisive for the evaluation (Fig. II, 39). Primary tuberculosis, which is found with increasing frequency in adults (Uehlinger, 1942), shows the bipolar image of a pulmonary focus and hilar adenopathy. Primarily in children, the adenopathy can be accompanied by perihilar epituberculous infiltrations (Eliasberg and Neuland, 1921) and perihilar atelectases (Roessle, 1935). Postprimary or reinfection tuberculosis appears as haematogenic dissemination (Fleischner, 1930; Neumann, 1930; Medlar, 1948), early infiltrate (Assmann, 1922, 1949; Redeker, 1927), subprimary initial foci (Malmros and Hedvall, 1938), pleuritis, bronchial tuberculosis (Engel and Pirquet, 1930; Goergeny-Goettche and Kassay 1947) and progressive pulmonary phthisis (Fig. II, 40). The early infiltrate, usually infraclavicular in location but occasionally found in the apical segment of the lower lobe (Assmann, 1922), is felt to be of particular importance in evolving postprimary tuberculosis. Survey chest radiographs of the general population and of persons who were in contact with tuberculous patients are considered mandatory for detecting postprimary or reinfection tuberculosis at its early stage (Kaiser-Petersen, 1924; Re-

deker, 1927; Brauning, 1938). Differentiating the radiological changes in tuberculosis remains difficult since productive and exudative lesions can be quite similar in appearance (Assmann, 1922; Ulrici, 1926; Neumann, 1930; Wurm, 1932; Policard, 1938; Caffey, 1945; Morgan, 1948). Pulmonary phthisis, which can arise from primary and postprimary manifestations, spreads through the bronchial system, typically in craniocaudal direction.

The spectrum of radiographic findings caused by disseminated pulmonary diseases has increased and expanded considerably. Boeck's sarcoid and its manifestation as hilar type and as perihilar type with fine and coarse nodularity, including its spontaneous regression and fibrotic development, were described by Hantschmann (1939), Longscope (1941), Leitner (1942) and Ricker and Clark (1950). Radiological patterns of silicosis, mixed stone-masons' lungs and silicatotis (asbestosis, talcosis), as well as benign types of pneumoconioses, such as siderosis, berylliosis, aluminosis and chromatosis, can be evaluated and followed (Pancoast and Pendergrass, 1926; Husten, 1931; Lochtkemper, 1932; Policard, Croizier and Martin, 1938; Saupe, 1938; Baader, 1942; Bruce, 1942; Koelsch, 1942; McLaughlin, Rogers and Dunham, 1949). Pulmonary fibrosis with discrete or massive radiographic abnormalities can be seen in scleroderma (Pugh, 1948; Church and Ellis, 1950) or represent an idiopathic or progressive-interstitial fibrosis (Hamman-Rich, 1935, 1944).

Diagnosing a central bronchial carcinoma that does present with a characteristic radiographic finding considerably improves with tomography and bronchography (Lenk, 1929; Chaoul and Greineder, 1936; Churchill, 1948; Stangl, 1949; Fischer, 1950; Lodge, 1950; Stutz, 1949/50). But neither method can differentiate between tumour tissue, atelectasis and obstructive pneumonia. In 1932, Pancoast described the unique pattern of a peripheral bronchogenic carcinoma at the lung apex with chest wall infiltration and rib destruction.

The radiographic findings of benign lung tumours, such as hamartomas, chondromas, leiomyomas, angiomas, bronchial adenomas and pulmonary adenomatosis, become usually known as published case reports.

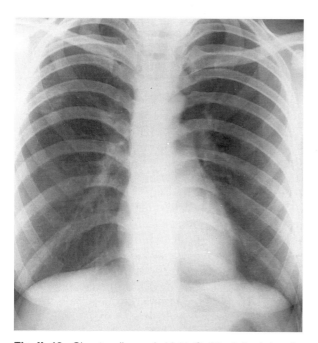

Fig. II, 40. Chest radiograph 1941. Soft indistinct density in the right upper lobe with larger density in the second intercostal space in an acute pulmonary embolus. Indistinct left cardiac border and pulmonary vessels in the left middle and lower fields. Motion unsharpness due to long exposure time.

Heart and large vessels

The radiographic findings of the heart and major thoracic vessels as seen during fluoroscopy and on radiographs obtained in various projections could be further validated by angiocardiography and cinematography. By correlating the phase analysis of the dextrogram and laevogram with the filling process and wall motions, Zdansky could, in 1949, show the inflow and outflow pattern of the ventricles and atria. While the dilatation of the ventricles causes enlargement of the heart, ventricular hypertrophy leads to characteristic changes of the cardiac configuration. The radiographic changes found in acquired cardiac defects also follow this pattern (Dedic, 1928; Dietlen, 1928; Hitzenberger, 1928; Kirch, 1929; Schwedel, 1936; Zdansky, 1939, 1962).

In addition to elementary cardiac parameters, attempts were made to record the heart volume as accurately as possible. The following calculation was formulated by Rohrer and Kahlstorf (1932):

$$V = A \times 1 \text{ max} \times 0.63$$

where A is the heart area in the sagittal-orthodiagram and 1 max the maximal depth of the heart in the frontal view. The constant 0.63 takes into account the parabolic or elliptical shape of the heart. The calculated values of the cardiac volume deviate between 10% and 15%. In 1934, Lysholm, Quarna and Nylin calculated the heart volume from teleradiographic images simultaneously taken in two planes with the patient standing, using Rohrer and Kahlstorf's formula.

Damage of the myocardium caused by myocarditis, infectious diseases, hyperthyroidism, myxoedema and metabolic disorders leads to enlargement of the heart. Athletic activities with considerable sustained cardiac stress can cause moderate cardiac enlargement (Deutsch and Kauf, 1924; Herxheimer, 1932). In the kymogram, the hearts of these athletes showed a reduced motion amplitude in the heart apex, which Reindell (1940) ascribed to an increase in the ventricular residual blood volume of the 'athletic heart'. Cardiac enlargement is also observed in arteriovenous intrapulmonary shunt with increased cardiac flow (Holzmann, 1952).

Angiocardiography provides a comprehensive radiographic conception of congenital cardiac anomalies. The conventional radiographic views of the entire chest are the foundation for evaluating the pulmonary vessels, revealing distended pulmonary vessels due to pulmonary fluid overload or hypovascularity secondary to pulmonary

or tricuspid valve disease. Calcifications seen within the heart can be in the valves, annulus fibrosis, ventricular wall aneurysms, cardiac tumours, coronary arteries and pericardium. Rotating fluoroscopy is valuable in determining the location of these calcifications (Klason, 1921/22; Lenk, 1929; Zdansky, 1931; Haubrich and Thurn, 1950).

After 1950

Technical developments

Technical developments after 1950 resulted in further improvements in chest radiology. The increased generator ratings with outputs of 30, 50 and finally 100 kW, with maximum voltage ratings of 150 kV and maximum currents of 1000 mA, and the high heat capacity of the rotating anode tubes enable exposure times of less than 20 ms. The short exposure times and the increased resolution of the intensifying screens improve the delineation of delicate lung structures. With the use of rare earth screens (1972), the radiation dose can be reduced by 25–50% without any loss of information and the exposure time shortened further. Early in this period, radiographs of the chest are generally obtained with tube voltages of 50-80 kV and without a scatter-reducing grid. In the 50s and 60s, the advantages of the high-voltage technique are increasingly recognized in chest radiography (Franke, 1926; Morgan, 1947; Ardran and Crooks, 1953; Fomin, 1953; W. Frik, 1954; Zanetti, 1955). The tube voltage is increased to 110-150 kV and a scatter-reducing grid or an air-gap technique is used (target-to-film distance 15 cm, Groedel and Wachter, 1926). This technique preserves the contrast between air-containing lungs and soft tissue structures, and small objects are still seen in regions of increased density (e.g. retrocardiac region or parenchymal densities) (Frik, 1961). The relative increase in attenuation of the mediastinum and chest wall declines, and the peripheral pulmonary structures can be followed to the lateral pleural space through the superimposed soft tissues of the chest wall. By retaining the detail contrast and reducing area contrast, chest radiographs obtained with the high-voltage technique appear more equalized and informative (Spiegler, 1957).

The use of image intensifiers (1952) connected to video monitors (1959) makes fluoroscopy considerably easier and improves diagnostic observations (Coltmann, 1948; Janker, 1956;

Stauffer et al., 1955; Noix, 1962). The spatial resolution of the systems and the visibility of details increase continuously. With the right choice of tube voltage and current and, respectively, correct setting of the automatic dose control, the radiation dose is considerably reduced in comparison with photofluorography.

Until the 70s, the radiographic examination of the chest film was usually preceded by fluoroscopy. It is now customary to obtain posteroanterior and lateral views of the chest first and to reserve fluoroscopy only to those cases with unclear radiographic findings. Fluoroscopy is also used to guide the taking of spot films and to study the movements of the thoracic organs (diaphragm, heart, mediastinum). Problem-oriented fluoroscopy often renders additional and more expensive examinations superfluous (Felson, 1960, 1973; Fraser and Paré, 1970, 1977). Chest radiographs obtained inspiration and expiration as well as in the lateral decubitus position provide additional information on lungs, diaphragm, pleura and mediastinum (Mueller and Loefstedt, 1945; Fraser and Paré, 1970, 1977; Felson, 1973).

Diagnostic developments – structural analyses of the lungs

The excellent radiographic delineation of the coarse and fine structures of the lungs enables the assignment of these structures to their respective anatomic-physiological structures or pathological changes. The individual radiographic image is analyzed for density, size, demarcation, extensions, detailed structure, calcium concentration and relationship to neighboring structures, as well as for spreading or regression (Simon, 1956, 1971; Teschendorf, 1939, 1975; Newell, Chamberlain and Rigler, 1954; Perrin and Fauré, 1974). The pulmonary vessels seen on the conventional chest radiograph can be assigned to the arterial or venous system on the basis of their position and course. The veins generally mark the segmental and subsegmental borders (Herrnheiser and Kubat, 1936; Kovats and Zseboek, 1953). Changes in the course of the vessels indicate parenchymal processes that affect the lung volume, which can be increased, as found in emphysema, or decreased, as found in fibrosis.

The classification of the pulmonary segments and subsegments as bronchopulmonary entities was laid down in an international nomenclature (1949). To evaluate the radiographic changes in the lungs, it is important to recognize and allo-

cate the smaller pulmonary entities. By comparing radiological and pathoanatomical observations, the characteristic patterns of intra-alveolar diseases in the lobulus and acinus (alveolar pattern) as well as changes in the intra- and extralobular interstitium (interstitial pattern) are recognized (Gould and Dalrymple, 1959; Felson, 1960; Fraser and Paré, 1970, 1977; Genereux, 1971; Anacker and Stender, 1963; Heitzman, 1973, 1984). Relating the patchy, reticular and linear densities to their anatomical substrate is considered important for a correct diagnosis. Differentiation into alveolar and interstitial patterns provides information relevant for the differential diagnosis (Table II, 1).

Table II, 1. Practical Application of Pattern Analysis to Differential Considerations in Diffuse Lung Disease

Pattern	Anatomical Site	Most Common Causes
Air space		
(1) Acute	Acinar air space	(1) Edema, hemorrhage, exudate
(2) Chronic		(2) Infectious edema, Neoplasia, Inhalation disease, Acute/chronic interstitial pneumonitis
Interstitial Reticular	Alveolar septum	Environmental diseases Sarcoidosis Collagen-vascular diseases Acute/chronic interstitial pneumonitis
Nodular	Alveolar septum	Granulomatous diseases Metastases
Reticulo-nodular	Alveolar septum	As per reticular unless definite nodulation is identified Certain members of COPD spectrum
Linear	Broncho-arterial Perienous Interlobular septum	Interstitial edema Lymphangitic malignancy Certain members of COPD spectrum

Cited from G.P. Genereuse, Radiologic Assessment of Diffuse Lung Disease, Page 9. In: J.M. Taveras, J.T. Ferrudi (Eds.), Radiology, Diagnosis-Imaging-Intervention, Lippincott Comp., Philadelphia, 1986

The intra-alveolar processes, which preferentially spread via the bronchioles and intra-alveolar pores of Kohn, are usually in the lobes, segments and subsegments, and, though less frequently, in the central pulmonary regions ('butterfly'). They consist of small or large, ill-defined densities and are likely to coalesce (Fig. II, 41).

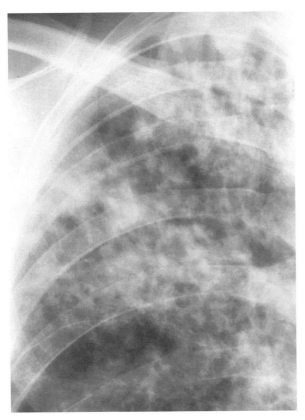

Fig. II, 41. Partial view of the right upper lung. Alveolar pattern. Confluent patchy densities, radiolucencies at the apex. Bronchial dissemination in cavernous pulmonary tuberculosis.

Air bronchograms (pneumobronchograms) or air alveolograms (pneumoalveolograms) can appear within these densities (Fleischner, 1927; Gough, 1955; Felson, 1960).

The interstitial processes lead to thickened peripheral interlobular septa (Kerley A and B lines, 1951) and subpleural tissues, and to a coarse reticular pattern of the more centrally located and superimposing interlobular septa (C lines), as well as to thickening of the axial peribronchial, perivascular and perihilar tissues (Grainger, 1958; Felson, 1960; Trapnell, 1964; Stender and Schermuly, 1961; Weibel, 1979; Fulmer and Crystal, 1979). If the changes in the alveolar septa are extensive, a fine reticular structure (reticular and reticulonodular), subtle opacities (ground glass) or minute nodular foci can be demonstrated radiographically (Friedman, 1973; Heitzman, 1973; Genereux, 1986) (Fig. II, 42).

Since tiny nodular densities often cannot be assigned to either alveoloacinar or alveoloseptal-interstitial changes, Heitzman (1973) proposes the additional term 'nodular pattern' (Fig. II, 43). Assigning pulmonary findings to one of these three patterns proves diagnostically valuable. Analysing the radiographic densities for a characteristic pattern must be carried out with great caution since it is fraud with errors due to the numerous factors that can interfere with a faithful presentation of pulmonary structures and densities (Heitzman, 1973, 1984; Felson, 1979; McLoud, 1986).

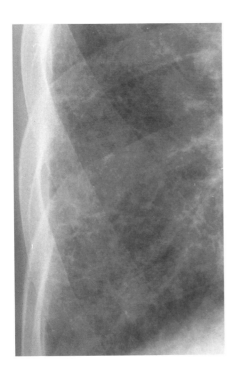
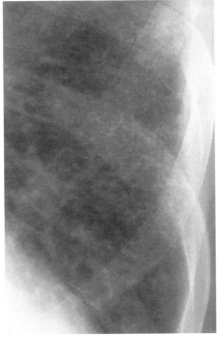

Fig. II, 42. Partial view of both lower lobes. Interstitial patterns. Reticular and fine-honeycombed structural densities with small patchy densities and thickened interlobular septal lines in pulmonary fibrosis.

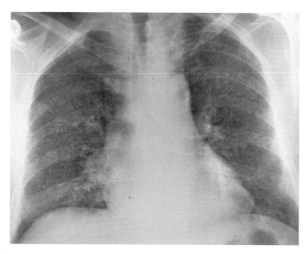

Fig. II, 43. Chest radiograph. Nodular pattern. Diffuse miliary densities of both lungs including apices in miliary tuberculosis.

Since 1930 (last revision published in 1980), lung changes in pneumoconioses are described and assessed according to a classification devised by the International Labour Organization (ILO). The radiographic features of small, round, irregular or large opacities as well as their extent and profusion are the basis of the description and the assessment. Since it is a descriptive classification, it is also adequate to describe other disseminated lung changes. McLoud, Carrington and Gaensler (1983) have generalized this classification for the description of all chest film findings. A nosologic classification is often possible by analyzing the structure of the individual foci, by assigning them to specific locations and by following their evolution, as well as by finding patterns of disseminated patchy and linear opacities and by recognizing structural change.

The differentiation of the pulmonary changes underlying the radiographic findings continues to be advanced by microbiological, serological and histological methods. To be mentioned in this context are acute respiratory distress syndrome, immunological, toxic and pharmaceutical pulmonary reactions, haemorrhages, changes in alveolitis, collagen diseases, granulomatoses, histiocytoses, the various types of interstitial pneumonia and fibroses, as well as lymphoproliferative lung diseases.

Conclusion

The most frequently performed radiographic examination is the chest film including fluoroscopically guided spot-films. In the last century, its diagnostic value has considerably increased through improved image quality made possible by technological advancements.

Until today, the elementary radiological examination of the chest holds its unique place in the early detection and follow-up of inflammatory and neoplastic pulmonary, pleural and mediastinal diseases as well as in finding their relationship to aging and the environment. It remains an important basis for evaluating cardiac disorders. Many special techniques, such as tomography, bronchography, pulmonary angiography, angiocardiography and computed tomography, represent a refinement of a simple roentgen examination and have immensely expanded the diagnostic possibilities.

References

Abreu, M. de: Verfahren und Apparatur zur kollektiven Röntgenphotographie (indirekte Röntgenaufnahme). Z. Tuberk. 80 (1938) 70

Albers-Schönberg, H.: Die Röntgentechnik. Hamburg, Lucas, Gräfe und Sillem 1903

Allbutt, T., H. Rolleston: A system of medicine by many writers (5 volumes). New York, MacMillan, 1909

Anacker, H., H.S. Stender: Krankheiten der Lunge. In: Klinische Röntgendiagnostik innerer Erkrankungen. Haubrick, Springer Berlin 1963

Ardran, G.M., H.E. Crooks: Comparison of radiographic techniques with special reference to dosage. Br. J. Radiol. 26 (1953) 352

Arnsperger, H.: Die Röntgenuntersuchung der Brusteingeweide und deren Ergebnisse für Physiologie und Pathologie. Leipzig 1909

Assmann, H.: Klinische Röntgendiagnostik der inneren Erkrankungen. 2. Auflage. F.C.W. Vogel, Leipzig 1922

Assmann, H.: Erfahrungen über die Röntgenuntersuchung der Lungen. G. Fischer, Jena 1914

Assmann, H.: Die klinische Röntgendiagnostik der inneren Erkrankungen. F.C.W. Vogel, Leipzig 1922/1949

Bade, P.: Über den Wert der Röntgenuntersuchung bei der Lungentuberkulose. Fortschr. Röntgenstr. 5 (1900) 193

Bader, E.W.: Gewerbekrankheiten. 2. Auflage 1943

Barden, R.P., D.A. Cooper: Roentgen appearence of the chest in diseases affecting the peripheral vascular system of the lungs. Radiology 51 (1948) 44

Béclère, A.: Les Rayons de Roentgen et la diagnostic des affections thoraciques. Paris, J.B. Baillière et fils, 1901

Béclère, A.: Zur Differentialdiagnose der Aneurysmen. Bul. et Mém. de la société de Radiologie médicale de Paris, Heft 14 (1910)

Béclère, A.: Les rayons de Roentgen et le diagnostic de la tuberculose. Actualités médicales 16 (1899) 1

Benedikt, M.: Das Röntgenlicht im Dienste der inneren Medizin. Kongr. inn. Medizin (1897) 307

Benedikt, M.: Die Herztätigkeit in Röntgenbeleuchtung. Dtsch. med. Wschr. Heft 28 (1896)

Berenroth, E.: Der Lungenechinokokkus. Erg. inn. Med. und Kinderheilk. 10 (1913)

Bergonié, J.: Nouveaux faits de radioscopie de lésions intrathoracique. Comptes rendus, 123 (1896) 1268

Bergonié, J., Carrière: Sur quelques résultats comparatifs des méthodes cliniques ordinaires et de l'examen fluoroscopique dans les épanchements pleurétiques. Comptes rendus, décembre 1897

Bouchard, Ch.: Les rayons de Roentgen appliqués au diagnostic de la tuberculose pulmonaire. Comptes-rendus, 14 décembre 1896

Bouchard, Ch.: Quelques pointes de la physiologie normale et pathologique du coeur révélées par l'examen radioscopique. La Semaine médicale (1898) 358

Bouchard, Ch.: Sur l'application de la radioskopie au diagnostic des maladies du thorax. Comptes rendus, décembre 1896, mai 1897

Bouchard, Ch., H. Guilleminot: De l'angle d'inclinaison des côtes étudiée à l'aide de la radioscopie et de la radiographie, en particulier dans la pleurésie sans épauchement. Comptes rendus (1899) 1429

Brauer, L.: Die Röntgendiagnose der Erkrankungen des Perikards. In: Groedel, F.M.: Grundriß und Atlas der Röntgendiagnostik. Lehmann, München 1921

Brauer, L.: Technik des künstlichen Pneumothorax. Beitr. Klin. Tbk. Bd. 15

Brauer, L.: Die Röntgendiagnostik der Pleuraerkrankungen. In: Groedel, F.M.: Grundriß und Atlas der Röntgendiagnostik 1921, 3. Aufl.

Brauning, H., F. Redeker: Die haematogene Lungentuberkulose des Erwachsenen. Tbk Bibl. 38 (1931)

Brauning, H.: Der Beginn der Lungentuberkulose beim Erwachsenen. Thieme, Leipzig 1938

Bruce, T.: Die Silikose als Berufskrankheit in Schweden. Acta med. Scand. Suppl. 129 (1942)

Brunner, A.: Erschwerung der Röntgendiagnostik der Lungen nach operativen Eingriffen im Bereich der Brustwand. Münch. med. Wschr. (1926) 21

Burghardt, H.: Röntgenbild von angeborenen Herzfehlern. Ver. inn. Med. Berlin 21.11.1898

Cabot, R.: Physical diagnosis of diseases of the chest. New York, William Wood 1901

Caffey, J.: Pediatric X-ray diagnosis. Vol. I, S. 249. Lloyd-Luke, London 1945, 6. Auflage 1973

Camp, O. de la: Was lehrt uns die radioskopische Untersuchung über die Lösungsvorgänge bei der croupösen Pneumonie? Fortschr. Röntgenstr. 8 (1904) 322

Camp, O. de la: Experimentelle Studien über die akute Herzdilatation. Z. Klin. Med. 51 (1903) H. 1 und 2

Carter, R.A.: Pulmonary mycotic infections. Radiology 26 (1936) 551

Carvalho, R.: A importancia da kymografia no estudo do coracao e pediculo vascular. Porto 1934

Cauley, J.H.: Results of the Boston Chest-X-ray survey. N. Engl. J. Med. 243 (1950) 631

Chaoul, H., E. Stierlin: Klinische Röntgendiagnostik der Erkrankungen der Brustorgane. In: Sauerbruch, F.: Die Chirurgie der Brustorgane. Berlin, Springer 1920

Chaoul, H., K. Greineder: Lungenkarzinom und Lungenabzeß im tomographischen Bild. Fortschr. Röntgenstr. 53 (1936) 232

Chaoul, H.: Über die Tomographie und insbesondere ihre Anwendung in der Lungendiagnostik. Fortschr. Röntgenstr. 51 (1935) 342

Chaoul, H.: Untersuchungen zur Frage der Lungenzeichnung im Röntgenbild. Dtsch. Zschr. Chir. 154 (1920) H. 5 und 6

Churchill, E.D.: Primary carcinoma of the lung. J. Am. Med. Ass. 137 (1948) 455

Cignolini, P.: Röntgenkymographie mit unterbrochnem Schlitz. Fortschr. Röntgenstr. 49 (1934) 224

Cocchi, U.: Die Lungensegmente und Segmentpneumonien. Fortschr. Röntgenstr. 75 (1951) 57

Cohn, M.: Die anatomische Substrate der Lungenröntgenogramme und ihre Bedeutung für die Röntgendiagnostik der Lungentuberkulose. Berl. med. Wschr. Heft 1 (1910)

Coltmann, J.W.: Fluoroscopy image brightening by electronic means. Radiology 51 (1948) 359

Cowl, W.: Eine Methode zur Gewinnung scharfer Röntgenbilder während der Atmung. Fortschr. Röntgenstr. 2 (1898) 169

Criegern, von: Aneurysmen der Brustaorta. Med. Ges. Leipzig 14.1.1902

Criegern, von: Über die Hiluszeichnung im Röntgenbild. Naturhistor. med. Ver. Heidelberg 1905

Criegern, von: Ergebnisse der Untersuchung des menschlichen Herzens mittels fluoreszierende Schirmes. Berl. Klin. Wschr. (1899) 422

Curschmann, H.: Die Verlagerung der Luftröhre und des Kehlkopfes als Folge von Veränderungen der Brustorgane. Münch. med. Wschr. Heft 48 (1905)

Da Costa, J.: A manual of modern surgery, general and operative. W.B. Saunders Philadelphia 1914

Dedic, S.: Das mitralstenotische und das mitralkonfigurative Herz im Profil. Fortschr. Röntgenstr. 38 (1928) 68

Delherm, P., H. Fischgold: Quatre années de radiokymographie cardio-vasculaire. Fortschr. Röntgenstr. 53 (1936) 223

Dessauer, F., B. Wiesner: Kompendium der Röntgenaufnahme und Röntgendurchleuchtung. 2. Auflage. O. Nemnich, Leipzig 1915

Dessauer, F., B. Wiesner: Über einen Fortschritt in der Technik der Röntgendurchleuchtung. Münch. med. Wschr. 1903

Deutsch, F., E. Kauf: Herz und Sport. Wien 1924

Dietlen, H.: Das Röntgenbild der Mitralstenose. J. Kreislaufforschung 20 (1928) 697

Dietlen, H., F. Moritz: Über das Verhalten des Herzens nach langdauerndem und anstrengendem Radfahren. Münch. med. Wschr. Heft 10 (1908)

Dietlen, H.: Die Röntgenuntersuchung von Herz, Gefäßen und Pericard. In: Rieder, H., J. Rosenthal: Lehrbuch der Röntgenkunde. J.A. Barth, Leipzig 1913

Dietlen, H.: Orthodiagraphie und Teleröntgenographie als Methode der Herzmessung. Münch. med. Wschr. Heft 32 (1913)

Dietlen, H.: Bemerkungen über das röntgenologische Verhalten der Pneumonie. Münch. med. Wschr. Heft 20 (1908)

Dietlen, H.: Die Röntgendiagnose der Lungenerkrankungen. In: Groedel, F.: Grundriß und Atlas der Röntgendiagnostik. 1921

Doub, H.P.: Roentgenologic aspects of bronchomycosis. Radiology 34 (1940) 267

Drüner, L.: Moderne Röntgenstereoskopie. Fortschr. Röntgenstr. 46 (1932) 142

Dumstrey, F, Metzner: Die Untersuchung mit Röntgenstrahlen. Fortschr. Röntgenstr. 1 (1898) 115

Durham, H.K.: The stereoscopic X-ray examination of the chest with special reference to the diagnosis of pulmonary tuberculosis. Bull. Johns Hopkins Hosp. 22 (1911) 229

Ebertz, E.H. Stürtz: Über abnorme Gestaltung des linken mittleren Herzschattenbogen bei Herzgesunden. Dtsch. Arch. Klin. Med. 107 (1912)

Engel, S., C. Pirquet: Handbuch der Kindertuberkulose. Thieme, Leipzig 1930

Engel, S.: Erkrankungen der Respirationsorgane. In: Handbuch der Kinderheilkunde. Hrg. Pfaundler und Schloßmann 3 (1924) 3

Engel, S.: Bronchialdrüsentuberkulose beim Kinde. Ergebn. inn. Med. und Kinderheilk. 11

Eppinger, H.: Allgemeine und spezielle Pathologie des Zwerchfells. Wien und Leipzig 1911

Esser, G.: Lungensegmente. Fortschr. Röntgenstr. 71 (1949) 395

Felson, B.: Fundamentals of chest roentgenology. Philadelphia, Saunders 1960

Felson, B.: Chest Roentgenology. Saunders, Philadelphia, London, Toronto 1973

Fischer, F.K.: Die Darstellung des Bronchialbaumes mit wasserlöslichem Kontrastmittel. Schw. med. Wschr. 42 (1948) 1025

Fischer, F.K.: Technik, Indikationen und Ergebnisse der Bronchographie mit wasserlöslichem viskösem Kontrastmittel (Jodium B). Schw. med. Wschr. (1950) 723

Fischer, F.K., H.R. Schinz: Zürcher Erfahrungen bei der kantonalen Schirmbildaktion bei über 65.000 untersuchten und abgeklärten Fällen. Schw. med. Wschr. 78 (1948) 217

Fleischner, F.G.: Heilungsvorgänge und Heilungsnachweis der Lungentuberkulose im Röntgenbilde. Ergebn. Tbk. Forschung 1 (1930) 195

Fleischner, F.G.: Der sichtbare Bronchialbaum, ein differentialdiagnostisches Symptom im Röntgenbild der Pneumonie. Fortschr. Röntgenstr. 36 (1927) 319

Foerster, A.: Über röntgenoskopisch feststellbare Zwerchfellbewegungsstörungen bei Bauchfelltuberkulose und Paranephritis. Münch. med. Wschr. Heft 38 (1920)

Fomin, G.B.: Die Bedeutung der Hartstrahlaufnahme für die Diagnostik des Lungenkrebses. Klin. Med. 31 (1953) 24. Fortschr. Röntgenstr. 79 (1953) 133

Fraenkel, E., A. Lorey: Das anatomische Substrat der sog. Hiluszeichnung im Röntgenbild. Fortschr. Röntgenstr. 14 (1909)

Fraenkel, E.: zit. nach P. Krause: Die Röntgendiagnose der Thoraxtumoren. In: Groedel, F.M.: Grundriß und Atlas der Röntgendiagnostik, Lehmann, München, (1921) 224

Fraenkel, E.: Über die Verknöcherung des menschlichen Kehlkopfes. Fortschr. Röntgenstr. 12 (1909) 15

Franke, H.: Ionometrische Bestimmung optimaler Belichtungszeiten. Fortschr. Röntgenstr. 40 (1929) 99

Franke, H.: Die Messung der bei der Aufnahme wirkenden Spannung und ihr Einfluß auf das Röntgenbild. Verh. Dtsch. Röntgenges. 17 (1926) 188

Fraser, R.G., J.A.P. Paré: Diagnosis of diseases of the chest. Saunders, Philadelphia, London, Toronto 1. Auflage 1970, 2. Auflage 1977

Friedman, P.G.: The concept of alveolar and interstitial disease. In: Potschen, E.J.: Current concepts in radiology. Mosby, St. Louis 1973

Frik, K.: Zur Deutung des Röntgenbildes im 1. schrägen Durchmesser. Fortschr. Röntgenstr. 29 (1922) 723

Frik, W.: Hartstrahltechnik. Thieme, Stuttgart 1961

Frik, W.: Die Ergebnisse der Erlanger Hartstrahlarbeitsgemeinschaft. Radiol. Austr. 8 (1954) 18

Fulmer, J.D., R.G. Crystal: Interstitial lung disease. Curr. pulmon. 1 (1979) 1

Garrigou: Radiographics du thorax. Comptes rendus, novembre 1897

Gebauer, A., E. Muntear, E. Stütz, H. Vieten: Das Röntgenschichtbild. Thieme, Stuttgart 1959

Gebauer, A., J. Lissner, O. Schott: Das Röntgenfernsehen. Thieme, Stuttgart. 1. Auflage 1965, 2. Auflage 1974

Genereux, G.P.: Radiologic assessment of diffuse lung disease. In: Taveras, J.M., J.T. Ferruci: Radiology, Diagnosis-Imaging-Intervention. Vol 1. 53. Lippincott, Philadelphia 1986

Gerhardt: Über interlobäre Pleuritis. Naturwiss. med. Ges. Jena, 14.2.1907

Gerhartz, H.: Die Fortschritte in der Diagnostik und Therapie. Med. Klin. Heft 37 (1912)

Gläßner, K.: Über Eventratio diaphragmatica. Fortschr. Röntgenstr. 24 (1917) 268

Gocht, H.: Lehrbuch der Röntgen-Untersuchung. Stuttgart, F. Enke 1898

Gocht, H.: Handbuch der Röntgenlehre. 2. Auflage. F. Euke, Stuttgart (1903) S. 10 Röntgentechnik und S. 315 Röntgenuntersuchung des Herzens.

Gocht, H.: Handbuch der Röntgen-Lehre. 2. Auflage, Stuttgart, F. Enke 1903 (Ausführliches Literaturverzeichnis)

Görgeny-Göttche, O., D. Kassay: Die Bedeutung der Bronchusperforation in der Tuberkulose der endobronchialen Lymphknoten. Ann. Paediatrici, 168 (1947) 245

Gough, J.: Correlation of radiological and pathological changes in some diseases of the lungs. Lancet 1 (1955) 161

Gould, D.M., D.J. Dalrymple: A radiological analysis of disseminated lung disease. Am. J. Med. Sc. 238 (1959) 621

Grainger, R.G.: Interstitial pulmonary oedema and its radiological diagnosis. A sign of pulmonary venous and capillary hypertension. Br. J. Radiol. 31 (1958) 201

Grangérard: Mensurateur radioscopique de l'indice du dévelopement ventriculaire en profondeur. J. radiol. et d'électr. (1920) 133

Greineder, K.: Die Tomographie der normalen Lunge. Fortschr. Röntgenstr. 52 (1935) 443

Groedel, F.M.: Die Dimension des normalen Aorten-Orthodiagramms. Berl. Klin. Wschr. Heft 14 (1918)

Groedel, F.M.: Die Röntgenuntersuchung des Herzens. In: Grundriß und Atlas der Röntgendiagnostik. Lehmann, München 1921

Groedel, F.M.: Grundriß und Atlas der Röntgendiagnostik in der inneren Medizin und den Grenzgebieten. 3. Auflage. J.F. Lehmann, München 1921

Groedel, F.M.: Roentgendiagnostik in der inneren Medizin und den Grenzgebieten. J.F. Lehmann, München (1909) 192

Groedel, F.M.: Über einige Fortschritte auf dem Gebiet der Röntgenuntersuchung der Lungenspitzen. Berl. Klin. Wschr. (1908) 674

Groedel, F.M.: Die normalen und pathologischen Herzformen im Röntgenbild. Röntgentaschenbuch, 4 (1912)

Groedel, Th., F.M. Groedel: Kombinierte röntgenkinematographie und elektrokardiographische Herzuntersuchung. Dtsch. Arch. Klin. Med. 109 (1912) 52

Großmann, J.: Tomographie. Fortschr. Röntgenstr. 51 (1935) 191

Grunmach, E.: Die Röntgenstrahlen im Dienst der inneren Medizin. Berl. Klin. Wschr. Heft 25 (1896)

Grunmach, E.: Diagnose eines Tumors mittels Röntgenstrahlen. Dtsch. med. Wschr. (1898) 260

Guilleminot, H.: Cinematographie du coeur. Arch. d'Electricité méd, exper. et clin. Heft 84 (1899)

Guilleminot, H.: Radiographie et Radioscopie cliniques de précision. La radiographie Heft 38 (1900)

Guilleminot, H.: Radiographie du coeur et de l'aorte aux différentes phases de la révolution cardiaque. Comptes rendus 17.7.1899

Hammer, G.: Die röntgenologischen Methoden der Herzgrößenbestimmung. Fortschr. Röntgenstr. 25 (1918) 510

Hasselwander, A.: Über die Verschieblichkeit der Brust und Bauchorgane nach Untersuchungen im Röntgenbild. Anatomische Hefte 46 (1912) 255

Hasselwander, A., C. Brügel: Anatomische Beiträge zur Frage der Lungenstruktur im Röntgenbild. Fortschr. Röntgenstr. 17 (1914)

Haubrich, R., P. Thurn: Zur Röntgensymptomatologie der Pericardverschwielung. Fortschr. Röntgenstr. 73 (1950) 288

Haubrich, R.: Der heutige Stand der Elektrokymographie. Ergebn. inn. Med. Kinderheilk. 6 (1955) 640

Hantschmann, L.: Über torpide sklerosierende Tuberkulose mit eigenartigem großzelligem histologischem Befund. Ergebn. Tbk. Forsch. 9 (1939) 3

Hawes, J.: Early pulmonary tuberculosis, Diagnostic prognosis and treatment. W. Wood, New York 1913

Heckmann, K.: Über Herzkymographie. Münch. med. Wschr. 82 (1935) 1079

Heckmann, K.: Elektrokymographie. Springer, Berlin 1959

Heitzman, E.R.: The mediastinum. Radiologic correlations with anatomy and pathology. Mosby, St. Louis 1977

Heitzman, E.R.: The lung, radiologic-pathologic correlations. Mosby, St. Louis 1973, 2. Auflage 1984

Herrnheiser, G., A. Kubat: Systematische Anatomie der Lungengefäße. Z. Anat. u. Entwicklungsgeschichte 105 (1936) 570

Herrnheiser, G.: Die Topik der Versorgungsgebiete der Lungenarterien und Bronchien erster Ordnung. Fortschr. Röntgenstr. 53 (1936) 251

Herxheimer, H.: Grundriß der Sportmedizin. Leipzig 1932

Hitzenberger, K.: Die Herzklappenfehler im Röntgenbild. Klin. Wschr. 7 (1928) 850

Hochsinger, K.: Ein Fall von Stridor thymicus congenitalis. Wien. med. Wschr. Heft 33 (1910)

Hofbauer, L., G. Holzknecht: Zur Physiologie und Pathologie der Atmung. Holzknecht Mitteilungen. 2. Heft. Jena, G. Fischer, 1907

Holfelder, H., F. Berner: Stand und Aussichten der Kleinbildphotographie vom Röntgenschirm. Münch. med. Wschr. 85 (1938) 1818

Holm, M., S. Holm, K. Winge: Results and experiences from mass examination for tuberculosis in Copenhagen. Acta tuberc. scand. 22 (1948) 97

Holm, J., M. Holm: National examination for tuberculosis. Acta tuberc. scand. 19 (1945) 71

Holzknecht, G., R. Kienböck: Zur Technik der Röntgenaufnahmen. Wien. Klin. Rundschau Heft 25 (1901)

Holzknecht, G.: Die röntgenologische Diagnostik der Erkrankungen der Brusteingeweide. Hamburg, Gräfe und Sillem 1901

Holzknecht, G.: Ein neues radioskopisches Symptom bei Bronchusstenose und Methodisches. Wien. Klin. Rundschau Heft 49 (1899)

Holzmann, M.: Erkrankungen des Herzens und der Gefäße. In: Schinz, H.R. et al: Lehrbuch der Röntgendiagnostik. Thieme, Stuttgart Bd III (1952) 2679

Hornykiewytsch, Th., H.S. Stender: Normale und pathologisch veränderte Lungengefäße im Schichtbild. Fortschr. Röntgenstr. 79 (1953) 639, 704

Hornykiewytsch, Th., H.S. Stender: Das Verhalten der Lungengefäße bei angeborenen und erworbenen Herzfehlern. Fortschr. Röntgenstr. 83 (1955) 26

Huizinga, E., E. Behr: On the division of the lung segments. Acta Radiol. 21 (1940) 314

Immelmann, M.: Kann man mittels Röntgenstrahlen Lungenschwindsucht schon zu einer Zeit erkennen, in der durch die bisherigen Untersuchungsmethoden noch nicht möglich. Fortschr. Röntgenstr. 3 (1899) 142

Immelmann, M.: Über die Bedeutung der Röntgenstrahlen bei der Pneumotherapie. Dtsch. med. Wschr. Heft 8 (1897)

Jacobsen, F.O.: Respiratorische Verschiebung des Mediastinums, ein Symptom einseitiger Bronchusstenose. Fortschr. Röntgenstr. 6 (1903) 242

Jaksch, R. von, H. Rotky: Die Pneumonie im Röntgenbilde. Fortschr. Röntgenstr. 1908

Jamin, F.: Zwerchfell und Atmung. In: Groedel, F.M.: Grundriß und Atlas der Röntgendiagnostik. Lehmann, München 1921

Janker, R.: Fernsehen in der Röntgendiagnostik. Röntgen-Bl. 9 (1956) 118

Janker, R.: Apparatur und Technik der Röntgenkinematographie zur Darstellung der Herzinnenräume und der großen Gefäße. Fortschr. Röntgenstr. 72 (1950) 513

Janker, R.: Leuchtschirmphotographie, Röntgenreihenuntersuchung. Barth, Leipzig 1938

Janker, R.: Die Leuchtschirmphotographie. Ein Bericht über eigene zwölfjahrige Erfahrungen. Fortschr. Röntgenstr. 58 (1938) 588

Kahlstorf, A.: Über eine orthodiagraphische Herzvolumenbestimmung. Fortschr. Röntgenstr. 45 (1932) 123

Kästle, C, H. Rieder, J. Rosenthal: Die Röntgenkinematographie (Bioröntgenographie) innerer Organe des Menschen. Z. Elektrol. und Röntgenk. Heft 1 (1909)

Kästle, C.: Röntgenologischer Beitrag zur Kenntnis der Tuberkulose. Münch. med. Wschr. Heft 50 (1921)

Kattentidt, B.: zit. n. Steinbrück, P., W. Angerstein: Die Röntgenschirmbild-photographie und ihre Anwendung in der Medizin. Verl. Volk und Gesundheit, Berlin 1971

Kerley, P.: Respiratory system. In: Shanks, S.C., P. Kerley: A textbook of X-ray diagnosis. Vol II. Saunders, Philadelphia 1951

Kienböck, R.: Über die intrathoracische Struma. Med. Klin. Heft 14 (1988)

Kienböck, R.: Über vorübergehende Verkleinerung des Herzens. Ref. in Fortschr. Röntgenstr. 12 (1908) 426

Kienböck, R.: Auf dem Röntgenschirm beobachtete Bewegungen in einem Pyopneumothorax. Wien. Klin. Wschr. (1898) 538

Kirch, E.: Über Größen- und Massenveränderungen der einzelnen Herzabschnitte bei Herzklappenfehlen, insbesondere bei Mitralstenose und Aortenstenose. Verh. Dtsch. Ges. inn. Med. 41 (1929) 324

Klason, T.: Pericarditis calculosa und Herzverkalkungen. Acta Radiol. 1 (1921/22) 162

Koelsch, F.: Die Lungenerkrankung durch Aluminium-staub. Beitr. Klin. Tbk. 97 (1942) 688

Köhler, A.: Kinematographische Röntgenvorführungen normaler und pathologischer Atmung. Deutscher Röntgenkongreß 1907

Köhler, A.: Teleradiographie des Herzens. Dtsch. med. Wschr. Heft 5 (1908)

Köhler, A.: Zur Röntgendiagnostik der kindlichen Lungendrüsentuberkulose. Hamburg 1906

Köhler, A.: Zur Röntgendiagnostik der intrathoracischen Tumoren. Fortschr. Röntgenstr. 17 (1914) 120

Kovats, F., Z. Zsebök: Röntgenanatomische Grundlagen der Lungenuntersuchung. Akadémia kiadó, Budapest 1953

Krause, P.: Die Röntgendiagnose der Lungentuberkulose. In: Groedel, F.M.: Grundriß und Atlas der Röntgendiagnostik, Lehrmann, München 1921

Krause, P.: Röntgenuntersuchung der Trachea und des oberen Mediastinums und Röntgendiagnose der Bronchialerkrankungen. In: Groedel, F.M.: Grundriß und Atlas der Röntgendiagnostik in der inneren Medizin und den Grenzgebieten. J.F. Lehmann, München 1921

Krause, P.: Zur Diagnosis der Lungentumoren. Zit. nach Krause, P.: Die Röntgendiagnostik der Thoraxtumoren. In: Groedel, F.M.: Röntgendiagnostik in der inneren Medizin und den Grenzgebieten. München, Lehmann, III, 1921

Kremer, W.: Die Deutung des Röntgenschichtbildes der Lungenobenfelder. Thieme, Leipzig 1945

Kremer, W.: Wert der Tomographie zur Erkennung von Restkavernen. Fortschr. Röntgenstr. 54 (1936)

Laubry, Ch., P. Cottenot et al: Radiologie clinique du coeur et des grande vaisseaux. Paris 1939

Leitner, S.: Morbus Besnier-Boeck-Schaumann. Schwabe, Basel 1942

Lenk, R.: Die Röntgendiagnostik der intrathorakalen Tumoren und ihre Differentialdiagnose. Handb. thor. und klin. Röntgenkunde Bd. I, Springer, Wien 1929

Levy, M.: Über Verstärkungsschirme und doppelseitig begossene Platten. Jahrbuch der Photographie und Reproduktionstechnik 1898

Levy, M.: Die Durchleuchtung des menschlichen Körpers zu medizinisch-diagnostischen Zwecken. Physiologische Gesellschaft zu Berlin, 1896

Levy, M.: Über Abkürzung der Expositionszeit bei Aufnahme mit Röntgenstrahlen. Fortschr. Röntgenstr. 1 (1897) 75

Levy, M.: Neues aus der Röntgentechnik. Fortschr. Röntgenstr. 2 (1898) 106

Levy-Dorn, M.: Asthmatischer Anfall. Berl. Klin. Wschr. Heft 47 (1896)

Levy-Dorn, M.: Verwertbarkeit der Röntgenstrahlen in der praktischen Medizin. Dtsch. med. Wschr. (1897) 119

Levy-Dorn, M.: Zur Untersuchung des Herzens mittels Röntgenstrahlen. Münch. med. Wschr. (1899) 572

Levy-Dorn, M.: Zur Untersuchung der Brust mittels Röntgenstrahlen. Münch. med. Wschr. (1900) 481

Levy-Dorn, M.: Zur Kritik und Ausgestaltung des Röntgenverfahrens. Dtsch. med. Wschr. (1897) 800

Levy-Dorn, M., J. Zadek: Zur Untersuchung mit Röntgenstrahlen bei Lungenechinococcus. Berl. med. Wschr. 36 (1899) 431

Levy-Dorn, M.: Röntgenuntersuchung der normalen Atmung. 4. Röntgen Kongreß 1908

Lewis, L., R.H. Morgan: The value of stereoscopy in mass radiography of the chest. Radiology 46 (1946) 171

Lissner, J., D. Hahn: Mediastinum und mediastinale Erkrankungen. In: Schinz: Radiologische Diagnostik in Klinik und Praxis. Bd I, 1, 387. Thieme, Stuttgart 1987

Lochtkemper, I.: Atlas der Staublungenkrankheiten. Arch. Gew. Path. 3 (1932) 153

Lodge, Th.: Primary bronchogenic carcinoma. J. Faculty Radiologists 2 (1950) 118

Löffler, W.: Zur Differentialdiagnose der Lungeninfiltrierungen. Beitr. klin. Tbk. 79 (1932) 368

Longcope, W.T.: Sarcoidosis of Besnier-Boeck-Schaumann. J. Am. Med. Ass. 117 (1941) 1321

Lorey, A.: Das Röntgenverfahren bei der Lungentuberkulose. Handbuch der Tuberkulose Bd. 1 (1914)

Lorey, A.: Die diagnostische Bedeutung der Bronchographie. Arztliche Rundschau Heft 7 (1927)

Lorey, A.: Das Röntgenverfahren bei der Lungentuberkulose. In: Brauer et al: Handbuch der Lungentuberkulose. J.A. Barth, Leipzig 1914

Luisada, A.A., G.G. Fleischner, M.B. Rappaport; Fluorocardiography (Electrokymography). Am. Heart J. 35 (1948) 336

Lysholm, E., G. Nylin, K. Quarra: The relative between heart volume and stroke volume. Acta Radiol. 15 (1934) 237

MacIntyre, J.: The application of the Röntgen rays in the medical and surgical departments of the Royal Infirmary of Glasgow. Glasgow Hospital Reports 1 (1898) 290

Malmros, H., E. Hedvall: Entstehung und Entwicklung der Lungentuberkulose. Tbk. Bibl. 68 (1938)

Marragliano, V.: Application de la radioscopie à l'examen des organes intrathoraciques à l'etat normal et pathologique. Semaine med. (1897) 50

Matthes: Die Diagnose der Miliartuberkulose. Med. Klin. Heft 44 (1912)

McLaughlin, A.J.G., E. Rogers, K.C. Dunham: Talk pneumoconiosis. Br. J. industr. Med. 6 (1949) 184

McLoud, T.C.: Chronic infiltrative lung disorders. In: Taveras, J.M., Ferucci, J.T.: Radiology-Diagnosis-Imaging-Intervention. Lippincott, Philadelphia 1986

McLoud, T.C., C.B. Carrington, E.A. Gaensler: Diffuse infiltrative lung disease. A new scheme for description. Radiology 149 (1983) 353

Medlar, E.M.: Pathogenesis of minimal pulmonary tuberculosis. An. Rev. Tuberc. 58 (1948) 583

Miller, Orton: A case of patent ductus arteriosis with skiagram. Br. J. Child. Dis. (1913) 109

Morales, O.: Further studies with Viscous Umbradil. Acta Radiol. 32 (1948) 317

Morales, O., H. Heiwinkel: A viscous water-soluble contrast preparation. Acta Radiol. 30 (1948) 257

Morgan, R.H.: Roentgen tube potentials in diagnostic roentgenology. Am. J. Roentgenol. 58 (1947) 211

Morgan, R.H.: The roentgenologic diagnosis of tuberculosis. Bull. Johns Hopkins Hosp. 82 (1948) 411

Morgan, R.H.: The control of diagnostic quality in roentgenograms of the chest. Am. J. Roentgenol. 50 (1943) 149

Moritz, F.: Zur Frage der akuten Dilation des Herzens durch Überanstrengung. Münch. med. Wschr. Heft 25 (1908)

Moritz, F.: Über orthodiagraphische Untersuchungen am Herzen. Münch. med. Wschr. Heft 1 (1902)

Moritz, F.: Über Veränderungen in der Form, Größe und Lage des Herzens beim Übergang von der horizontalen zur vertikalen Körperstellung. Dtsch. Arch. Klin. Med. 82 (1905)

Mueller, P.: Perikarditische Verkalkungen. Fortschr. Röntgenstr. 25 (1917) 17

Müller, R., S. Löfstedt: The reaction of the pleura in primary tuberculosis of the lungs. Acta med. Scand. 122 (1945) 105

Munk, F.: Grundriß der gesammten Röntgendiagnostik innerer Krankheiten. G. Thieme, Leipzig 1914

Neumann, W.: Die Klinik der Lungentuberkulose Erwachsener. Springer, Wien 1930

Newell, R.R., W.E. Chamberlain, L. Rigler: Descriptive classification of pulmonary shadows. Am. rev. Tuberc. 69 (1954) 566

Noix, M.: La television radiologique, la problemes physiques, physiologiques, pathologiques. Doin, Paris 1962

Orton, G.: The diagnosis of thoracic aneurysm by means of the Roentgen rays. Archiv of the Roentgen ray 1905

Otten, M.: Die Röntgendiagnose der Lungengeschwülste. Fortschr. Röntgenstr. 15 (1910)

Otten, M.: Zur Röntgendiagnostik der primären Lungenkarzinome. Fortschr. Röntgenstr. 9 (1906) 369

Oudin, P., Barthélemy: Applications de la méthode de Roentgen aux sciences medicales. La France 11 + 18 decembre 1896

Paget, S.: The surgery of the chest. New York, E.E. Treat 1897

Palmieri, G.: Über meine Methode der plastischen Darstellung des Herzens am Lebenden. Acta Radiol. 10 (1920) 127

Pancoast, H.K., E.P. Pendergrass: Pneumoconiosis (Silicosis), a roentgenological study with notes on pathology. Hoeber Inc. New York 1926

Perrin, L.F., U. Fauré: Le poumon. In: Buffard, P., U. Eauré, M. Bochu: Radiologie clinique II. Flammarion, Paris 1974

Pfahler, J.: The X-rays in the diagnosis of pulmonary tuberculosis. Proc. Phil. Co. Med. Soc. 26 (1905) 249

Pfahler, J.: The Roentgen ray in medical diagnosis. In: Anders, H.: Physical Diagnosis with Case Examples of the Inductive Methods, New York, D. Appleton 1907

Pfeiffer, G.: Über die Röntgenuntersuchung der Trachea bei Tumoren und Exsudat im Thorax. Münch. med. Wschr. Heft 8 (1906)

Policard, A., L. Croizier, E. Martin: La fibrose pulmonaire des mineurs. Masson, Paris 1938

Policard, A.: Le Poumon. Masson, Paris 1938

Redeker, F.: Über das Frühinfiltrat und die Irrlehre vom gesetzmäßigen Zusammenhang der sogenannten Spitztuberkulose und der Erwachsenenphtisis. Dtsch. med. Wschr. 53 (1927) 97

Redeker, F., O. Walter: Entstehung und Entwicklung der Lungenschwindsucht des Erwachsenen. Kabitzsch, Leipzig 1929

Reindell, H.: Größe, Form und Bewegungsbild des Sportherzens. Arch. Kreislaufforschung 7 (1940) 117

Ricker, W., M. Clark: Sarcoidosis, a clinicopathologic review of 300 cases, including 22 autopsies. Am. J. Clin. Path. 190 (1950) 725

Rieder, H.: Zur Diagnose der chronischen Lungentuberkulose durch das radiologische Verfahren. Fortschr. Röntgenstr. 7 (1903) 1

Rieder, H.: Die Untersuchung der Brustorgane mit Röntgenstrahlen in verschiedenen Durchleuchtungsrichtungen. Fortschr. Röntgenstr. 6 (1902) 115

Rieder, H.: Die Untersuchung der Brustorgane mit Röntgenstrahlen in verschiedenen Durchleuchtungsrichtungen. Fortschr. Röntgenstr. 6 (1902) 115

Rieder, H., J. Rosenthal: Momentaufnahmen des Thorax mit Röntgenstrahlen. Münch. med. Wschr. (1899) 1048

Rieder, H.: Die Röntgenuntersuchung der Lungen und Bronchien. In: Rieder, H., J. Rosenthal: Lehrbuch der Röntgenkunde. Barth, Leipzig 1913

Rieder, H.: Panzerherz. Fortschr. Röntgenstr. 20 (1913) 50

Rieder, H.: Der Wert der Röntgenuntersuchung für die Frühdiagnose der Lungentuberkulose. Verh. dtsch. Röntgenges. 4 (1908)

Rieder, H.: Über den Wert der Thoraxdurchleuchtung bei der Pneumonie, namentlich bei zentraler Lokalisation. Münch. med. Wschr. (1906) 1945

Rienzo, S. di, H.H. Weber: Radiologische Exploration des Bronchus. Thieme, Stuttgart 1960

Rollins, W.: Notes on X-Light. Cambridge, The University press 1904

Romberg, E. von: Lehrbuch der Krankheiten des Herzens und der Blutgefäße. 1915

Rosenfeld, G.: Die Diagnostik innerer Krankheiten mittels Röntgenstrahlen. Wiesbaden 1897

Rumpf: Demonstration von Röntgenbildern. Kongr. für Innere Medizin 1897 S. 534

Sabat, B.: Zur Geschichte der Röntgenkymographie und Ausarbeitung der Modifikation der Methode. Fortschr. Röntgenstrahlen 50 (1934) 309

Sante, L.R.: Lobar pneumonia. Hoder, New York 1928

Sante, L.R.: Acute consolidation of the lungs. Their recognition and differential diagnosis. Radiology 4 (1925) 221

Sauerbruch, F.: Chirurgie der Brustorgane. Berlin 1920

Sauerbruch, F.: Die Beeinflussung von Lungenerkrankungen durch künstliche Lähmung des Zwerchfells. Münch. med. Wschr. (1913) 625

Saupe, E.: Röntgenatlas der Asbestosis. Thieme, Leipzig 1938

Schieffer: Über Herzvergrößerung infolge Radfahrens. Dtsch. Arch. Klin. Med. 89 (1906) H. 5 und 6

Schinz, H.R., R. Blangley: Generalisierte Akinomykose. Röntgenpraxis 6 (1934) 169

Schinz, H.R.: Lehrbuch der Röntgendiagnostik. Thieme, Leipzig 1928

Schjerning, O. von, Kranzfelder: Zum jetzigen Stand der Frage nach der Verwertbarkeit der Röntgenschen Strahlen für medizinische Zwecke. Dtsch. med. Wschr. (1896) 541

Schröder, G.: Über Lungentyphilis. Münch. med. Wschr. (1919) 401

Schwarz, G.: Die Röntgenuntersuchung des Herzens und der großen Gefäße. F. Deutike, Wien, 1911

Schwedel, J.B.: Clinical Roentgenology of the cardiovascular system. New York, 1936

Sicard, J.A., J. Forestier: Méthode générale d'exploration radiologique par l'huile jodée (Lipiodol). Bull. Soc. méd. hôp. 38 (1922) 463

Simon, G.: Principles of chest X-ray diagnosis. Butterworths, London, 1. Auflage 1956, 3. Auflage 1971

Sluka: Die Hilustuberkulose des Kindes im Röntgenbild. Wien. klin. Wschr. Heft 7 (1912)

Spiegler, G.: Physikalische Grundlagen der Röntgendiagnostik. Thieme, Stuttgart 1957

Stauffer, H., M.J. Oppenheimer et al: Practical image amplifier technics, fluoroscopy, cinefluoroscopy, spot-film radiography and use with closed circuit television. Radiology 65 (1955) 784

Stechow: Über Technik und Resultate der Röntgenphotographie mit Demonstrationen. Stockholm, 5.8.1897

Stender, H.S., W. Schermuly: Das interstitielle Lungen-ödem im Röntgenbild. Fortschr. Röntgenstr. 95 (1961) 461

Stumpf, P.: Die Flächenkymographie. Fortschr. Röntgenstr. 56 (1937) 143

Stumpf, P.: Zehn Vorlesungen über Kymographie. Leipzig 1937

Stumpf, P., H.H. Weber, G.A. Weltz: Röntgenkymographische Bewegungslehre innerer Organe. Leipzig 1936

Stürtz, E.H.: Die lymphangitische Entstehung des Lungenspitzenkatarrhs von den Hilusdrüsen aus. 4. Ver. der Tuberkulose-Ärzte, Berlin 1907

Stutz, E.: Bronchographische Beiträge zur normalen und pathologischen Physiologie der Lungen. Fortschr. Röntgenstr. 72 (1949/50) 129, 309, 447

Stutz, E., H. Vieten: Die Bronchographie. Thieme, Stuttgart 1955

Teschendorf, W.: Lehrbuch der röntgenologischen Differentialdiagnostik (Erkrankungen der Brustorgane). Thieme, Leipzig, 1. Auflage 1939, 2. Auflage 1950, 5. Auflage 1975

Teubern, K. von: Orthodiagraphische Messungen des Herzens und des Aortenbogens bei Herzgesunden. Fortschr. Röntgenstr. 24 (1916) 549

Thomson, J.: The practical application of the Roentgen rays in diseases of the heart and great vessels. Lancet II (1896) 1676

Thomson, J., J.H. Campbell: The estimation of the size and shape of the heart by the Roentgen rays. Lancet II (1896) 1011 a. 1605

Trapnell, D.H.: Radiological appearance of lymphangitis carcinomatosa of the lung. Thorax 19 (1964) 251

Tuffier: De la difficulté de localiser les lésions pulmonaires par les signes stéthoscopiques. Société médicale des hôpitaux, 27.1.1899

Tuffier, Aubourg: Angiom du poumon. Soc. du Radiol. de Paris 34 (1904) 887

Uehlinger, E.: Die tuberkulöse Spätestinfektion und ihre Frühevolution. Schweiz. med. Wschr. (1942) 701

Ulrici, H.: Die Formen der Lungentuberkulose. Klin. Wschr. (1926) 969

Vallebona, A.: La stratigraphie pulmonaire. J. Radiol. 21 (1937) 211

Vaquez, H., F. Bordet: Le coeur et l'aorte. Bailliere et fils, Paris 1913

Vaquez, H., E. Bordet: Radiologie du coeur et des vaisseaux de la base. Baillière. Paris 1928

Vaquez, H., E. Doucetot: Dextrocardie et Dextroversion. Presse méd. Heft 5 (1920)

Vieten, H.: Die gezielte Bronchographie mit wasserlöslichen Kontrastmitteln. Fortschr. Röntgenstr. 72 (1949/50) 270

Vogl, J.: Miliartuberkulose im Röntgenbild. Prager med. Wschr. Heft 40 (1912)

Volhard, E.: Internistenkongreß 1930

Walsh, D.: The Roentgen rays in medical work. Ballière, Tindall and Cox 1897

Walsham, H., G. Orton: The Roentgen rays in the diagnosis of diseases of the chest. London, H.K. Lewis, 1906

Walsham, H: On the diagnosis of pleural effusion - the Roentgen rays. Br. Med. J. (1901) II, 8

Warembourg, H., P. Graux: Pathologie des Zones pulmonaires. Paris, Masson et Cie, 1947

Wassermann, J.: Zur Diagnose innerer Krankheiten mittels Röntgenstrahlen. Wien. Klin. Wschr. 10 (1897) 86

Wegelius, C., K. Noschis: Screen photography equipment for easier photography with routine roentgen diagnosis work. Acta Radiol. 29 (1948) 101

Weibel, E.R.: Looking into the lung: what can it tell us? Am. J. Roentgenol. 133 (1979) 1021

Weinberger, M.: Atlas der Radiographie der Brustorgane. E.M. Engel, Wien und Leipzig 1900

Williams, F.H.: Roentgen ray examinations in incipient pulmonary tuberculosis. Trans Am. Clin. Assoc. 15 (1899) 68

Williams, F.H.: Frühdiagnose der Lungentuberkulose mittels Röntgenstrahlen. Boston Med. and Surg. J. 140 (1899). Ref. Dtsch. med. Wschr. (1899) 27, 175

Williams, F.H.: The Roentgen rays in medicine and surgery. London, MacMillan, 1901

Williams, F.H.: The Roentgen rays in thoracic diseases. Am. J. med. sci. 114 (1897) 665

Wurm, E.: Über die Grenzen der Röntgendiagnostik für die Beurteilung der Krankheitsanfänge bei Lungentuberkulose Erwachsener. Beitr. Klin. Tbk. 81 (1932) 707

Zanetti, E.: Primi resultati della tecnica dei raggi duri applicata alla diagnostica pulmonare. Med. d. Lavoro 46 (1955) 441

Zdansky, E.: Beiträge zur Kenntnis der kardialen Lungenstauung auf Grund röntgenologischer, klinischer und anatomischer Untersuchungen. Wien. Arch. inn. Med. 18 (1924) 461

Zdansky, E., E. Ellinger: Röntgenkymographische Untersuchungen am Herzen. Fortschr. Röntgenstr. 47 (1933) 648

Zdansky, E.: Über das Röntgenbild des Lungenoedems. Röntgenpraxis 5 (1933) 248

Zdansky, E.: Zur Diagnose der Concretio und Accretio cordis. Fortschr. Röntgenstr. 44 (1931) 48

Zdansky, E.: Röntgendiagnostik des Herzens und der großen Gefäße. Springer, Wien, 1. Auflage 1939, 2. Auflage 1949, 3. Auflage 1962

Zehbe, M.: Beobachtungen am Herzen und an der Aorta. Dtsch. med. Wschr. Heft 11 (1916)

Ziedses des Plantes, B.G.: Eine neue Methode zur Differenzierung in der Röntgendiagnostik (Planigraphie). Acta Radiol. 13 (1932) 182

Soft tissues - mammography

W. Hoeffken

As early as 1895, the 'new kind of rays' was used for medical applications to visualize the interior of the body. The emphasis was mainly on bone injuries and diseases of the joints: for the first time, fractures could be seen and corrected by non-invasive reposition and optimal fixation. Subsequently the internal organs and the digestive tract were investigated using X-rays.

At first, there was hardly any interest in using X-rays for the diagnosis of soft-tissue diseases, because these, usually superficial, changes were accessible for inspection, palpation and clinical assessment: palpable nodes were removed, abscesses and infectious soft-tissue diseases were treated surgically.

However, a special situation existed for the diagnosis of changes in the female breast: a wide range of breast diseases with infection, chronic inflammatory changes, cysts and benign nodes, as well as the necessity for early diagnosis of breast cancer, needed better diagnostic methods than inspection, palpation and operative biopsy alone.

It took another 18 years after the discovery of X-rays before the first publication on radiographs of breast diseases appeared: in 1913 the surgeon Albert Salomon (Fig. II, 44), of the Royal Surgical University Clinic in Berlin (Medical Superintendent Professor A. Bier) published 'Contribution to the pathology and clinical medicine of breast cancer'.

This study included radiographs of surgical specimens of the breast for the first time. On the basis of eight cases, Salomon demonstrated the radiomorphological changes in various types of breast cancer.

These first 'mammographs' already provided satisfactory information on tumour spread and the edges of the tumour. The different types of

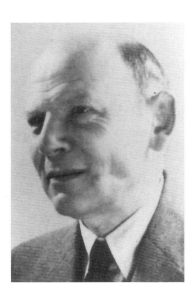

Fig. II, 44. Albert Salomon (born 1883). Surgeon. Medical education under Bier in Berlin. Assistant professor at the University of Berlin in 1921, full professor in 1927. Discharged in 1933 and emigrated to The Netherlands in 1939. First radiographic examination of a specimen of a breast carcinoma in 1913. Later only surgical and medical publications.

growth of solid nodular carcinomas or scirrhous tumours, with central tumour nodes and radial spicula formation, could be recognized. Notably, on a radiograph of one of the surgical specimens with a large cyst, Salomon had found a neighbouring small scirrhous carcinoma, which had not been detected by histopathological examination (Fig. II, 45).

Thus, historically, Salomon is the first to have reported on a 'clinical occult mammary carcinoma', found by radiographic examination. Salomon summarized his findings: *'The radiographs of excised mammary glands demonstrate satisfying survey views of the spread and type of cancer. By combining the results of these pictures with the histological examination of suspicious tumour boundaries, it becomes necessary to make excisions at a distance of at least three fingers away from the peripherally palpable border of a tumour.'*

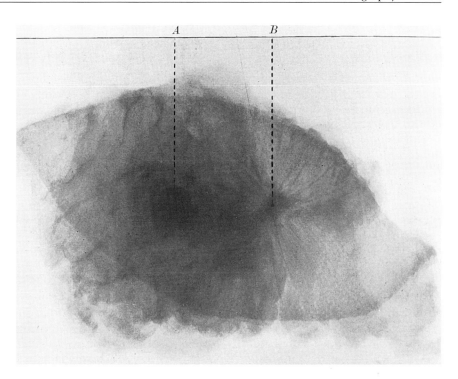

Fig. II, 45. Radiograph of a surgical specimen of the female breast with a large cyst (A) and a small carcinomatous lesion (B) with linear densities radiating from its margin to the edge of the specimen (Salomon, 1913).

Mammography only won clinical recognition many years later. In 1913, the radiographic techniques to examine patients with breast diseases *in vivo* were not available. Furthermore, there was no immediate clinical need for radiographs because the standard rule in diagnosing breast diseases was *'every palpable node should be removed.'* Assessment of its malignancy or otherwise was provided by histopathological examination. Moreover, in those days, the efforts concentrated mostly on the improvement of treatment results, to overcome resignation and despair.

In 1863, Sir James Paget wrote: *'I am not aware of a single clear instance of recovery; that is, if the patient should live for more than ten years free from the disease. . . . In deciding for or against the removal of a cancerous breast in any individual case, we may, I think, dismiss all hope that the operation will be the final remedy for the disease.'*

In 1856, the Frenchman Velpeau wrote with a similarly gloomy viewpoint: *'The surgical destruction of a carcinomatous tumour is usually simple. However . . . the disease always recurs after the operation, its course is even accelerated by the operation and the fatal end quickened.'* In America, D.H. Agnew (1883) expressed the hope: *'I have no doubt that cancer will be curable one day, but I do not think that the surgeon's scalpel will perform this deed.'*

In 1891, William Halsted marked a new epoch in breast surgery. As a result of radical mastectomy, with excision of the musculus pectoralis and axillary lymph nodes, Halstedt was the first to achieve a 4-year survival rate of 41% with a local recurrence rate of only 10%. The initial optimism diminished after the presentation of the first statistics on late results, but was renewed by Steinthal in 1905. He gave a new impetus to radical mammary surgery with his more precise differentiation of the tumour stages (Steinthal I to III) and his recommendation to restrict radical surgery procedures to stages Steinthal I and II. Attempts to improve the prognosis by ultraradical surgical methods did not lead to further improvement of cure rates. An improvement could thus only be expected from earlier diagnosis of malignant breast diseases.

In 1927, Otto Kleinschmidt reported on his long-standing experience of radiological examinations of the female breast at Payr's University Clinic in Leipzig, Germany. For many years, preoperative radiographs had been taken in any patient with an uncertain diagnosis. In addition, radiographs were taken postoperatively of the surgically removed tissue. Thus, the first papers on radiographic diagnostics of the female breast, in patients with problematic clinical findings, were published by Kleinschmidt. With the introduction of radiographic examination in preoperative evaluation, the first step had been taken towards the early recognition of breast cancer.

In 1932, Walter Vogel reported in his publication 'Die Roentgendarstellung von Mammatumoren' [Roentgenography of Breast Tumours] on further experiences at Payr's Clinic. He wrote: *'In our clinic all breast tumours are radiographed pre-operatively for many years. By comparing these radiographs with the pathoanatomical findings of the operative sample, we obtained insight into the meaning of alterations in patterns and structures seen on the film. Our procedure is now: roentgen apparatus – Transverter (Koch and Sterzel), Doneo-Film, 43 kVp, 22 mA, 55–65 cm focus-film distance. Exposure time four to six seconds'* (Fig. II, 46).

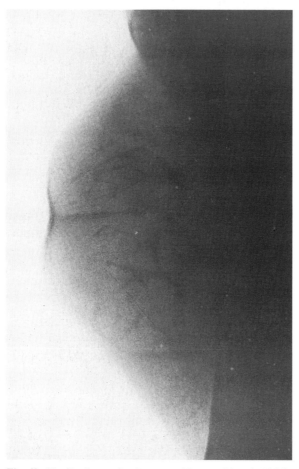

Fig. II, 46. Radiograph of a normal breast (Vogel, 1931).

In the early thirties, studies on mammography were published in South America first by Dominguez (1930) and Baraldi (1935), as well as by Goyanes et al (1931). Almost simultaneously, papers were published in Paris by Espaillat (1933) and in North America. A pioneering feat had been attributed to Stafford L. Warren (1930). He published a report on 119 female patients of whom 48 women had breast cancer. Except for four false interpretations, all cancers were di-

agnosed correctly using mammography. Images of the most advanced stages of the tumours were indeed shocking. Warren's roentgen technique was: Potter–Bucky grid and double screens: 50–60 kVp tube voltage; oblique views only. Fray and Warren had already attached great importance to comparing images with the healthy breast and postulated stereoscopic images for spatial assessment (1932).

During those years there was only one publication of German origin, which was by R. Finsterbusch and F. Gross (1934) of the Leipzig University (Medical Superintendent Professor Payr) and Professor W. Baensch's Roentgen Institute. It reported on the radiological evidence of calcifications in both breasts, in mastopathy, with cystic widened lactiferous ducts.

Meanwhile in the USA, extensive knowledge was compiled on structural changes of the mammary glands during pregnancy and throughout the menstrual cycle, as well as on menopausal processes later in life (Seabold, 1931; Reimann and Seabold, 1933).

Lockwood (1931, 1933; Lockwood and Stewart, 1932) had also taken a keen interest in the physiological changes of breast structures and proposed the differentiation between 'mazoplasia' and 'cystiphorous desquamative epithelial hyperplasia.' In the following decades, this classification has been abandoned and is now combined under the term 'mastopathy'.

In 1935, Raoul Leborgne had begun his radiological examinations of breast diseases in Montevideo, Uruguay. It is admirable to see, time and again, the results Leborgne compiled to differentiate between microcalcifications in mastopathic changes and those in malignant formations. He furthered his studies in the following years and became particularly dedicated to the anatomy and pathology of the mammary glands and lactiferous ducts and the visualization of the main lactiferous ducts using contrast medium. He described the results of these investigations in a 1943 monograph 'Die Radiologie des Milchgangssystems der normalen und pathologischen Brustdrüse' [The Radiology of the Lactiferous Duct System in the Normal and Pathological Mammary Gland].

He specifically pointed out that a perfect radiographic technique is imperative to recognize slight differences in the opacity of normal and pathological tissues. Leborgne expressly drew attention to the importance of adding a craniocaudal view to the mammogram, which, until then, consisted of a lateral–oblique projection only. It was remarkable that Leborgne had, although without specific evidence and only based on his vast experience, anticipated the differential diagnostic contribution of microcalcifications. As early as 1951, Leborgne accurately described intramammary calcifications in malignant tumours as *'countless punctated calcifications that are arranged like clustered grains of salt in the breast.'* He found such calcifications, *'which look like film defects'*, inside tumour nodes and their periphery, but also as single radiological signs of malignancy (Fig. II, 47).

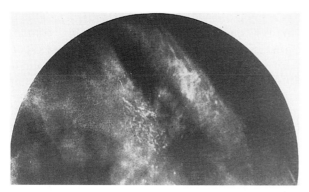

Fig. II, 47. Intraductal carcinoma with a group of microcalcifications (R. Leborgne, 1951).

Leborgne classified calcifications without visible tumour mass as 'canalicular type' of tumor growth, indicating a comedocarcinoma: *'This is the anatomic type that often presents calcifications, even without the existence of palpable tumour.'*

Through his investigations, Leborgne proved that mammary carcinoma can also grow and expand relatively far throughout the breast without a palpable nodular resistance. In those days he had already promoted 'systematic prophylactic roentgen examinations of all women with a family history of breast cancer.'

As early as 1951, Leborgne outlined the following requirements for mammographic techniques:

1 Survey view in craniocaudal direction, entire breast with long cone (60 cm), slight compression of the breast, 30 kVp, 5 mA/6 s, film without intensifying screens.
2 Additional lateral views if the upper part of the breast is not clearly visible.
3 Selective view: 20 kVp, 30-cm focus-film distance, cone opening as small as possible.

With this radiological technique (low kilovoltage, short focus-film distance and selective views, no-screen films and breast compression), Le-

borgne attained optimal results to demonstrate microcalcifications.

In 1937, Gershon-Cohen, at first with Colcher and in 1938 with Strickler, reported on 'Roentgenologic examination of the normal breast', and, later, in numerous publications together with the pathologist Helen Ingelby, on comparative studies of anatomy and pathology of breast diseases in the roentgen image.

In his book, 'Comparative Anatomy, Pathology and Roentgenology of the Breast' (1960), Gershon-Cohen, in collaboration with Helen Ingelby, summarized the extensive knowledge gained so far on mammography (Fig. II, 48). They had already mentioned clinically occult lactiferous duct carcinomas, the carcinoma *in situ*, adenosis, as well as the nonpalpable scirrhous carcinoma, and discussed the relationship between the radiographic findings and the corresponding pathoanatomic structures.

Gershon-Cohen also described the differential diagnosis of radiologically smooth, rounded structures in the breast. However, further diagnostic procedures, such as cyst puncture and pneumocystography, were not yet known. We should be grateful to Gershon-Cohen and Helen Ingelby for compiling, for the first time, a standard work on mammography.

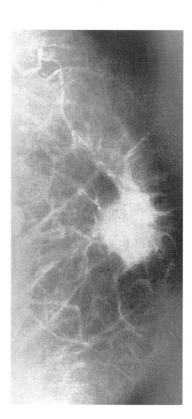

Fig. II, 48. Mammogram of a scirrhous carcinoma (Gershon-Cohen, 1970).

In an extensive study Gershon-Cohen determined that the accuracy of clinical examination with palpation and inspection alone was only 48%, while the radiological examination gave a diagnostic certainty of 90%. He continued: *'In a combination of clinical and radiological findings it should be feasible to detect more than 95% of malignant breast lesions. . . . Hopefully the introduction of routine mammography will lead to a reduction in the mortality statistics as a result.'*

Galactography

In 1930, Ries, from Chicago, was the first to write on galactography. By filling the lactiferous duct system with Lipiodol contrast medium, pathologically dilated lactiferous ducts were proved to be the cause of postweaning bleeding.

In 1937, N. Frederick Hicken, Russel Best and J.P. Tollman, Departments of Surgery and Pathology, University of Nebraska, again reported on the diagnostic role of galactography in diagnosing lactiferous duct diseases (Fig. II, 49).

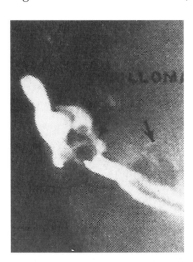

Fig. II, 49. Galactography (Hicken, 1937).

In the same year, Hicken also wrote on the introduction of galactography with contrast media in cases of breast tumours and further on 'aeromammography': a mammographic visualization of breast tumours after insufflation of air into the lactiferous duct system. Hicken pointed out: *'A haemorrhage or serosanguineous secretion may occur in malignancy, lactiferous duct papilloma, Paget's disease of the breast, after trauma, in fibroadenoma, tuberculosis, chronic-cystic mastitis and senile parenchymal hypertrophy. The diagnostic differentiation of the various pathoanatomic causes of bloody breast secretions can be attained by galactography.*

Thorotrast is used as a contrast medium which has proved particularly suitable and well tolerated in more than 375 cases.'

He encouraged the use of stereoscopic radiographic views to obtain a better perspective of the spatial arrangement of abnormal lactiferous ducts. Thorium-dioxide (Heyden), Lipiodine (Ciba), Hippuran (Mallinckrodt), Diodrast (Winthrop), bismuth, oxychloride (Mallinckrodt), 15% sodium iodide as well as Thorotrast and air have been tried as contrast media. Thorotrast proved to be the best tolerated. Many years later, however, the first reports on the relationship between the diagnostic application of Thorotrast and possible development of breast cancer later in life was published (Brody and Cullen, 1957; Ahmed and Steele, 1972, Kingston in Ontario).

Additionally, after a high-dose radiation burden, for instance, as a result of multiple fluoroscopies necessary during pneumothorax treatment of pulmonary tuberculosis in young women, an increased incidence of breast cancer had been observed (Myrden and Hiltz, 1969). The same was found after previous radiotherapy of immature or adolescent mammary tissue in cases of Hodgkin's disease. Despite all this, the result of a life-saving treatment through medical measures, such as additional radiodiagnostic or radiotherapeutic methods, certainly outweighed the risk of a possible carcinomatous disease later in life.

In 1960, a new stimulus to improve radiographic techniques came from Robert L. Egan (Tumor Institute, Department of Radiology, University of Texas, M.D. Anderson Hospital, Houston). He reported on variations of technical factors that would be required for optimal mammographic examination: high milliamperage (300 mA/6 s), low kilovoltage (22–28 kVp), and the use of industrial films (Kodak Industrial M). In addition, he reported the first attempts using fine-granularity intensifying screens: *'With a single intensifying screen–film combination most details are captured, with double intensifying screen–film combination, details of the soft tissues are sacrificed.'* The quality of the image attained by this technique gave him excellent diagnostic accuracy as early as 1960.

Egan also deserves the credit of first using the term 'mammography' for roentgenological examination of the breast; Hicken had only used this name to visualize the lactiferous duct system with contrast medium. In the course of the ensuing technical development of mammography, Egan gave ample attention to the reduction of radiation exposure in mammography as a prerequisite for screening.

Under the sponsorship of the Breast Cancer Detection Demonstration Project (BCDDP), Egan emphatically proposed mammographic screening for early detection of breast cancer since 1973. This was preceded by the Health Insurance Plan's (New York City) mammographic study comprising 64 000 women. The results showed that, in the screening group, the mortality rate of breast carcinoma could be reduced by 30% compared with the control group. This study as well as the BCDDP study (Georgia Baptist Medical Centre and Memorial University in Atlanta) greatly contributed to the acceptance of mammography as a screening method in the early detection of breast cancer. This was later followed by studies in Canada, in The Netherlands and in Sweden (Penn, Hendriks and Tabar, 1987).

In view of the radiation exposure to a large number of healthy women undergoing mammographic screening, all these studies were carried out with a low dose of less than 0.5 rad 5 mSv per examination, which increases the natural risk of carcinoma from 7.0 to 7.07% (at the age of 35 years), with a lower risk in higher age groups.

This dose was a tenth of the annual permitted total body dose in professional exposure to radiation (5.0 rad, 50 mSv). The results of all screening studies carried out in America, Canada and Europe showed a distinct improvement in the early diagnosis of breast cancer and a reduction in the number of radical operations, as well as better recovery and long-term survival rates.

In Europe, it was not until the early 50s that Charles Gros (Fig. II, 50) initiated a new phase in mammography in Strasbourg. The first publication by Gros and Sigrist 'La Radiographie de la Mamelle' [Radiography of Breast] dates back to 1951. The second publication, 'Radiographie de la Glande Mammaere' [Radiography of the Mammary Gland], followed, and thereafter, in rapid succession, Gros wrote a total of 55 publications on diagnostic radiology of the breast. In his book, 'Les Maladies du Sein' [Diseases of the breast], Gros (1963) described, in an elegant French style, the interrelationship of pathology, clinical examination, histology and radiology.

Gros also described the typical carcinomatous configuration of microcalcifications in intraductal comedocarcinoma and pointed to the irregularity of the separate microparticles, their density and their dimension within the pathologically altered tissue. This expanded the basis for the future recognition of differences between malignant and benign microcalcifications of the breast (Lanyi, 1977).

In addition, Gros differentiated very precisely between the various types of growth of breast carcinoma and their radiomorphology (Fig. II, 51). His observations on the development of intracystic carcinoma deserve particular attention. Furthermore, his dealings with benign changes of the female breast, particularly the physiological structural changes of the mammary gland during the course of life, such as hormonal influences due to the menstrual cycle and pregnancy,

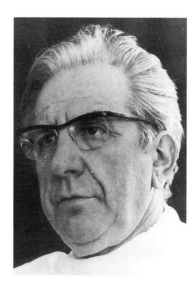

Fig. II, 50. Charles Gros (1910–1984). Worked in Strasbourg/France. Developed with CGR the Senograph, the first device dedicated to mammography. Molybdenum anode with 0,7 mm focal spot. Continued to work on the detection of clinically occult mammary carcinomas.

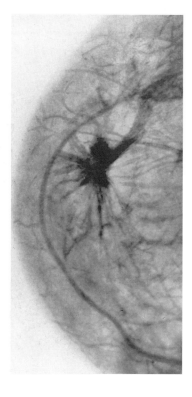

Fig. II, 51. Scirrhous carcinoma of the breast in a mammogram (Gros, 1963).

are of particular importance. Based on radiological and histological findings, he described the various types of mastopathy and the technique of galactography and pneumocystography. Gros began to localize clinically nonpalpable, occult findings by implanting wire hooks preoperatively, and also performed fine-needle aspiration of cysts and firm nodes for cytological examination.

Gros's revolutionary achievement (1966) was the technical improvement of mammography by using a molybdenum-anode tube, which was originally applied for material testing in industry. Resorting to an X-ray tube with a beryllium window fitted with a molybdenum filter for the absorption of the inconsequential low energy radiation that does not contribute to the image, he developed the SENOGRAPH, the first X-ray unit dedicated to mammography (Fig. II, 52).

The improved image quality expanded the knowledge of the fine structures of breast tissue, forming the basis of today's mammography which has become indispensable for the early diagnosis of breast carcinoma in its *in-situ* stage.

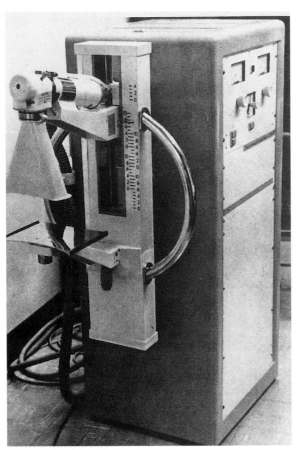

Fig. II, 52. SENOGRAPH, Molybdenum technique according to Gros 1965.

Using a molybdenum anode combined with a molybdenum filter takes advantage of the characteristic radiation of molybdenum at 17.4 and 19.6 keV (in contrast to the previously used tungsten, which has its characteristic radiation lines around 60 keV) for mammographic imaging. Despite the superimposed *Bremsstrahlung*, molybdenum enables a low-energy X-ray technique that is ideally suited to breast tissue.

In Europe, a few Austrian radiologists, encouraged by Gros's experiences and the preceding American publications, adopted mammography and published their results.

The first papers were published by Muntean (1954) 'Early radiological diagnosis and treatment of breast carcinomas', Kratochvil (1954) 'Early surgical diagnosis and treatment of breast carcinomas following preoperative radiotherapy', and Seyss (1957) 'Roentgen diagnostics of breast tumours'. Seyss specifically addressed refinements of the mammographic technique and emphasized the importance of a small focal spot of 0.3 x 0.3 mm necessary to obtain magnification views for improving the detectable details in problematic findings. Attempted tomograms of the female breast (the first by Fugazzola, 1954) failed to improve the diagnostic findings.

Interest in the radiographic examination of the female breast was renewed in Germany in the 50s: the first publications were by Reinhardt (1953), Kuebler (1955), and Dohrmann and Labusch (1958) at the Radiation Institute of the Free University of Berlin (Chairman Professor Oeser). The accuracy of mammography was still viewed rather skeptically: *'The high percentage of erroneous interpretation of benign alterations – in our own material, 20% had been identified as malignant – should be a warning against preoperative radiation therapy without prior histological confirmation by tumour excision.'* On the other hand, the researchers pointed out that carcinomas could be discovered by mammography even in the absence of clinical palpation. However, the idea of breast-screening programs, as proposed by Gershon-Cohen, was still treated with reserve as to its usefulness.

In 1958, Werner, Buttenberg and Zeitz (Radiologic Clinic, Heidelberg, Chairman, Professor Becker, and Heidelberg University Gynecologic Clinic, Chairman Professor Runge) published a paper entitled: 'Roentgen examination of the breast'. Reference was made to the log-etron method, which was developed for military aerial survey photography by Log-Electronics, Washington, after the Second World War. Significant contrast enhancement was provided by this method.

Applying this method, which provides a equalized general density together with an impressive contrast enhancement, Keiling could, at the 39th German Roentgen Congress in 1957, demonstrate remarkable images acquired by Gros in Strasbourg. At the same time, Bischoff and Schott, working for Siemens-Reiniger, studied a contrast enhancement method that was clinically tested by Parschwitz in Bonn, Germany. This method applied television technology using magnification, size reduction, and contrast enhancement as well as negative or positive image display. This method still could not delineate very fine structural details adequately for diagnostic purposes.

In The Netherlands, von Ronnen published an in-depth article on the method and results of mammography in 1956.

In 1962, the first German book on mammography, 'Die Mammographie', was published by Buttenberg and Werner. This book, although just a small contribution compared with the impressive world literature in the field of mammography, was the first in its kind. It is amazing how many diagnoses could be made by the mammographic imaging technique of those days, but only in advanced cases and in context with the clinical findings.

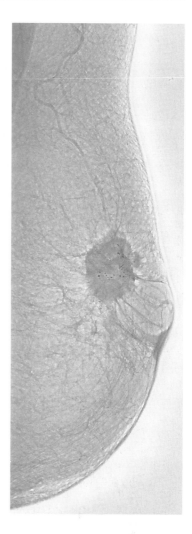

Fig. II, 53. Xerox mammography.

Technical developments

The search for a more reliable diagnostic method was pursued by increasing the image latitude to improve the visualization of the compact structures in the central parenchyma without compromising the visualization of the delicate structures in the fatty peripheral parenchyma and subcutaneous regions of the breast.

In the USA, Gould had tested xeroradiography in the visualization of the female breast since 1960, a technique subsequently used intensively in a clinical setting by John Wolfe of Detroit (Fig. II, 53). The xerographic technique of those days improved the image quality enormously, not only because of its wider latitude, but also because of its intrinsic edge-effect with better demarcation of differences in tissue densities. However, a faithful delineation of microstructures as obtained with today's film-screen combinations, grid techniques and specially designed tubes cannot be achieved by xeroradiography. The equalizing effect of the Xerox technique can interfere with the visualization of fine tissue structures and

the detection of early ductal microcarcinomas. Xeromammography remains advantageous for large breasts and for visualizing breast structures that have substantially different absorption (e.g. after augmentation with silicon implants).

In 1965, Dobretsberger took a different route to improve the mammographic technique: he introduced the isodense method for breast examination to homogenize the different tissue densities. In a special apparatus (FLUIDOGRAPH), the breast was submerged into an alcohol containing Plexiglas receptacle, with the alcohol used as an agent of fat-equivalent attenuation, to obtain an even image of the entire breast, including its subcutaneous fatty tissue and skin (Fig. II, 54). He used a X-ray tube voltage of 40–50 kVp and film–screen combinations, with either one or two screens in a plastic cassette.

Van der Plaats and Nievelstein (1967), as well as Gajewski and Hoeffken (1966), obtained further improvement in image contrast by lowering the X-ray tube voltage to 35–40 kVp and by

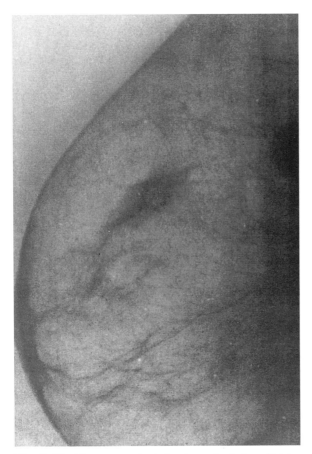

Fig. II, 54. Mammography in isodense technique/fluidography (Dobretsberger, 1965).

using a grid. This isodense method was not developed any further due to its cumbersome operation and inadequate delineation of the more delicate structures, though the obtained isodense images were quite impressive for those days.

Throughout the world, research was undertaken to improve the standard low-radiation technique. In Erlangen, Gajewski's work was a considerable step forward. As early as 1967, he had already indicated the advantages of a specialized X-ray tube with a rotating anode and thinner glass window (abraded). The inherent absorption was reduced to 0.5–0.6 mm aluminium-equivalent. Connected to a 2-pulse generator and a maximum tube voltage of 28 kVp (later also with three-phase generators and a lower voltage), and fitted with special compression devices without additional filtration and without a light beam indicator, these dedicated X-ray tubes could achieve good differentiation of even low attenuation differences in the female breast.

Phototimer

Investigating the relationship between the measurable thickness of the breast and the mAs product revealed no reliable correlation between both values. The adequate exposure times for breast of the same thickness can vary by a factor of three to five.

This called for the construction of a phototimer to obtain reproducible image quality.

Such an automatic exposure control for mammography was the "IONTOMAT" with an ionization chamber developed by Siemens and tested on a large number of patients by Hoeffken, Heuss and Roedel in 1970. Phototiming is now available on all mammographic units.

The next major improvement in mammographic technique can be attributed to M. Friedrich (1977). Using meticulous scientific analyses and practical trials, he laid the foundation for the construction of grids suitable for low-energy X-rays. His work with film densitometry could show that about 44% of the total radiation in mammography was scattered radiation. Friedrich studied the ratio of scattered-to-primary radiation in mammography by investigating the relationship of film gradation, scattered radiation, spatial resolution, and contrast. He realized that collimation and compression alone will not achieve a significant reduction in scattered radiation and that grids are necessary to overcome this problem. He wrote in 1975: 'The technical problems are unresolved as for now.' Friedrich found the solution together with Weskamp.

At first, they tested the physical components of then widely used radiographic units used for mammography: direct exposure industrial film, low-dose system (both Dupont), a combination of industrial film and low-dose intensifying screen.

Investigations of the geometry of radiographic systems and its effect on total unsharpness and detail-recording capability revealed that appreciable differences in the resolution are eroded by the geometric unsharpness and that with an average film-object distance of approximately 3 cm the total resolution of the different systems is about equal. After it was established that the resolution can only be improved by reducing scattered radiation, elaborate investigations followed to determine the relationship between scattered radiation and image size. It could be found that collimation and breast compression, the generally recommended measures for reducing scattered radiation, decrease the proportion of scattered radiation from 45% to 36% at the most.

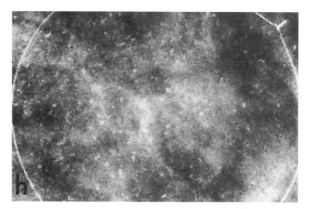

Fig. II, 55. Reduction of scattered radiation by means of the grid technique after Friedrich in 1975. Left (g): mammogram without grid; right (h): mammogram with grid.

Only by halving the amount of scattered radiation, a diagnostically significant improvement of the image quality can be expected. This is only feasible by using the low-kV grid technique (Fig. II, 55).

An 'optimal' low-kV grid requires:

1 high penetration of the primary radiation for the low-energy radiation between 25–35 kVp;
2 low absorption (20% at the most) of the primary radiation in the grid medium (grid ratio 5:1), which still absorbed 30% of the primary radiation. The thickness of the lead strips was reduced from 30 μm (1978) to 16 μm (1983);
3 fewer strips per grid area (strip density of approximately 30 to 35 per centimeter;
4 replacing the aluminum cover and interspace medium with carbon fiber (maximal grid thickness of 3 mm).

The focusing of the grid had to be adapted to the necessary increase in the object–film distance as well as to the increase in focus–film distance from 45 to 60 cm, to accommodate the grid between the breast and film–screen system.

Grid mammography was introduced in 1978.

Figure II, 56 shows the prototype of grid a mammography unit with molybdenum-tube system as proposed by Gros and with a Plexiglas compression plate and grid device after Friedrich, and with a carbon fibre tray and cassette holder.

With a total grid excursion of 18 mm and a travel time of 1 to 4 seconds, the transmission of scattered radiation could be markedly reduced.

To offset the increased radiation dose and the higher kVp setting with the use of grids, a search for dose-reducing screen systems of high image quality began. Friedrich found the Cronex system 70 (Dupont) on MR-50-screen (Agfa Gaevart) to be the best image producing system, which could even capture microcalcifications as small as 100 μm in diameter.

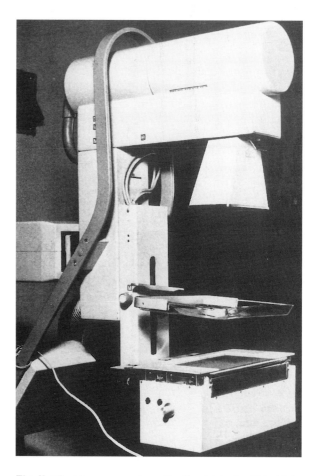

Fig. II, 56. Mammography unit with grid device (Friedrich, 1978).

Initially, it was recommend that the radiological technique be adjusted to the breast thicknesses:

1 up to 3 cm breast thickness: industrial film;
2 between 3 cm and 5 cm breast thickness: industrial film with screen;
3 thicker breasts of considerable density: low-kV grid and industrial film with screen.

At first, there were many objections to the general use of the grid technique and film–screen systems because of cassette-related artifacts and difficulties with the film loading and unloading.

Nevertheless, the grid technique has now been fully adopted worldwide and, used together with film–screen combinations, is the standard mammographic method for any type of breast and tissue density. The considerable reduction of the non-image forming scattered radiation has attained a superb improvement in detecting details in microcalcifications and fine soft tissue structures, resulting in a definite progress of the diagnostic assessment.

Apart from Friedrich and Weskamp, numerous other scientists studied the optimization of radiographic conditions in mammography, the reduction of scattered radiation and the improvement of radiographic systems. We would like to mention the names of a few:

Barnes, G.T. and Brezovich, J.A. (1976)
Deichgräber, E. et al (1974)
Deichgräber, E. et al (1975)
Dutreix, J. et al (1966)
Haus, A.G. et al (1977)
Hüppe, J.R. and Schneider, H.J. (1977)
Kuhn, H. (1977)
Ledin, S. and Wasser, E. (1966)

Miller, E.R. et al (1963)
Ostrum, B.J. et al (1973)
Price, J.L. and Butler, P.D. (1970)
Rossmann, K. (1966)
Stanford, R.W. et al (1959)
Spiegler, G. (1966)
Tonge, K.A., Davis, R. et al (1976)
Trout, E.D. and Kelley, J.P. (1965)
Wagner, R.F. and Weaver, K.E. (1976)
Weissleder, H. and Kiefer, H. (1977).

Innumerable improvements have since been formulated on film sensitivity, optical film density and gradation as well as on screen sensitivity and granulation.

The design of the X-ray tubes has also improved considerably. The initial focal spot size of 0.6 x 0.6 mm could be reduced to 0.4 x 0.4 mm, which has become the maximal permissible focal spot size in the meantime. Currently, almost all mammographic X-ray tubes have a focal spot size of maximal 0.3 x 0.3 mm.

Microfocus magnification technique

Friedrich and Weskamp had already drawn attention to the importance of magnification mammography. Experimental studies and investigations on a large number of patients revealed the advantage of magnification mammography using a small focal spot in recording fine structural details (Fig. II, 57) (Hoeffken, Joetten and Richter, 1977).

In 1987, Teubner, Lenk, Wentz and Georgi refined these conclusions through meticulous scientific work. Their results have since been ver-

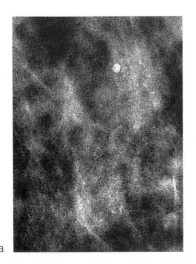
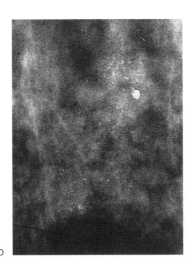
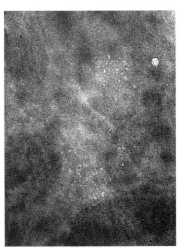

a   b   c

Fig. II, 57a-c. Different detectability of microcalcifications in an intraductal cribriform carcinoma in relation to the focal spot of the X-ray tube **a)** 0.6 mm, **b)** 0.3 mm and **c)** 0.1 mm.

ified and confirmed by several mammographic centres. This has led to the design of the needed bifocal tubes with a 0.3 x 0.3 mm focal spot and an additional 0.1 x 0.1 mm focal spot. By visualizing fine tissue structures not seen before, mammography could considerably increase its diagnostic accuracy.

Today, microfocus magnification is, without question, an asset in recognizing fine structures in mammography and indispensable for the early diagnosis of breast cancer and for decisions about the use of invasive diagnostic procedures. An important technical detail remains to be solved: the geometric, not the projected (apparent), focal spot has to be square in shape instead of rectangular and reduced to 0.1 x 0.1 mm. Only such a focal spot can attain a faithful visualization of microstructures when a magnification factor is applied to the average breast with its inherent object–film distance. The polymorphism of microcalcifications, which provides information about the growth of intraductal carcinomas, can only be discerned under these conditions.

The technical developments of the last four decades and, particularly, the microfocus magnification techniques could improve the recognition of detail, first attempted by Leborgne.

In 1977, Marton Lanyi pointed to the typical arrangement of clusters of microcalcifications and to the polymorphism of the individual microcalcification as essential in the differential diagnosis of carcinomatous calcifications. He published his findings in 1986 in his book, 'Diagnostik und Differentialdiagnostik der Mammaverkalkungen' [Diagnosis and Differential Diagnosis of Breast Calcifications].

Lanyi had reviewed earlier reports by Leborgne, Egan and Gershon-Cohen and other authors on the diagnostic importance of microcalcifications in mammograms and, together with the pathologist P. Citoler, performed comparative analyses of mammographic images with histological sections in a sophisticated scientific analysis of approximately 300 surgical cases with microcalcifications. These comparative analyses revealed that a differentiation between 'benign' calcifications and 'malignant' calcifications can be made: in benign mastopathic changes (Figs II, 58 and fig. II, 59) the individual microcalcification is round and the clustering is round or ovoid as well.

Malignancy is characterized not only by punctate microcalcifications but also by longitudinal, linear, V-shaped or Y-shaped arrangements of the microcalcifications according to their intraductal locations, corresponding to the branching

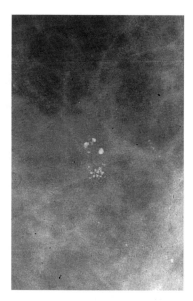

Fig. II, 58. Microcalcifications with a group individual circular particles and a group formation of circular-elliptical particles: microcysts in mastopathy.

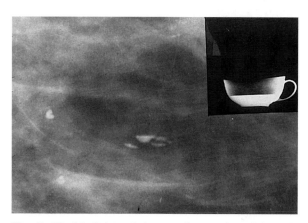

Fig. II, 59. Mediolateral view: sedimentation of the calcium contents in microcysts ("tea-cup phenomenon" after Lanyi).

course of the lactiferous ducts ('triangular phenomenon' (Lanyi); Fig. II, 60). Actually, such a 'triangle' is only seen in the true lateral projection of the intraductal calcifications. Lanyi, together with this chapter's contributor, Lanyi's colleague for many years and coauthor of the book 'Roentgenuntersuchung der Brust' [Roentgenological Examination of the Breast] (Hoeffken and Lanyi, 1973), deserves great merit for the analysis of microcalcifications in the mammogram.

It was not until 1992 that a new and significant technical improvement was achieved through the design of a bimetallic X-ray tube with a rotating molybdenum and rhodium focal track. In addition, molybdenum, rhodium and aluminum fil-

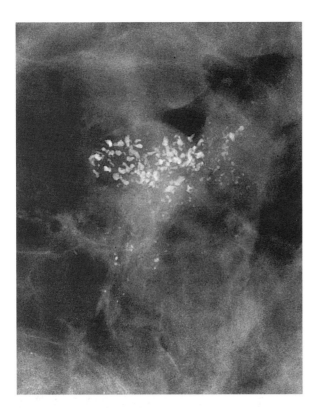

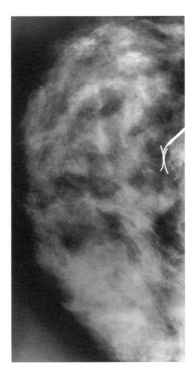

Fig. II, 62. Pre-operative stereo-tactic localization by means of a hook wire in a problem case to facilitate the surgical resection.

Fig. II, 60. Typical group of carcinomatous polymorphic microcalcifications ("triangle phenomenon" after Lanyi): intraductal carcinomatous growth with polymorphism of the group and of the individual particles.

ters can now be exchanged. Following a short test exposure, the system automatically selects the optimal radiation necessary for tissue density. For objects of high density, the rhodium-anode with an aluminum filter or the combination of the rhodium-anode with a rhodium filter is chosen; for lower tissue densities, the molybdenum-anode with molybdenum filter is chosen. This achieves an optimal image quality for all measured density differences of the breast parenchyma. The automatically selected combination is indicated and printed. This results in an optimal image quality and improved diagnostic confidence, as well as the maximally achievable dose reduction.

In 1993, Küchler and Friedrich have published the underlying physics, improvement of image quality and dose reduction of the optimal adjustment of the anode-filter combination.

In the future, attention will be directed towards digital imaging.

First reports of digital mammography go back to Smathers et al. (1986) and Asage (1987). In Germany, Krahmann (1988) and Friedrich (1989), later also Johnen, published their experi-

ence with mammography using a digital luminescence radiographic system with high resolution storage plate and laser beam scanning. Currently, the advantage of a wide image latitude, elimination of incorrect exposure and standardized digital processing must be balanced against an inferior resolution due to the width of the laser beam of 100 µm and the still inadequate resolution of the storage plate, video display systems and hard copy. Work on improvements is already in progress.

In the field of mammography, a first attempt at introducing digital imaging in stereotactic puncture has been made. Visualizing the fine structures of soft tissues and microcalcifications with a diameter of 100–200 µm is not yet possible with the current digital imaging systems.

References

Agnew, D.H.: The Principles and Practise of Surgery. Lippincott philadelphia, Bd. III (1883).

Ahmed, M.Y., H.D. Steele: Breast Carcinoma 30 Years after Thorotrast Mammography. The Canadian Journal of Surg. 15 (1972) 45–49.

Baraldi, A.: Roentgen neumo-mastia. Rev. de cir. des Buenos Aires 14 (1935) 321–342.

Barnes G.T., J.A. Brezovich: The Intensity of Scattered Radiation in Mammography. 4th Internat. Confer. Medical Physics, Montreal, 1976.

Fig. II, 61. a) The stereotactic principle of localization of nonpalpable lesions in the breast. **b)** Stereotactic examination table for prone patient (after Nordenstroem/now manufactured by Fischer) **c)** Stereotactic supplement attached to modern mammography unit for examinations with the patient sitting. **d)** Stereotactic views obtained for documenting the position of the needle in a problem case. **e)** Stereotactically obtained tissue core exposed in the biopsy window by retracted outer cannula of the Tru-Cut needle.

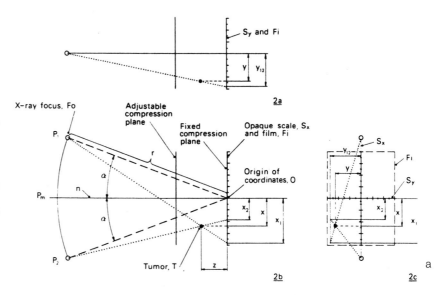

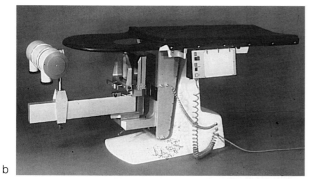

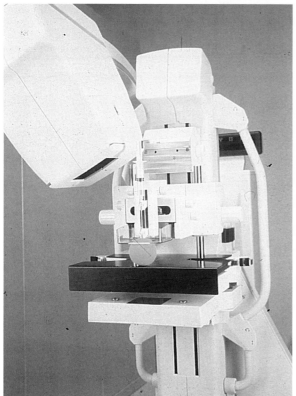

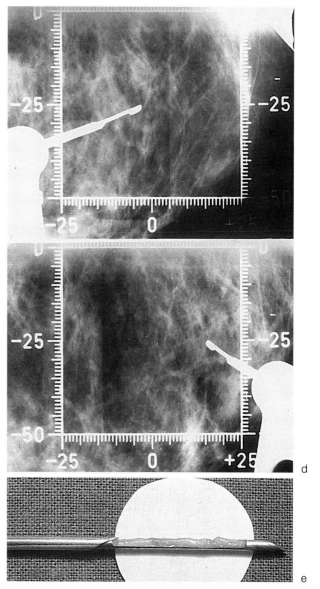

Brody, J.L., M. Cullen: Carcinoma of breast seventeen years after mammography with Thorotrast. Surgery 42 (1957) 600.

Buttenberg, D., K. Werner: Die Mammographie. Schattauer Verlag, 1962.

Deichgräber, E., S. Reichmann, M. Buren: Film Quality in Mammary Radiography. Acta Radiol. Diagnosis 15 (1974) 93–103.

Deichgräber, E., S. Reichmann, K.G. Strid: Intensifying Screens in Soft Tissue Radiography. Acta Radiol. Diagnosis 16 (1975) 54–64.

Dobretsberger, W.: Mammadiagnostik mittels Isodens-Technik. Radiol. Austriaca 13 (1962) 239.

Dobretsberger, W.: Die Fluidographie der weiblichen Brust. Electromedica 4 (1967) 12.

Dobretsberger, W.: Die isodensische Weichteilaufnahme (Fluidogramm). Radiologe 5 (1965) 28.

Dohrmann, R., R. Labusch: Über den Wert der röntgenologischen Mammadiagnostik. Chirurg 29 (1958) 3.

Dominguez, C.M., A. Lucas: Investigacion radiografica y quimica sobre el calcio precipitado en tumores del aparato genital feminino. Bol. de la Soc. Anatomia Patologica I (1930) 217–226.

Dutreix J., R. Riby, Y. Fernandez: Die Bedeutung der Streuung für das Röntgenbild. Anwendung auf die Fernröntgenographie. In: Stieve, F.E., C. Fischer: Bildgüte in der Radiologie. Stuttgart (1966) 180–190.

Egan, R.L.: Experience with mammography in tumor institution: evaluation of 1000 studies. Radiology 75 (1960) 894–900.

Egan, R.L.: Mammography. Thomas, Springfield 1964.

Egan, R.L.: Fundamentals of Technique and Positioning in Mammography. Oncology 23 (1969) 99–112.

Egan, R.L., M.B. Sweeny, C.W. Sewell: Intramammary calcifications without an associated mass in benign and malignant diseases. Radiology 137 (1980) 1.

Espaillat, A.: Contribution a létude radiographique de sein normal et pathologique. These de Paris (1933) 417.

Finsterbusch, R., F. Gross: Kalkablagerungen in den Milch- und Ausführungsgängen beider Brustdrüsen. Röntgenpraxis 6 (1934) 172.

Fray, W.W., S.L. Warren: Stereoscopie röntgenography of the breasts and aid in establishing diagnosis of mastitis and carcinoma. Ann. Surg. 95 (1932) 425–432.

Friedrich, M.: Der Einfluß der Streustrahlung auf die Abbildungsqualität bei der Mammographie. Fortschr. Röntgenstr. 123 (1975) 556–566.

Friedrich, M., P. Weskamp: Bildgütefaktoren bei der Filmmammographie. I Mitteilung. Fortschr. Röntgenstr. 125 (1976) 269–279.

Friedrich, M., P. Weskamp: Bildgütefaktoren bei der Filmmammographie. II Mitteilung. Fortschr. Röntgenstr. 125 (1976) 461–471.

Friedrich, M.: Bildqualität in der Mammographie. Einfluß der Streustrahlung und der Bildaufzeichnungssysteme. Röntgenstrahlen 36 (1977) 4–11.

Friedrich, M.: Neuere Entwicklungstendenzen in der Mammographie Technik: die Raster Mammographie. Fortschr. Röntgenstr. 128 (1978) 2.

Friedrich, M., P. Weskamp: Komplexe Bewertung filmmammographischer Abbildungssysteme. Teil I: Methodische Grundlagen. Fortschr. Röntgenstr. 140 (1984) 585.

Friedrich, M., P. Weskamp: Komplexe Bewertung filmmammographischer Abbildungssysteme. Teil II: Vergleich von 18 Systemen mittels Signal-Rausch-Matrix. Fortschr. Röntgenstr. 140 (1984) 707.

Friedrich, M.: Folien-Raster-Kombinationen in der Mammographie. Lymphol., 1983.

Friedrich, M.: Schlitzblendentechnik für die Mammographie. Fortschr. Röntgenstr. 141 (1984) 574.

Fugazzola: Radiol. med. Torino 40 (1954) 643–652.

Gajewski, H., W. Hoeffken: Vergleichungsuntersuchung zur Mammographie mit Weichstrahltechnik und Isodensmethode. Radiologe 6 (1966) 407.

Gajewski, H.: Aufnahmetechnik bei der Mammographie. Röntgenpraxis 20 (1967) 177.

Gajewski, H., H.P. Heilmann: Experimentelle Untersuchungen zur optimalen Aufnahmetechnik bei der Mammographie. Fortschr. Röntgenstr. 11 (1971) 248.

Gershon-Cohen, J., A.E. Colcher: Evaluation of roentgen diagnosis of early carcinoma of breast. J. Am. Med. Ass. 108 (1937) 867–871.

Gershon-Cohen, J., A. Strickler: Roentgenologic examination of normal breast; its evaluation in demonstrating early neoplastic changes. Am. J. Roentgenol. and Rad. Therapy 40 (1938) 189–210.

Gershon-Cohen, J., H. Ingleby: Roentgenography of Cancer of the Breast. Am. J. Roentgenol. 68 (1952) 1–7.

Gershon-Cohen, J., H. Ingleby, M.B. Hermel: Roentgenographie Diagnosis of Calcification in Carcinoma of the Breast. J. Am. Med. Ass. 29 (1953) 676–677.

Gershon-Cohen, J., H. Ingleby: Carcinoma of the breast. Roentgenographic Technik and Diagnostic Criteria. Radiology 60 (1953) 68–76.

Gershon-Cohen, J., H. Ingleby, M.B. Hermel: Accuracy of preoperative x-ray Diagnosis of Breast Tumor. Surg. St. Louis 35 (1954) 766–771.

Gershon-Cohen, J., H. Ingleby, M.B. Hermel: Occult carcinoma of the breast. Arch. Surg. 70 (1955) 385.

Gershon-Cohen, J., H. Ingleby, M.B. Hermel: Calcification in secretory disease of the breast. Am. J. Roentgenol. 76 (1956) 132.

Gould, H.R., F.F. Ruzicka, R. Sanchez-Ubeda, J. Perez: Xeroradiography of the breast. Am. J. Roentgenol. 84 (1960) 220–223.

Gros, Ch.M., M. Sigrist: La radiographie de la mamelle. Annuel Congres des Medecins Electro-Radiologique de Culture latine, Brussel 1951.

Gros, Ch.M., M. Sigrist: La radiographie et la transillumination de la mamelle. Strasbourg (1951) 451.

Gros, Ch.M., L. Fruhling, R. Sigrist, R. Keiling: Des calcifications de la glande mammaire tumorale. Congres des Med. Electro-Radiol. C.R., Madrid (1952) 6.

Gros, Ch.M.: Les maladies du sein. Masson, Paris (1963).

Halsted, W.S.: A clinical and histological study of certain adenocarcinomata of the breast. Ann. Surg. 28 (1898) 557

Haus, A.G., C.E. Metz, J.T. Chiles, K. Rossmann: The effect of X-Ray spectra from Molybdenum and Tungsten target tubes on image quality in mammography. Radiology 118 (1976) 705–709

Hicken, N.F.: Mammography: roentgenologic diagnosis of breast tumors by means of contrast media. Surg. Gynec. and Obst. 64 (1937) 593–603

Hicken, N.F.: Mammography: preoperative visualization and diagnosis of breast tumors by contrast roentgenograms. Nebraska Med. J. 22 (1937) 211–213

Hicken, N.F., R.R. Best, J.P. Tollman: Mammographic recognition of intracystic papilloma of the breast. Am. J. Surg. 36 (1937) 611–617

Hicken, N.F., R.R. Best, H.B. Hunt: Discharges from nipple; their clinical significance and mammographic interpretation. Arch. Surg. 35 (1937) 1079–1094

Hoeffken, W., C. Hintzen: Die Diagnostik der Mammazysten durch Mammographie und Pneumozystographie. Fortschr. Röntgenstr. 112 (1970) 9

Hoeffken, W., E. Heuss, E. Rödel: Die Notwendigkeit einer Belichtungsautomatik für die Mammographie. Radiologe 10 (1970) 154

Hoeffken, W., M. Lanyi: Röntgenuntersuchung der Brust. Thieme Verlag 1973

Hoeffken, W., G. Jötten, D. Richter: A new method for reducing radiation exposure and improving the image quality in mammography. Medicamundi 22 (1977) 2

Hüppe, J.R., H.J. Schneider: Zur Frage des richtigen Mammographiefilms. Radiologe 17 (1977) 195–196

Kleinschmidt, O.: Brustdrüse. In: Die Klinik der bösartigen Geschwülste. Edited by Zweife, P., E. Payr (Hrsg.), S. Hirzel, Leipzig (1927) 5–90

Kratochvil, K.: Zur chirurgischen Frühdiagnostik und Therapie des Mammacarcinoms unter Berücksichtigung der präoperativen Bestrahlung. Fortschr. Röntgenstr. 81 (1954) 727–734

Kreuzer, G., E. Roquot: Die Triple-Diagnostik gut- und bösartiger Mammatumoren. Geburtsh. und Frauenheilk. 34 (1974) 279

Kübler, E.: Über die Differentialdiagnose des pathologischen Mammabildes. Fortschr. Röntgenstr. 82 (1955) 789–799

Küchler, M., M. Friedrich: Fortschritte in der Mammographie-Technik, Bi-Metall-Anodenröhren und selektive Filtertechnik. Fortschr. Röntgenstr. 159 (1993) 91–96

Kuhn, H.: Optimierung der Aufnahmebedingungen in der Mammographie. Elektromedica 45 (1977) 32–27

Lanyi, M.: Differentialdiagnose der Microverkalkungen. Die verkalkte mastopathische Microzyste. Radiologe 17 (1977) 217

Lanyi, M.: Differentialdiagnose der Microverkalkungen. Röntgenbildanalyse von 60 intraductalen Carcinomen, das "Dreieckprinzip". Radiologe 17 (1977) 213

Lanyi, M., P. Citoler: Differentialdiagnostik der Microverkalkungen. Die kleinzystische (blunt duct) Adenose. Fortschr. Röntgenstr. 134 (1981) 225

Lanyi, M.: Formanalyse von 153 Microverkalkungsgruppen maligner Genese. Das "Dreiecksprinzip". Fortschr. Röntgenstr. 136 (1982) 77

Lanyi, M.: Formanalyse von 136 Microverkalkungsgruppen benigner Genese. Fortschr. Röntgenstr. 136 (1982) 182

Lanyi, M.: Formanalyse von 5641 Microverkalkungen bei 100 Milchgangskarzinomen: Die Polymorphie. Fortschr. Röntgenstr. 139 (1983) 240

Lanyi, M., K.F.R. Neufang: Möglichkeiten und Grenzen der Differentialdiagnostik gruppierter intramammärer Microverkalkungen. Fortschr. Röntgenstr. 141 (1984) 4

Lanyi, M.: Diagnostik und Differentialdiagnostik der Mammaverkalkungen. Springer, Heidelberg, New York, Tokyo 1986

Leborgne, R.: Diagnostico de los procesos pathologicos de la mama por la radiografia con la inyeccion de medios de contraste. Obst. y. ginec. latino-am. 2 (1944) 551–561

Leborgne, R.: Estudio radiologico del sistema canalicular de la glandula mamaria normal y patologica. Monografia, Montevideo 1943

Leborgne, R.: Biopsia por nia endocanalicular en los procesos patologicos de la glandula mamaria. Obst. y. ginec. latino-am. 2 (1944) 605–614; Arch. de ginec. y obst. 3 (1944) 331-346

Leborgne, I., R. Leborgne: Endoscopia de los canales galactofores. V.J. Rioplatenses de obst. y. ginec. 4 (1945) 107–114

Leborgne, R.: Estudio radiologico de la glandula mamaria. Bol. soc. de cir. 17 (1946) 336–364

Leborgne, R.: Diagnostico de los tumores de la mama por la radiografia simple. Bol. Soc. cir. d. Urugay, 20 (1949) 407–422

Leborgne, R.: Diagnosis of tumors of the breast by simple roentgenography, calcifications in carcinomas. Am. J. Roentgenol. 65 (1951) 1–11

Leborgne, R.: Esteatonecrosis quistica calcificata de la mama. Thorax 16: 172

Ledin, S., E. Wasser: Bekämpfung der Streustrahlung. In: Handbuch der medischen Radiologie III (1966) 305

Lockwood, I.H.: Radiation in carcinoma of the breast. J. Arkansas med. ass. 28 (1931) 51–55

Lockwood, I.H., W. Stewart: Roentgen study of physiologic and pathologic changes in mammary gland. J. Am. Med. Ass. 99 (1932) 1461–1466

Lockwood, I.H.: Roentgen-ray evaluation of breast symptoms. Am. J. Roentgenol. and Rad. Therapy 29 (1933) 145–155

Miller, E.R., E.D. Nickel, N. Scotfield, C. Mott: Radiographic density and contrast versus quantity and quality of radiation. Radiology 80 (1963) 668–685

Muntean, E.: Zur radiologischen Frühdiagnose und Therapie des Mammacarcinoms. Fortschr. Röntgenstr. 81 (1954) 201–205

Myrden, J.A., J.E. Hiltz: Breast cancer following multiple fluoroscopies during artificial pneumothorax treatment of pulmonary tuberculosis. Ca. Med. Assoc. J. 100 (1969) 1032

Nordenström, B.E.W.: Biologically closed electric circuits. Nordia Med. Publ. 1983

Ostrum, B.J., W. Becker, H.J. Isard: Low-dose mammography. Radiology 109 (1973) 323–326

Plaats, G.J. van der, J.T.K.G. Nievelstein: Die Mammographie nach Dobretsberger. J. Radiol. Electrol. 48 (1967) 656

Price, J.L., P.D. Butler: The reduction of radiation and exposure time in mammography. Br. J. Radiol. 43 (1970) 251–255

Reimann, S.P., P.S. Seabold: Correlation of x-ray picture with histology in certain breast lesions. Am. J. Cancer 17 (1933) 34–41

Reinhardt, K.: Die Bedeutung der Mammoaufnahmen für Diagnostik und Verlaufsbeobachtung des Brustkrebses. Fortschr. Röntgenstr. 78 (1953) 714–718

Ries, E.: Diagnostic lipiodol injection into milkducts followed by abscess formation. Am. J. Obst. and Gynec. 20 (1930) 414–416

Ronnen, J.R. von: Plain roentgenography of the breast. Amsterdam Academic Press, (1956) 229

Rossmann, K.: Comparison of several methods for evaluation image quality of radiographic screen-film systems. Am. J. Roentgenol. 97 (1966) 772–775

Salomon, A.: Beiträge zur Pathologie und Klinik der Mammakarzinome. Arch. klin. Chir. 103 (1913) 573

Seabold, P.S.: Diagnosis of breast diseases by x-ray. Ann. Surg. 94 (1931) 443–444

Seabold, P.S.: Roentgenographic diagnosis of diseases of breast. Surg. Gynec. and Obst. 53 (1931) 461–468

Seabold, P.S.: Procedure in roentgen study of breast. Am. J. Roentgenol. and Rad. Therapy 29 (1933) 850–851

Seyss, R.: Zur Röntgendiagnostik von Mammatumoren. Fortschr. Röntgenstr. 86 (1957) 356–363

Spiegler, G.: Bildgüte und Dosis in der Röntgenologie. In: Bildgüte in der Radiologie. Hrsg. F.E. Stieve, G. Fischer, Stuttgart 1966

Stanford, R.W., R.D. Moore, T.H. Hills: Comparative performance of grids in relation to their stated ratio. Br. J. Radiol. 32 (1959) 106–113

Steinthal, C.P.: Zur Dauerheilung des Brustkrebses. Beitr. z. klin. Chir. 47 (1905) 226

Teubner, J., J.Z. Lenk, K.U. Wentz, M. Georgi: Vergrößerungsmammographie mit 0,1 mm Mikrofokus. Radiologe 27 (1987) 155–164

Trout, E.D., J.P. Kelley: Scattered radiation in a phantom from diagnostic quality radiation. Radiology 85 (1965) 546–554

Velpeau, A.: The diseases of the breast and mammary region. Zit. n. Haagensen, C.D.: Diseases of the breast. Saunders, Philadelphia 1856

Vogel, W.: Die Röntgendarstellung von Mammatumoren. Arch. klin. Chir. 171 (1932) 618–626

Wagner, R.F., K.E. Weaver: Prospects for X-ray exposure reduction using rare earth intensifying screens. Radiology 118 (1976) 183–189

Warren, S.L.: A roentgenologic study of the breast. Am. J. Roentgenol. and Rad. Therapy 24 (1930) 113–124

Weissleder, H., H. Kiefer: Mammographie mit minimaler Strahlendosis. Fortschr. Röntgenstr. 126 (1977) 520–529

Werner, K., D. Buttenberg, H. Zeitz: Zur Röntgenuntersuchung der Mamma. Fortschr. Röntgenstr. 88 (1958) 690–698

Wolfe, J.N.: Mammography: errors in diagnosis. Radiology 87 (1966) 214

Wolfe, J.N.: Xerography of the breast. Radiology 91 (1968) 231–240

Chapter 3

The invisible light captured

Diagnostics of organs by means of artificial absorption changes

Introduction

G. Rosenbusch, M. Oudkerk, E. Ammann

At the end of the nineteenth century, medicine expanded enormously following advances in physical recording methods, chemical analyses, bacteriology, serology and pathology. Furthermore, surgery benefited through anesthesia, antisepsis and asepsis.

After the Hungarian Philipp Ignaz Semmelweis (1818–1865) could reduce the death-rate of puerperal fever by hand washing with a chlorinate lime solution and by taking general hygienic measures, the Englishman Joseph Lister (1827–1912) could lower the mortality of his operations to 2% after he had introduced carbolic acid as an antiseptic in 1865. To appreciate the role of antisepsis and asepsis, it should be remembered that before their introduction 70 of 100 patients used to die after amputation.

After Robert Koch (1843–1910) had proved that bacteria cause wound infections, antisepsis was accepted almost immediately, followed by asepsis, in several European countries, including Germany, and in the USA.

Before the nineteenth century, measures for alleviating pain were rather limited. For inevitable limb amputations, compression of the nerve plexus or hypothermia were tried. Opium, cocaine or alcohol were also used to reduce the sensation of pain.

In the first half of the nineteenth century, laughing gas, ether and chloroform were discovered and introduced as narcotics by Horace Wells (1815–1848), Thomas W. Morton (1829–1869), and James Y. Simpson (1811–1870). Already in 1871, the first endotracheal narcosis was successfully performed. Further improvements affected lumbar and local anesthesia and intravenous narcosis. Work on improving and refining anesthetic measures continues to this day.

After it had become possible at the beginning of the second half of the nineteenth century to operate without pain and under sterile conditions, surgical procedures of the abdomen, urogenital system, lungs and heart were developed.

In 1881, Theodor Billroth (1829–1894) performed the first gastrectomy on a woman with a gastric carcinoma. Appendicitis, if timely diagnosed, was no longer invariably fatal after surgery since opening of the peritoneal cavity had become a procedure of low risk. In 1882, Carl Langenbuch (1846–1901) was the first to remove a gallbladder because of cholelithiasis. Thoracic surgery was introduced around the turn of the century: the first heart sutures after an injury were placed by Ludwig Rehn in 1896, soon followed by lung surgery performed by Ferdinand Sauerbruch (1875–1951), who developed the negative-pressure method, which was soon surpassed by the positive-pressure method.

The preoperative diagnostic evaluation was of great importance for these and many other surgical procedures. Previously, the diagnosis had been based on case history, palpation, auscultation, percussion and laboratory findings. Exploratory laparotomy was often necessary. An early or timely diagnosis could not be made for many operable changes of the thoracic or abdominal cavity. Endoscopy of the oesophagus and stomach was in its very early stages and several decades had to go by before the flexible scope became available. The discovery of X-rays and their application in the diagnostic process was therefore of vital importance: roentgenology or, as it is generally referred today, radiology became an indispensable and reliable partner of surgery.

Radiographs of the lungs and skeleton provided much valuable information. This was true only to a lesser degree for the soft tissues, such as the intestines and retroperitoneal cavity. Although calcifications could be recognized in the abdominal cavity and classified according to their position, proof remained absent unless confirmed by subsequent surgery. On the basis of the intestinal distribution of air, only assumptions as to the condition of the intestines were possible. It is therefore not surprising that in the early days attempts were made to visualize organs or organ systems by means of administered substances. These substances had to be of different absorption coefficients for X-rays than for the organs to be demonstrated. They should be low, as in gas and air, or considerably higher. In January 1896, the angiography of a cadaver hand was, surprisingly, the first investigation undertaken with a contrast medium. Both E. Haschek and T.O. Lindenthal from Vienna had apparently scrutinized Roentgen's articles, in which he had pointed out that substances with a higher absorption coefficient exist. Haschek's and Lindenthal's contrast media, however, could only be used for a non-living specimen (s. Fig. III, 96).

The process of developing contrast substances for living patients depended on the differing properties needed to visualize internal organs. Water-insoluble, nonabsorbable contrast media were necessary for the alimentary tract. For the visualization of the biliary tract, contrast media had to be excreted by the liver, and for visualization of the urinary tract, they had to be filtered and excreted by the glomeruli and/or tubuli. They should not be toxic or allergenic and should not affect the circulatory system, and, of course, produce an adequate contrast in the organs to be examined. The pharmaceutical industry accepted this challenge and until today strives for constant improvement in the development of substances with more contrast and better tolerance.

While radiographs of the thorax and skeleton could be taken without fluoroscopy, the radiographic examinations of the alimentary tract, urogenital tract, and vessels require fluoroscopy as an essential part.

Fluoroscopy allowed: analysis of the function of many organs; localization for spot-film radiography; introduction of catheters for subsequent contrast-medium injection; and insertion of protheses.

How was fluoroscopy carried out in those first decades? In 1908, Gocht (s. Fig. I, 23) wrote that in addition to the photographic plate, there was a second medium, the fluorescent screen, which

could also 'look' through the body without 'time-consuming machinations'. But even today, barium platinocyanide, as Roentgen had used, has maintained its place. He wrote:

'The carrier of the screen consists of a good, even, white piece of cardboard. The aim is to make barium platinocyanide from a very pure platinum chloride without any foreign metals; this is purified by repeated recrystallization and appropriate further treatment until it possesses the necessary fluorescence. The salt is repeatedly sieved to obtain the most regular grain possible, because this is the only way to attain a satisfactory illuminating power. The separate barium platinocyanide particles should not become too small either, so that the fluorescent quality does not suffer. It is further of great importance that the salt is applied to the paper evenly. Particularly in the past, when they did not have machines especially built for this purpose, dark, light and cloud-like patches were seen on the fluorescent screen, which, if not evaluated properly, could lead to false diagnoses or at least give grounds to an aggravation of the interpretation. This is no longer true today.

The layer side of the plate is covered with a colourless varnish to protect against stains and damage, In addition, a transparent, very thin celluloid plate is drawn tight on top of this.

Usually wooden frames were used in which the screen was drawn tightly and were therefore easier to manage. . . . The screens were custom-made and this serves an important role in two respects. Firstly, a screen is needed to cover a general view of the part of the body. To cover the largest body region a screen of 30 x 40 cm is sufficient. However, because the parts of the screen next to the object to be fluoroscoped are hit directly by the X-rays, they appear particularly bright and blind the eyes; in this respect the bright parts disturb the exact screening of the shadow image. Secondly, therefore, the screen should be as large as the part of the body to be radiographed, or a larger one should be used first for topographic orientation, followed by a smaller one to enter into the interpretation of the respective details. One should therefore be availed of several screens. This can be avoided by ordering some black cardboard frames of various central apertures together with a 30 x 40 cm screen at the same time. The screen is always stored in a dark place; it is therefore best to hang it in a 50-cm-long binding sling which has been attached to the broadside of the screen and facing the wall.

In case only a survey or radioscopy is needed, without the necessity for others to view it, or when radioscopy takes place in a partly darkened room, a smaller sized screen consisting of a black paste or thin black varnished wood can be made at the bottom of a stereoscopic type of box. Such apparatuses, called fluoro-

scope or cryptoscope, were manufactured in appropriate mountings.

The handle serves for easy use, and the opening for the eyes is padded with fur so that daylight is completely shut off from the screen when the face is put against it; the radiographic screen can be taken from the bottom. It is also practical to have a cardboard frame with an aperture of 6 x 8 or 6 x 10 cm, e.g. to account for the very small dimensions in incidental screening of the eye sockets.

As tempting as such an instrument looks, few could claim to have been used by serious investigators in difficult roentgenoscopy....

Fluoroscopy is performed in the upright, sitting and supine positions, depending on the particular part of the body and depending on how we wish to take the radioscopy and measurement, e.g. of the heart ratio in the upright or supine position.

For all fluoroscopies in a supine position we need a table top penetrable for roentgen rays and where the tube can easily be placed under the table. . . .

All fluoroscopes are furnished with collimators and the investigator who operates them properly does not, of course, need the above described collimator devices of the fluorescence screen. Two points of view are decisive in the lead-scanner-collimator technique, both equally important: firstly there is the objective to obtain really clear images, and secondly the protection of the investigator against roentgen rays. . . .

The roentgen tube is securely fixed inside the box, with its front covered by a 4–5-cm-thick lead plate. In the middle is a circular opening 12 cm in diameter, which can be enlarged or narrowed with lead collimator rings. This heavy box hangs from a special iron construction and can be moved up, down and sideways. Levy-Dorn placed an additional glass plate on top of the layer side of the fluorescent screen to protect the investigator against the roentgen rays that traverse the body of the patient and the fluorescent screen.

Albers-Schoenberg described similar lead screens in his book on roentgen technique; these have the advantage that the entire box is covered by lead so that tube radiation outside the box is impossible. The real collimator device consists of a sliding lead screen; the entire box rests on a heavy iron stand and can be moved up and down. This set-up also ensures that the roentgen rays passing through the lead diaphragm can leave the box. . . .

The tube does not need to have such a small focus because the screen never has, or is expected to have, such finely detailed images as are present in the high-sensitive photographic plate. In addition, we should always use tubes of a certain weakness to achieve a good contrasting image. Tubes with the capacity to generate a male pelvis on the plate are not suitable for fluoroscopy due to their considerable pene-

trative power. In such cases, the bones would be radiographed so strongly that the hand, arm and knee would show too little contrast with the soft tissues; in the thorax it is particularly necessary to protect oneself against the all-penetrating light. With very hard tubes nothing can be differentiated, exact observations are only possible in good differential light. . . .

Because it is often required to maintain the image, a transparent piece of paper is fixed onto the glass plate, on which the image is copied with a pencil or directly onto the glass with an "oily glass pen"'.

Everybody engaged in radiographic examinations had to be mechanically and technically inclined. Alone the facts that before the examination the quality of the tube had to be tested by hand and the eyes adjusted to the dark for several minutes – a physician could easily be recognized as roentgenologist by the red goggles (Fig. III, 1) until well into the sixites – are witness to the enormous technical progress achieved between then and now.

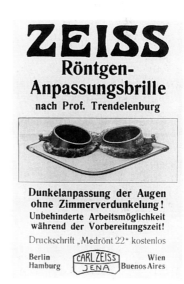

Fig. III, 1. Advertisement for Zeiss-Roentgen adaptation goggles.

High-voltage was first conducted through blank wires from the inductor to the tube. This was of great danger, and protective measures against electric shock and radiation had to be taken. In the early thirties, patient positioning was improved and devices introduced that could place either fluoroscopic screen or cassette device in a radiation-protected standby position, allowing a rapid change from fluoroscopy to radiography. This phase in the development was pursued by engineers with great enthusiasm. Each movement, such as moving the cassette from the park position to the exposure position, is associated with vibration, leading to motion unsharpness on the film. Proper balancing of its components determined quality and ease of the control of its component. Three approaches were taken: counter weights over pulleys, springs or electromechanical devices.

The X-ray tube had a low performance and radiated continually. The mode of operating the X-ray tube had to be switched between fluoroscopy and photography since not only the applied voltage had to be changed but also the current required to increase the output for adequate exposure per unit time. X-ray tubes manufactured according to Coolidge's design could be operated with voltage and current that can be varied over a wide range. The increased output was made pos-

sible by the rotating anode. Rotation was not needed for fluoroscopy, thus the bearing of the rotating anode could rest and the X-ray tube's lifetime prolonged. Many functions had to be performed before a film could be exposed. Radiologist and assistants had to perform all these operations by hand. Later, technical advancements helped automate the operations. With automatic exposure control, incorrect exposure times were avoided since it was no longer necessary to guess the radiolucency or, respectively, absorption of the organ to be radiographed.

Switching the roentgen equipment back from film exposure to fluoroscopy also took time; the temperature of the cathode cooled only slowly to the lower output needed for fluoroscopy.

Only after the fluorescent screen had been superseded by the image intensifier (Fig. III, 2), it was possible to work in an undimmed examination room.

The image intensifier represented one of the most important developments in diagnostic radiology. The adaptation goggles, the roentgenologist's trade mark, disappeared. In the sixties, the overtable unit was added to the conventional undertable fluoroscopic unit. The X-ray tube is suspended from the ceiling above patient and table, and spot-film device with image intensifier, light distributor, video and 70/100-mm camera below the table. This arrangement had the advantage of easy access to the patient, who no longer was squeezed between spot-film carriage and table. Furthermore, the same X-ray tube could be used for spot-film exposures and Bucky radiography. It was even possible to obtain oblique projections and to perform linear tomography. As a re-

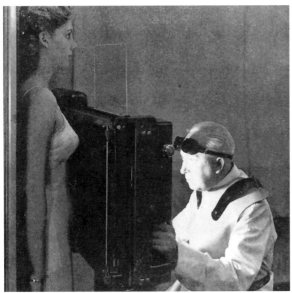

Fig. III, 2a. Fluoroscopy with fluoroscopic screen in the dark.

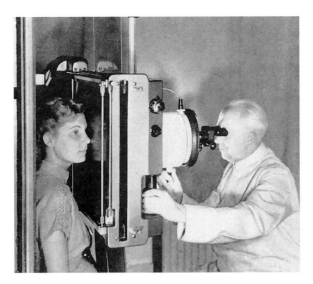

Fig. III, 2b. Image intensifier.

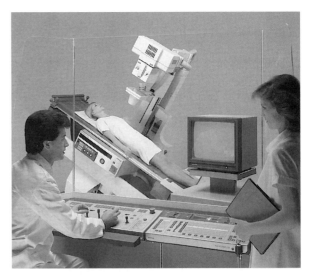

Fig. III, 2c. Image intensifier coupled to a television chain.

sult, a single examination room sufficed for contrast medium examinations in the morning and Bucky radiographs in the afternoon. Only the image geometry of the spot-film device is inferior for the overtable unit because of the increased film-focus distance of one meter or more. The patient is also subjected to a higher radiation dose due to the added absorption of the table top and the inevitable increase in exposure. This could be compensated by obtaining 70/100-mm films from the image intensifier, which only required about one-third of the previous dose. Eventually, sensitive screens, mechanical film processing, and automatic exposure control reduced the radiation exposure. Both overtable and undertable units are still supported today. The overtable units require generators and X-ray tubes of stronger performance and higher energy rating.

X-ray tubes with energy ratings of 100 kW and more were necessary. The heavy workload of the overtable units over many hours required air cooling since the entire work had to be done by only one tube. The undertable unit is equipped with two or even three tubes: a tube under the table to be used with the spot-film device and a tube over the table to be used with the built-in Bucky grid as well as with a tomographic device and Bucky wall stand.

Rationalization and simplification led to cassetteless systems at the end of the sixties and beginning of the seventies, and carrying the heavy cassettes from the dark room and examination room was no longer necessary.

Finally, television has enabled instant replay of recorded sequential images (MEMOSPOT). This opened up the possibility to decide whether contrast medium examinations are adequate or not, even before the film has been developed.

Interventional radiology, which could flourish in the eighties and nineties through the widely used image amplifier television systems, has its specific demands for the equipment manufacturer: better patient accessibility, but also multidirectional fluoroscopy to project lesions without interfering superimposed structures as well as instant high-quality images.

This meant that the engineers had to design a tilting table attached to a C-arm mounted with the X-ray tube and image intensifier. The television system, analogue or digital (CCD), transmits the signal of the image intensifier for further processing, such as storage, fast transmission, filtering, magnification, oscillation-free fluoroscopy, subtraction, and quantitative analysis. By saving films and time, the total cost can be lowered despite the required expensive equipment.

Angiography could improve the diagnostic information by using multipurpose and customized catheters of the smallest diameter but also required longer fluoroscopy time. To reduce the radiation exposure pulsed fluoroscopy using low-frequency oscillation was introduced. This could be achieved with digitally stored images, which display high-contrast, flicker-free images on the monitor, but only after 1990 when the flickering was eliminated by a high enough refresher rate. This has been the most important improvement in fluoroscopy since the introduction of the image intensifier television system.

Recording the image on individual cassettes, cassette changers, roll-film changers and then cut-film changers had always been governed by the inherent film properties and by film processing. For various reasons related to the mechanical film transport problems, it was not possible to increase the image sequence from 6 to 12 images per second.

At the beginning, the patient was placed on a moving table top. The X-ray tube was suspended form the ceiling and had to be correctly positioned over the patient aligned with the film changer. Generator performance, control frequency and operation had to be mastered for this new exposure technique.

Overloading X-ray tubes could initially be avoided solely by a well-trained, dedicated staff and only later be eliminated by increasingly sophisticated protection devices. Organ programs with stored relevant examination data prevented incorrect exposures. Through improved and expanded control and safety functions, the contrast-medium injector had been integrated into the radiographic equipment, contributing to increased patient safety.

The contribution of U. Speck, who has been involved in improving and developing contrast media, reviews the evolution of radiographic contrast media, which are insusceptible for many radiographic studies.

Johan Sellink developed the enteroclysis or high enema for imaging the small intestine. Until then, only the beginning and the end of the small intestine had been accessible with endoscopy. The radiographic examination of the oesophagus and stomach has been replaced almost entirely by endoscopy in many countries, although a high level of gastrointestinal radiology can be found in the literature through the work of H. Rieder, G. Holzknecht, H.H. Berg, R. Prévôt, B. Swart and W. Frik.

In J.H.J. Ruijs' and E. Loehr's contributions, the extreme pressure on visualizing the biliary tract and urinary tract for diagnostic evaluation becomes apparent. E. Boijsen, the teacher and master of abdominal angiography, illustrates the technical developments of angiography. E. Zeitler, who promoted the treatment of peripheral vascular disease by using the Dotter technique, shows the historical path of peripheral angiography, and J. W. Ludwig relates the development of cardiac and coronary angiography, with which he was intimately involved. P.H. Heintzen continues along this line by describing digital angiocardiography and angiocardiometry. Finally, L. Beltz introduces us to the origin of lymphography and describes its current indications.

These contributions emphasize the interrelation between conventional imaging techniques, such radiography and fluoroscopy, and newer imaging modalities, such as ultrasonography, CT, and MRI.

Development of intravascular contrast media

U. Speck

Today's diagnostic radiology has originated from a number of different disciplines:
- Radiation physics and technique
- Development of contrast media
- Application of medical techniques
- Establishing diagnostic strategies
- Therapeutic resources

The development of contrast media depends on four disciplines: The radiographic technique, for instance, determines the lowest attenuation difference necessary to visualize a specific structure in the body. If an intrinsic difference is absent or cannot be achieved by administration of an oral or intravenous contrast medium, special techniques have to be developed to deliver the contrast medium to the site to be visualized. This only is meaningful if the diagnosis cannot be made simpler or better by other than radiographic methods, and if the radiographic diagnosis achieves an acceptable degree of accuracy and certainty. Finally, application and usefulness of the method depends on the therapeutic consequences of the established diagnosis or, at least, on its prognostic implication. A change of any of these contributing factors can, in addition to any progress in chemistry, pharmacology and the clinical application of contrast media, provide new impulses to the development of contrast agents but also can make products already marketed or under development superfluous.

Roentgenology without contrast media

The value of contrast media can be appreciated by looking at the spectrum of radiological examinations without contrast enhancement. Is con-fined to the assessment of bones, chest, abdomen and breast. Changes affecting blood vessels, different body cavities (stomach, intestines, joints, subarachnoidal cavity) and tracts (urinary tract, biliary tract, lymphatics) cannot or only inadequately evaluated, and many parenchymal organs and tissues and the fine tissue structures are not visualized.

Computed tomography is more suited to visualize the contours of soft tissue organs than projectional radiography, particularly when the organs are surrounded by fat. Due to its improved contrast resolution, computed tomography also can, in part, visualize the internal structures of the soft tissue organs as well as small calcifications. However, vascular structures, cardiac cavities, gastrointestinal lumen, many other body cavities, and the majority of pathological tissue changes cannot be recognized without contrast.

An additional, recently introduced radiographic technique, digital subtraction angiography, depends entirely on contrast media.

Without contrast, the nature of radiology would be completely different. Not only the contribution of radiology to medical care would be severely limited, but also its technically demanding aspect would be lost. Though angiography, which is entirely dependent on contrast media, does not contribute greatly to the number of radiological examinations performed, it represents an essential part of the many radiology departments. Like computed tomography, it has considerably increased the reputation of radiology and its contribution to medical care. A correct diagnosis obtained through sophisticated catheter techniques often is the basis of many interventional radiological procedures, which are continuously advanced.

Contrast medium for functional diagnosis

The term 'contrast medium' refers to the original purpose of this category of pharmaceutical substance: to enhance contrast in the radiographic image between otherwise isodense structures.

In the course of the development of contrast media, recognizing function has always been of great importance, for instance:
- assessment of gastrointestinal peristalsis;
- excretory function of kidneys and liver;
- blood flow and perfusion;
- permeability of blood vessels and barrier function (blood–brain barrier).

In this respect, contrast media remain useful despite the increasing quality of diagnostic imaging. By displaying function, they add a new dimension to the image. It is a unique feature of diagnostic imaging that the functional information is superimposed on an anatomical image of high spatial resolution.

Development of contrast media

Soon after the discovery of X-rays, several investigators independently conceived the basic principle of using contrast media. Almost simultaneously with the *in vitro* observation of attenuation of X-rays in various substances, body cavities and anatomic specimens were *in vivo* investigated with photon-absorbing media. By visualizing blood vessels of an amputated hand, Haschek and Lindenthal [1] performed the first radiographic examination on an anatomic specimen. The achieved vascular opacification was satisfactory, but the paste to fill the vessels was based on particulate matter contained in petroleum jelly, unsuitable for use *in vivo*. In the first few years after the discovery of X-rays, works with contrast media concentrated on the hollow viscera, that is, the gastrointestinal tract and bladder, which were less prone to adverse reactions.

The almost immediate adoption of contrast substances by radiology was amazing. There were discussions about the pros and cons of individual substances, their manufacture and route of administration, their clinical application and toxicity, with the objective of finding better and more efficient methods of contrast enhancement. Never questioned, however, was the principle of a 'contrast medium' to be administered from the outside and to be retained only for a short time inside the body.

The choice of appropriate elements

In the first few years after the discovery of X-rays, the radiographic contrast properties of almost all known elements and chemicals were investigated. These early investigations (Table III, 1) included:

Table III, 1. First use of contrast media

Lead acetate:	Gastrointestinal tract of guinea pigs, Becher, 1896 [2]
Bismuth nitrate:	Gastrointestinal tract of cats, Cannon, 1896 [3]
Calcium sulphate (gypsum):	Blood vessels, anatomical preparations, Dutto, 1896 [4]
Mercuric sulphide:	Blood vessels, amputated hand, Haschek and Lindenthal, 1896 [1]
Halogens, iodide:	In vitro, Sehrwald, 1896 [6]

Already in the first year following the discovery of x-rays, significant knowledge of radiographic contrast media and their application could be gathered. The heavy elements were identified as radiopaque, the use of iodide as a nonmetallic element was described and the principle of filling vessels and body cavities was established.

During the following 30 years, the spectrum of effective substances had significantly increased. However, there were few fundamental contributions of importance (Table III, 2):

Table III, 2. Use of contrast media until 1928

Air:	Stomach, Bade, 1899 [7]
Silver (as iodide also):	Pyelography, Voelcker & von Lichtenberg, 1905 [8]
Barium sulphate:	Gastrointestinal tract, Bachem & Guenther, 1910 [9]
Thorium (nitrate):	Pyelography, Burns, 1915 [10]
Strontium (bromide):	Venography, arteriography, Berberich & Hirsch, 1923 [11]
Sodium iodide/bromide:	Pyelography, Urography Cameron, 1918 [12]
Thorium dioxide:	Angiography, Bluehbaum et al., 1928 [13]

In 1899, air had been described as a negative contrast medium. Air and gases remain important in filling the body cavities, often in combination with positive contrast media as double-contrast technique. Recently, the use of resorptive gases (carbon dioxide, oxygen) have been described as contrast media for digital subtraction angiography [14]. The heightened contrast sensitivity of this method also permits the visualization of relatively small vessels. Good tolerance and low costs are considered advantageous, while the inability of gases to mix with blood and the problems of regulating their contrast intensity are seen as disadvantages.

The use of silver iodide [8] and strontium bromide [11] is interesting in that a high contrast density can be expected with salts made up of radiopaque cations (silver, strontium) and radiopaque anions (iodide, bromide). A 20% solution of strontium bromide had been used in patients for venography and angiography, producing good radiological findings. Its trade name was 'Strontium bromatum purissimum pro Röntgen' and 'Dominal X'. On the basis of modern, tri-iodinated, organic contrast media, the work on salts of radiopaque cations and radiopaque anions was resumed several years ago, evaluating their use for angiography [16]. This approach became obsolete with the introduction of non-ionic contrast media.

Introducing the use of barium sulphate in gastrointestinal radiology in 1910 [9] did not follow a new principle of diagnostic radiology, but is an example of a good contrast medium that has found its suitable indication. The virtually insoluble barium sulphate is unsuitable for parenteral and intravascular use.

In 1915, thorium was used as a nitrate [10] in retrograde pyelography. Sodium citrate was added to the 10–15% preparation in order to improve tolerance. Thorium forms complex salts with citric acid, and metal complexes were later proposed and tested as radiographic contrast media [15]. Thorium was successfully introduced as Thorotrast in the late twenties and early thirties [13]. Colloidal thorium oxide in concentrations of up to 25% was used to visualize blood vessels, liver and spleen. Initially, this contrast medium seemed to have very favorable properties: it hardly had any adverse reactions, was very radiopaque, and accumulated in the liver and spleen to such a level that the outline of both organs could be seen in the radiographic image. The low osmolality of its colloidal solution allowed arteriography without adverse reactions. Several manufacturers offered thorium-oxide preparations as radiographic contrast media.

As early as 1932, numerous papers reported a complete lack of excretion of thorium particles and mentioned the radiation risks due to its radioactivity. It was found that thorium oxide is stored in the liver, spleen and bone marrow for life and that its radioactivity leads to radiation-induced tumours following a latent interval of several decades.

In 1989, van Kaick et al. examined over 5000 patients, who underwent an angiography with Thorotrast between 1937 and 1947. They found a statistically increase in cases of malignant liver tumors, myelogenous leukemia, cirrhosis and bone marrow aplasia [13a].

The soluble and eliminative salts of halogens (sodium iodide, potassium iodide, sodium bromide) were only introduced into pyelography [12, 17] in 1918, and then soon thereafter also in angiography (sodium iodide) [18, 19]. In 1921, Schering-Kahlbaum Co. presented lithium iodide as a urographic agent [20]. The 15–25% solution of halogen salts was not as radiopaque as Thorotrast. Its high osmolality caused pain and other adverse reactions, but contrary to all heavy metal preparations, it was excreted rapidly and completely. Pioneers in angiography like E. Moniz used sodium iodide.

Organic molecules as iodine carrier

In the twenties, work on the radiographic visualization of blood vessels converged on iodine salts and organic compounds suitable as iodide carriers. Visualizing brain vessels by injecting 5–6 ml of a 25% sodium iodide solution in the surgically exposed and clamped internal carotid artery, as developed by Moniz, caused temporary cramps in some patients [21]. The low iodide concentration of the solution and its patient intolerance posed problems. Sodium iodide was also used for the first successfully performed excretory urography [22]. The method could be improved by adding urea [23] and using compression to some extent, but overall the results were unreliable and inadequate. It is remarkable that visualized renal pelves and ureters have been mentioned even after oral administration of 8–10 g of sodium iodide and 10 g of urea [24]. None of these methods had been adopted for routine use, but indicated the clinical potential of using intravascular contrast media based on iodine. Halogenated organic molecules have been tried early as intravenous or oral biliary contrast media [25, 26], and already in 1927 Schering marketed a di-iodinated compound under the trade name Biloptin.

Even earlier, in 1921, iodized oils had been used for various purposes in individual cases and also for visualizing blood vessels in patients [27]. 'Lipiodol' was introduced and its name is still well known. To use iodized oils as contrast media was limited by their inability to be dissolved in blood and the high risk of oil emboli [28].

The development of appropriate intravascular contrast media owes its real breakthrough the goal of finding an agent for excretory urography. In the search for chemotherapeutics to be used against infectious diseases in domesticated animals, A. Binz (Fig. III, 3) and C. Raeth of the Agricultural College in Berlin synthesized a series of iodinated compounds, among them, in December 1926, 5-iodide-2-pyridon-N-acetate, later known as Uroselectan. Schering had just taken over the financial support of this investigation, after an unknown large chemical manufacturer had lost interest following many years of research. In October 1927, the substance was sent by Schering to Dr Hryntschak, in Vienna, whose tests on rabbits revealed no significant advantages of the preparation.

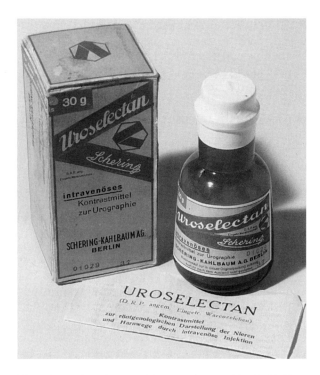

Fig. III, 4. Uroselectan vial, manufactured in 1929. Uroselectan was marketed as dry powder to be dissolved on use, just like the first non-ionizing radiographic contrast medium Amipaque.

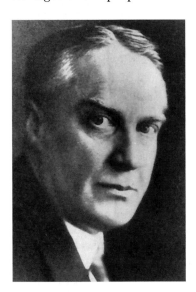

Fig. III, 3. Arthur Binz (1868–1943). Worked as pharmacologist in Bonn, Berlin and Frankfurt am Main. Syntheses of dyes and pharmaceuticals. Discovered in animal experiments with pyridines that iodine-containing substances are excreted by the kidneys in high concentration.

It was not until the summer of 1929 that Uroselectan was again tested, this time by the American Dr M. Swick, who worked as a visiting physician in Professor von Lichtenberg's department of St Hedwig Hospital in Berlin. The tests were immediately successful and the results published in two articles by von Lichtenberg and Swick in November 1929 [29, 30]. In the same year, the production of Uroselectan began. An original vial (Figs III, 4 and 5) found in Leipzig was given to me by Dr. B. Kunz from the radiological department of the 'Charité'. The history of Uro-

selectan has been described many times [31, 32, 33].

Uroselectan was supplied as a dry powder in 40-g vials. It had to be dissolved and sterilized before use. The recommended dose of 30 g or 12 g of iodide produced good results, although Uroselectan only has one atom of iodide, and the iodine content of the molecule was relatively low, amounting to only 42% of its weight. By selecting Uroselectan, Binz had to compromise, passing over substances with a higher iodine content, which he preferred, because of inadequate solubility and compatibility.

Over a short period of time, reports on di-iodinated products with approximately 50% iodine content were published in 1930 and 1931. These products provided, for the first time, solutions with more than 350 mg iodine/ml desirable for the visualization of vessels. Uroselectan-B was the di-sodium salt of a dicarbonic acid. Indeed, the iodine content had been increased but so too had its osmolality. Bayer Co. succeeded in finding a di-iodinated derivative of pyridon that only contained one carboxyl group and therefore twice as much iodine per molecule and had the same osmolality as Uroselectan. Under the label Diodone or Perabrodil, this contrast

UROSELECTAN

(D. R. P. angem. Eingetr. Warenzeichen)

Kontrastmittel
zur röntgenologischen Darstellung der Nieren
und Harnwege durch intravenöse Injektion

Gebrauchsanweisung

Bereitung der Lösung: Man trägt den Inhalt einer Packung Uroselectan (40 g) unter Umrühren portionenweise in etwa 110 ccm redestillierten Wassers ein, filtriert die erhaltene Lösung in ein Becherglas, erhitzt sie sodann zum Sieden (Achtung vor Siedeverzug!) und läßt 10 Minuten kochen. Nach dem Abkühlen auf Körpertemperatur verwendet man die möglichst frische Lösung, die nunmehr 100 ccm betragen soll, zur Injektion. Man kann aber auch so vorgehen, daß man den Inhalt einer Packung (40 g) zunächst in 80 ccm sterilem redestillierten Wasser löst und die Lösung auf 100 ccm auffüllt. Das Wasser soll vorher leicht angewärmt und die zu lösende Substanz langsam zugeschüttet werden. Die Lösung wird zweimal filtriert und im Dampfsterilisator oder auf dem Wasserbade 20 Minuten lang sterilisiert, wodurch etwas von der Menge verloren geht.

Die filtrierte und sterilisierte Injektionslösung muß vollständig klar sein. Sie hat eine leicht gelbe Färbung, die, wie die Untersuchungen zeigten, keineswegs durch Jodabspaltung bedingt ist.

Ausführung der Injektion: Die körperwarme Lösung soll man möglichst langsam, in etwa 10—15 Minuten in die Cubitalvene injizieren; vorher wird die Injektionsstelle mit Alkohol desinfiziert. Man injiziert am besten die eine Hälfte und nach einer Unterbrechung von 2—3 Minuten die andere Hälfte der Lösung, eventuell in zwei Venen.

Dosierung bei Kindern: Die Menge des zur Anwendung gelangenden Uroselectan richtet sich nicht nach dem Körpergewicht, sondern ist nur eine Funktion der Nierenschwelle, die mit 5% ohnehin begrenzt bleibt.

Kinder jedoch müssen naturgemäß mit Rücksicht auf das Fassungsvermögen ihres Gefäßapparates kleinere Mengen erhalten, und zwar:

Säuglinge u. kleine Kinder   20 ccm der 40%igen Lösung
Kinder bis zu 6 Jahren . 40 „ „ 40% „ „
„ „ „ 12 „ . 60 „ „ 40% „ „
Jugendliche . . . . 60—100 „ „ 40% „ „
Erwachsene . . . . . 100 „ „ 40% „ „

Aufnahme des Pyelogramms:

Für gewöhnlich macht man die erste Aufnahme $^1/_4$ Stunde, die zweite Aufnahme $^3/_4$ Stunden und die dritte Aufnahme $1^1/_4$ Stunde nach erfolgter Injektion. Vor der zweiten und dritten Aufnahme muß die Blase entleert werden, damit der Schatten den Beckenteil des Harnleiters nicht verdeckt. Bei normaler Nierenfunktion ist in der zweiten Stunde die Höhe der Ausscheidung erreicht. In Fällen von erheblicher Störung der Nierenfunktion treten die Bilder erst später hervor und können 6—24 Stunden nach der Injektion erst die für die bildliche Darstellung notwendige Dichtigkeit erreichen. Ist die Niere zerstört oder im Stadium einer momentanen Sperre, so wird kein Uroselectan ausgeschieden. Eine bildliche Darstellung der Niere ist dann nicht möglich.

Im allgemeinen ist Vorsicht mit Uroselectan bei Patienten am Platze, bei denen eine Schädigung der Leberfunktion sowie akute und chronische Urämie besteht.

Originalpackung: Für sichere Bildwirkung ausreichende maximale Einzeldosis 30 g
Klinikpackung: Karton mit 10 Flaschen zu je 40 g.

SCHERING-KAHLBAUM A.G.
BERLIN

St. 4. 30. 20 000

Fig. III, 5. Package insert of Uroselectan.

medium became the standard contrast medium for urography for the next 20 years.

After the benefit of organic compounds with chemically firmly-linked iodide had clearly been established, iodine-containing substances other than those of the pyridon group (Uroselectan, Uroselectan-B, D iodone) were tested for clinical applicability [31]. Abrodil (iodomethyl-sulphonic acid, Methiodal) and the corresponding di-iodinated compound were used in urography. The tri-iodinated substance, however, was unstable.

O-iodohippuric acid has been known since 1906. Swick [32] recommended the corresponding iodinated compounds (1933) as a urographic contrast medium since hippuric acid was rapidly excreted by the kidneys. There was little interest in iodohippurate, but it contained a forward looking concept as the first iodinated derivative of benzoic acid used as urographic agent.

Between 1944 and 1950, Wallingford [5] succeeded with the synthesis of the first tri-iodinated derivative of benzoic acid in the research laboratories of Mallinckrodt, St Louis. The objective was to improve the properties of o-iodohippuric acid. Acetrizoate was selected and marketed in 1950 under the name of Urokon as the first tri-iodinated benzoic acid derivative for urography and angiography. This laid the basis of the water-soluble contrast media still in use today.

Urokon itself was short-lived. As early as 1953, diatrizoate had been synthesized in Berlin by Schering [34] and, independently, in New York in 1954, by Sterling Winthrop [35], and was introduced shortly afterwards. Finally, a nearly universal contrast medium for urography, angiography and, later, computed tomography was available. The basic structure of tri-iodinated benzol was copied from acetrizoate, and its compatibility was improved by adding a side-chain to its molecule. Diatrizoate became the first urographic contrast medium that has negligible binding to plasma proteins and also is virtually biologically inert otherwise. The preparation introduced by Schering under the trade name 'Urografin' contained the better-tolerated meglumine salt with low sodium, which later proved to be essential in angiocardiography.

Contrast media on the basis of diatrizoic acid became very popular. For more than 30 years, they were the most frequently used contrast media and still hold a prominent place in many countries. Numerous variations of its structure were marketed between 1960 and 1980, but no major improvements were accomplished.

Urokon not only succeeded in paving the way for urography and angiography. Linking two acetrizoic-acid molecules created iodipamide [36], which represents the basic structure of the intravenously injected biliary contrast media until today. By forming one complex out of two acetrizoate molecules

– the binding to plasma protein (albumin) is increased and consequently the glomerular filtration reduced, and
– the molecular dimension has the size necessary for biliary excretion.

After 1950, hardly any attempts were made to use structures other than tri-iodobenzoic-acid derivatives. The tri-iodobenzoic acids optimally satisfy the most important requirements:
– very high iodine content;
– firm binding of contrast-producing elements with the organic structure;
– high chemical and metabolic stability;
– considerable chemical variability with the potential of modifying pharmacokinetics and compatibility to a large extent;
– production in large quantities at acceptable cost.

Because of their high radio-opacity, heavy metals are still of fundamental interest. In particular,

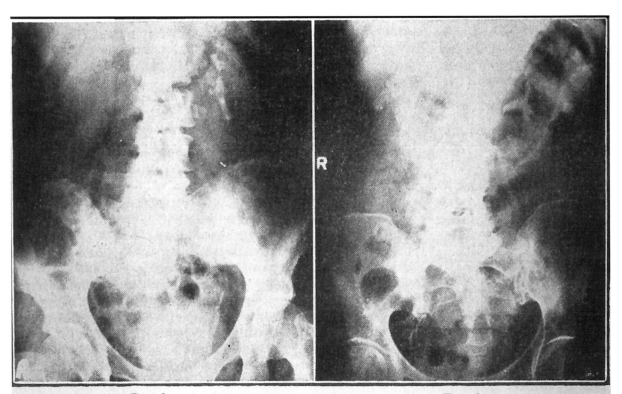

FIG. 2   FIG. 3

FIG. 2.—Case 1. Radiograph showing the kidneys and the left calices and ureter, six minutes after intravenous injection of 15 ml. of lead complex 50% solution. FIG. 3.—Case 3. Radiograph showing both kidneys and renal pelves twenty minutes after injection of 18 ml. of lead complex 50% solution.

Fig. III, 6. Lead compound as urographic contrast medium.

the lead used for protection against X-rays promises more contrast than the iodine-containing agents. Following the introduction of chelating agents, several in vestigators believed that heavy metals are no longer toxic after they are bound to organic molecules just like iodine. The simultaneously accelerated elimination of heavy metals was also seen as beneficial. July 1955, Sapeika [15] even published the clinical application of such a compound (lead EDTA) in urography, which was performed with intravenous administration of more than 5 g of lead per patient (Fig. III, 6). In the same year, Clark and Tomich [37] described animal experiments with lead EDTA and unequivocally opposed its use on patients.

Since then, intravascular radiographic contrast media have remained derivatives of tri-iodobenzoic acids.

Low-osmolality and non-ionic contrast media

Diatrizoate, which was available as meglumine, sodium salt or mixed salts, was used in the fifties and sixties as a very satisfactory intravascular contrast medium for most radiological examinations. With the number of radiographic examinations growing and the expected diagnostic quality rising, more attention turned to the relatively infrequent adverse reactions. Vast statistics were gathered to learn more about the frequency of cardiovascular and allergic reactions and, in particular, about the rare deaths attributed to contrast media. At the same time, selective angiographic procedures increased in number and significance and, depending on the nature of the procedure, could be beset with frequent and characteristic adverse reactions. In contradistinction to such reactions as

(a) nausea, vomiting, urticaria and a sudden fall in blood pressure, many of the adverse reactions seen in angiography were related to dose and concentration. They could be evoked in nearly every patient and reproduced in animal experiments. These adverse reactions include

(b) vasodilatation, endothelial damage, pain, impaired microcirculation. The cause and mechanism of the adverse reactions mentioned under (a) are still not or only incompletely understood. The relationship between the effects mentioned under (b) and the high osmolality of the contrast media was soon recognized.

In 1969, Almen [38] proposed the synthesis of low-osmolar contrast media. His publication anticipated the principles followed in subsequent years by various research groups and pharmaceutical firms for the synthesis of water-soluble, low-osmolar contrast media:
- non-ionic contrast media;
- the use of tri-iodinated cations to form salt with the usual tri-iodobenzoic acid;
- linking two or more tri-iodinated benzoic acids.

The ensuing development took an unforeseen course in more than one respect. A new type of contrast medium, the non-ionic metrizamide, developed by the Nycomed Company in Oslo, was introduced in 1975. Initially, it was only used in myelography, and for the first time, thoracic and cervical myelography could be performed with a water-soluble contrast medium. The good tolerance found with this application is less related to the lower osmolality of Metrizamide than to the non-ionic nature of the molecule and its lack of dis sociating into cations and anions. The general use of Metrizamide or Amipaque was restricted by its instability in solution and its high costs. The goal of finding a 'low-osmolar contrast media to visualize vessels' was barely achieved. Instead, the low neurotoxicity of non-ionic contrast media was discovered and utilized.

The goal of 'a better-tolerated contrast medium for angiography' was reached first by the French company Guerbet. In 1979, Hexabrix (sodium meglumine ioxaglate) was introduced, an ionic dimeric contrast medium that, like a monomer, only contains one carboxyl group. Its solution was sufficiently stable to be marketed as a ready-to-inject product, and it was less expensive than Amipaque. Its osmolality of approx imately 600 mOsm/kg H_2O at 320 mg iodine/ml was still hypertonic but considerably less than that of angiographic agents used so far. The experience gained through the use of Hexabrix led to fundamentally new insights. It proved to have excellent vascular tolerance and to be painless, but despite its low osmolality similar to that of Amipaque, its neurocompatibility was inferior and it was not developed further for myelography. Finally, it was found that the good vascular tolerance and particularly the low pain potential did not imply an overall satisfactory tolerance. Adverse reactions, as described above under (a), were even more frequent with Hexabrix than with the conventional hypertonic ionic contrast media [39]. It could also be shown that the intravenous cholegraphic agents, which are of low-osmolality and considerably more toxic, hardly cause any pain. The painfulness of contrast media observed in angiography is primarily related to hypertonicity and bears no relationship of the contrast media's toxicity.

Felder at the Bracco company was the first to succeed in developing a non-ionic contrast medium (Iopamidol) suitable for angiography. Iopa midol has been marketed under the trade names Solutrast, Niopam, Iopamiro and Isovue since 1981. It was also developed for myelography and had an improved general tolerance compared to Hexabrix (see (a) above). So on thereafter, Iohexol (Nycomed) and Iopromide (Sch ering) followed. The new non-ionic contrast media (Iopamidol, Iohexol, Iopromide) were disappointingly more painful than Amipaque and, to certain extent, Hexabrix. This can be explained by their slightly higher osmolality.

During the clinical tests of the non-ionic contrast media, an unexpected positive quality was noted: the poorly understood adverse reactions, which are largely unrelated to dose and osmolality, such as nausea, vomiting, urticaria etc. were strikingly less frequent, especially after intravenous administration. Elaborate studies in Germany, Japan, Australia and USA [40, 41, 42, 43] showed a reduction of the adverse reactions by a factor two to ten, including serious reactions leading to shock and unconsciousness. It can therefore be assumed that fatal reactions from non-ionic contrast media are rare, but this has not been confirmed yet.

For the intravascular administration, the advantages of non-ionic contrast media over low-osmolar ionic contrast media (Ioxaglate) are so convincing that new ionic contrast media have not been developed since 1979, while the number and quantities of available non-ionic products continue to increase (Iopamidol, Iohexol, Iopromide, Ioversol, Iopentol).

Schering finally succeeded in binding two non-ionic, tri-iodinated contrast-medium molecules, producing the first water-soluble contrast medium of high iodine concentration and isotonicity with blood and CSF [44]. A first preparation on the basis of Iotrolan (Isovist) was introduced in 1988 [45]. H.W. Fischer [47] has compared the development of the radiographic contrast media with a tree, with dead branches that include Thorotrast, iodomethyl sulphonic acid, and ionic dimers, a trunk of tri-iodinated ionic substances, and a crown comprising the non-ionic contrast media. Figure III, 7 shows a recent overview of contrast media currently available

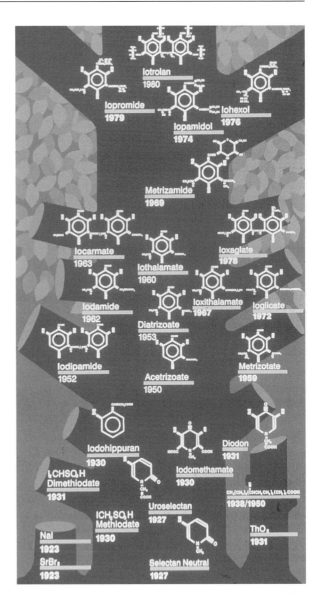

Fig. III, 7. Development of contrast media according to H.W. Fischer [47]. Most of numbers refer to the year of patent application.

and under development for angiography, urography and computed tomography.

Organ-specific or pathology-specific contrast media?

Urographic contrast media, used for continuously changing and expanding numbers of indications, are quite unspecific. They are almost biologically inert. After intravascular injection, they diffuse through pores from the capillaries into the extracellular space and are finally excreted through unspecific glomerular filtration. Undoubtedly, there seems to be a correlation between the inert behavior of urographic agents and their comparatively good tolerance.

Biliary contrast media, introduced at an early date, have lost their importance after the development of ultrasound. Their hepatic concentration was even insufficient to enhance the liver for computed tomography. Many other developments of organ-specific contrast media failed because of problems with adverse reactions.

In the meantime, the unspecific urographic agents have been adopted through dynamic computed tomography for the selective visualization of organs and their internal structures as well as of certain pathological processes. After bolus injection of contrast medium, a different distribution occurs within seconds to a few minutes. The tissue concentration of contrast media increases with the blood flow to the tissue and with tissue's capillary permeability, blood volume and extracellular space.

New developments of specific contrast media should be critically judged by comparing it with the information content of the early distributive phase of the urographic media and their excellent tolerance.

Change in the application of contrast media

In general, new contrast media are developed with very specific objectives in mind, but it should be kept in mind that the development of most products continues after they have been introduced. Through innovations in technique and radiology, many already existing products have found new applications, as it happened to Lipiodol and Urografin.

In 1953, Urografin – as the name implies – was mainly developed for urography. Because of the serendipitously optimal ratio of sodium and meglumine salts, it was until recently also the contrast agent of choice for angiocardiography. Urografin (Renografin, Hypaque) has found widespread use in computed tomography and intravenous digital subtraction angiography, applications that had not been fore seen at the time Urografin was introduced in the early fifties, while its use in urography decreased.

Lipiodol has initially been used for many procedures, including angiography and myelography, and later found a prominent place in lymphography. After lymphography was largely replaced by computed tomography in the mid-eighties, Lipiodol was injected into the hepatic artery for the diagnosis and, combined with cytostatic agents, treatment of liver tumours.

These and similar instances illustrate that the availability of different contrast media is an asset for radiology, allowing it to react quickly to new technical developments and changed expectations. The response to a new situation is shorter by having already commercially a vailable contrast media at one's disposal than by waiting for the development of new pharmaceutical products (Table III, 1).

Expectation

Immediately after the discovery of X-rays, the concept of utilizing pharmaceutical substances to obtain additional information from the body was investigated and considered useful. Today, it affects important specialities within radiology and is still undergoing further development [46]. Applying this concept to other imaging modalities, such as ultrasound and magnetic resonance imaging, was the most important innovation in the last decade. Despite entirely different image-forming principles, contrast media seem to be as valuable in these modalities as in conventional radiology. It is important to keep in mind that each method has specific advantages and limitations, which have to be taken into account in the development of contrast media.

References

1. Haschek, E., O.T. Lindenthal: Ein Beitrag zur praktischen Verwertung der Photographie nach Röntgen. Wien. klin. Wschr. 9 (1896) 63
2. Becher, W.: Zur Anwendung des röntgenischen Verfahrens in der Medizin.#Dtsch. med. Wschr. 22 (1896) 202
3. Cannon, W.B.: The movements of the stomach studied by means of the roentgen ray. Am. J. Physiol. 1 (1898) 359
4. Dutto, U.: Fotografi del sistema arterioso ottenute con raggi Röntgen. Rendic. Reale Acad. Lincei 5 (1896) 129
5. Wallingford, V. H.: The development of organic iodine compounds as X-ray contrast media. J. Am. Pharmaceut. Ass. Sci. Ed. 42 (1953) 721–728
6. Sehrwald, E.: Das Verhalten der Halogene gegen Röntgenstrahlen. Dtsch. med. Wschr. 22 (1896) 477
7. Bade, P.: Eine neue Methode der Röntgenphotographie des Magens. Dtsch. med. Wschr. 25 (1899) 627
8. Völcker, F., A. von Lichtenberg: die Gestalt der menschlichen Harnblase im Röntgenbild. Münch. med. Wschr. 52 (1905) 1576
9. Bachem, C., H. Günther: Bariumsulfat als schattenbildendes Kontrastmittel bei Röntgenuntersuchungen. Z. Röntgenk.-Radiumforsch. 12 (1910) 369

10. Burns: The use of thorium in urology and roentgenology. Am. J. Roentgenol. 3 (1916) 482
11. Berberich, J., S. Hirsch: Die röntgenographische Darstellung der Arterien und Venen am lebenden Menschen. Klin. Wschr. 2 (1923) 2226
12. Cameron, D.F.: Aqueous solutions of potassium and sodium iodids as opaque mediums in roentgenography. J. Am. Med. Ass. 70 (1918) 754
13. Blühbaum, Th., K. Frik, H. Kalkbrenner: Eine neue Anwendungsart der Kolloide in der Röntgendiagnostik. Fortschr. Röntgenstr. 37 (1928) 18
13a. Van Kaick, G., H. Wesch, H. Lührs, D. Liebermann, A. Kaul, H. Muth: The German thorotrast study – report on 20 years follow-up. BIR report 21 (1989) 98
14. Hawkins, I.F.: Carbon dioxide digital subtraction arteriography. Am. J. Roentgenol. 139 (1982) 19–24
15. Sapeika, N.: Radiographic use of lead E.D.T.A. in man. Brit. Med. J. 2 (1955) 167–169
16. Speck, U., W. Mützel: Two new classers of low-osmotic contrast agents: triiodinated cations and nonionic dimers. In Amiel (ed): Contrast Media in Radiology. Springer Verlag, 1982
17. Weld, E.H.: The use of sodium bromide in roentgenography. J. Am. Med. Ass. 71 (1918) 1111
18. Heuser, O.: Pieloradiografia con iodur potásico y las inyecciones intravenosas de iodura potásico en radiografia. Sem. méd. (B. Aires) 26 (1919) 424
19. Dünner, L., A. Calm: Die Röntgenologie der Gefässe, insbesondere Lungengefässe am lebenden Menschen. Fortschr. Röntgenstr. 31 (1923) 635
20. Joseph, E.: Ein neues Kontrastmittel für die Pyelographie. Zbl. Chir. 49 (1921) 707
21. Jacobi, W.: Studien zur röntgenographischen Darstellung der Kopfarterien des lebenden Hundes. Arch. Psychiatr. 86 (1929) 240–248
22. Osborne, E.D., C.G. Sutherland, A.J. Schell, L.G. Rowntree: Roentgenography of urinary tract during excretion of sodium iodide. J. Am. Med. Ass. 80 (1923) 368
23. Roseno, A.: Die intravenöse Pyelographie: II. Mitteilung. Klinische Ergebnisse. Klin. Wochenschr. 8 (1929) 1165
24. Ziegler, J., H. Köhler: Perorale Pyelographie. Med. Klinik 1 (1930) 10–11
25. Graham, E.A., W.H. Cole, G.H. Copher: Visualization of the gallbladder by the sodium salt of tetrabromphenolphthalein. J. Am. Med. Ass. 82 (1924) 1777
26. Pribram, B.O.: Über ein neues Kontrastmittel zur röntgenologischen Darstellung der Gallenblase. Dtsch. med. Wschr. 31 (1926) 1291–1292
27. Sicard, J.A., J. Forestier: Méthode radiographique d'exploration de la cavité épidurale par le lipiodol. Rev. neurol. 28 (1921) 1264
28. Sicard, J. A., G. Forestier: Injections intravasculaires d'huile iodée sous controle controle radiologique. C.R. Soc. Biol. (Paris) 88 (1923) 1200
29. Swick, M.: Darstellung der Niere und Harnwege im Röntgenbild durch intravenöse Einbringung eines neuen Kontraststoffes, des Uroselectan. Klin. Wochenschr. 8 (1929) 2087–2089
30. Lichtenberg, A. v., M. Swick: Klinische Prüfung des Uroselectans. Klin. Wochenschr. 8 (1929) 2089–2091
31. Binz, A.: Geschichte des Uroselectans. Z. Urologie (1937) 73-84
32. Swick, M.: The discovery of intravenous urography: historical and developmental aspects of the urographic media and their role in other diagnostic and therapeutic areas. Bull. N.Y. Acad. Med. 42 (1966) 128–151
33. Grainger, R.: Intravascular contrast media - the past, the present and the future. Brit. J. Radiol. 55 (1982) 1–18
34. Langecker, H., A. Harwart, K. Junkmann: 3,5-Diacetylamino-2,4,6-trijodbenzoesäure als Röntgenkontrastmittel. Arch. exp. Path. u. Pharmakol. 222 (1954) 584–590
35. Hoppe, J.: The evaluation of iodinated organic compounds as radiopaque media. J. Am. Pharm. Ass. Sci. Ed. 48 (1959) 368–379
36. Langecker, H., K. Junkmann: 2,4,6-Trijod-3-acetaminobenzoesäure-Abkömmlinge als Kontrastmittel. Arch. exp. Path. u. Pharmakol. 220 (1953) 195–206
37. Clark, B.J., E.G. Tomich: Pharmacological studies on lead E.D.T.A. Brit. Med. J. 2 (1955) 831–832
38. Almen, T.: Contrast agent design. J. Theoret. Biol. 24 (1969) 216–226
39. Brismar, J., B.F. Jacobsson, H. Jorulf: Miscellaneous adverse effects of low- versus high-osmolality contrast media: A study revised. Radiology 179 (1991) 19–23
40. Schrott, K.M., B. Behrends, W. Clauss, J. Kaufmann, K. Somasundaram: Drug monitoring für 50 bzw. 100 ml Omnipaque-300 in der Ausscheidungsurographie. Urologe (B) 25 (1985) 24
41. Katayama, H., K. Yamaguchi, T. Kozuka, T. Takashima, P. Seez, K. Matsuura: Adverse reactions to ionic and nonionic contrast media. Radiology 175 (1990) 621–628
42. Palmer, F.J.: The RACR survey of intravenous contrast media reactions final report. Australasian Radiology 32 (1988) 426–428
43. Wolf, G.L., M.M. Mishkin, S.G. Roux, E.F. Halpern, J. Gottlieb, J. Zimmerman, J. Gillen, C. Thellman: Comparison of the rates of adverse drug reactions: ionic contrast agents, ionic agents combined with steroids, and nonionic agents. Invest. Radiol. 26 (1991) 404–410
44. Speck, U., W. Mützel, G. Mannesmann, H. Pfeiffer, H.-M. Siefert: Pharmacology of nonionic dimers. Invest. Radiol. 15/Suppl. (1980) 317–322
45. Sovak, M., R. Ranganathan, U. Speck: Nonionic dimer: development and initial testing of an intrathecal contrast agent. Radiology 142 (1982) 115–118
46. Fritzsch, T., W. Krause, H.J. Weinmann: Status of contrast media research in MRI, ultrasound and X-ray. Eur. J. Radiol. (1992) 2–13
47. Fischer, H.W.: Historical aspects of contrast media development. In Felix et al. edts: Contrast media from the past to the future, pp 3–18, Georg Thieme Verlag Stuttgart New York, 1987

Digestive tract

J.L. Sellink

In the year 1896, radiographic examinations were limited to fluoroscopy of the limbs and the lungs. The image was faint, allowing only limited conclusions, and was often documented as a sketch. Only after a few months, the fluoroscopic image had improved to the level that abdomen and pelvis became accessible, and size and position of the stomach and colon, as long as they contained air, became visible. If innate air was absent, air was introduced via a rectal or gastric tube. Later, gas-forming substances were administered. Physicians with a special interest in surgery or internal medicine and a physicotechnical aptitude devoted themselves to this type of investigation [8].

As early as in the beginning of 1896, first attempts were made to visualize the stomach by means of lead acetate as contrast medium. Becher [9] worked with a dead guinea-pig and, 6 months later, Hemmeter [10] had a man swallow an essentially stomach-shaped balloon, which he subsequently distended through an attached tube. The navel was usually marked with a coin. After completion of the examination, the lead acetate was drained and balloon and tube pulled from the stomach. Wegele [11] had a thin metal spiral spring swallowed until it lay along the greater curvature. By making use of respiratory movements, he could determine the displacement of the stomach, using the navel as the point of reference.

Six months later, Lindemann [12] repeated this experiment but used a rubber tube whose lumen contained a copper mesh. By using a carbon inductor and a Siemens and Halske X-ray tube, he was able to make two photographs of it, each with an exposure time of approximately 20 min. A publication dated from early 1897 shows a radiograph taken by Rumpel [13] with a distended oesophagus, filled with a 300 ml 5% bismuth-nitrate solution. This solution was considered harmless because it was a well-known remedy in the treatment of stomach ache. Already previously, Rumpel had performed several experiments with all kinds of contrast solutions, even with ordinary milk, which casts slightly more of a "shadow" than water.

Publications by the Frenchmen Roux and Balthazard [14, 15] on observed gastric peristalsis in a frog, a dog, and a young, thin human – in that order – became famous. It was only possible to take photographs of the frog; drawings had to be made from the fluoroscopic findings of the dog and man. These investigations showed that in all three subjects the top part of the stomach (corpus) functioned mainly as a reservoir and that the lower, distal part (prepyloric and antrum) had an emptying function.

Even more famous became the article 'The Movements of the Stomach Studied by means of the Roentgen Rays' published a year later by the American W.B. Cannon [16] (Fig. III, 8). Fasting female cats were given a mixture of bismuth nitrate and food. The carefully sketched observations of the fluoroscopic findings corresponded rather well to those of Roux and Balthazard [17] and also to those of the German Rossbach [18], who had made those drawings in 1890 before the discovery of X-rays. Cannon's conclusions read as follows:

'The stomach consists of two physiologically distinct parts: the pyloric part and the fundus; over the pyloric part, while food is present, constriction-waves are seen continually coursing towards the pylorus; the fundus is an active reservoir for the food, and squeezes out its contents gradually into the pyloric part.

The stomach is emptied by the formation, between the fundus and the antrum, of a tube along which con-

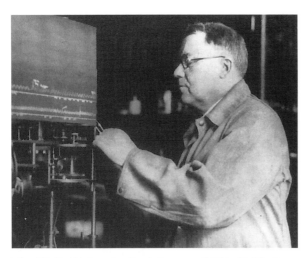

Fig. III, 8. Walter Bradford Cannon (1871–1945). From 1900 to 1945 as physiologist at the Harvard Medical School in Boston. Worked with F.H. Williams on radiographic examinations and physiology of the stomach by means of bismuth salts.

strictions pass. The contents of the fundus are pressed into the tube and the tube and antrum slowly cleared of food by the waves of constriction.

The food in the pyloric portion is first pushed forward by the running wave, and then by pressure of the stomach wall is returned through the ring of constriction; thus the food is thoroughly mixed with gastric juice, and is forced by an oscillating progress to the pylorus.

The food in the fundus is not moved by peristalsis and consequently it is not mixed with the gastric juice; salivary digestion can therefore be carried on in this region for a considerable period without being stopped by the acid gastric juice.

The pylorus does not open at the approach of every wave, but only at irregular intervals. The arrival of a hard morsel causes the sphincter to open less frequently than normally, thus materially interfering with the passage of the already liquefied food.

Solid food remains in the antrum to be rubbed by the constrictions until triturated, or to be softened by the gastric juice, or later it may be forced into the intestine in the solid state.

At the beginning of vomiting the gastric cavity is separated into two parts by a constriction at the entrance of the antrum; the cardiac portion is relaxed and the spasmodic contractions of the abdominal muscles force the food through the opened cardia into the oesophagus.

The stomach movements are inhibited whenever the cat shows signs of anxiety, rage, or distress.'

Cannon pointed out that a disturbance in the blood supply caused hyperperistalsis. In 1901,

Williams [19] published an identical examination on two children of 7 and 10 years of age, which was in direct agreement with Cannon's previous results. They observed the course of the food bolus mixed with contrast medium through the small bowel and colon, and found that the radiopaque bolus was in continuous motion between the corpus ventriculi and the most distal part of the colon.

In 1898, Cannon and Moser [20] also published their investigation on the movements of swallowing, and the passage of both liquid and solid food in geese, cats, horses and humans. In the same year in Vienna, Holzknecht [21] investigated the oesophagus with a watery bismuth subnitrate solution.

In 1901 and during the following years, the Dutchman Eijkman [22] investigated the behavior of the larynx during the swallowing process by means of radiographs, but for another 10 years, investigations of the pharynx and esophagus showed hardly any progress.

The first stage of investigating the colon was extremely difficult. Initially, it was tried to visualize the colon locally with a contrast medium instilled into the rectum through a tube.

Schuele [23] published a study in which he had reached Bauhin's valve by means of a 400-ml oily suspension, possibly with the patient in a knee–elbow position. He reported that Stegmann [24] had already pointed this out in a lecture held July 1903 in Freiburg. Schuele was of the opinion, that it would be feasible to use air as a contrast medium in routine examinations instead of the expensive oily bismuth suspension. But he was rather disappointed with the results.

The colon examination had the advantage, compared to the stomach examination, that radiographs could be obtained, though requiring long periods of breath-holding. The photographs of the colon showed acceptable motion blurring for that time (1904). This was definitely not true of the stomach, which is subject to stronger peristalsis. While only a few years earlier the exposure time of films was 10–25 min, in 1904 an exposure time of 10–25 s sufficed as a result of improvements of the X-ray tube and the use of intensifying screens.

In 1904, interest in examinations of the stomach increased as a result of the remarkable improvement in image quality, which Rieder [25] (Fig. III, 9) together with his engineer Rosenthal had achieved in Munich. Rieder used the improved fluoroscopic technique to study all functional aspects of the stomach in detail as well as to study the small bowel and colon transit. Among

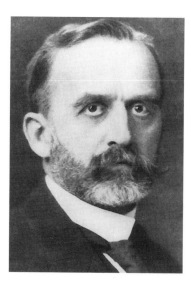

Fig. III, 9. Hermann Rieder (1858–1932). Worked in Munich. Diagnostic radiology of the gastrointestinal tract and lungs. Introduction of barium sulfate. Also numerous technical improvements, often together with the Engineer Joseph Rosenthal.

other things, he determined that the more fat the food contained and the less the stomach was filled, the slower was the rate of gastric emptying. As a contrast medium, he administered the famous 'Rieder meal', a substance that enjoyed extensive use for many years.

To apply a graded compression to the stomach, Holzknecht [26] developed a spoon, which was named after him and remains an indispensable instrument in every gastroenterological fluoroscopy room until today.

In 1906, Hemmeter [27] surgically induced local lesions in the gastric mucosa in cats, dogs and rabbits, and subsequently observed these radiographically with a bismuth subnitrate suspension. He noted that these artificial 'ulcera' healed within two hours. Using the same contrast medium on patients, he could also visualize an ulcer niche after the patient had been placed for half an hour in a position in which the bismuth could pool in the ulcer crater. He therefore recommended that the patient should lie on his back for half an hour since gastric ulcers are found in the posterior wall of the stomach. In this way, the examination could well take two hours and might not even produce any result.

Together with and under the driving force of the internist Kaestle, also in Munich, Rieder and Rosenthal [28] published cinematographic studies of the stomach ("bio-roentgenography") in 1911, which made a great impression.

Since long exposure times were an obstacle to obtaining radiographs in sequence, as it is done today, several radiographs were taken at long intervals, with lead markers used to ensure mounting of the images in the right order. These investigations revealed that the gastric peristalsis was

different from what had been previously believed.

While the roentgen cinematography had found limited recognition in Europe, it received attention in the USA, though modified, under the leadership of the pioneer Cole [2] and his collaborators. Technical advancement enabled them to take several radiographs in sequence, at a few seconds' interval and with a very short exposure time. They called it 'serial roentgenography'. Using this technique for the examination of the stomach required 8–12 films per position, both standing and lying, with the entire examination consisting of up to 50 radiographs.

In 1906, Holzknecht and Brauner [29] replaced the viscous bismuth meal with a more liquid bismuth suspension, which improved and simplified the representation of the gastric mucosal folds. They also accomplished a double-contrast effect by giving the patient a gas-producing mixture of tartaric acid and sodium bicarbonate. But the importance of this phenomenon was not recognized at the time.

The differences in the orientation of the folds around a benign or malignant ulcer niche could now be demonstrated through carefully graded compression. This diagnostic refinement, which originated in about 1910 and to which Haudek, Plakler and Holzknecht [30] contributed greatly, had far reaching effects. Publications about contrast-media poisoning caused by chemical transformation of bismuth-nitrate into the poisonous nitrite appeared by Groedel and Meyer [31] in 1908. As a result, bismuth nitrate was replaced almost everywhere by the harmless and just as good bismuth bicarbonate, but this compound was not used for long either.

In 1910, Kaestle, Kraus, Bachem and Guenther [32] replaced bismuth bicarbonate with barium sulphate, which was indeed superior. It was not so heavy and did not show rapid sedimentation. Both the fluoroscopic images and the radiographs were improved further. As early as 1904, Cannon [33] referred to the excellent properties of this contrast medium.

In 1911, von Elischer [34] tried to reintroduce the double-contrast technique to examine the stomach, but this time using a small dose of viscous zirconium oxide as contrast medium. Through a tube, the stomach was filled with this contrast medium as well as with air. Despite good results, von Elischer's method, like the one by Holzknecht and Brauner five years earlier, was not taken up. Following these refinements of the radiographic images and the elimination of interfering motion blurring, the roentgenographic exploration using direct signs was developed in the USA, primarily under the influence of Cole [2] and his collaborators, with diagnostic evaluation exclusively based on the radiographic findings as seen in various radiographic projections.

The well-known researcher Carman [7] was not a follower of this direct-sign method. He used the symptom-complex method, recommended by Holzknecht [35]. This method gives the fluoroscopic findings great importance. It is known that Carman fluoroscoped meticulously, intensively using manual palpation. On the advice of Leonard [36], he wore lead gloves and a lead apron for protection of the body. Carman did not succeed in drawing more attention to the information found on the radiographic film.

Nobody could have better put into words the original mistrust in the usefulness of perfect documentation of the radiographic findings than the American 'Godfather' of radioscopy, Carman in his publication of 1913 [37]. Among other things, he wrote:

'1. The radiological diagnosis of the duodenal ulcer, not substantiated with clinical data, is in most cases nothing but a suspicion.
2. Compression of the stomach between the vertebrae and cassette produces a clear filling defect or even a manifest hourglass phenomenon.
3. What in the photographs looks like kinking, narrowing or obstruction of the small or large intestines, very seldom reflects such disorders. Even serial photography shows elements of doubt.
4. The representation of stomach cancer or ulcer has, unfortunately, in certain centres, given the impression that roentgen rays were already capable of surpassing the ordinary diagnostic methods. This impression must be contradicted.
5. The roentgen-ray findings should, together with case history, the laboratory results, and the clinical data, and always with a sound mind, be brought into line'.

This quotation provides an insight into the practice and opinions of Carman. It is tragic that he had to discover his own stomach carcinoma in 1914. As reflection of his conservative attitude, he continues to use bismuth carbonate instead of barium sulphate as a contrast medium. Carman's description of his method of stomach examination published in 1913 under the title: 'The technique of roentgen-ray examination of the gastrointestinal tract and the interpretation of screen and plate findings', is excellent, and almost identical with the ways learned by the writer of this article in 1957 from his teacher, Bartstra

[38], who was specialized in gastroenterology. Bartstra's book on the roentgen examination of the digestive organs published at that time makes it clear that, in a somewhat modified form, he was one of the last followers of the symptom-complex method.

Although Carman always wore lead gloves, his hands were visibly branded by this examination method. Today, the symptom-complex method belongs to times past as a result of the double-contrast technique imported from Japan in 1969, and has been replaced by procedures and diagnostic evaluation in accordance with the direct-sign principle. The number of followers of the direct-sign method has increased rapidly, in the USA even faster than in Europe.

It is obvious that observing radiographic findings depends on the image quality of the radiographs taken during the examination. The number of publications on the various techniques for the visualization of the gastric mucosa and duodenal bulbus and their radiographic findings was considerable. The reduction in exposure time by using the much improved Coolidge tube, the introduction of the Potter–Bucky grid to absorb scattered radiation, and the continuous advancements of the intensifying screens have contributed to the improvement of image quality.

To illustrate the image quality of gastrointestinal radiology as practiced around 1920, several figures found in publications of several important authors are shown (Figs III, 10–20). Illustra-

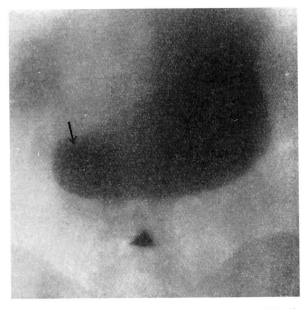

Fig. III, 10. Small carcinoma of the pylorus (arrow)(1916).

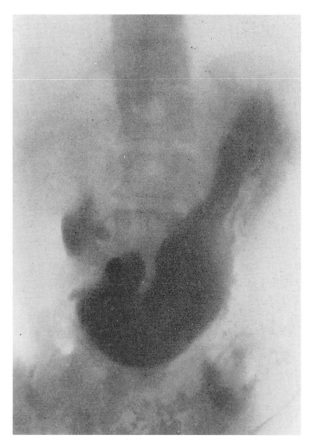

Fig. III, 11. Adhesive periduodenitis. Comment: in my opinion a deformed duodenal bulb (1916).

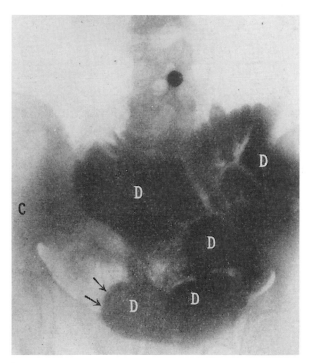

Fig. III, 12. Tuberculous strictures of the small intestine. Photograph after eight hours. Arrow = distal stricture. D = dilatated intestinal loops. C = cecum, not visible (1916).

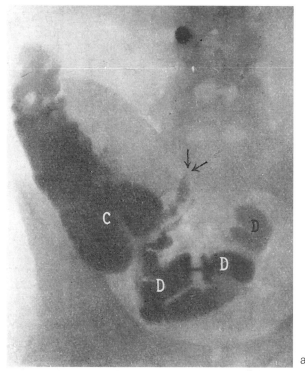

a

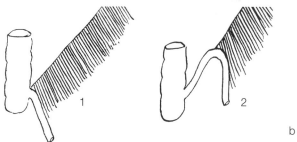

b

Fig. III, 13a, b. Lane's kink. Photograph after eight hours. Arrow = fixed upward displacement of an intestinal loop (1916). **a)** = normal situation, **b)** = situation shown in the figure.

tions III, 10–16 are taken by E. Stierlin, from the book, 'Klinische Roentgendiagnostik des Verdauungskanals', J.F. Bergmann, Wiesbaden, 1916. Illustrations III, 17 and 18 are taken from H. Assmann, 'Klinische Roentgendiagnostik der inneren Erkrankungen', 2nd edn, F.C.W. Vogel, Leipzig, 1922. Illustrations III, 19 and 20 from R.D. Carman, 'The Roentgen Diagnosis of Diseases of the Alimentary Canal', 2nd edn, Saunders, 1921.

It is remarkable that all reproductions found in the German literature are reversed with respect to the original radiographs that show the contrast medium as not black but white. This probably cheap display is extremely irritating and also pre-

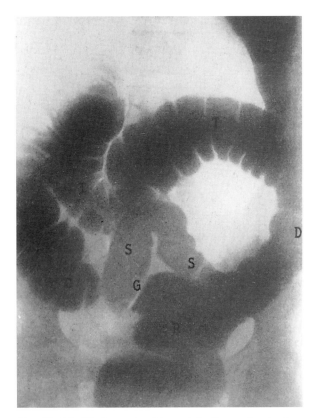

Fig. III, 14. Photograph of large intestines after barium enema (normal image) (1916).

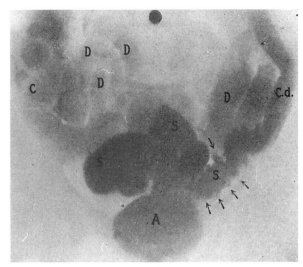

Fig. III, 15. Multiple diverticula of the sigmoid colon (arrow) (1916).

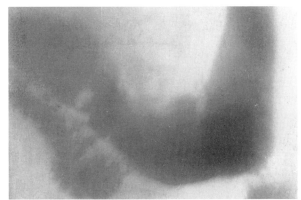

Fig. III, 17. Gastric polyp (1922).

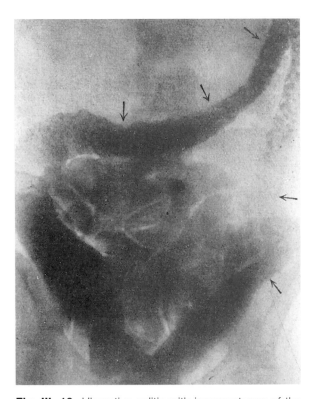

Fig. III, 16. Ulcerative colitis with incompetence of the ileocecal (Bauhin's) valve resulting in retrograde filling of the small intestine (1916).

vailed in The Netherlands for quite a long time, actually until this author's thesis in 1971. It is striking that Carman already recognized the psychological necessity of this extraphotographic procedure; today, this is the standard procedure everywhere.

In 1908, the famous Swedish researcher Goesta Forsell [39] began the long series of improvements of the details with his publication on small 'spot-film radiography', showing details of the mucous membrane with a specially designed fluoroscope, in which a translucent compression tube was mounted in front of the fluoroscopic screen. Other means of compression were inflatable rubber balloons in various sizes and cushions filled with textile or cork. In the mid-twenties

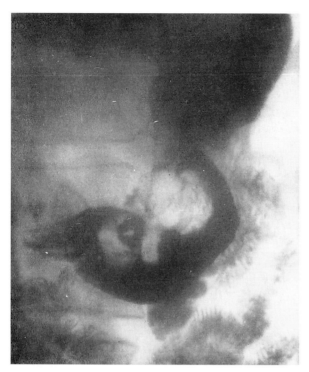

Fig. III, 18. Large filling defect as a result of gastric carcinoma in supine position (1922).

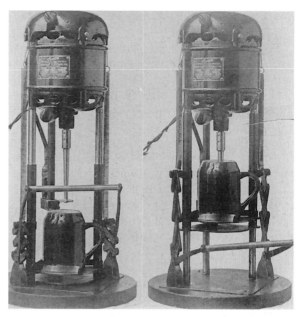

Fig. III, 20. The machine used to mix the ingredients of the contrast medium and to keep the suspension until the examination (1921).

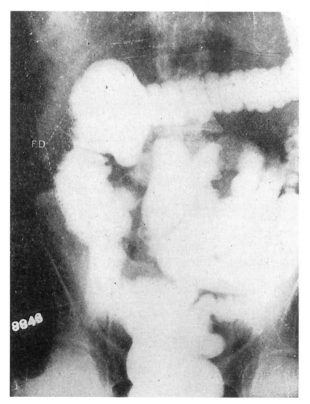

Fig. III, 19. Filling-defect (F-D) corresponding to a palpable tumor. A large retrocecal abscess was found at surgery (1921).

similar types of procedures were also used by Vallebona, Hilpert and Pribram and Kleiber [40].

In 1921, Åkerlund [41] compressed the partly filled duodenal bulb in such a manner that a contrast depot only remained when an ulcer niche was present. The patience and skill that many a physician mustered in those days, with a much inferior fluoroscopic quality than today, is commendable. A striking example of this can be found in the publication by Schatzki, at that time still in Leipzig, and the internist Henning [42]. Without making use of the double-contrast technique and by using, compared to today, a qualitatively inferior barium suspension, Schatzki showed compression films with distinctly visible erosions, in which even the flat central niche could be identified. This is the unabridged summary of their article:

'*A description of a case of gastroscopically and roentgenologically recorded gastric ulcer. The stomach erosions could be determined by means of spot-film photography of the stomach. Contrary to the general opinion, it is possible to record the ulcerative gastritis roentgenologically.*

We find here round and egg-shaped lentil- to green-pea-sized radiolucencies (infection ridges) with a central deposit of contrast medium (erosion). One can usually find these radiolucencies in the course of the rugae, which seem locally elevated. The folds themselves were widened in the case discussed. At the same time a severe hypersecretion exists, hampering the examination.

The majority of erosions, and probably the largest part, has, according to our own roentgenological investigations, not been recognizable until now.

Once the image of ulcerative gastritis is satisfactory, it is one of the few absolute roentgenological proofs of the presence of a clinical gastritis.'

Furthermore, the work published by Kaufman and Kienboeck (1911) [43] is interesting. They administered a small amount of viscous contrast medium, followed by a large amount of fluid of low viscosity and without radiopacity. They observed that the nonradiopaque fluid left the contrast medium in the spaces between the folds and progressed through the central lumen distally.

In 1923, Rendich [44] used the same method, which is based on the same principle, followed by giving a methylcellulose solution after a viscous barium suspension has been administered, as introduced by Herlinger [45] for the examination of the small bowel. The intestinal mucosa is covered with a thin, visible layer of contrast medium and the intestinal lumen distended, resulting in excellent double-contrast radiographs.

In contrast to the radiographic examinations of the stomach and duodenum, the colon examination developed in a less spectacular way until about 1930. As early as 1910 and again in 1923, Haenisch [46, 47] pointed out that an enema with retrograde rectal administration of bismuth suspension took less time and provided better results than the natural filling of the colon via oral administration of a bismuth meal. As late as 1933, he admitted to being a passionate supporter of fluoroscopy, and stated that a definite diagnosis on the basis of a filling defect without additional fluoroscopy was absolutely impossible. He palpated manually and warned against compression with the fluoroscopic screen. According to him, a short interruption in the administration of contrast medium could spoil the whole examination, a judgement almost incomprehensible today. He was puzzled by the image of a smooth, narrowed segment of colon, measuring 10–15 cm in length, possibly an old local ischemia. He also described an apparent 'stop' to the flow of administered contrast medium if a loop runs parallel to the direction of the X-rays. Finally, he also suggested that fluoroscopy should be kept short and that the patient should be given the opportunity to empty as much contrast medium as possible after the examination since constipation might result otherwise.

Carman reported in 1913 [37] that using barium sulphate as a contrast medium provided better results and that the colon can be cleansed thoroughly with laxatives, such as castor oil, and a cleansing enema shortly before the colon examination. In 1923, Haenisch [47] followed this approach, but still used bismuth carbonate as contrast medium, solved in aluminum oxide and water. For reasons unknown, he also took radiographs in the upright position. In those days, it was adequate to diagnose a megacolon, large polyps, diverticulosis, and tuberculosis. The differentiation between benign and malignant was already a very demanding task.

Carman could distinguish a true colitis from an irritable colon. He also noted that, completely contrary to what had previously been assumed, ileocecal reflux was unimportant.

In 1921, Laurel [48] had for the first time applied the double-contrast method, in which he insufflated air into the rectum, after the colon had been filled with a barium meal. It is not surprising that this method was not pursued further.

In the years 1923 and 1925, publications by Fischer [49] appeared. He instilled the smallest possible amount of barium suspension into the rectum and then filled the colon with air. When he needed a large amount of contrast medium to reach the cecum, air was insufflated only after the patient had emptied the surplus of the contrast medium in the toilet.

Although Fischer was now able to detect smaller polyps, his clearly improved procedure found only a few followers. Fischer pointed out that radiographs of complete luminal filling should not be obtained since they were useless. On the other hand, by obtaining double-contrast radiographs only, stenoses can easily be missed. The specific gravity of his contrast medium was apparently very high. Besides Fischer, a number of other investigators, such as Pansdorf, Frik, Cole and Knothe [50] considered the postevacuation radiographs very valuable. This author is of the opinion that the same holds true even today. Unfortunately, this is unjustly neglected by most radiologists.

At the same time, Weber [51] improved the double-contrast technique by making the barium suspension a little more viscous. He also deserves credit for having proposed criteria for malignancy and chronic ulcerative colitis.

In 1933, Ledoux-Lebard and Garcia-Calderon [52] tried to improve the diagnostic results of the complete filling technique by making the contrast medium more transparent for X-rays. It failed since the specific gravity was definitely too low. Gelfland and collaborators [53] use the correct specific gravity today.

In 1936, Rigler and Erikson [54] again tried to improve the complete filling technique. They decided against the reduction of the contrast medium's specific gravity, but for overexposure of the radiographs instead. At the same time, Gianturco [55] was able to increase the information of radiographs obtained with colon completely filled by applying the 'high-kV technique'. He even went as far as using 120 kV. It is unfortunate that he did not report this until 1950, possibly because of the increasing international tensions resulting from Second World War.

In the thirties and for some time thereafter, the colon examination was conducted as follows: first, radiographs of the completely filled colon following rectal administration of a barium suspension, which invariably had a specific gravity that was too high; subsequently, after evacuation, one or two radiographs to assess the colonic mucosa; and finally – but this was not universal – a few double-contrast radiographs after rectal air insufflation.

In the thirties, the radiographic evaluation of the colon lacked far behind that of the stomach, but this applies even more to the small bowel.

Even 17 years later, little had changed. The book 'Kurzes Handbuch der gesamten Roentgendiagnostik und Therapie', published in 1928 by S. Karger, Berlin, and edited by G. Kohlmann, showed the different attention given to the various regions of the gastrointestinal tract by the number of pages devoted to them: oesophagus, 28 pages; stomach, 52 pages; resected stomach, 25 pages; small bowel, 6 pages; and colon, 18 pages.

Ten years later, some changes had been made, mainly in favor of the colon, but the small bowel still remained a largely unexplored area. The book published in 1938 by H.K. Lewis Ltd., London, 'Textbook of X-Ray Diagnosis by British Authors', covers the various gastrointestinal regions as follows: pharynx and oesophagus, 33 pages; stomach and duodenum, 163 pages; small bowel, 16 pages; and appendix, colon and rectum, 92 pages.

It was not until 30 years later, in 1969, that a fundamental change took place in favor of the small bowel.

The book, published by Williams and Wilkins, Baltimore, 'Golden's Diagnostic Radiology' with Laurence L. Robbins as editor, showed the following distribution: oesophagus, 120 pages; stomach and duodenum, 380 pages; small bowel, 220 pages; and colon 122, pages. The small bowel had by now surpassed the colon, with the spread widening further in the future.

In 1915, exactly 20 years after the discovery of X-rays, no less a man than Carman had found obvious differences in motility, without drawing usable diagnostic or therapeutic consequence, at least none have been described. Carman did determine that the intestinal loops were dilated proximal to an obstruction and that tuberculosis could well be the cause of narrowing and spasms of the distal end of the ileum.

Initially, Rieder [57] took radiographs of the intestines with the patient upright because of constraints related to the examination table. To image the mucosal folds he used a quick-settling quality of bismuth to fill the spaces between the folds. In 1911, Gottwald Schwarz [58], one of the oldest collaborators of Holzknecht, complained that in the six months following Rieder's publications on gastrointestinal radiology, only four cases of an abnormality in the small bowel had been described in the bibliography, in contrast to many publications on the colon and even more on the stomach.

In 1928, Loichinger [59] tried to improve Rieder's results by administering a larger amount of a suspension with a lower bismuth ratio and, later, by using the much slower settling bismuth sulphate.

In 1932, Cole [2] advocated the use of a rather viscous suspension of barium sulphate in water, which passed slowly through the small bowel, but was quickly emptied from the stomach. He took radiographs at 0.5, 2, 4 and 6 hours after administration of the contrast medium. Interestingly, he already stated that the contrast medium should not contain any nutritional substances and that milk should not be used as a solvent.

Since 1927, Pansdorf [60] had administered the contrast medium in intervals, a big swallow every 10 to 15 minutes. Cole did not agree with this method, because he considered the degree of intestinal filling inadequate. From a publication by Pansdorf in 1937, 10 years after his first publication, we learn that he had good results with this method. He found that giving cold contrast media caused, among other things, artificial hypermotility, and he recommended that contrast medium should be given at body temperature.

Agreeing with Kuhlmann [61], Pansdorf was of the opinion that it is better to examine the distal ileum loops via a retrograde colon filling, thus acknowledging the diagnostic superiority of the complete filling. We further learn from his article that he was able to observe motility changes in either direction. Moreover, a rather pronounced flocculation as well as a locally swollen mucosa and stenoses of the intestinal lumen did not escape his attention.

One of the frequently occurring infection processes in those days was tuberculosis. In this context, the well-documented files by Boles and Gershon-Cohen (1934) [62], which contain 1000 autopsy examinations of the intestines performed in 1933, deserve special attention. They recommended the double-contrast technique to detect the often subtle superficial lesions, which in the early stages could present only as local flocculation and as mosaic structure of the covering barium. This corresponds to irritability and hypermotility observed fluoroscopically.

One of the most significant publications of this period was the one by Crohn, Ginzburg and Oppenheimer in 1932 [63]. It concerned a regional enteritis, which was different from tuberculosis and for which no cause could be found. Tuberculosis was widespread, contrary to the present situation. It had largely given way to the very similar findings of Crohn's disease.

Until the fifties and even later, Pansdorf's method of administering contrast medium had, although occasionally modified, found general use. Nevertheless, efforts were being made to improve the examination technique of the small bowel, but with little notable success.

The figures III, 21 (in 'Roentgenuntersuchungen am Innenrelief des Verdauungskanals', by H.H. Berg, 2nd edn, Thieme, Leipzig 1931) and III, 22 (in 'Lehrbuch der roentgenologischen Differentialdiagnostik der Erkrankun-

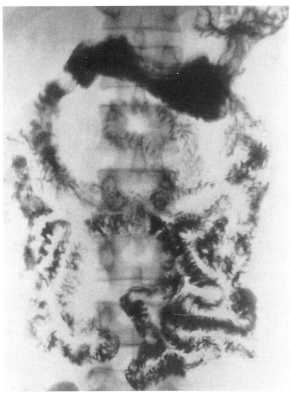

Fig. III, 21. Thickened gastric folds. Mottling of the contrast-filled stomach (mucous). Accelerated emptying. A 35-year-old man with achylia gastrica. Leukocytic gastric sediment with eosinophilia (1931).

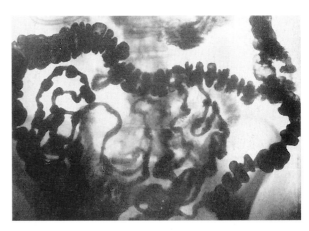

Fig. III, 22. Radiograph of opacified small intestines and colon without any abnormalities (1937).

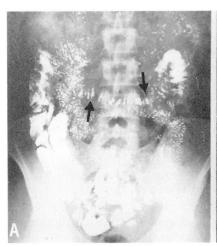
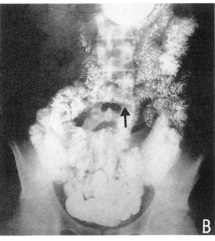

Fig. III, 23a, b. a) Extreme flocculation of contrast medium in the jejunum and ileum and also in the transverse colon due to worm infestation. **b)** Return to an almost normal intestinal mucosa two months later (1945).

gen der Bauchorgane', by W. Teschendorf, Thieme, Leipzig 1937) could be considered representative for the period 1930 to at least 1950. This also applies to the figure III, 23 (in Golden's "Radiological Examinations of the Small Intestine", Lippincott, Philadelphia 1945).

As seen in all publications now, the barium-filled colon is already shown as white structure.

Golden's examination of a 2-day-old baby (Fig. III, 24) can be considered to be representative of the familiar images seen until at least 1970. Only flocculated barium is seen, without visualization of the intestinal wall or lumen – a finding given the most absurd interpretations. Golden's book indicates that he was certainly familiar with the considerable better results of the enteroclysis, but apparently did not dare risk such an ex-

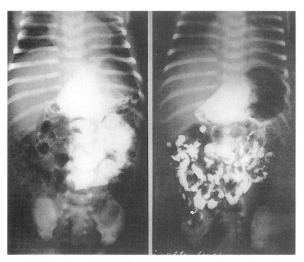

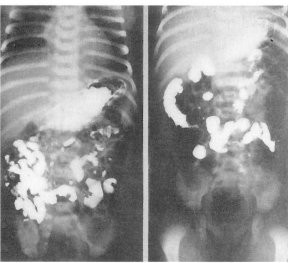

Fig. III, 24. Upper GI-series in a two-day-old infant. Complete fragmentation of the contrast medium in all four radiographs, taken at 15 minutes, 45 minutes, two hours and five and a half hours after the oral administration of the contrast medium (1945).

amination on a 2-day-old baby. It is unfortunate that the author also did not have the chance to perform a similar examination at Indiana University, even in 1977!

In his publication in the American Journal of Roentgenology of September 1929, Pesquera [64] expressed his dissatisfaction that lesions were often not clearly visible due to poor filling of the small bowel. He referred to the superior results of Einhorn and collaborators [65], who, directly through a tube, filled the duodenum with a mixture of $BaSO_4$, gum arabic and water. In a patient suffering from intestinal obstruction, Pesquera succeeded to fill the entire small bowel, after previous conventional small bowel series had given an unsatisfactory result. Encouraged by the outcome, he recommended this technique in certain cases. He stated that such an examination did not take more than half an hour. The time saving did hardly impress anyone, and no reason was seen to change established examination methods. Moreover, the very limited clinical knowledge of the diseases of the small bowel had led to a lack of interest to improve the image quality, which would have been achieved with Pesquera's method. Pesquera himself did not recommend his method as a routine examination.

In 1934, five years after Pesquera's publication, a very remarkable contribution appeared in the Archives of Internal Medicine by Snell and Camp [66] from Rochester, presenting the clinical symptomatology of a 'chronic idiopathic steatorrhea' together with the corresponding radiographs. They saw dilated small bowel loops and colon as well as an effaced mucosal relief in the small bowel, as proximal as in the duodenum. They attributed this to a chronic infection with mucosal edema and mural infiltration, leading to a reduced motility and flocculation of the barium suspension. They also found that the atrophy of the mucosal relief improved, though only slightly, after medical treatment.

In retrospect, these mentioned interpretations of radiographs belong to one of the most tenacious errors in the history of radiology.

One year later, Mackie, Miller and Rhoads [67] from New York describe in their article 'Roentgenologic changes in the small intestine' observations similar to those of Snell and Camp, affecting both the small bowel and the colon. In their view, it represents a marked motility disorder, not associated with increased transit. The following sentence from their article is noteworthy, *'The absence of specific and significant morphologic changes in postmortem examination is a distinctive characteristic'*. It is even more noteworthy that they did not address the question how this could be possible, but were satisfied with the statement, *'There are basic contradictions in the statements on pathological changes and in the interpretations based on this.'*

Again 5 years later, a publication by Kantor [68], also from New York, showed that nothing had changed. Kantor was also impressed by the smooth, sausage-like 'barium tube', which, especially in the duodenum and proximal jejunum, was most distinct and became known under the name he gave it, 'moulage sign'.

He was of the opinion that this finding was the best indicator for diagnosis, severity and prognosis of idiopathic steatorrhea. Kantor believed, not quite unjustifiably, that this impressive finding could be ascribed to be specific for an impaired fat resorption. He reported, however, that Camp had 'suggested' that it had also been found in a number of other diseases. Subsequently, Kantor pointed out that steatorrhea was the only grave, chronic diarrhoea in which a dilated instead of a narrowed colon was found. Many failed to appreciate how much the diagnosis of the 'moulage sign' in patients with steatorrhea depended on the examiner.

In 1939, 10 years after Pesquera's publication [64] on the administration of contrast medium via a probe, Gershon-Cohen and Shay [70], in Philadelphia, tried to reintroduce this method and gave it the name 'barium enteroclysis'. After the direct administration of 800–1200 ml, they reached the ileocecal (Bauhin's) valve in 8–15 min. They found that contrast medium refluxes into the stomach if instilled too fast. To overcome the interference of superimposed intestinal loops, they took radiographs whenever 200 ml was administered. Subsequently, they often injected air in small increments of 5 ml and observed that it moves quickly through the small bowel. But the origin of the 'moulage sign' remained unclear to them.

Several authors, among them Bouslog (1935) [71] and Henderson (1942) [72], drew attention to the identical 'moulage sign' that were visible on the intestinal radiographs of babies and infants, more severe the younger the age.

Golden wrote in 1945 [73] that the sedimentation of the barium suspension in babies was caused by the inability of the intestinal wall to relax, because of the immaturity of the 'nervous reflex control mechanism'. Although having already ascribed it in 1941 to a vitamin-B-complex deficit, Golden advocated the need for further radiological investigations as to the cause of this problem. Two years earlier in 1943, Zwerling and Nelson [74] had expressed serious doubts about the radiological diagnosis of coeliac disease (Gee-Herter) in a number of small children without corresponding symptoms. They therefore performed a small bowel series on 77 healthy children, varying between 3 months and 11 years of age, and found that half of the children showed a 'deficiency pattern' and the other half various transitional stages up to the normal adult pattern. They also often observed abnormal findings in the same children who had normal findings 30 min after the onset of the examination. On the grounds of this excellent study, the authors came to the conclusion that a 'deficiency pattern' was not proof of a "nutritional deficiency state".

In 1949, Frazer, French and Thompson [74a] confirmed Zwerling and Nelson's observations, not only in children but also in adults. Within a short interval, they observed the change of barium-filled loops with a normal mucosal relief to segments devoid of folds and containing smooth, elongated masses of barium, the 'moulage sign', in steatorrhea, but also following addition of acetic acid, lactic acid, fatty acid, bile and mucus to the contrast medium. Furthermore, they noticed that this phenomenon had nothing to do with the so-called 'disordered motor function' of the small bowel but that it did occur in jaundice, pancreatic fibrosis, food allergy and coeliac disease. Apparently, this pioneering article by Frazer, French and Thompson [74a] had not been read or understood. In any case, its paramount implication was not realized.

Schatzki [75], who in the forties no longer worked in Leipzig but in Boston, concluded in 1943 that small intestinal radiology had, until then, been a stepchild of diagnostic radiology. Maybe it was a stroke of luck that Schatzki did not know Pesquera's [64] and Gershon-Cohen's [70] earlier investigations. His study was in many respects much more elaborate. He pointed out, among other things, that a preceding cleansing of the colon is of great value to the outcome of the examination, in addition to using a contrast medium of low specific gravity and placing the patient in the right lateral position.

In 1912, the Dutch roentgenologist van der Haer [76] opened his address at a meeting of colleagues with the soothing announcement that the radiological examination of the alimentary tract was rather simple. He had a patient swallow a few spoonfuls of a viscous-bismuth meal since a bismuth containing milk 'plunged' down too quickly. Only by means of strong thermic or chemical stimuli causing cardiospasm, the time necessary to reach the cardia – normally between 2 and 8 s – was lengthened slightly. If the time was 30–60 s, one should immediately suspect an obstruction.

He then showed four cases in which his suspicion was proved correct. Answering a question from his colleague Eykman concerning the difference between a purely spastic and a carcinomatous stricture, van der Haer stated that the radiographic examination is not in a position to resolve this issue.

Eight years later, Carman [77] reported in the second edition of his book, 'The Roentgen Diagnosis of the Alimentary Canal' that some improvement had been accomplished, particularly in the diagnosis of cardiospasm, tumors, stenoses and diverticula, but that the differentiation between a benign and malignant stricture remained difficult. In 1932, Cole [2] stated that for an esophageal image he used to administer a barium-sulphate and water mixture of such viscosity that it could only be swallowed after thorough mixing with saliva in the mouth. He preferred to administer the paste with the patient supine to delay, as was assumed in those days, the passage through the oesophagus for optimal filling. In reality, the oesophagus examination was only performed for a better assessment of the outlines of the heart. Thus, the esophageal examination remained the stepchild of gastrointestinal radiology.

Nevertheless, Barclay's [78] publication on 35 years of diagnostic evaluation of the oesophagus deserves special attention. He performed pioneering cinematographic studies on the pharyngeal swallowing mechanism and further transport of liquids and solid food through the oesophagus. His work was far ahead of his time. Barclay's observations contributed to the challenge of the concept that gravity influenced food transportation through the oesophagus.

He could also confirm the assumption expressed by Schreiber in 1911 and later supported by Laurell [79] that negative pressure plays an important part in the transport from pharynx to oesophagus. In case of a dysfunction in this mechanism, peristalsis can take over this function.

Until the end of the Second World War, the radiologic evaluation of esophageal disorders was confined to the following changes:
- malignant and benign tumors, including submucosal tumors with interluminal spreading;
- varicose changes of some consideration;
- diaphragmatic hernia with limited characterization;
- different types of perforation, including the Mallory–Weiss syndrome and the Boerhaave syndrome;
- scleroderma and myasthenia;
- oesophagitis with solitary or superficial ulcerations.

It was not until after the Second World War, since about 1950, that knowledge and diagnostic evaluation of oesophageal disorders would undergo a major progress, soon followed by a similar development in the evaluation of the swallowing mechanism and its disorders.

Unfortunately, the number of radiologists who specialized in this field was very limited and most countries had only one or two specialized centres.

The development of diagnostic radiology came to a standstill during the Second World War and its postwar period of approximately 5 years. It is remarkable that almost all important improvements initially encountered a great deal of resistance for a longer or shorter period. This began already with Hamilton's publication in 1946 [80]. He was the first to add tannic acid to the barium meal to improve mucosal coating, but even such an authority as Weber could not appreciate the value of this improvement.

The resistance to this was not overcome until Christie and collaborators in 1950 [81] announced that they had examined 4225 patients in this manner and concluded that it was indeed a 'valuable addition to previous methods'. Still in the same year, the manufacturers of contrast-media also contributed to the progress with the discovery of a considerable refinement of the adhesive power of barium suspension by using smaller barium particles. However, it appeared that the micro-particles increased the toxicity through resorption, and the particle size could not be too small. The mucosal adhesiveness was further improved by increasing the viscosity of the contrast medium by adding not only acids but also gelatin and gum arabic. An additional benefit was a contrast medium that did not flocculate easily.

Until the end of the Second World War, most radiology departments were equipped with vertically mounted systems for examinations of the stomach and horizontal tables for examinations of the colon. These tables were excellent for colon examination, but taking a radiograph in the Chassard–Lapiné projection, valuable for a long and tortuous sigmoid, meant an extremely strenuous procedure for elderly, ill or immobile patients. The patient had to sit on the table edge and bend over as far as possible, the X-ray tube was disengaged, and a radiograph of the pelvis region was obtained with a vertically oriented central beam. Frequently, this led to a rather underexposed radiograph and a very dirty table. A better result was often achieved by taking a radiograph with the x-ray beam in ±45° craniocaudal angulation and the patient placed in the prone position.

Universal tables had been developed in the first few years after the Second World War. With electric motors, the tables could be tilted from the horizontal to the vertical position during examination. This was of great importance to improve the quality of the examination and facilitate its performance.

The specific gravity of the contrast medium remained a matter of controversy. In past 50 years, a small number of physicians, among them Gianturco [82] and this author [83], stood up, time and again, for a lower than customary specific gravity. Moreover, the value of a postevacuation radiograph, as part of the colon investigation was not generally acknowledged. Its supporters were, among others, Robinson [84], Marshak and Lindner [85], Kabakian and Massabni [86], and this author. These radiographs delineate the abnormal colonic mucosa considerably better than the radiographs obtained with the colonic lumen completely filled with barium. In addition, the rectosigmoid usually returns to its normal position in the small pelvis, from which it is displaced during complete luminal filling. Also the frequently present internal haemorrhoids are only visible in postevacuation films.

Even long before the Second World War, the German surgeon Fischer [87] and Kirklin and Weber [88] from the Mayo-Clinic, and later after the war, Bell and Morson [89], Stevenson [90], Douglas [91] and Moreton [92] obtained good results with a double-contrast colon examination, but it was not sufficiently accepted as a routine method. Gianturco even thought it ridiculous. Robinson [84], on the contrary, found the postevacuation radiographs outstanding, and Marshak was of the opinion that these radiographs show the radiographic changes of Crohn's disease better than the double-contrast technique. The prevailing opinion was that a double-contrast investigation was labour intensive and unpleasant for the patient. Using the high-voltage technique for the demonstration of polyps was even preferred over the double-contrast examination by Peister and Gilchrist [93]. Jarre and Fiegel (1961) [94] expressed a similar opinion and applied a very comprehensive

compression technique. In contrast, the author's teacher Bartstra [95] required his students to obtain double-contrast radiographs as the final phase of the examination after defecation (1958). Welin [96] in Malmö succeeded in introducing the double-contrast technique as a generally accepted examination (1953), undoubtedly, helped by his detailed attention to all aspects of this method.

The most important factor was an extremely thorough cleansing of the colon by means of a 'peroral lavage', developed in his institute. Polyps of 2-mm in size can only be detected in an absolutely clean colon [97]. Acknowledged as authority, Welin [6], together with his daughter, could report their experience with this technique on more than 50000 patients.

A statistical investigation conducted by Thoeni and Margulis [98] among radiologists revealed that in the USA in 1976, 17% of all the patients had a completely unprepared colon examination and only 6% had a double-contrast examination. In 1987, these figures had improved to 3% and 56%, respectively [99].

Many physicians, including the author, share the view that all three phases of the colon examination have their own specific value. In particular, a completely filled elongated, redundant sigmoid colon can detect space-occupying processes better, revealing them as defects, than the double-contrast visualized colon, where they produce extra lines that might not be appreciated amidst the already confusing interplay of normal lines. It is, however, mandatory that the contrast medium is of lower specific gravity than that used for a standard double-contrast examination. The author has shown in a series of experiments that a contrast medium of low specific gravity of ± 1.3 increases the possibility of demonstrating lesions in the vertical projection in comparison with the horizontal projection, which requires a higher specific gravity.

It is clearly apparent that improving examination techniques and improving radiographic equipment through the efforts of the industry are closely interrelated. This also applies to the clinical demands posed by internists and surgeons and to the efforts of radiologists to provide appropriate solutions. As a result, outstanding clinical articles were published in the sixties and seventies, covering a wide range of diagnoses and their differential diagnoses. A few examples, not confined to the colon, are found in the references 100–109.

Cummings (1974) [109] reported on a smoothly outlined, ahaustral colon found in a psychologically unstable, thin woman with anorexia nervosa and who was on multiple medications, including laxatives. But the author of this article noted that a similar type of colon is almost normal in the indigenous population of Curaçao, without apparent emaciation. As its cause, he could find the old-established habit of using laxatives to prevent and treat parasitic worm infestations.

Another very important publication was by Morton A. Meyers (1971) [110] of New York. On the basis of an anatomical study of the mesenteric attachments and a series of peritoneograms to determine the flow of intra-abdominal fluids, he arrived at the conclusion that metastatic spread follows predictable paths, which depend on the patient's position and are rather different between the upright and supine position. The increased incidence of metastases in certain known sites is predestined by the blind-ending peritoneal pouches in the mesenteric folds [111]. These publications set aside the obsolete ideas that intra-abdominal fluids are stationary. More than any other publication, it contributed to a better understanding of the intra-abdominal fluid currents and related intra-abdominal metastatic spread, which is completely independent from the already known hematogenous and lymphatic spread.

Not all complaints and disorders of the anorectal area could be detected or explained by radiologic examinations of the colon, supplemented by colonoscopy. Among other conditions, this applies to constipation and incontinence, as well as to such complaints as the feeling of incomplete evacuation of the bowls, too frequent bowel movements, and the necessity for strong and continued straining. Although Brown [112] and Brodén and Snellman [113] had already drawn the attention to the defecation mechanism from cinematographic studies in the sixties, limited interest only arose as late as in the eighties. The contributing physicians included Ekberg, Nylander and Fork [114], and Mahieu, Pringot and Bodart [115]. In The Netherlands, these defecation studies were introduced by Ottens and Janssen [116], a radiologist and electronics engineer, and adapted for clinical use by Goei [117] in his thesis. Mueller-Lissner [118] introduced these studies in Germany.

The investigation is easy to perform and takes 10–15 min at the most. It may seem drastic but in reality it is not, and with a modern remote-controlled table is even easier. The following treatable disorders can be detected:
– intra-anal rectal invagination;
– extra-anal rectal invagination (prolapse);
– rectocele;
– spastic pelvic floor syndrome;
– descending perineum syndrome;
– solitary rectal ulcer syndrome, often as a result of a rectum prolapse.

This relatively young method deserves a great deal more attention than we have seen so far. But it should be emphasized that such an investigation is only indicated if it can be followed by the necessary surgical treatment. Not all hospitals have a surgeon on staff with expertise in this field.

Radiologic examinations of the stomach and duodenum were already performed before the Second World War and, essentially unchanged, for the next 15 years afterwards, except for a little more attention paid to the diagnosis of hiatal hernias. The double-contrast technique, which invaded the world of radiology, did not remain limited to examinations of the colon but was also applied to examinations of the stomach. It is understandable that the extraordinary diagnostic quality of this technique was first proved in Japan, where gastric carcinomas are four times more frequent than in Western countries. Consequently, the interest in an early diagnosis of cancer, as first described by Gutman and Prèvot (1937) [119], was greater in Japan than elsewhere.

Shirakabe and Ichikawa [120, 121] had worked on the development of an improved double-contrast technique for the stomach since about 1955, followed a few years later by their compatriot Kawai [122]. In 1961, the two physicians mentioned above presented their results at a convention but, as it happens so often with new ideas, their Japanese colleagues showed hardly any interest. Frik and Hesse [123] from Erlangen and Buecker [124] from Hamburg showed great enthusiasm and they helped their Japanese colleagues in 1963 to make this technique better known throughout the world. As early as 1958, Amplatz [125] had his patients drink the barium suspension through a straw punched with a hole so that they swallowed air with the contrast medium.

Some physicians use Amplatz's method, but most radiologists use the bubbly-barium method according to Pochaczevsky [127], promoted by Op den Orth [126]. The barium meal is under CO_2 pressure in a soda siphon. After pouring, the gaseous barium meal must be drunk quickly, but the examination should not commence before the gas production has ceased. Buscopan, or even better glucagon, injected before the examination paralyses the stomach and prevents premature and potentially interfering filling of the duodenum.

It is well known that the double-contrast study shows the posterior gastric wall noticeably better than the anterior gastric wall, necessitating a complementary second phase of the examination following administration of more barium solution and graded compression, as described by Op den Orth [128] in his thesis 'Standard biphasic contrast examination of the stomach and duodenum.' A hypotonic agent administered prior to the double-contrast study of the stomach might conceal a sliding gastro-oesophageal hernia that might be observed endoscopically.

While remote-control equipment is suitable for examinations of the small bowel and colon, this is certainly not true for examinations of the stomach. The patient's position often needs very subtle adjustments that cannot be easily accomplished by verbal instructions and are achieved more quickly and efficiently by the physician himself, requiring a direct contact between patient and physician.

Today, the radiographic examination of the stomach has reached such a high degree of perfection that, if performed correctly, further improvement seems neither possible nor necessary. The duodenum is usually so well visualized that the 'hypotonic duodenography' as an additional examination, common in the sixties, is hardly ever performed nowadays. The hypotonic duodenography is performed by injecting both contrast medium and air via the so-called Bilbao tube into the duodenum and was mainly used for the indirect visualization of the pancreatic head. Another fundamental reason for the disappearance of the hypotonic duodenography as well as for the more recent decline in the number of upper gastrointestinal series, which is also observed in the USA, is the enormous evolution of the gastroduodenoscopy, including retrograde cholangiopancreatography. These endoscopic examinations are performed by gastroenterologists. This has created a very dynamic competitive environment in many hospitals but, in the end, professional expertise of each specialist should prevail.

Whenever required, the double contrast examination of the stomach can be followed (or preceded) by a double contrast examination of the oesophagus, which can detect even the smallest lesions. The best technique to obtain a double contrast esophagram has been described by Brombart (1961) [129] and has also been promoted in the USA since 1976 by G.J. Dodd [130]. A large swallow of a barium solution

with good adhesive properties is immediately followed by several large swallows of water or methylcellulose solution from a different cup. This produces a good double contrast image of the distended oesophagus over an extended period, which is only rarely achievable after the more difficult procedure of swallowing air. This method can differentiate mucosal from submucosal lesions, can visualize both reflux oesophagitis and varices, and can detect cancer at an early stage.

At the end of the sixties and the beginning of the 70, the knowledge of the multitude of oesophageal disorders increased commensurate with the improved examination methods, yet the number of radiologists with expertise in this area remains surprisingly low in all countries. In the early days, Barclay [131] and Ardran and Kemp [132] were great pioneers in this field, and later, among others, Dodds [133] and Donner [134] in the USA, and Pringot and Ponette [135] in Belgium. Already 1962, Klinkhamer [136], 137] in the Netherlands could describe pathological and normal vascular esophageal impressions in detail.

Standard works covering the wide range of diseases in this field and the various examination techniques were published by Brombart [138], Huepscher [139], Dodds [140] and most recently by Levine and Laufer [141].

In 1965 and in the following years, Dodds [142, 143, 144], Donner [145, 146, 147] and Jones [148] concentrated on oesophageal motility disorders and anomalies of the very complex swallowing mechanism affecting the pharyngo-oesophageal transition zone, the most complicated field in radiology of the alimentary tract. Dahm [149] in Germany, must be given the honor to have been the first to have gained more insight into this field by using kymographs as early as 1941. Nowadays, this has been considerably improved by cinematography or video recording, preferably with simultaneous pressure recording.

A very thorough investigation of the normal swallowing mechanism and its changes with cinematography was performed on 400 individuals by Olle Ekberg [150, 151] from Malmö, partly in collaboration with Nylander. According to Donner and Siegel [134], the most frequently occurring swallowing complaints result from a paralysis of the pharyngeal muscles. Repeated swallowing movements supported by head and lower jaw movements are characteristically observed. With this condition as well as with laxity of the pharyngeal wall, and with mechanical obstruction or in cachectic and elderly patients, stasis of food residues or aspiration may occur. The most frequent diseases that can be accompanied by swallowing complaints are: poliomyelitis, amyotrophic lateral sclerosis, multiple sclerosis, syringomyelia, myasthenia, sarcoidosis, dermatomyositis, systemic lupus erythematosus and diphtheria. Anaesthesia of the throat can also cause swallowing problems.

During the Second World War and certainly for many years afterwards, patients undergoing a small bowel series drank 200 or, at most, 300 ml of barium solution, initially in small increments but after 1945, as Golden recommended [73], the entire amount at once. It is worth mentioning that in 1945, in a short but articulate thesis, the Chilean Manuel Concha Urra [152] (Fig. III, 25) demonstrated better results by administering the contrast medium via a probe rather than by drinking, as the illustrations in his booklet show. Because this thesis was published in Spanish, it was denied the wider readership it deserved. As far as this author could verify, Urra performed his investigation on more than 50 patients and administered approximately 500 ml contrast medium at a somewhat higher infusion speed. A slight gastric reflux and a decreased peristalsis of the intestinal loops were often found. To compare this method with the conventional examination of the small bowel, he only administered 200 ml contrast medium orally, which does not allow a valid comparison.

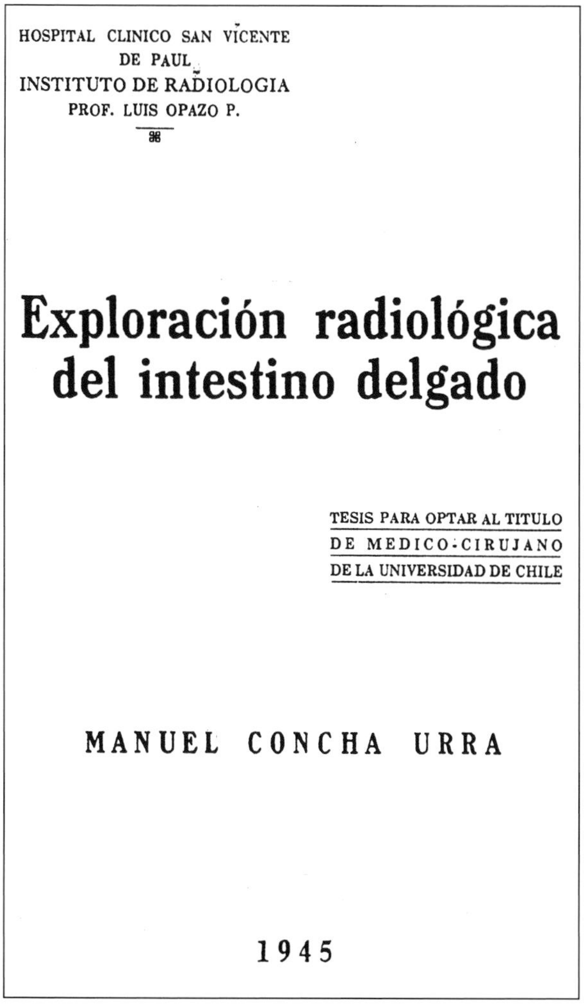

Around 1955, Marshak [153] improved the conventional method considerably by increasing his already high dose of 450 to 600 ml, if necessary. Nevertheless, in those days flocculation of contrast medium was frequent and the list of diseases to be taken into consideration was impressive. In their publication on Whipple's disease in 1967, R.P. Rice and collaborators [154] pointed out that the cause of disintegration of the contrast medium lay with the radiologists and was lowest when micropulverized barium powder was used. Weltz [155] deserves the credit to have, as early as 1937, drawn attention to the fact that the quality of the radiographs improved when the amount of contrast medium was increased. Incorrectly interpreting the flocculation of the barium suspension, the thickening of the mucosal folds and, finally, the complete mucosal effacement (moulage sign) as the result of oedema and anomalous motor function continued into the fifties, sixties and seventies. Actually, everybody could see that these broad folds appear normal for a brief period of time at the beginning of the examination, confirmed by fluoroscopy and autopsies. Moreover, it could be shown that the transit time was completely normal in cases of suspected impaired motility.

Wherever hypertrophy of the intestinal musculature was suspected, autopsy showed atrophy. Even the 'deficiency pattern' that J. Friedman (1954) [156] thought to have proven in four patients by provoking their emotions remained unproven. To be exact, the flocculation of the contrast medium was already clearly visible in all four patients on radiographs obtained before the emotions were released, but was not recognized as such at that time. In the period 1955–1975, publications on the sprue syndrome were numerous, as were those on several other diseases related to the flocculation of barium, such as Whipple's disease, giardiasis, Zollinger–Ellison syndrome, and a countless variety of deficiency syndromes. Many types of tumors, infection processes, vascular anomalies and thesaurosis were presented in numerous publications. The most striking publication in this fruitful period of in-

HOSPITAL CLINICO SAN VICENTE
DE PAUL
INSTITUTO DE RADIOLOGIA
PROF. LUIS OPAZO P.
98

Exploración radiológica del intestino delgado

TESIS PARA OPTAR AL TITULO
DE MEDICO-CIRUJANO
DE LA UNIVERSIDAD DE CHILE

MANUEL CONCHA URRA

1945

Fig. III, 25. Cover page of M.C. Urra's thesis.

testinal radiology was provided by Richard Marshak [157], partly in collaboration with Lindner, an internist.

Despite Marshak's profound work, the applied radiographic techniques remained inadequate compared to the excellent clinical and radiological knowledge of intestinal diseases achieved in the interval. Although competitiveness and pressure to publish are extremely strong in the USA, several European authors also contributed to this publication avalanche.

In 1966, this author was fortunate enough to be working as a rather young radiologist at the Leiden University clinic with Prof. van Ronnen. In addition to the responsibility for radiology in the surgical clinic, he was to direct, from 1968, the roentgen discussions on gastroenteric patients who had been transferred to the surgical department. With respect to this function, the professor of gastroenterology soon assigned the author to deliver a 30-min address about the radiological contribution to the diagnosis and differential diagnoses of coeliac disease at an international coeliac symposium in Leiden in 1969. The review of the patient material available from previous years and a critical evaluation of the radiological literature published on this disease enabled the author to conclude that it was impossible to arrive at the diagnosis of this illness by means of radiology as it was at that time. This well-documented, but potentially provoking information was introduced to the shocked audience in a fraction of the allotted time. The author was called to his superior's office the next morning, as was whispered, to receive an immediate dismissal. On that particular morning the two angry professors had decided, after a good night's sleep, to offer the author an alternative instead of dismissal. They demanded that he should not be satisfied with his devastating criticism, but should investigate how this diagnosis might be obtained otherwise.

After accepting the challenge, the first few months were wasted on trying to convince some manufactures of contrast medium to produce a more stable and less quickly flocculating barium suspension. Financial means and the necessary time appeared to be obstacles. Moreover, the author was unknown and the only one criticizing. All other users were satisfied, among whom were a few authorities. Convinced of the impossibility of the quest, no other solution remained than to ponder how the contrast medium could win the fight with the secretions present in the stomach and small bowel. He had never heard or read anything on the subject previously,

neither did he know of Pesquera, Gershon-Cohen, or Schatzki, not to mention the Chilean Urra(1945) [152]. But he was aware of the good results obtained by Marshak with his high-dose barium meals. The aim was to get a high dose of contrast medium into the small bowel as quickly as possible.

At first, it was tried to get the patient to drink as much of the barium meal as possible, and to accelerate the gastric emptying with a peristalsis-enhancing drug, but then the approach was changed to a quick administration via a tube directly into the duodenum. At first the Rehfuss tube with metal nozzle was used in the right lateral position, but it took long for the tube to pass through the pylorus. A few months later this tube was replaced by an extended Bilbao tube [158], which could be moved into the right place by means of a guide wire. When this method proved to be successful and the survey radiographs of the small bowel taken in the prone position were obviously better than the ones taken in the supine position, a remote-control unit could be obtained for the department, tough with some difficulty.

For a thesis, it was necessary for the sake of completeness to research the historic literature. It was only then that the author, much to his surprise, was confronted with the work of his colleagues who long ago had pursued the same line of thought, but without lasting results at that time.

Even in my own clinic it was problematic to accept the consequences of such an unfamiliar subtle diagnosis. This was also the case with an approximately 35-year-old patient without even the slightest abdominal complaints, where by coincidence, some irregular thickening of mucosal folds and a number of lymph follicles were discovered, which we took for a lymphoreticular malignancy with a near 100% certainty, so that at least an exploratory laparotomy was indicated (Fig. III, 26). After an incredibly heated discussion, a limited intestinal resection took place and our pathologic-anatomic diagnosis was confirmed. A follow-up examination of the patient 10 years later was unremarkable.

Because many physicians found, undeservedly, intubation awkward and time consuming, enteroclysis encountered considerable opposition in small and medium-sized hospitals for many years. It often happened that radiologists, asked by gastroenterologists to perform such an examination, telephoned the author to ask for 2 min of instruction in the method. The results obtained in this way were in most cases pathetic and probably only meant to make the gastroenterologists change their minds. Nolan and Cadman [159] from Ox-

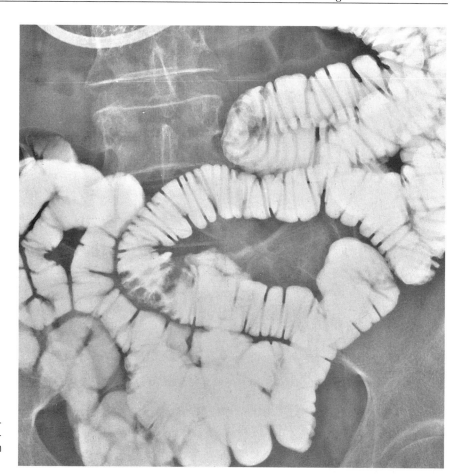

Fig. III, 26a. In the mid-jejunum, four or five thickened mucosal folds and a few swollen lymph follicles.

ford, who promoted the enteroclysis technique in England, made the insertion of the tube more acceptable by introducing a somewhat thinner tube that could be passed through the nose, as done later by Maglinte [160] from Indianapolis.

At the beginning, cold contrast medium was administered with the aim of stimulating peristalsis to reach the cecum fast and with the lowest possible amount. At first, the infusion speed between 100 and 120 ml/min was only determined empirically. It has been a considerable contribution from Oudkerk [161] to solve this fundamental problem through a very systematic study. With a specially constructed and very accurately adjustable infusion pump having a deviation of no more than 3 ml/min, he determined that the most favorable infusion speed for adults without medication was 75 ml/min, and that, under no circumstances, should exceed 100 ml/min. An increase of the infusion speed paralyses the intestinal motility and lengthens the duration of the examination. In addition, it becomes quite impossible to achieve good details with compression spot films.

An enteroclysis performed with professional skill should have no flocculation of the contrast

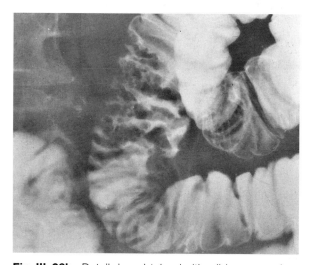

Fig. III, 26b. Detail view obtained with mild compression.

medium before it reaches the cecum, and a correct morphologic diagnosis is guaranteed each time. This is even true in infants, where now for the first time, mucosal folds can be found that were previously impossible to detect (Fig. III, 27). In infants, the flocculation of the barium

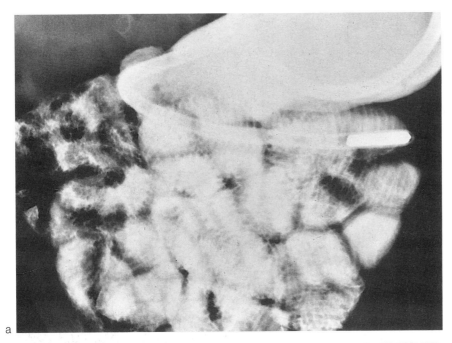

a

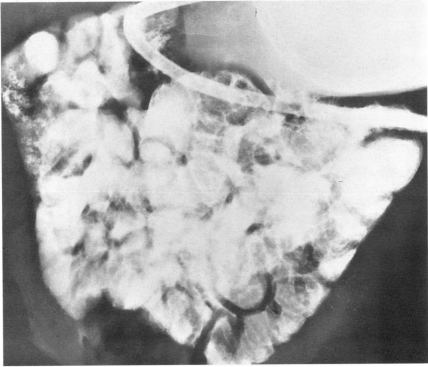

b

Fig. III, 27a, b. a) Plain radiograph of a three-month-old baby after barium has just reached the cecum. **b)** Due to extremely rapid disintegration of the barium suspension, the mucosal relief still visible in **a)** had already disappeared on this radiograph obtained approximately one minute later.

solution is so quick, even in an enteroclysis, that only a few minutes remain to perform the examination and to obtain the required radiographs. As soon as the contrast fluid flow stops after reaching the cecum, flocculation sets in. All radiographs should therefore be taken before this point in time; it is not possible to take additional radiographs thereafter.

A further considerable asset is that by standardizing the infusion speed and by excluding the gastric emptying, a reliable insight has been gained in motility disturbances that accompany a narrowed, a normal or distended intestinal lumen. This is a field where previously hardly any knowledge was available. The most frequently occurring diseases in this group are hypomotility and dilatation of the small bowel caused by medication [162]. Sedatives and soporifics are the worst offenders. In many cases, this may lead to a nonobstructive ileus. The recovery phase of this serious illness, after medication is stopped, is almost as long as the period the patient had taken the drug. Also long and continuous use of laxatives leads to the same serious effects, in this case, however, originating in the colon, and later progressing to the small bowel. A very good study on 'Laxative abuse' was undertaken by Cummings [109].

In all these cases of severely impaired intestinal motility and also in the presence of a mechanical ileus (obstruction), the intestinal lumen was dilated and it was therefore impossible to reach the cecum with approximately 600 ml barium suspension. In such cases, the amount of the barium solution was increased to a maximum of 1200 ml, possibly followed by a slow infusion of a maximum of 1200 ml water and the administration of a peristalsis-increasing drug. By quickly administering water after each normal examination, a better filling of the small bowel could be obtained as well as a more stretched course of the mucosal folds. But water increased the speed of barium flocculation, which is not the case with a methylcellulose solution. In addition, this technique produces a mediocre, long lasting double-contrast image [45].

After the contrast medium infusion, air can also be insufflated to obtain a double-contrast effect. The smallest mucosal lesions can be detected when the previously administered contrast-medium infusion was performed with a barium solution of a definitely higher specific gravity.

In 1976, the American radiologist R.E. Miller (Fig. III, 28) of Indianapolis visited the author's department in Leiden for a few weeks. It was typical for his personality that he wanted to take part in enteroclysis, including the intestinal cleansing, and the additional examinations, such as double-contrast and water infusion. One outcome of Miller's visit was that the author spent a few months in Indianapolis in 1977, to introduce the intestinal infusion or small bowel enema there. This cooperation resulted in the book, 'Radiology of the Small Bowel' [163].

With unrelenting energy and great enthusiasm, R.E. Miller [164] had always tried to raise the quality of gastrointestinal radiology to the highest possible level in his country. He had a strong sense of humor and relished giving people very difficult or preferably impossible assignments, and thus confronting them with their lim-

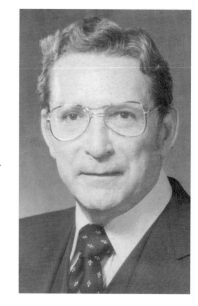

Fig. III, 28. R.E. Miller (1918–1984). Leading gastroenterologic radiologist, worked in Indianapolis. Improvements and standardization of the examination techniques of the Gastrointestinal tract in the USA.

itations. That is why the author, who came to Indianapolis with the strict instruction that a conventional upper gastrointestinal series should never take place again, will forever remember the very first patient he was confronted with, and who had been especially reserved for him; it was by far the most difficult task in his entire career. The patient was a woman of 200 kg, who 2 weeks previously had a bypass operation to divert the food via the proximal jejunum directly somewhere into the ileum. The patient was in a bad condition and absolutely inaccessible for clinical examination, so that an upper gastrointestinal series was requested, its indication hard to understand for the author. The patient could not lie on the examination table and had to be hoisted slightly with a special crane to get the cassette with film and grid into place. The tube had to be inserted without the help of fluoroscopy. The subsequently taken survey radiograph (Fig. III, 29) after contrast-medium infusion was fortunately very good as far as clarity was concerned.

The author could hardly have wished for a better way to introduce the enteroclysis in the USA. In the author's memory also linger the many discussions he had with R.E. Miller about the question of which colon examination method was best: the double-contrast method, which Miller had brought with him from his stay with Welin in Malmö, or the one promoted by the author, the conventional three-phase method. Neither of us succeeded in convincing the other. In a completely surprising manner, Miller once ended the discussion permanently by acknowled-

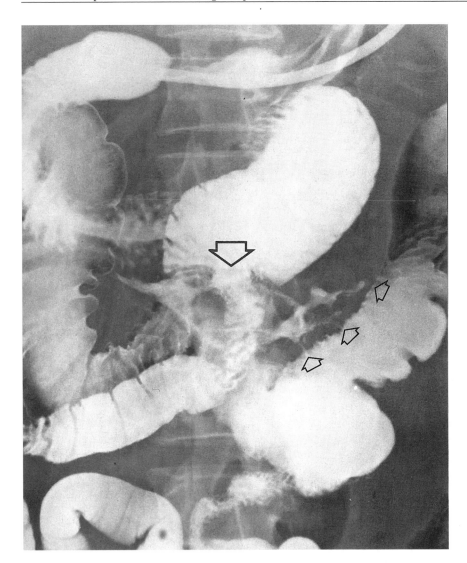

Fig. III, 29. Bedside entero-clysis performed in Indiana-polis on a female patient, weighing more than 200 kg, after bypass surgery because of morbid obesity. Anasto-motic leak (large arrow) be-tween the dilatated proximal jejunum and mid-ileum, with infiltration and fistulous tracts to the distal transversal colon (small arrows).

ging that it might be possible that the three-phase colon examination was the best method, but that he, after 20 years of campaigning to replace a less satisfactory method by the superior Welin method, could hardly be expected to abandon it now. The sudden death of the author's dear personal friend and fellow radiologist after a minor operation when this book was published some 10 years ago affected him deeply.

In the meantime, for more than six years, a treasure of experience of all sorts was collected, proving that not following the instructions or making impromptu changes could result in a poorly conducted or even failed examination. This was the reason for two very fundamental review articles, published in the USA together with R.E. Miller [164] and in Germany together with G. Rosenbusch [165]. In 1987, the veterinarian Wolvekamp [166] of Hilversum took his doctor's degree at Utrecht University with the subject 'Enteroclysma in dogs.' In 270 investigations on an-imals with suspected small-intestinal changes, a diagnostic accuracy of 98% was achieved.

The workload of radiologists continued to increase, leaving no time to consult voluminous standard works when reading films. This motivated the author, after having retired, to write a very concise booklet on how to arrive quickly at a differential diagnosis and a probability diagnosis [167].

In the mid-fifties, the water-soluble iodine-containing contrast medium Urokon had been introduced in Canada, and in the following years other water-soluble agents, such as Urografin, Gastrografin and Hypaque, which all became well known [168, 169].

After initial enthusiasm found among many radiologists and specialists in other disciplines, such as surgeons, paediatricians, gastroenterologists and ENT specialists, they gradually discovered the considerable disadvantages of these water-soluble preparations [170], namely:

- Hyperosmolarity, causing severe dehydration, dangerous in children and cachectic patients, and possibly leading to shock or death.
- Marked intestinal dilution distally, rendering the contrast medium absolutely useless.
- Inability to adhere to the intestinal mucosa, producing no or only faint coating of the mucosal folds.
- Low viscosity, allowing passage through stenoses, which can be easily overlooked and remain undetected.
- With prolonged intraluminal retention, a severe mucosal reaction may result.

It has been stated that Gastrografin was useful in differentiating a mechanical (obstructive) from a paralytic ileus, as well as in resolving a meconium ileus and in demonstrating fistulous tracts. Today, we know that these two types of ileus can be differentiated in the first minutes of a conventional small bowel series and that better methods are available for treating a meconium ileus.

Low-viscous, water-soluble contrast media are absolutely useless in visualizing the gastrointestinal tract and for injection into fistulous tracts since they pass rapidly without leaving any trace of mucosal coating. A modest place in the diagnostic evaluation with water-soluble contrast media can be given to agents of a slightly higher viscosity, such as Dionosil, which is used in bronchography. This agent has also proved to be more suitable in delineating swallowed foreign bodies in the oesophagus than Gastrografin-dipped cotton wool. Dionosil is also better than a barium solution in detecting suture leaks since in case of extravasation the contrast medium can be removed by suction during the surgical intervention. Finally, using the viscous Dionosil for fistulograms has the advantage that it adheres to the wall of the fistulous tract and is visible as a white liquid when it exits the fistula at its cutaneous opening.

Recapitulating, it can be stated that in the past 40 years, water-soluble contrast media in gastrointestinal radiology have hardly ever been necessary and were largely unjustifiable.

References

1. Bruwer, A.J.: Classic descriptions in diagnostic roentgenology. C.C. Thomas Publischer, Springfield, Illinois, USA 1964
2. The Cole collaborators: Roentgenologic exploration of the mucosa of the gastro-intestinal tract. Radiology 18 (1932) 221–244, 471–485, 886–941
3. Margulis, A.R., R.R. Eisenberg: Gastrointestinal radiology from the time of W.B. Cannon to the 21st century (Diamond Jubilee Lecture). Radiology 178 (1931) 297–302
4. Stevenson, C.A.: The development of gastrointestinal roentgenology. Am. J. Roentgenol. 75 (1956) 230–237
5. Berg, H.H.: Röntgenuntersuchungen am Innenrelief des Verdauungskanals. Georg Thieme Verlag, Leipzig 1931
6. Welin, S., G. Welin: The double contrast examination of the colon – Experiences with the Welin modification. Georg Thieme Publishers, Stuttgart 1976
7. Brown, P.: The inception and development of fluoroscopy: the influence of Carman on its status in America. Radiology 38 (1942) 414–425.
8. Van Iterson, J.E.: De ontwikkeling der Heelkunde (voordracht voor KNMG te Arnhem, 4-7-1899. NTvG 43 (1989) 87–94
9. Becher, W.: Zur Anwendung des röntgen'schen Verfahrens in der Medizin. Dtsch. med. Wschr. 22 (1896) 202–203. In: Brewer [1] S. 1787–1789
10. Hemmeter, J.C.: Photography of the human stomach by the Roentgen method, A suggestion. Boston Med + Surg.I. 134 (1896) 609–610. In: Bruwer [1] S. 1793–1795
11. Wegele, C.: Ein Vorschlag zur Anwendung des röntgen'schen Verfahrens in der Medizin. Dtsch. med. Wschr. 22 (1896) 287
12. Lindemann, E.: Demonstration von Röntgenbildern des normalen und erweiterten Magens. Dtsch. med. Wschr. 23 (1897) 266–267. In: Bruwer [1] S. 1798–1799
13. Rumpel, Th.: Die klinische Diagnose der spindelförmigen Speiseröhrenerweiterung. Med. Wschr. 44 (1897) 420–421. In: Bruwer [1] S. 1796–1797
14. Roux, J.Ch., V. Balthazard: A note on the motor function of the dog's stomach. C.R. Soc. Biol. (Par) 10 (1897) 704–706. In: Brewer [1] S. 1806–1807
15. Roux, J.Ch., V. Balthazard: A study of the contractions in man through the use of Roentgen rays. C.R. Soc. Biol. (Par) 10 (1897) 785–787. In: Bruwer [1] S. 1808–1809
16. Cannon, W.B.: The movements of the stomach studied by means of the Roentgen rays. Am. J. Physiol. 1 (1898) 359–382. In: Bruwer [1] S. 1811–1827
17. Roux, J.Ch., V. Balthazard: The use of Roentgen rays for the study of gastric mobility (1897). C.R. Soc. Biol. (Par) 10 (1897) 567–569. In: Bruwer [1] S. 1804–1805
18. Rossbach, M.J.: Beiträge zur Lehre von den Bewegungen des Magens, Pylorus und Duodenums. Dtsch. Arch. Klin. Med. 46 (1890) 296–322
19. Williams, F.H.: Methods for observing the stomach – the Roentgen rays in medicine and surgery, as an aid in diagnosis and as a therapeutic agent. MacMillan Company, New York, 1901. In: Bruwer [1] S. 1837–1849
20. Cannon, W.B., A. Moser: The movements of food in the oesophagus. Am. J. Physiol. 1 (1898) 435–444. In: Bruwer [1] S. 1828–1835
21. Holzknecht, G.: Roentgenologic exploration of the mucosa of the gastro-intestinal tract. In: the Cole collaborators [2]
22. Eijkman, P.H.: Bewegungsphotographie mittels Röntgenstrahlen. Fortschr. Röntgenstr. 5 (1901/02) 347

23. Schüle, A.: Über die Sondierung und Radiographie des Dickdarms. Arch. Verdauungskr. 10 (1904) 111–118. In: Brewer [1] S. 1943–1949

24. Stegman, R.: Eine neue Darstellungsart der Gangsysteme des menschlichen Körpers mittels Röntgenstrahlen. Vortrag in Freiburg, Juli 1903. Zit. in Bruwer [1] S. 1947

25. Rieder, H.: Radiologische Untersuchung des Magens und Darmes beim lebenden Menschen. Münch. med. Wschr. 51 (1904) 1548–1551. In: Bruwer [1] S. 1849–1858

26. Holzknecht, G.: Zit. in: Bruwer [1] S. 1780

27. Hemmeter, J.C.: Neue Methoden zur Diagnose des Magengeschwürs. Arch. Verdauungskr. 12 (1906) 357–363. In: Bruwer [1] S. 1858–1860

28. Kaestle, C., H. Rieder, J. Rosenthal: Über kinematographisch aufgenommene Röntgenogramme (Bio-Röntgenographie) der inneren Organe des Menschen. Münch. med. Wschr. 56 (1909) 280–282. In: Bruwer [1] S. 1866–1869

29. Holzknecht, G., Brauner: Zit. in The Cole collaborators [2]

30. Haudek, M., G. Holzknecht: Zit. in: Bruwer [1] S. 1780

31. Groedel, F.: Zit. in The Cole collaborators [2]

32. Bachem, C., H. Günther: Bariumsulfat als schattenbildendes Kontrastmittel bei Röntgenuntersuchungen. Zeitschr. für Röntgenkunde 12 (1910) 369–376. In: Bruwer [1] S. 1875

33. Cannon, W.B.: The passage of different foodstufs from the stomach and through the small intestine. Am.J. Physiol. 12 (1904) 387–418

34. Elischer, J. von: Über eine Methode zur Röntgenuntersuchung des Magens. Fortschr. Röntgenstr. 18 (1911) 332–340

35. Holzknecht, G.: Zit. in The Cole collaborators [2]

36. Leonard, L.: Siehe Stevenson [4]

37. Carman. R.D.: The technic of Roentgen-ray examination of the gastro-intestinal tract, and the interpretation of screen and plate findings. J. Am. Med. Ass. 61 (1913) 321–326

38. Bartstra, D.S.: Het röntgenonderzoek van de spijsverteringsorganen uit "De ziekten van de spijsverteringsorganen". Elsevier publishing company, Amsterdam, 1945

39. Forssell, G.: Studies of the mechanism of movement of the mucoses membrane of the digestive tract. Am. J. Roentgenol. 2 (1923) 87–104. In: Bruwer [1] S. 1900–1916

40. Vallebona, A., Hilpert, Pribram, Kleiber: Zit. in The Cole collaborators [2]

41. Åkerlund, A.: Zit. in The Cole collaborators [2]

42. Henning, N., R. Schatzki: Gastrophotographisches und röntgenologisches Bild der Gastritis ulcerosa. Fortschr. Röntgenstr. 48 (1933) 177–181

43. Kaufman, R. Kienböck: Zit. in The Cole collaborators [2]

44. Rendich, R.A.: The roentgenographic study of the mucosa in normal and pathological states. Am. J. Roentgenol. 10 (1923) 526–537. In: Bruwer [1] S. 1918–1929

45. Herlinger, H.: A modified technique for the double contrast small bowel enema. Gastroint. Radiol. 2 (1978) 397–400

46. Haenisch, G.F.: The value of the Roentgen ray in the early diagnosis of carcinoma of the bowel. Am. Quart. Roentgenol. 3 (1911) 175–180. In: Bruwer [1] S. 1966–1967

47. Haenisch, G.F.: Der Röntgenuntersuchung bei Verengungen des Dickdarms. Röntgenologische Frühdiagnose des Dickdarmkarzinoms. Münch. med. Wschr. 58 (1923) 2375. In: Bruwer [1] S. 1951–1965

48. Laurell, H.F.: Zit. in The Cole collaborators [2]

49. Fischer, A.W.: Über eine neue röntgenologische Untersuchungsmethode des Dickdarms: Kombination von Kontrasteinlauf und Luftaufblähung. Klin. Wschr. 2 (1923) 1595–1598. In: Bruwer [1] S. 1970–1977

50. Pansdorf, H., K. Frik, L.G. Cole, W. Knothe: Zit. in The Cole collaborators [2]

51. Weber, H.M.: Zit. in Welin [6] S. 2, 88

52. Ledoux-Lebard, G., J. Garcia-Calderon: Zit. in Welin [6] S. 2

53. Gelfland, D.W., Y.M. Chen, D.J. Ott: Detection of colonic polyps on single-contrast barium enema study: Emphasis on the elderly. Radiology 164 (1987) 333–337

54. Rigler, L.G., L.G. Erikson : Zit. in: Welin [6] S. 2

55. Gianturco, C.: Zit. in Welin [6] S. 2

56. Carman (see 37.)

57. Rieder, H.: Radiologische Untersuchungen des Magens und Darmes beim lebenden Menschen. Münch. med. Wschr. 51 (1904) 1548–1551. In: Bruwer (1) S. 1849–1858

58. Schwarz, G.: Die Erkennung der tieferen Dünndarmstenose mittels des Röntgenverfahrens. Wien. Klin. Wschr. 40 (1911) 1386–1390. In: Bruwer (1) S. 1930–1942

59. Loichinger, C.: Zur Geschichte der röntgenologischen Magendarmuntersuchung. Fortschr. Röntgenstr. 38 (1928) 1067

60. Pansdorf, H.: Die fraktionierte Dünndarmfüllung und ihre klinische Bedeutung. Fortschr. Röntgenstr. 56 (1937) 627

61. Kuhlman, F.: Zit. in Pansdorf (60)

62. Boles, R.S., J. Gershon-Cohen: Intestinal tuberculosis – Pathologic and roentgenologic observations. J. Am. Med. Ass. 103 (1934) 1841–1848

63. Crohn, B.B., K. Ginzburg, G.D. Oppenheimer: Regional ileitis. A pathologic and clinical entity. J. Am. Med. Ass. 99 (1932) 1323–1329

64. Pesquera, G.S.: A Method for the direct visualization of lesions in the small intestines. Am. J. Roentgenol. 22 (1929) 254–257

65. Einhorn, M.: The duodenal tube and its possibilities. W.B. Saunders Co, Philadelphia 1920

66. Snell, A.M., J.D. Camp: Chronic ideopathic steatorrhea – Roentgenologic Observations. Arch. Int. Med. 53 (1934) 615–629

67. Mackie, T.T., D.K. Miller, C.P. Rhoads: Roentgenologic changers in the small intestine. Am. J. Trop. Med. 15 (1935) 571–589

68. Kantor, J.L.: The Roentgen diagnosis of idiopathic steatorrhea and allied conditions – Practical value of the "Moulage Sign". Am. J. Roentgenol. 41 (1939) 758–778

69. Golden, R.: The small intestine and diarrhea. Am. J. Roentgenol. 36 (1936) 892–901

70. Gershon-Cohen, J., H. Shay: Barium Enteroclysis – A method for the direct immediate examination of the small Intestine by single and double contrast Techniques. Am. J. Roentgenol. 42 (1939) 456

71. Bouslog, J.S.: The gastro-intestinal tract in children. Radiology 28 (1937) 683–692

72. Henderson, S.G.: The gastro-intestinal tract in the healthy newborn infant. Am. J. Roentgenol. 48 (1942) 302–335

73. Golden, R.: Radiological examination of the small intestine. J.B. Lippincott, Philadelphia (1945) Chapt. 4

74. Zwerling, H., W.E. Nelson: The roentgenologic pattern of the small intestine in infants and children. Radiology 40 (1943) 277–282

74a. Frazer, A.C., J.M. French, M.D. Thompson: Radiographic studies showing the induction of a segmentation pattern in the small intestine in normal human subjects. Br. J. Radiol. 22 (1949) 123–135

75. Schatzki, R.: Small intestinal enema. Am. J. Roentgenol. 50 (1943) 743–751

76. Van der Haer, Ph.M.: Demonstratie van Röntgenopnamen van de slokdarm. NTvG (1912) 864

77. Carman, R.D.: The Roentgen diagnosis of diseases of the alimentary canal. 2nd Edition, 1920

78. Barclay, A.E.: Der normale Schlingmechanismus. Acta Radiol. 13 (1932) 87–90

79. Laurell, H.: Zur Frage der Entstehung kardionaher Magendivertikel und Zenkerscher Oesophagusdivertikel. Zugleich ein Beitrag zum Schluckmechanismus. Acta Radiol. 12 (1931) 455–478

80. Hamilton, J.B.: zit. in: Welin (6)

81. Christie, A.C. et al: Zit. in: Welin (6)

82. Gianturco, C.: Fast radiological viceral survey. Radiology 54 (1950) 59–64

83. Sellink, J.L.: Radiological Examination of the Colon. Radiologia Clin. 45 (1976) 155

84. Robinson, J.M.: Zit. in: Welin (6) S. 3

85. Marshak, R.H., A.E. Lindner: Zit. in: Welin (6) S. 3

86. Kabakian, H.A., S.R. Massabni: The value of the postevacuation view of the colon in the detection of pelvic pathology. Am. J. Roentgenol. 11 (1973) 393–403

87. Fischer, A.W.: Über eine neue röntgenologische Untersuchungsmethode des Dickdarms: Kombination von Kontrasteinlauf und Luftaufblähung. Klin. Wschr. 2 (1923) 1595–1598

88. Weber, H.M.: Roentgenologic demonstration of polypoid lesions and polyposis of large intestine. Am. J. Roentgenol. 25 (1931) 577–589

89. Bell, J.C.: General consideration in the roentgen examination of the colon. Radiology 55 (1950) 20–23

90. Stevenson, C.A.: The development of the colon examination – Indications for double contrast colon examination. Am. J. Roentgenol. 71 (1954) 385–403

91. Douglas, J.B.: The double contrast examination of the colon. Radiology 60 (1953) 490–495

92. Moreton, R.D.: Zit. in: Welin (6) S. 3

93. Peister, F.A. de, R.K. Gilchrist: Zit. in: Welin (6) S. 3

94. Jarre, H.A., S.J. Fiegel: Zit. in: Welin (6) S. 3

95. Bartstra, D.S.: Persönliche Information des Autors.

96. Welin, S.: Zur Darstellung der Kolonpolypen mit der Doppelkontrastmethode. Fortschr. Röntgenstr. 82 (1955) 341–344

97. Welin, S.: Examination and cleansing of the large bowel. J. Belge Radiol. 54 (1971) 1–6

98. Thoeni, R.F., A.R. Margulis: The state of radiographic technique in the examination of the colon: a survey. Radiology 127 (1978) 317

99. R.F. Thoeni, A.R. Margulis: The state of radiographic technique in the examination of the colon: a survey. Radiology 167 (1988) 1

100. Nicolette, C.C., T.E. Tully: The duodenum in celiac sprue. Am. J. Roentgenol. 113 (1971) 248–254

101. Balthazar, E.J., M. Ferrante Gade: Gastrointestinal edema in cirrhosis. Gastroint. Radiol. 1 (1976/77) 215–223

102. Rogers, L.F., H.M. Goldstein: Roentgen manifestations of radiation – Injury to the gastrointestinal tract. Gastroint. Radiol. 2 (1977/78) 281–291

103. Ghahremani, G.G., M.A. Meyers, J. Farman, R.B. Port: Ischaemic disease of the small bowel associated with oral contraceptives. Gastroint. Radiol. 2 (1977/78) 221–228

104. Hyson, E.H., M. Burrel, R. Toffler: Drug induced gastrointestinal disease. Gastroint. Radiol. 2 (1977/78) 183–212

105. Dodds, W.J.: Clinical and Roentgen features of the intestinal polyposis syndromes. Gastroint. Radiol. 1 (1976/77) 127–142

106. Bancks, N.H., H.M. Goldstein, G.D. Dodd: The roentgenologic spectrum of small intestinal carcinoid tumors. Am. J. Roentgenol. 123 (1975) 274

107. Osborn, A.G., G.W. Friedland: A radiological approach to the diagnosis of small bowel disease. Clin. Radiol. 24 (1973) 281–301

108. Nelson, S.W.: Extraluminal gas collections due to diseases of the gastrointestinal tract. Am. J. Roentgenol. 115 (1972) 215–248

109. Cummings, J.H.: Laxative abuse – Progress report. Gut 15 (1974) 758–766

110. Meyers, M.A.: Distribution of intra-abdominal malignant seeding: Dependancy on dynamics of flow of ascites fluid. Am. J. Roentgenol. 111 (1971) 189–206

111. Meyers, M.A.: Clinical involvement of mesenteric and antimesenteric borders of small bowel loops. Gastroint. Radiol. 1 (1976/77) 41–47

112. Brown, B. Defecography or anorectal studies in children including cinefluorography observations. J. de l'association canadienne des radiologistes 16 (1965) 66–76

113. Brodén, B., B. Snellman: Procidentia of the rectum studied with cineradiography – a contribution to the discussion of causative mechanism. Dis. Colon Rectum 11 (1968) 330–347

114. Ekberg, O., G. Nylander, F.T. Fork: Defecography. Radiology 155 (1985) 45–48

115. Mahieu, P., J. Pringot, P. Bodar: Defecography. I Description of a new procedure and results in normal patients. II Contribution to the diagnosis of defecation disorders Gastroint. Radiol. 9 (1984) 247–261

116. Ottens, D.E., L.W.M. Janssen: Defaecografie – Röntgenonderzoek bij anorectale dysfunctie. In: Reeders, J.W.A.J. Gastro-enterologische Radiodiagnostiek. Uitg. Post Acad. Onderw. Gen. K. A'dam. 1990

117. Goei, R.: Defecography – A radiological study on anorectal function and related disorders. Thesis University of Maastricht 1990

118. Goei, R., S.A. Müller-Lissner: Radiologische Methoden (Defäkographie, Transitmessung). In: Müller-Lissner, S.A., L.M.A. Akkermans: Chronische Obstipation und Stuhlinkontinenz. Springer Verlag 1989

119. Gutman, R.A., R. Prévôt: Gastroenterologen Kongr., Paris 1937

120. Shirakabe, H., H. Ischikawa, et al: Frühkarzinom des Magens – Atlas der Röntgendiagnostik. Georg Thieme Verlag Stuttgart 1966

121. Shirakabe, H., H. Ischikawa: Early gastric cancer. In: The esophagus and stomach, an atlas of tumor radiology. Hrsg. von Stein, Finkelstein, Yearbook Medical Publishers 1973, 277–283

122. Kawai, K. In: Early gastric cancer, current status of diagnosis. Hrsg. von Grundmann, Grunze, Witte, Springer Verlag 1974

123. Frik, W., R. Hesse: Die röntgenologische Darstellung von Magenerosionen, verbesserte Ergebnisse mit Doppelkonstrast-Aufnahmen und Bildverstärker. Dtsch. med. Wschr. 81 (1956) 1119–1121

124. Bücker, J.: Die Antrumgastritis. Radiologe 6 (1966) 264–270

125. Amplatz, K. A new and simple approach to air-contrast studies of the stomach and duodenum. Radiology 70 (1958) 392–394

126. Op den Orth, J.O., S. Ploem: The standard biphasic contrast gastric series. Radiology 122 (1977) 530–532

127. Pochaczevsky, R.: Bubbly barium, a carbonated cocktail for double contrast examination of the stomach. Radiology 107 (1973) 461–462

128. Op den Orth, J.O., S. Ploem: The standard biphasic contrast examination of the stomach and duodenum method, results and radiological atlas. Series in Radiology, Martinus Nijhoff publishers 1979

129. Brombart, M.: Clinical radiology of the esophagus. John Wright, Bristol 1961

130. Goldstein, H.M., G.J. Dodd: Double contrast examination of the esophagus. Gastroint. Radiol. 1 (1976) 3–6

131. Barclay, A.E.: Der normale Schlingmechanismus. Acta Radiol. 13 (1932) 91–110

132. Ardran, G.M., F.H. Kemp: Closure and opening of the larynx during swallowing. Br. J. Radiol. 29 (1956) 205–208

133. Dodds, W.J.: Current concepts of esophageal motor function: Clinical implications for radiology. Am. J. Roentgenol. 128 (1977) 549–561

134. Donner, M.W., Ch.I. Siegel: The evaluation of pharyngeal neuromuscular disorders by cinefluography. Am. J. Roentgenol. 94 (1965) 299–307

135. Pringot, J., E. Ponette: Radiological Examination of the Esophagus. In: Diseases of the Esophagus: pp 119–203. Ed. by G. Vantrappen and J. Hellemans. Springer Verlag 1974

136. Klinkhamer, A.C.: Het vaststellen van aberrante arteriën in het bovenste mediastinum door middel van het oesophagogram. Thesis Leiden 1962

137. Klinkhamer, A.C.: Aberrant right subclavian artery, clinical and roentgenologic aspects. Am. J. Roentgenol. 97 (1966) 438–446

138. Brombart, M.M.: Gastrointestinal radiology – a functional approach to radiological investigation and diagnosis. Georg Thieme Publishers 1980

139. Hüpscher, D.N.: Radiology of the esophagus. Georg Thieme Verlag 1988

140. Dodds, W.J.: Radiology of the esophagus. In: Alimentary tract radiology. Ed. by Margulis and Burhenne. The CV Mosby Cy, St. Louis (1983)

141. Levine, M.S., I. Laufer: Radiology of the esophagus In: Diseases of the esophagus: pp 51–74. Ed. by S. Cohen, R.D. Soloway. Churchill Livingstone, New York 1984

142. Dodds, W.J. et al: Effect of esophageal movement on intraluminal esophageal pressure recording. Gastroenterology 67 (1974) 592

143. Dodds, W.J. et al: Radial distribution of esophageal peristaltic pressure in normal subjects and patients with esophageal diverticulum. Gastroenterology 69 (1975) 584

144. Dodds, W.J., W.J. Hogan, J.F. Helm, J. Dent: Pathogenesis of reflux esophagitis. Gastroenterology 81 (1981) 376–394

145. Donner, M.W., G.P. Saba, C.R. Martinez: Diffuse diseases of the esophagus – a practical approach. Seminars in Roentgenology 16 (1981) 202–212

146. Donner, M.W.: Advances in diagnostic imaging of esophageal disease. In: Esophageal disorders: pathophysiology and therapy Ed. by Skinner, De Meester, Raven Press, New York, 1985

147. Donner, M.W., J.F. Bosma, D.L. Robertson: Anatomy and physiology of the pharynx. Gastrointest. Radiol. 10 (1985) 196–212

148. Jones, B., S.S. Kramer, M.W. Donner: Dynamic imaging of the pharynx. Gastroint. Radiol. 10 (1985) 213–224

149. Dahm, M.: Schluckstörungen und Schlucklähmungen. Fortschr. Röntgenstr. 64 (1941) 167–202, 241–281, 309–353

150. Ekberg, O.: Cineradiography in normal and abnormal pharyngo-esophageal deglutition. Thesis Malmö 1981

151. Ekberg, O., G. Nylander: Dysfunction of the cricopharyngeal muscle. Radiology 143 (1982) 481–486

152. Urra, M.C.: Exploración radiológica del intestino delgado. Thesis, Santiago, Chile (1945)

153. Marshak, R.H., B.S. Wolf, D. Adlersberg: Roentgenstudies of the small intestine in sprue. Am. J. Roentgenol. 72 (1954) 380–400

154. Rice, R.P., W.M. Roufail, R.J. Reeves: The Roentgen diagnosis of Whipple's disease (Intestinal Lipodystrophy). Radiology 88 (1967) 295–301

155. Weltz, G.A.: Der kranke Dünndarm im Röntgenbild. Am. J. Roentgenol. 72 (1954) 380–400

156. Friedman, J.: Roentgen studies of the effects on the small intestine from emotional disturbances. Am. J. Roentgenol. 72 (1954) 367–379

157. Marshak, R.H., A.E. Lindner: Radiology of the small intestine. W.B. Saunders Company 1970

158. Bilbao, M.K., L.H. Frische, Ch.T. Dotter, J. Rösch: Hypotonic duodenography. Radiology 89 (1967) 438–443

159. Nolan, D.J., P.J. Cadman: The small bowel enema made easy. Clin. Radiol. 38 (1987) 295–301

160. Maglinte, D.D.T., J.C. Lappas, S.M. Chernish, J.L. Sellink: Intubation routes for enteroclysis. Radiology 158 (1986) 553–554

161. Oudkerk, M.: Infusionrate in enteroclysis examination. Thesis Leiden (1981)

162. Achterberg, J.R., J.L. Sellink: Medicamenteuze atonie van de dunne darm. NTvG 118 (1974) 1743–1753

163. Sellink, J.L., R.E. Miller: Radiology of the small bowel – modern enteroclysis technique and atlas. Martinus Nijhoff Publishers 1982

164. Miller, R.E., J.L. Sellink: Enteroclysis: the small bowel enema – how to succeed and how to fail. Gastroint. Radiol. 4 (1979) 269–283

165. Sellink, J.L., G. Rosenbusch: Moderne Untersuchungstechnik des Dünndarms oder die 10 Gebote des Enteroklysmas. Radiologe 21 (1981) 366–376

166. Wolvekamp, W.Th.C.: Enteroclysis in the dog. Thesis at Utrecht 1987

167. Sellink, J.L.: X-Ray differential diagnosis in small bowel disease – a practical approach. Kluwer Academic Publishers 1988

168. Lessman, F.P., R.M. Lilienfeld: Gastrografin as water soluble medium in roentgen examination of the G.I. tract. Acta Radiol. 51 (1959) 170–178

169. Shehadi, W.H.: Studies of the colon and small intestine with water soluble iodinated contrast media. Am. J. Roentgenol. 89 (1963) 740–751

170. Harris, P.D., E.B.D. Neuhauser: The osmotic effect of water soluble contrast media on circulating plasma volume. Am. J. Roentgenol. 91 (1964) 694–698

Gallbladder and biliary tract

J.H.J. Ruijs

'The real summit in the histories of adventures of discoveries is the visualization of the human gallbladder by means of X-rays following the intravascular administration of an agent that accumulates in the gallbladder, rendering it opaque to X-rays...'

This paraphrased statement of the American pharmacologist B. Fantus (1874–1940) reflects the seriousness of the pursuit to visualize diseases of the gallbladder and biliary tracts by X-rays.

Thanks to the progress in surgery at the end of the last century [1, 2], the first gallbladder operation took place in 1878, but it was a long search to find methods of obtaining more information of diseases of the gallbladder and biliary ducts, to be available before the patient is referred to the surgeon. Though this necessity was clearly recognized around the turn of the century, most clinicians were reluctant to use the "modern" X-rays, which indeed were of limited value.

This attitude is clearly reflected in the 'Textbook on diseases of the liver and biliary tracts' published in 1910 by the Dutch authority on internal medicine Dr. P.K. Pel (1852–1919) [3]: on the one hand, the various syndromes were exceedingly well described in great detail, under special consideration of inspection, palpation and physical examination; on the other hand, new methods, such as laboratory test and diagnostic radiology, were completely ignored.

Nevertheless, the need for a more direct examination was expressed in the course of the first two decades of this century after it had become apparent that the information obtained from survey radiographs was only valuable in a few exceptional cases [4, 5]. Meanwhile, the diagnostic approach propagated by Pel and his contemporaries still prevailed.

Radiological examinations remained limited to postmortem studies that were performed to visualize organs, among other attempts, by means of contrast media. (Fig. III, 30) [6, 7].

It was also discovered that certain 'halogens' [9], including iodine-containing substances

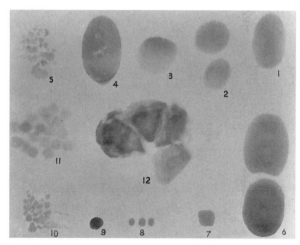

Fig. III, 30a. Surgically recovered gallstones: cholesterol stones, lamellated stones, mixed stones (1909).

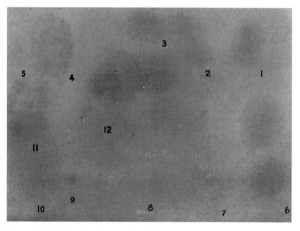

Fig. III, 30b. Radiograph of the same stones arranged the same way and placed under an adult (1909).

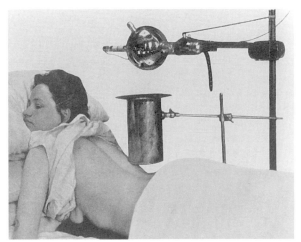

Fig. III, 31. Radiograph of a gallstone obtained with a tubular collimator. The main purpose is the absorption of secondary radiation and not the compression (C. Beck, 1909).

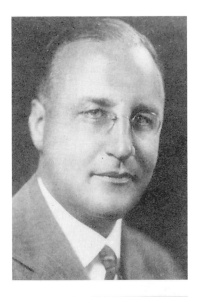

Fig. III, 32. Evarts Ambrose Graham (1883–1957). American Surgeon in St. Louis. Together with Cole, he reported the radiographic visualization of the gallbladder in 1924. Numerous surgical contributions.

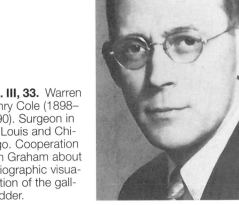

Fig. III, 33. Warren Henry Cole (1898–1990). Surgeon in St. Louis and Chicago. Cooperation with Graham about radiographic visualization of the gallbladder.

such as Lipiodol, were visible on preoperative [8] radiographs. These investigations, however, were mainly performed on very severe and chronic cases.

It was the exception when an examination was performed preoperatively (Fig. III, 31) [10]. Mueller's related studies and his remarks [11] at the end of one of his publications should be mentioned here:

'In this context, we have in mind not so much the obvious long-standing and severe cases of diseases of the biliary system but rather the early cases of a diseased gallbladder in which a definitive diagnosis and direct treatment is still not possible at present time.'

From this, it is apparent that diseases of the gallbladder and biliary tract were regarded as important and surgically treatable and that a lack of adequate preoperative radiological visualization had to be conquered.

In mid-November of 1923, a radiograph was taken of a dog that, for the first time, showed a gallbladder filled with contrast medium. That was quite unexpected after studies performed on more than 200 dogs had been all unsuccessful.

The basis for this result was a clever concept, coinciding with an incidental finding (serendipity). The hypothesis assumed an almost exclusive excretion of phenoltetrachlorophthalein by the biliary tract. In 1871, the pharmacologist Bayer (the 1905 Nobel Prize Winner) had already discovered that the gallbladder has a concentrating action through water resorption of its mucosa [12]. This concept was further developed by Abel and Rowntree [13] in 1910 and again later

by Rous and McMaster [14] in 1921. Graham (Fig. III, 32) and Cole (Fig. III, 33) may take the credit having made this method suitable for radiology [15]. The exhilarating moment when it became clear that it was possible to visualize the gallbladder of a laboratory animal exited the investigators. Their radiological assistant who had helped with the research called (according to Dr Cole in 1960) [16] on the telephone one stormy November night to tell them that it was now really visible, upon which both gentlemen hurried to the dark room of the roentgen department. Let us hear Dr Cole's own report:

'We both stood there admiring the dripping film with a white shadow in the centre as if we had discovered the famous pot-of-gold at the end of the rainbow … .'

But at that moment it was not yet clear why, after so many fruitless attempts, a cholecystogram was successful in this dog. Therefore, the investigators decided to review the study protocol thoroughly, but no answer was forthcoming. Later, they learned by chance that the keeper had forgotten to feed the dog. Because of the dog's fasting state, the contrast medium – calcium tetrabromophenolphthalein – was in a higher concentration in the excreted bile and the gallbladder was not contracted. This led to a radiographically visible gallbladder. Very soon thereafter, the intravenous cholecystography (first examination February 12, 1924) and later the oral cholecystography [17] (period 1925–1940) became established in the preoperative diagnostic investiga-

tion. Initial problems, such as toxicity and dosage, were solved and the visualization of the biliary system was performed in every radiological practice throughout the world (Fig. III, 34–36).

After initially investigating the pharmacokinetics of the contrast medium [18, 19], research later turned to defining the criteria used in the differential diagnoses of cholelithiasis, acute cholecystitis, and chronic cholecystitis.

In 1962, Jutras [20]) made a major step forward by connecting the various (degenerative)

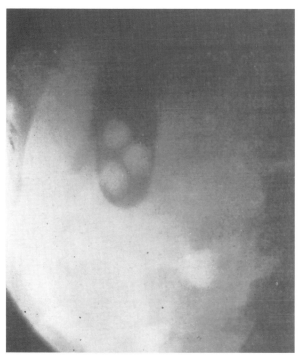

Fig. III, 34. Three stones in a gallbladder, 16 hours after ingestion of contrast medium (Schinz et al, 1928).

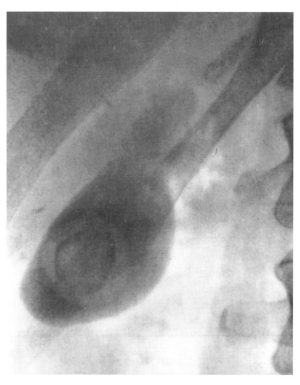

Fig. III, 35. "Cockade stone" (lamellated, mixed cholesterol stone) five hours after ingestion of contrast medium administration (W. Frommhold, 1965).

Fig. III, 36a, b. Normal opacified gallbladder **(a)** and 20 minutes after a fatty meal **(b)**. Satisfactory contraction of the gallbladder. Cystic and bile ducts are well visualized (W. Frommhold, 1952).

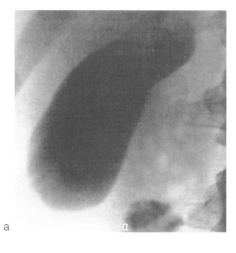

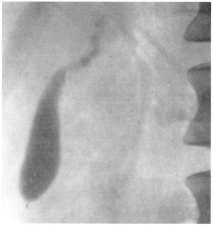

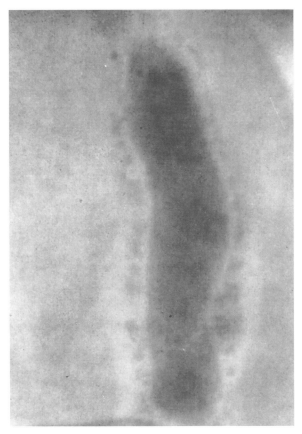

Fig. III, 37. Diffuse adenomyomatosis (W. Frommhold, 1965).

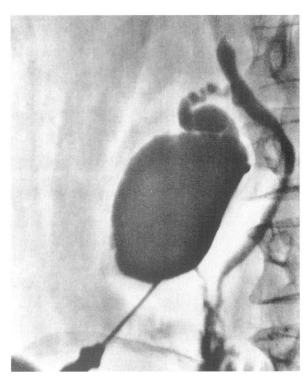

Fig. III, 38. Hepatic carcinoma. Intraoperative transvesical cholecystangiography. Irregularly outlined termination of the opacified duct (W. Frommhold, 1965).

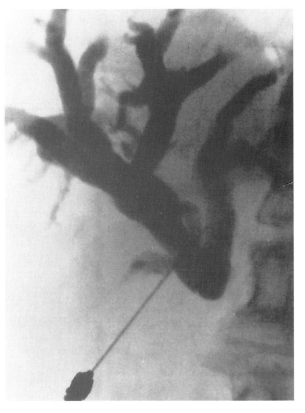

Fig. III, 39. Adenocarcinoma of the proximal bile duct. Percutaneous transhepatic cholangiography (W. Frommhold, 1965).

gallbladder diseases, which he called cholecystoses (Fig. III, 37), with the underlying histological findings. His work made it not only possible to diagnose or exclude cholelithiasis but also to recognize acalculous gallbladder diseases [21]. The subsequent developments in radionuclide imaging, CT and ERCP added new material to these investigations [22, 23].

The contrast-medium examination also had its limitation. Diseases of the biliary ducts were rarely detected, and, in particular, carcinomas of the liver, gallbladder and pancreas could not be inadequately diagnosed. For these reasons, more invasive investigation methods were increasingly used. Direct intraoperative cholangiography (Fig. III, 38) was introduced in 1931, followed by transhepatic puncture (Fig. III, 39) in 1937, and direct and safe puncture techniques of the biliary tract via the liver in 1952. A considerable improvement of gallbladder examination was achieved in 1953 by the development of safe contrast media without major adverse reactions (Fig. III, 40) [24, 25].

In summary, the biliary examination developed very rapidly after the development of safe

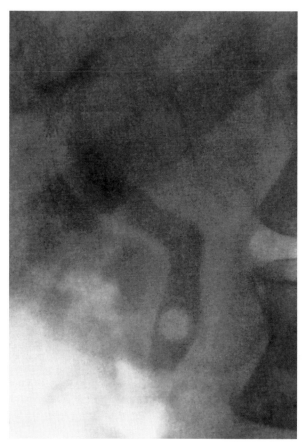

Fig. III, 40. Choledocholithiasis after cholecystectomy: ovoid defect in the opacified bile duct, i.v. cholangiography (W. Frommhold, 1965).

contrast media and particularly after improving their effect and tolerance.

The introduction of ultrasound had a considerable influence on the further development in the diagnosis of diseases of the liver, biliary tract and pancreas.

In 1980, Cooperberg and Burhenne [26] published in the New England Journal of Medicine that the properly performed real-time ultrasound examination is superior as to sensitivity and specificity in diagnosing gallstones than the classic oral cholecystography. Though a scientifically inadequate study (the false-negative findings were not verified; the conclusions were exclusively based on the positive and false-positive groups), this article changed the evaluation of the gallbladder. Both the intravenous and the oral cholecystography quickly lost grounds and today, the nineties, they are rarely performed. In essence, the intravenous cholangiography can be considered obsolete, while the oral cholecystography is now reserved for patients selected for nonsurgical gallstone treatment [27].

In addition to advancing the diagnosis of gallstones, ultrasound improved the diagnosis of acute and chronic cholecystitis, and has even become indispensable in evaluating the right upper-section of the abdomen for the detection or exclusion of malignant diseases [22].

Ultrasound proved to be too unspecific for the diagnosis of degenerative gallbladder disorders, and these diagnoses are only rarely made today [23].

Thus, an important discovery made in 1923 had a rapid expansion, achieved a secured position, and, eventually, became obsolete, replaced by another technique. The invasive examinations and the more recently introduced ultrasound examinations have maintained their position in clinical medicine.

What does the future hold?

There always will be a need for an imaging study of the gallbladder, but cholecystography probably will completely disappear one day, except for selecting patients for extracorporeal lithotripsy of gallstones.

For the diagnostic evaluation of the biliary tract, ultrasound has become the first examination of choice, and transhepatic, intraoperative and endoscopic cholangiography will continue to have a place.

New imaging modalities have been added, most importantly CT and MRI. So far, it has not become clear what role they will play in the evaluation of the biliary tract. It is obvious that further research should be pursued systematically. The discovery of 1923 may play a part again.

References

1. Lyon, A.S., R.J. Petrucelli: Geschiedenis van de Geneeskunde. Standaard Uitgeverij
2. Whittaker, J.T.: Detection of gall-stones by the exploring needle. Medical Record, 21 (1882) 568–569
3. Pel, P.K.: De ziekten van lever en galwegen en de poortader, mede op grond van eigen waarneming. De Erven F. Bohn - Haarlem, Nederland (1910) 298–304, 319–381
4. Burckhardt, H.: Experiments on puncture of the gallbladder and its visualization with roentgen rays. Dtsch. Ztschr. Chirurgie, 162 (1921) 168–197
5. Carman, R.D.: Roentgen observation of the gallbladder and hepatic ducts after perforation into the duodenum. J. Am. Med. Ass. 65 (1915) 1812
6. Reich, A.: Accidental injection of bile ducts with petrolatum and bismuth paste. J. Am. Med. Ass. 71 (1918) 155
7. Otte, G.: Examination of the bile ducts with lipiodol in cases of fistula. Bull. Soc. nat. Chir. 51 (1925) 759–767

8. Mirizzi, P.L., C. Quiroga Losada: Exploration of the principal biliary pathways during the course of operation. Congreso Argentino de Cirurgia. Session of October 17 (1931) 694–703

9. Sehrwald, E.M.C.: The behavior of the halogens toward röntgen rays. Dtsch. med. Wschr. 30 (1896) 477–480

10. Huard, P., Do-Xuan-Hop: Transhepatic puncture of the biliary ducts. Bull. Soc. Méd.-Chir. de l'Indochine, 15 (1937) 1090–1100

11. Burckhardt, H., W. Müller: Experiments on puncture of the gallbladder and its visualization with roentgen rays. Dtsch. Ztschr. Chirurgie, 162 (1921) 168–197

12. Pallardy, G., M.J. Pallardy, A. Wackenheim: Histoire illustrée de la radiologie. 1989. Les Éditions Roger Dacosta - Paris, France

13. Abel, J.J., L.G. Rowntree: On the pharmacological action of some phthaleins and their derivatives, with especial reference to their behaviour as purgatives. J. Pharmacol. Exper. Ther. 1 (1909/10) 231–264

14. Rous, P., P.D. McMaster: The concentrating activity of the gallbladder. J. Exp. Med. 24 (1921) 47–73

15. Graham, E.A., W.H. Cole: Roentgenologic examination of the gallbladder. Preliminary report of a new method utilizing the intravenous injection of tetrabromphenolphthalein. J. Am. Med. Ass. 82 (1924) 613–614

16. Cole, W.H.: Historical features of cholecystography. Radiology, 76 (1961) 354–375

17. Menees, T.O., H.C. Robinson: Oral administration of tetraiodophenolphthalein for cholecystography. Radiology, 5 (1925) 211–221

18. Dohrn, M., P. Diedrich: A new X-ray contrast agent for the gallbladder. Dtsch. med. Wschr. 41 (1940) 1133–1134

19. Kleiber, N.: The problem of peroral representation of the gallbladder. Dtsch. med. Wschr. 41 (1940) 1134–1135

20. Jutras, J.A., J.M. Longtin, H.P. Lévesque: Hyperplastic cholecystoses. AJR 83 (1960) 795

21. Ruijs, J.H.J., S.G.Th. Hulst: Diagnosis of cholecystoses. 1977 Martinus Nijhoff Medical Division – The Hague, The Netherlands

22. Hatfield, Ph.M., R.E. Wise: Radiology of the gallbladder and bile ducts. Golden's diagnostic radiology. Section 22. 1976. The Williams and Wilkins Company – Baltimore, USA

23. Berk, R.N., J.T. Ferrucci Jr, G.R. Leopold: Radiology of the gallbladder and bile ducts. Diagnosis and intervention. 1983 W.B. Saunders Company – Philadelphia, USA

24. Frommhold, W.: A new contrast agent for intravenous cholecystography. Fortschr. Röntgenstr. 79 (1953) 283–291

25. Langecker, H., A. Harwart, K. Junkmann: 2, 4, 6-Triiodine-3-acetaminobenzoic acid derivates as contrast media. Arch. Exper. Path. u. Pharmakol. 220 (1953) 195–206

26. Cooperberg, P., H. Burhenne: Real time ultrasonography. Diagnostic technique of choice in calculous gallbladder disease. N. Eng. J. Med. 302 (1980) 1277

27. Brakel, K.: Radiological aspects of nonsurgical therapy of gallbladder stones. 1992. Thesis Rotterdam. CIP-gegevens Koninklijke Bibliotheek – Den Haag, Nederland.

Urinary tract

E. Löhr

One or two fathers of modern cystoscopy: Karl Nitze and Thomas Edison

As early as 1868, the French surgeon Antoinin Jean Desormaux constructed the first cystoscope. The illumination, however, was poor because of the use of candles. Employing prisms for the optics and placing a carbon filament lamp at the tip of the cystoscope, Max Nitze and the Viennese instrument maker Joseph Leiter achieved a breakthrough in cystoscopy in 1886. Decisive for the new illumination was Thomas Edison's invention of the incandescent lamp. Because of the illumination, the bladder could now be observed directly and evaluated.

In the following years, the cystoscopes were developed further and equipped with channels (Maluf 1956). This meant that urine could be collected from the ureters through an inserted catheter to evaluate each kidney separately for pathology and to take biopsies from suspicious areas under visual guidance. Indeed, it was already possible to perform small therapeutic procedures, such as polypectomies.

Despite such an important progress, the diagnostic evaluation of the kidneys and ureters for stone disease, tumors, ureteral obstruction, or infections remained far from being satisfactory.

New diagnostic modalities needed

In 1893, shortly before the discovery of X-rays, Franz Koenig wrote in his famous three-volume textbook on surgery about the diagnostic evaluation for renal calculi:

'The diagnostic investigation has to determine, apart from questioning the presence of renal stones, the involvement of one or both kidneys and the kind of concrements.

To diagnose a renal colic is not always easy. Because of the neuralgic complaints, other neuralgias may be questioned, such as biliary colic or bladder complaints. The symptoms are often so uncertain that further diagnostic means seem desirable. Sometimes the stones, if there are many, can be recognized by characteristic crepitation in bimanual examination, with one hand on the stomach and the other in the lumbar region... The diagnosis before the operation is, of course, of utmost importance. If one considers the side confirmed without having been ascertained of the tumor, crepitation, etc, the kidney is exposed first and palpated, possibly also along the course of the ureter. If the kidney is exposed, it is touched and searched for the stone. A small stone may easily escape detection.'

This illustrates how uncertain and inaccurate the examination methods were and how imperative the need for more exact techniques.

First attempts to show renal stones radiographically

The interest of urologists in X-rays was immediate. It was known that these rays could penetrate the soft tissues, but not osseous structures. It might even be possible to demonstrate stones in the collecting system with these rays. In 1896, the English physician McIntyre had conducted a successful experiment with X-rays on a resected kidney. He had *'an excellent negative of the specimen after a three-minute exposure, showing the structure and contours of the organ with the stone in the centre'*, previously put by him in the renal pelvis.

Soon thereafter, he could detect a calculus in the kidney of a patient, and the calculus was actually found during surgery.

As early as 1898, Ringel attributed the different densities of the renal calculi to differences in their chemical compositions and stated that a negative radiograph does not exclude the presence of stones. This led to revising many too optimistic opinions as to the diagnosis of concretions. As we now know, uric acid stones are indeed not radiopaque and cannot be seen on plain radiographs of the abdomen.

In the early years, the exposure times of radiographs obtained to detect renal stones were usually 30–50 min and only seldom less. McIntyre, for instance, used an exposure time of only 12 min. The spark gap, therefore, must have been wide and the voltage correspondingly high.

To reduce the exposure time, Kuemmel (1898) called for a better vacuum of the X-ray tubes, thus making them harder, and for increasing the spark gap from 8 to 25 cm, predicting a shortening of the exposure time from the 30–50 min to 3 s.

Setback and progress

Diagnosing calculi of the urinary tract had failures of various causes, such as long exposure times with corresponding blurring, scattered radiation with corresponding poor contrast, superimposed intestinal contents, and misinterpretations since the normal radiographic image was unknown or only vaguely known. The correct interpretation of radiographs had still to be learned first (Fig. III, 41).

To improve the radiograph, R. Kienboeck (1902) recommended a lead collimator and positioning of the tube close to the abdominal wall but in a way that no skin reaction occurs. The colon should be evacuated to avoid interference from intestinal contents.

In 1903, H.E. Albers-Schoenberg stated that a good image could only be obtained with a reliable tube fitted with the proper collimator. The collimator was necessary to absorb interfering secondary radiation. In addition, he introduced the compression cone to compress the soft tissues, to reduce the thickness of the object and to displace interfering superimposed intestinal structures. It may not have been known yet that reducing the radiation volume decreases the amount of scattered radiation, ultimately improving the image quality.

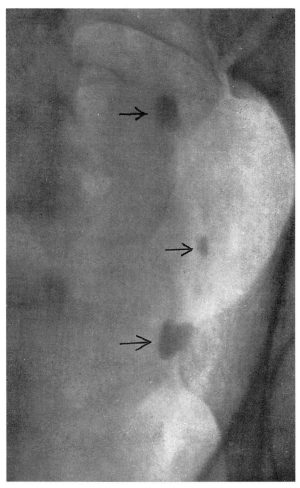

Fig. III, 41. Plain radiograph of left kidney: Ureter stone (from Joseph, 1928).

Can instrumental cystoscopy be combined with radiographic examinations?

It was indeed possible to introduce a catheter via the cystoscope into the ureters, but nothing could be said about their course since the catheters were not radiopaque. Ureteral catheters with a metal guide wire had been used in cadavers and, eventually, with a lead or silver wire in patients, whereby the wire was somewhat shorter than the catheter to avoid a perforation (Tuffier, 1897; Illeys, 1901; Klose, 1904; Schmidt and Kolischer, 1901). The catheterized section of the ureter was delineated by the wire. Eventually, radiopaque material was added to the ureteral catheter. A stone in the catheterized ureter could now easily be distinguished from an extrinsic calcification.

Failures in detecting stones but also the need for evaluating the morphology of the pelvicaliceal system and ureters led to the idea of using contrast agents to delineate the collecting system. This was possibly encouraged by the successful results of using contrast medium for the examinations of the gastrointestinal tract (Fig. III, 42–45).

As early as 1903 and 1906, respectively, Voelcker (Fig. III, 46) and von Lichtenberg (Fig. III, 47) succeeded in obtaining a good contrast visualization of the ureters and pelvicaliceal system via a

ureteral catheter by retrograde injection of a 5% Collargol solution (Collargol = colloidal argentum), which was a radiopaque substance. At the end of the examination, they rinsed the renal pelvis carefully with boric acid to avoid or at least

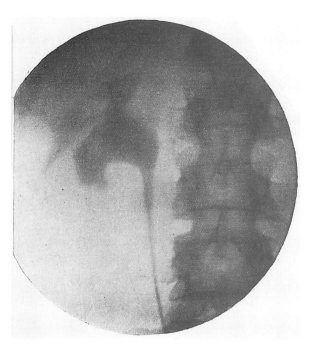

Fig. III, 42. Opacification of the right pelvicaliceal system by retrograde administration of Kollargol (from Voelcker and von Lichtenberg, 1906).

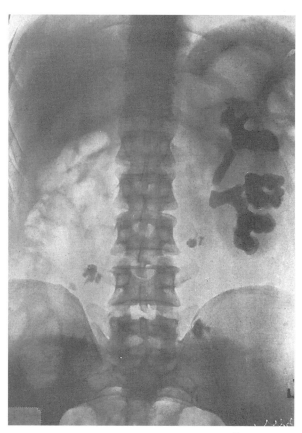

Fig. III, 44. Staghorn calculus in the left renal pelvis on plain radiograph, in addition, calcified abdominal lymph nodes (from Schinz et al, 1928).

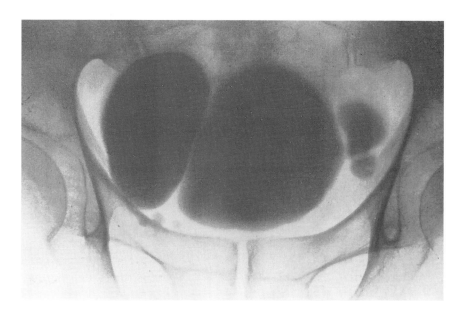

Fig. III, 43. Three bladder diverticula (from Joseph, 1926).

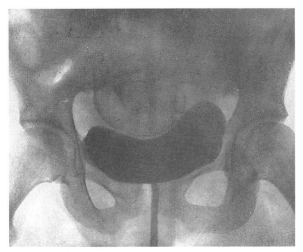

Fig. III, 45. Cystogram during pregnancy visualizing the engaged head in the lesser pelvis (from Schinz et al., 1928).

reduce damage to the epithelium. They described their normal findings: the course of the ureters, particularly as found in wandering kidneys, a caliceal stone, and ureteral obstruction by an ovarian tumor as manifestation of an extrinsic compression on the ureter. The era of the visualization of the collecting system by means of contrast media had commenced.

In 1908, Albarran and Ertzbischoff described a cavernous tuberculosis in a kidney, which was seen as hydronephrosis after the resected kidney was injected with bismuth. In addition, they were able to demonstrate a communication with the kidney after injection of Collargol into a lumbar fistula.

Braasch (Fig. III, 48), a urologist at the Mayo Clinic, USA, developed retrograde pyelography further and in 1909 and 1910 he described various pathologic findings, such as hydronephrosis, solitary kidneys, nephrolithiasis and tumors.

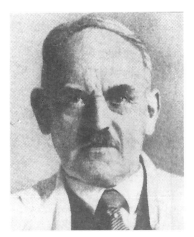

Fig. III, 46. Fritz Voelcker (1872–1955). Surgeon in Heidelberg and Halle, primarily urologic interest. Development of renal excretion tests. Together with von Lichtenberg, work on Cystography and Pyelography.

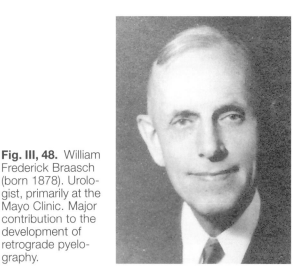

Fig. III, 48. William Frederick Braasch (born 1878). Urologist, primarily at the Mayo Clinic. Major contribution to the development of retrograde pyelography.

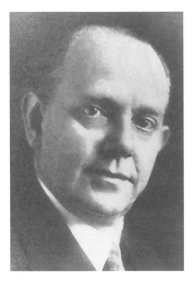

Fig. III, 47. Alexander von Lichtenberg (1880–1949). Born in Budapest. Surgeon in Heidelberg, Straßburg, Budapest, Berlin. Cooperation with Voelcker and Swick. Work on intravenous urography.

Furthermore, retrograde visualization of the ureters and pelvicaliceal system had to be performed for accurate localization of calcifications to avoid unnecessary surgery.

Since the retrograde injection of Collargol had complications, including deaths, a different and less dangerous contrast medium was sought.

In 1911, von Lichtenberg and Dietlen filled the pelvicaliceal system with oxygen, a radiolucent contrast medium. The method did not improve the visualization of the pelvicaliceal system; it even had fatal complications due to excessive distension of the pelvicaliceal system and injury of the renal vein, leading to air emboli (Cohn, 1927; Koehler, 1927).

By using a larger syringe to avoid a high injection pressure, Voelcker countered the criticism that pyelography would lead to ruptures and other injuries due to high pressure.

Because plate errors could also simulate concretions, Koehler developed the double-plate method. Two photographic plates, one on top of the other, were exposed at the same time; a concretion was seen in both plates and a plate error only in one.

In his monograph on radiology of the kidneys in the form of an "atlas of typical actinograms", Grunmach (1914) stressed the importance of radiographic localization of renal calculi. He recommended that several actinograms of film plates or films be obtained to distinguish plate errors from concretions and other formations.

Albers-Schoenberg (1903) and Haenisch (1910) were of the opinion that three to six radiographs are necessary to establish the presence of concrements in the kidneys and ureters. Depending on the clinical indication, a retrograde filling of the pelvicaliceal system with Collargol solution should follow. The calculi were surrounded by the radiopaque solution and seen as defects.

The radiographically diagnosed calculi were not always found surgically. Therefore, attempts were made from the very beginning to obtain intraoperative radiographs for the exact localization of stones so that they could be easily found and removed.

Nephroptosis – over-diagnosed? A fashionable diagnosis?

In the early literature, nephroptosis plaid a role that, according to our current thinking, is no longer justified. This can be attributed to the fact that with radiographic examinations functional and positional changes of internal organs could be seen for the first time in the living. Many organs were found to be less strongly attached and immobile as thought previously. Thus, radiographic examinations opened entirely new aspects, most certainly overemphasizing the role of nephroptosis.

The lagging diagnosis of renal tumors

Before the discovery of X-rays, tumors could only be attributed to the kidneys by assessing their respiratory and palpable mobility. In addition, it was determined how the audible intestinal peristaltic activities changes with a change of the patient's position. To obtain gaseous intestinal distension, it was even proposed to fill the colon with carbon dioxide. Furthermore, bimanual palpation was performed with the abdominal muscles relaxed under chloroform narcosis, particularly to detect small tumor of the kidney.

Early percutaneous intervention

As early as 1893, Franz Koenig pointed out that a puncture was needed to obtain histological material in cases that are uncertain as to representing a cyst or a solid tumor. Retrograde pyelography provided information about the pelvicaliceal system. Displacement and destruction of calyces were interpreted as tumor signs (Braasch, 1910; Haenisch, 1910). Of course, tumors in the renal periphery could not be found by this method which does not visualize the contours and parenchyma of the kidneys. Oehlecker's work (1908) should be mentioned here since he was the first to investigate carefully the polycystography with large survey radiographs of the entire urogenital system, combining cystourethroscopy and radiology.

Barium sulphate and air to outline the kidneys

During the first two decades, an oral contrast medium was administered to classify space-occupying processes in the renal fossa, to determine a few hours later location and site of origin of the tumor by the position of the adjacent contrast-filled colon. While large renal tumors, which generally displace the neighboring organs, could be found, this method, being an indirect method, was doomed to be inaccurate.

In 'coelioscopy', as laparoscopy was at first called, filtered air was introduced into the abdominal cavity before insertion of the cystoscope. Rautenberg used this principle of peritoneal air injection also for radiographs of the abdominal organs.

It outlined not only spleen and liver, but also the kidneys. For this pneumography, 1.5–3 liters of sterile air or oxygen was instilled through a 5-cm-long cannula into the peritoneal cavity. After changing the patient's position to distribute the gas more evenly, radiographs were taken.

Because of the extraperitoneal position of the kidneys, they were less well outlined than liver and spleen. Concrements, however, could be seen better. Goetze, who expanded this method,

Fig. III, 49a-e.

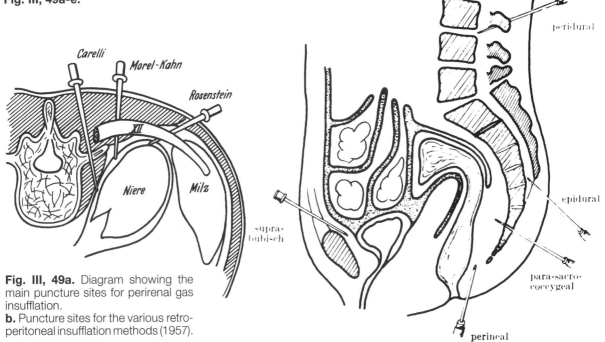

a

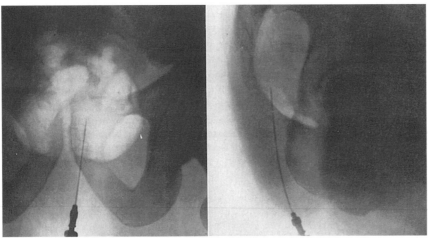

Fig. III, 49a. Diagram showing the main puncture sites for perirenal gas insufflation.
b. Puncture sites for the various retroperitoneal insufflation methods (1957).

b

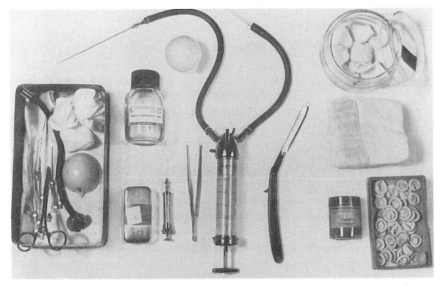

Fig. III, 49c. Instruments for presacral insufflation.

Fig. III, 49d. Needle position for presacral insufflation.

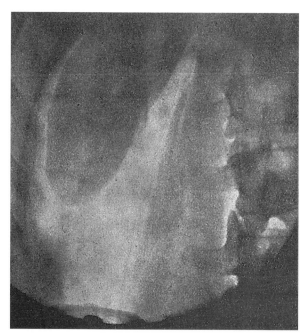

Fig. III, 49e. Image of a normal kidney as seen in pneumogram (from Rosenstein, 1921).

senstein – was the separate injection, requiring a separate puncture, for each kidney. Rosenstein even performed the examination on both sides on outpatients! He mentioned acute abscesses as a contraindication. He emphasized that his pneumoradiography of the kidneys could not replace any of the other methods and should be considered complementary to them. The direct combination with pyelography often proved especially valuable.

However, even this method had complications, such as meningeal symptoms, apnea and even cardiac arrest, though reversible.

In the chapter on uroradiology in the first edition of his textbook of diagnostic radiology, Schinz (1928) emphasized the importance of retroperitoneal gas insufflation in the detection of renal tumors (Fig. III, 50).

The retropneumoperitoneum was still used even after the introduction of the intravenous pyelogram, not so much for the kidneys but more for the adrenal glands. It was superseded only by newly developed diagnostic methods such as angiography (Seldinger, 1953, Boijsen, 1961, Olsson, 1964) and, later, sonography, CT and MRI.

witnessed one death of 200 examinations performed in this manner, probably caused by intestinal puncture and the subsequent peritonitis.

To overcome the unsatisfactory visualization of the renal contours, Rosenstein (1921) injected approximately a 0.5–1 litre of oxygen directly into the perirenal space (Fig. III, 49) A disadvantage of this retropneumoperitoneum – or 'pneumoradiography of the renal bed' as called by Ro-

Physiology and pharmacology applied – intravenous pyelography

Despite tremendous progress, retrograde pyelography remained rather strenuous for the patients. Moreover, the risk of an infection could not be entirely eliminated, even by using a gentle

Fig. III, 50a-c. Tumor of the left kidney (from Schinz, 1928).

Fig. III, 50a. Pneumoperitoneum: clear delineation of a lobulated mass of the left kidney, outlined by the insufflated oxygen in the peritoneal space.

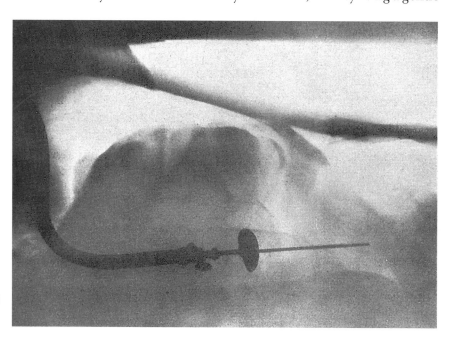

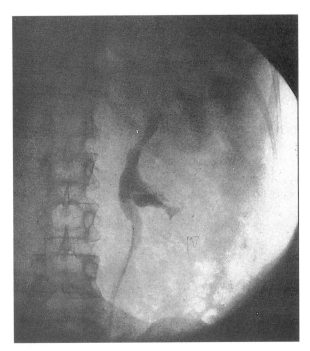

Fig. III, 50b. Retrograde pyelogram: Spreading and displacement of the upper and medial calyceal group due to a central mass representing a tumor.

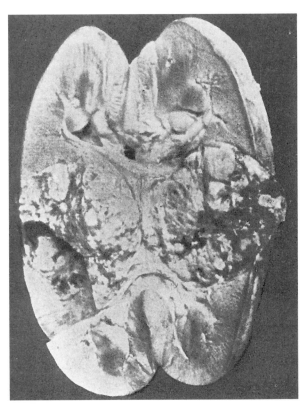

Fig. III, 50c. Surgical specimen showing the renal tumor (hypernephroma).

technique and aseptic conditions. The risk to the patient was even higher if a 'pneumoradiography' was performed at the same time.

Would it not be possible to see the morphology and function of the kidneys in a more physiological way, that is, by using the excretory function of the kidneys? Contrast agents were needed that were almost exclusively excreted by the kidneys, were harmless and nontoxic, and that could be given intravenously or, better still, orally,. Such contrast media would also be suitable for retrograde pyelography. But as early as 1916, Zindel had warned about the renal damage caused by heavy metal salts used for the retrograde ureteropyelography (in addition to Collargol, silver iodide and thorium dioxide were used) (see also Pendergrass et al, 1942).

In 1922, Rowntree observed that patients in the Department of Dermatology and Syphilology at the Mayo Clinic, USA, who had been injected intravenously with 50–250 ml of a 10 % sodium-iodide solution to investigate the iodine metabolism, showed an opacification and outline of the bladder approximately 1.5 h later. In many cases, the kidneys and even the ureters were visible as well. Osborne and coworkers recommended and tried the oral application of sodium iodide to visualize the urinary tract if only the bladder had to be seen.

The oral method could not be developed further since no absorbable contrast medium became available. In 1923, Osborne and coworkers, including Rowntree, measured the iodine levels in the urine at certain time intervals after intravenous administration of iodine and concluded that radiographs should be obtained 0.5, 1, 2 and 3 h later. This was the beginning of intravenous urography, pointing the way to be pursued for the morphological evaluation of the kidneys.

While Volkmann (1924), K. Frik and Bluehbaum (1928) described further studies performed with colloids, first reports were published by Casper (1927), but above all by Hryntschak (1929) and Fraenkel (1930), on the intravascular application of contrast media excreted by the kidney. Von Lichtenberg and Swick (Fig. III, 51a) (1929) and, at the same time, Roseno (1929) and Swick (1929) achieved a breakthrough with the introduction of Uroselectan, which was excreted by the kidneys and well tolerated. In 1931, the chemist Binz deserves credit for contributing to the synthesis of this contrast medium. The state of the art at that time was well presented in the known textbooks of Boehminghaus (1927) and Schinz, Baensch and Friedl (1928).

Fig. III, 51a.
Moses Swick (born 1900). After graduation from medical school, fellowship in Hamburg and Berlin. Cooperation with Binz and Raeth, later also with Lichtwitz and von Lichtenberg. Worked as urologist for more than 30 years in New York.

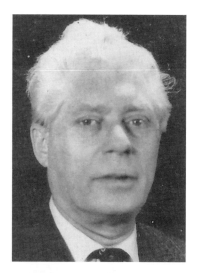

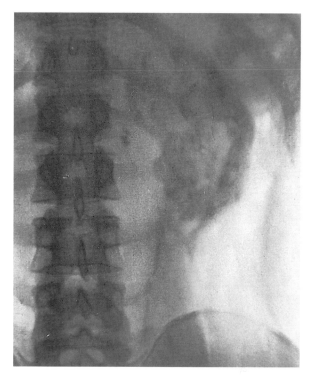

Fig. III, 52. Plain radiograph: Extensive diffuse calcified lesions in urotuberculosis (from Boehminghaus, 1927).

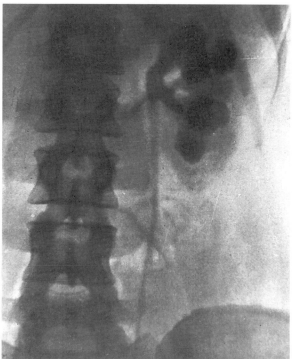

Fig. III, 51b. Primary pyelonephrosis with generalized dilatation of the pelvicaliceal system and parenchymal atrophy. Retrograde pyelogram (from Boehminghaus, 1927).

Not until the introduction of water-soluble intravenous contrast media, the diagnosis of inflammatory and neoplastic renal diseases could improve. The new contrast media produced an adequate, often even excellent, opacification of the pelvicaliceal system, enabling a direct correlation between radiographic morphology and pathoanatomic morphology, as found in pyelonephritic changes and in space-occupying lesions (Fig. III, 51–54) (Alken, 1938; Hornykiewytsch, 1963; Prevôt 1964, Bosniak 1972).

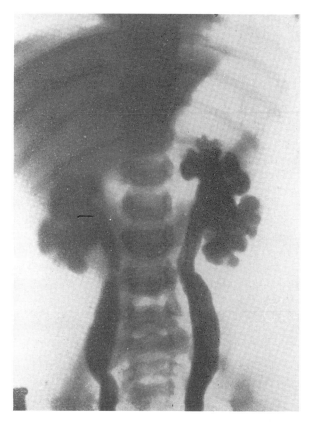

Fig. III, 53. Radiograph showing bilateral vesicoureteral reflux in pyelitis, primarily affecting the right kidney (from Joseph, 1926).

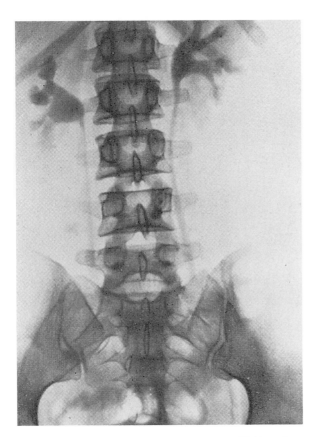

Fig. III, 54. Intravenous excretory urogram with Uroselectan showing pyelitic changes of the right kidney (from Swick, 1929).

In the following years, intravenous urography became of great importance to demonstrate obstruction, whether by stones, tumors or exogenic processes, and to assess the excretory renal function.

Diagnosing hypertension caused by renal artery stenosis was attempted by rapid sequence urography, performed by obtaining a sequence of films within minutes following bolus injection of the contrast agent. The renal perfusion was deduced by assessing parenchymal opacification and pelvicaliceal concentration of contrast. Later, angiography became the standard method to assess the renal arteries. The performance of the intravenous urogram was tailored according to the clinical question. For better filling of the pelvicaliceal system, the proximal ureters were compressed with a specially developed compression device to cause a temporary obstruction. It was often imperative to modify the technique during examination for better evaluation of the pathological processes. Despite standardization, each examination had to be individualized for each patient.

Incorporating many years of experience, intravenous urography, now also referred as pyelography, has gained a central place in diagnosing diseases of the kidneys and ureters.

New methods were introduced to increase the diagnostic information that can be obtained from intravenous urography. Kymography was performed to evaluate the motility of the kidneys during inspiration and expiration, with limited respiratory motion attributed to perirenal inflammations, and to analyze the peristalsis of the ureters. Kymography was short-lived in intravenous pyelography and replaced by the respiration pyelogram, in which one radiograph of the kidneys was exposed twice, in inspiration and expiration, often using half the exposure each. The kidneys were imaged twice, in a higher and lower position corresponding the respiratory excursion. This allowed an indirect conclusion as to the kidneys' motility. In contrast, tomography, which eliminates interfering superimposed intestinal structures, has become part of the standard protocol used for intravenous pyelography today.

Recently, the electronic harmonizing was found to improve the resolution of the pelvicaliceal system and the renal parenchyma as seen on the i.v. pyelogram, improving the diagnostic evaluation for inflammatory changes in the kidneys (Fig. III, 55) (Loehr and Mellin, 1957, 1976).

Well into the sixties, excretory urography also played a major role in evaluating and following urogenital tuberculosis (Elke et al, 1967, Rodeck and Bethge, 1976).

Another mode of intravenous contrast-medium administration – infusion urography

In the last two decades, 'infusion urography' was added to the conventional intravenous pyelogram. Infusing the contrast-medium was meant to obtain a better contrast enhancement of the renal parenchyma by prolonging the parenchymal phase and to achieve an even opacification of the ureters in their entire length.

Infusion urography, however, also has disadvantages due to potential misinterpretation, such as calling calyceal distension and deformity pathologic though these changes are caused by the massive excretion of contrast medium and its solution. This is also true for pyelorenal reflux, which is often mimicked in infusion urography due to massive accumulation of contrast medium in the collecting tubules. This can even be mistaken for papillary necrosis.

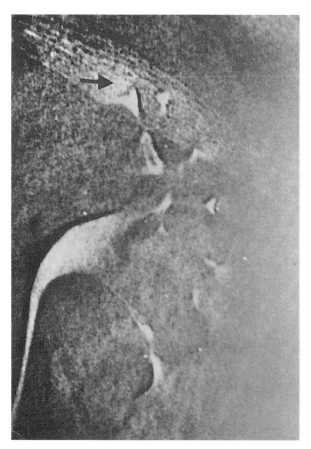

Fig. III, 55. I.v. urogram during an acute attack of chronic pyelonephritis, with marked opacification of the left kidney, which shows generalized swelling and narrowing of the pelvicaliceal system. The magnification and applied electronic harmonization technique enhance the visualization of the generalized renal swelling and reveal caliceal defects with extravasation of contrast medium (from Loehr and Mellin, 1976).

Not infrequently, infusion urograms, if performed during a renal colic, have shown pelvicaliceal ruptures due to increased pressure in the collecting system. General clinical experience suggest that it is better to avoid an urogram during an acute renal colic.

Other urinary organs also accessible for roentgen examination?

Kidneys, pelvicaliceal system, and ureters were in the foreground so far since they were the least accessible by other investigations. The radiographic examination of the bladder (Loewenhardt, 1901; Wulff, 1904) has become important to detect diverticula and stones as well as to evaluate its function. The latter includes verification of vesicoureteral reflux causing pyelonephritis

and evaluation of the bladder floor with possible pathological descend, resulting in incontinence.

The cystographic evaluating of the bladder carcinoma has not advanced much, despite great efforts. It was tried to assess the carcinomatous infiltration of the bladder wall by polycystography. A radiographic film was exposed at various stages during filling of the bladder, resulting in multiple superimposed images of the bladder. Segments of absent or impaired distension and contraction of the bladder were equated with tumor infiltration and penetration. By means of the double-contrast method, using either barium sulphate or water-soluble contrast medium and air, it was tried to diagnose smaller, particularly superficial carcinomas. However, cystoscopy remained the basis for the diagnostic evaluation of the bladder. Only recently, this has changed somewhat as to the staging of bladder carcinoma by the introduction of the new imaging modalities.

By combining cystoscopy and urethrography, strictures of the urethra had been described only a few years after Roentgen's discovery (Edebohls, 1898; Leonard, 1900; Illeys, 1901; Cunningham, 1910).

Antegrade and retrograde urethrography are still used today and represent a central examination method to clarify various urethral conditions.

What remained from the conventional roentgen examination?

Although sonography and computed tomography have changed and reduced the indications for i.v. urography and infusion urography, the excretory urography has remained a standard examination of great value in urologic radiology and, so far, has not been entirely replaced by the newer imaging modalities. Other conventional radiographic examinations, only briefly mentioned, also remain an essential part of the morphological evaluation in urology.

References

Albarran, J., P. Ertzbischoff: Radiography of normal and pathologic pelves and ureters. Assoc. Fanc. d'Urol. Proc-Verb. 12 (1908) 282–294.

Albers-Schönberg, A.: Zur Technik der Nierenaufnahmen. Fortschr. Röntgenstr. 3 (1901) 210–211

Alken, C.E.: Die Papillennekrose. J. Urol. 32 (1938) 433–438

Binz, A.: The chemistry of Uroselectan. J. Urol. 25 (1931) 297–301

Binz, A.: Geschichte des Uroselectans. J. Urol. 31 (1937) 73–84

Böhminghaus, H.: Urologische Diagnostik und Therapie für Ärzte und Studierende. G. Fischer, Jena 1927

Boijsen, E.: Selektive renale Angiographie. Radiologe 1 (1961) 170–173

Bosniak, M.A., R.D. Schweizer: Urographic findings in patients with renal failure. Radiol. Clin. N. Amer. 10 (1972) 433–445

Braasch, W.F.: Deformities of the renal pelvis. Ann. Surg. 51 (1910) 534–540

Casper, L.: Pyelo-Uretrogramme, eine kritische Studie. Verh. Dtsch. Ges. Urol. (1927) 106–111

Cohn, Th.: Die Aufblasung des Nierenbeckens für das Röntgenbild. Zbl. Chir. 54 (1927) 1988–1995

Cunningham, J.H. Jr: The diagnosis of stricture of the urethra by the roentgen rays. Trans Am. Ass. Genitour. Surg. 5 (1910) 369–371

Edebohls, G.M.: The other kidney in contemplated nephrectomy. Ann. Surg. 27 (1898) 425–435

Elke, M., G. Rutishauser, I. Baumann: Vorschlag einer einfachen Stadieneinteilung der Nierentuberkulose aufgrund röntgenologischer und therapeutischer Gesichtspunkte. Urologe 6 (1967) 40

Fränkel, W.K.: Ein neues reizloses Kontrastmittel zur pervesikalen ambulanten Pyelographie. Münch. med. Wschr. 77 (1930) 1447–1448

Frik, K., T. Blühbaum: Eine neue Anwendungsart der Kolloide in der Röntgendiagnostik. Fortschr. Röntgenstr. 38 (1928) 1111–1119

Goetze, O.: Die Röntgendiagnostik bei gasgefüllter Bauchhöhle. Münch. med. Wschr. 65 (1918) 1275–1280

Grunmach, E.: Die Diagnostik mittels der Röntgenstrahlen in der Inneren Medizin und den Grenzgebieten im Atlas typischer Aktinogramme. Engelmann, W.: Krankheiten des Urogenitalapparates. Leipzig, Berlin 1914, s.bes. S. 39–40

Haenisch, A.: Hydronephrose infolge Ureterabknickung. Z. Röntgenk. (1910) S 12.

Hornykiewytsch, Th.: Röntgenologische Symptomatologie der Pyelonephritis. Acta Radiol. Austriaca 13 (1963) 215–237

Hryntschak, T.: Studien zur röntgenologischen Darstellung von Nierenparenchym und Nierenbecken auf intravenösem Wege. Z. Urol. 23 (1929) 893–904

Illeys, G.: Ureteral catheterization and roentgenography. Oro Hetil 45 (1901) 659–662

Klose, B.: Radiography of a case of complete ureter duplication diagnosed by cystoscopy. Dtsch. Z. Chir. 72 (1904) 613–617

Kienböck, R.: Zur radiographischen Diagnose der Nierensteine. Wien. Klin. Wschr. 15 (1902) 1324

Kienböck, R.: Über Blitzfiguren auf Röntgenplatten. Zbl. Röntgenstr. 2 (1911) 162

Köhler, A.: Zur Plattenfrage. Z. Elektrol. Röntgenk. 9 (1907) 141

Köhler, H.: Über das Indikationsgebiet der Pneumoradiographie der Niere und Blase. Verh. Dtsch. Ges. Urol. (1927) 119–122, 129–131

König, F.: Lehrbuch der speziellen Chirurgie. 2. Bd., 6. Aufl. Berlin 1893.

Kümmel, H.: Die Bedeutung der Röntgenstrahlen für die Chirurgie. Zbl. Chir. 24 (1898) 18–33

Leonard, C.L.: The x-ray diagnosis of nephrolithiasis. A resumé of its development and value. Philadelphia Med. J. 5 (1900) 50–55

Leonard, C.L.: Technique of positive and negative diagnosis of ureteral and renal calaili by aid of roentgen rays. Ann. Surg. 31 (1900) 349–355

Lichtenberg, A. von, H. Dietlen: Die Darstellung des Nierenbeckens und Ureters im Röntgenbilde nach Sauerstofffüllung. Münch. med. Wschr. (1911) 1341

Lichtenberg, A. von, M. Swick: Klinische Prüfung des Uroselectans. Klin. Wschr. 8 (1929) 2089–2091

Löhr, E., P. Mellin: Zur Diagnose und Differentialdiagnose entzündlicher Nierenveränderungen im Röntgenbild. Intern. Praxis 13 (1957) 73

Löhr, E., P. Mellin, G. Rodeck, J.W. Rohen: Atlas der urologischen Röntgendiagnostik. Schattauer Verlag, Stuttgart-New York 1976.

Loewenhardt: Determination of the position of the ureter before operation. Jahresbericht der Schlesischen Ges. vaterl. Kultur 79 (1901) 136–137

MacIntyre, J., C.H. Glasg, F.R.S. Edin: Roentgen Rays. Photography of renal calculus; description of an adjustable modification in the focus tube. Lancet (London) 2 (1896) 118

Maluf, N.S.R.: Role of roentgenology in the development of urology. Am. J. Roentgenol. 5 (1956) 847–854

Oehlecker, R.A.: Übersichtsaufnahmen vom uropoetischen System. Fortschr. Röntgenstr. 17 (1908) 195–207

Olsson, O.: Selektive Nierenangiographie. In: Schinz, H.R., R. Glauner, Rüttimann: Ergebnisse der medizinischen Strahlenforschung. Thieme Stuttgart 1964, s.bes. S. 201–414

Osborne, E.D., C.G. Sutherland, A.J. Scholl, L.G. Rowntree: Roentgenography of urinary tract during excretion of sodium iodid. J. Am. Med. Ass. 80 (1923) 368–373

Pendergrass, E.P., G.W. Chamberlin, E.W. Godfrey, E.D. Burdick: A survey of deaths: an unfavorable sequelae following the administration of contrast media. Am. J. Roentgenol. 48 (1942) 741–762

Prevôt, R.: Röntgendiagnostik der Pyelonephritis. Radiologe 4 (1964) 29–37

Rautenberg, E. Pneumoperitoneale Röntgendiagnostik. Z. Urol. 13 (1919) 318

Ringel, T.: Beitrag zur Diagnose der Nephrolithiasis durch Röntgenbilder. Zbl. Chir. 25 (1898) 1217–1220

Rodeck, G., H. Bethge: Urogenitaltuberkulose. In: Löhr, E., P. Mellin, G. Rodeck, J.W. Rohen: Atlas der urologischen Röntgendiagnostik. Schattauer Verlag, Stuttgart, New York 1976

Roseno, A. Die intravenöse Pyelographie. II. Mitteilung Klinische Ergebnisse. Klin. Wschr. 8 (1929) 1165–1170

Rosenstein, P.: Pneumoradiology of kidney position. A new technique for the radiological representation of the kidneys and neighboring organs (suprarenal gland, spleen, liver). Z. Urol. 15 (1921) 447–458

Schinz, H.R., W. Baensch, E. Friedl: Lehrbuch der Röntgendiagnostik. Thieme Verlag Leipzig 1928, 1. Auflage, S. 1077–1118

Schmidt, L.E., G. Kolischer: Radiography of catheterized ureters and kidneys. Mschr. Urol. 6 (1901) 427–431

Seldinger, S.I.: Catheter replacement of the needle in percutaneous arteriography. Acta Radiol. 39 (1953) 368–376

Swick, M.: Visualization of the kidney and urinary tract on roentgenograms by means of intravenous administration of a new contrast medium – Uroselectan. Klin. Wschr. 8 (1929) 2087–2089

Tuffier, T.: Course of ureter outlined with catheter. In: Duplay et Reclus: Traite de Chirurgie (2. Ed.). Masson et Cie, Paris (1897–99) VII: 412–413

Voelcker, F., E. Joseph: Funktionelle Nierendiagnostik ohne Ureterenkatheter. Münch. med. Wschr. 50 (1903) 2081–2089

Voelcker, F., Lichtenberg, A. von: Die Gestalt der menschlichen Harnblase im Röntgenbild. Münch. med. Wschr. 52 (1905) 1576–1578

Voelcker, F., Lichtenberg. A. von: Pyelography (roentgenography of the renal pelvis after filling with Kollargenol). Münch. med. Wschr. 53 (1906) 105–106

Volkmann, J.: Zur röntgenographischen Darstellung der Harnwege durch intravenöse Verabreichung schattengebender Mittel. Dtsch. med. Wschr. 50 (1924) 1413–1414

Wulff, P.: Applicability of X-rays in the diagnosis of bladder deformities. Fortschr. Roentgenstr. 8 (1904) 193–194

Zindel, L.: Kritische Sichtung der Fälle von Nierenschädigung nach Pyelographie. Z. Urol. Chir. 3 (1916) 359–404

Heart and blood vessels – evolution of angiography

E. Boijsen

Angiography is the general term for radiographic visualization of vessels after injection of a contrast medium; or more correctly, it was before the new non-invasive imaging techniques ultrasonography, computed tomography, and MR imaging took over most of the vascular imaging. In this presentation, we discuss only the radiographic method of angiography. To perform angiography, radiopaque or radiolucent contrast media are injected into arteries, veins, lymphatics, or into the heart. We most often use the term 'angiography' when contrast medium is injected on the arterial side and then followed through the vascular system of an organ to the venous side, utilizing a series of exposures and a recording system for documentation. For instance, we talk about cerebral, pulmonary, coronary, renal, hepatic, pancreatic etc. angiography. We also use it less consistently for cardioangiography or femoral angiography when we mean cardiography and femoral arteriography. Thus, when we exclusively study the arterial system we usually talk about arteriography, the venous system – venography, and the lymphatic system – lymphography.

Two different methods have been developed for angiographic studies. One is by means of direct needle puncture either after a local surgical exploration of a vessel or as a percutaneous puncture. Contrast medium is then injected at the puncture site. The second is by catheterization when the contrast medium is deposited at a distance from the site of introduction of the catheter after a cutdown or percutaneous puncture.

The first arteriography (s. Fig. III, 96) was performed only a few months following Roentgen's discovery. Teichman's mixture was injected into the arteries of an amputated hand with excellent anatomical demonstration of the vessels. It became obvious that arteriography of cadavers gave good information of vascular anatomy, and textbooks on the subject soon appeared.

The first three decades (1900–1930)

There was certainly a great desire for in-vivo arteriography during the first two decades of the 20th century, but there was a great obstacle to this: the lack of a suitable contrast medium. The second great obstacle was of course the First World War. As a consequence, no angiography on living humans was performed during the first two decades of this century. Various contrast media were, however, tested in animals and the twenties became a fascinating period in the history of angiography. After extensive studies on animals utilizing intravenous administration of Lipiodol, Sicard and Forestier [1] were the first to perform angiography in humans. They followed oil droplets fluoroscopically from the antecubital vein to the pulmonary vessels in humans, but the small amount injected and the slow injection rate prevented radiographic documentation. The same year Berberich and Hirsch [2] documented in man injection of strontium bromide in arteries and veins of the upper extremity, and in 1924 Brooks [3], for the first time, used sodium iodide for femoral arteriography in vivo with quite good results in terms of vascular anatomy and pathology. During the twenties, sodium iodide became the preferred contrast medium in intravascular studies.

It is obvious that these investigations stimulated further studies, which appeared during the second half of the twenties. The first reports were on cerebral angiography in humans by Moniz (s. Fig. IV, 38) [4]. Before exploring the human cardiovascular system, he and coworkers tested the contrasting effect of arterially injected media on cadavers in various concentrations of bromides and iodides. Finally, they used 70% strontium bromide for cerebral angiography. They were, however, not successful with the first few cases of carotid artery injection and therefore switched to sodium iodide 25%, which they knew was well tolerated by intravenous injection.

Sodium iodide was also used by the second pioneer of the twenties, Dos Santos (s. Fig. III, 69) [5]) who considered it to be a safe and reliable contrast medium for abdominal aortography.

Vascular approach

All arteriographic studies of cerebral and peripheral arteries during these two decades were performed with a needle after exploration of a vessel. Moniz attempted at first percutaneous puncture, but was not successful and therefore his neurosurgeon (Lima) assisted him in finding the carotid artery by a surgical incision. Dos Santos, stimulated by Moniz' work, explored the brachial and femoral arteries for extremity arteriography and showed excellent radiographs of various arterial lesions. Most important, however, was his pioneering work in lumbar aortography. He punctured the lumbar aorta from behind with a long needle and was successful in demonstrating not only the lumbar aorta and its visceral branches but also the iliac and femoral artery systems. After percutaneous puncture of the lumbar aorta, 30–35 ml of sodium iodide 100% was injected, first by hand, but later with a kind of pump as rapidly as possible. One radiograph was obtained about 0.8 s after the beginning of the injection. Coordination of exposure and injection was made and the amount of contrast medium could be reduced. To improve the information of the aorta and abdominal arteries, he applied tourniquets on both thighs, thus reducing the flow in the femoral arteries.

Dos Santos et al. did not find any complications with the percutaneous technique for lumbar aortography, but subsequent reports stated that the method could cause thrombosis of the superior mesenteric as well as of renal arteries with infarctions. Also paraplegia was reported. The method did therefore not receive immediate wide acceptance.

Forssmann (s. Fig. III, 76) [6] in 1929 passed a catheter from his cubital vein to his heart and when he felt the catheter in position he went to the fluoroscopy room for documentation. La-

ter he made attempts at visualizing the right heart and the pulmonary circulation by this technique. He was successful in animals but not when contrast medium was injected into the human heart. Nevertheless, Forssmann's pioneer work with catheters was a new angiographic technique, but it became the method of choice only after more than two decades.

Contrast media

As mentioned, the main contrast media used were strontium bromide and sodium iodide. Even though the pioneers considered sodium iodide acceptable, with no serious consequences for the patients, others had an opposite opinion in the twenties. It is therefore understandable that technical and clinical development was hindered by toxic contrast media, usually injected by hand through narrow tubes.

Late in the twenties, two new contrast media appeared. They were not initially intended for angiography. One was Thorotrast, a 25% solution of thorium dioxide, introduced for imaging of the spleen and liver by Radt in 1929 [7]. Thorotrast was soon found to be a safe medium for intra-arterial use. A few years later, however, it was considered unsuitable because of its radioactivity with serious effects both local and distant. Thorotrast was nevertheless used in many centers, in particular for cerebral angiography after recommendation by Moniz among others [8]. Thorotrast was not abandoned completely for arteriography until late in the forties.

The second contrast medium was an organic iodide, later known as Uroselectan, introduced for urography by Swick in 1929 [9]. This product as well as its organic iodide containing successors inaugurated a new, safer method for angiography during the subsequent two decades.

Documentation

The radiographic documentation during the twenties was limited to obtaining one radiograph only for each injection. Understandable enough with the contrast medium used and the low injection rate, the diagnostic information was poor. Nevertheless, a number of new observations were made and they stimulated further research in angiography.

The thirties and forties

Contrast media

Soon after the introduction of Uroselectan, it was realized that its use for urography by intravenous injection also visualized vessels. This stimulated research to find new, less toxic and less irritating contrast media. Methiodal sodium (Abrodil, Skiodan) with one iodine atom in the molecule was first developed and tested in peripheral arteriography and venography. It was soon followed by a contrast medium with a higher density, iodopyracet (Perabrodil, Diodrast, Diodon), with two iodine atoms. It was found to be less toxic and irritating and had better contrasting effect than previously used media. For the following two decades iodopyracet was the contrast medium of choice for angiography. However, Thorotrast was also frequently used during this period, particularly for cerebral angiography.

Vascular approach: veins

After the early description of peripheral venography by Berberich and Hirsch in 1923 [2], the new less toxic contrast media opened up the way for more systematic studies in the thirties [10, 11]. The superior and inferior venae cavae were also demonstrated during these two decades. The superior vena cava was observed repeatedly during the many cardioangiographic studies subsequently performed but was also evaluated for the analysis of mediastinal lesions.

Forssmann's [6] catheterization of himself, and his intention to visualize the cardiac chambers and the pulmonary circulation in man, received, despite his own failures, much attention, and many other attempts were made. Moniz et al. [12], still using sodium iodide in various concentrations in experimental work, punctured the right chamber or injected the contrast medium into the jugular vein and obtained good visualization of the pulmonary vessels. Using Forssmann's method in man, they were able to demonstrate the pulmonary vessels better than by peripheral injection, but the documentation was poor since only one radiograph was obtained in each injection.

In the following years, several attempts were made to demonstrate the cardiac chambers in humans from the venous side. Castellanos et al. [13] used peripheral venous injection of contrast medium in children and were successful in demonstrating a number of congenital cardiac malformations. However, the technique was only successful in children and only for the right heart and pulmonary arteries. In 1939, Robb and Steinberg [14] improved the technique remarkably without using a catheter. Diodrast was injected via a wide-bore needle into the basilic or cephalic veins. After determination of the circulation time, with the patient sitting upright with the arm elevated, contrast medium was injected by hand. With this technique, Robb and Steinberg were able to demonstrate not only the right heart and pulmonary vasculature, but also the left heart and the aorta in adults for the first time.

Soon after the important contribution of Robb and Steinberg, the Second World War began, restricting further technical development in angiography for a number of years. A new radiopaque catheter for heart catheterization was, however, developed in 1941, the Cournand catheter, which is still used. It eventually replaced the ureteral catheters. In 1947, Chavez et al. [15] refined the angiocardiographic information by direct intracardiac deposition of the contrast medium. Joensson et al. [16] improved this technique further with what they called 'selective angiocardiography'.

Arteries

When we entered the thirties, angiography of the peripheral and cerebral arteries was relatively well documented in humans. Surgical exploration of the vessels was the most commonly used technique during this period despite the fact that Loman and Myerson [17] and Shimidzu [18] showed percutaneous puncture of the carotid artery to be a simple, reliable technique. The latter was also first to puncture the vertebral artery for angiography.

The left heart, the thoracic aorta, and the coronary arteries were only incompletely observed radiographically. In 1933, Rousthöi [19] explored the carotid artery in rabbits and monkeys and placed ureteral catheters into the aorta and the left ventricle. An ECG was recorded simultaneously. He obtained remarkably good left ventriculograms, aortograms and coronary arteriograms (Fig. III, 56). Independently, and in the same year, Reboul and Racine [20] punctured the left ventricle in dogs and obtained a good demonstration of both the left ventricle and the aorta. The first attempts at thoracic aortography in humans occurred 3 years later when Nuvoli [21] penetrated the sternum and the anterior wall of the ascending aorta to demonstrate syphilitic aor-

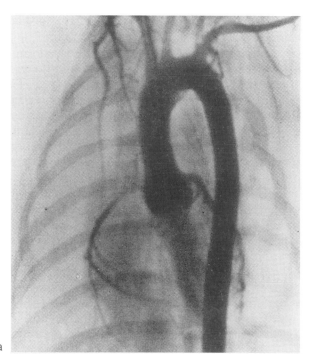
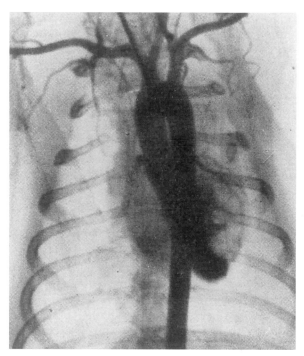

a

b

Fig. III, 56. Rousthoi's experimentally performed left ventriculography **(a)** and aortography **(b)**, which also visualized coronary arteries [19] (1933).

titis in one patient, and punctured and injected contrast medium into the left ventricle in another patient. It took almost 10 years before Radner [22] performed transsternal aortography in five patients in an attempt to demonstrate the coronary arteries. Thorotrast was used and incomplete information of the coronary arteries was obtained. Furthermore, a high rate of complications (2 of 5) prevented further attempts at coronary angiography with this technique.

The first arterial catheterization in human was reported by Ichikawa [23] and by Fariñas [24]. The femoral artery was surgically exposed and a ureteral catheter inserted and advanced into the lumbar aorta. Radner (1947) [25] introduced arterial catheterization from the radial artery. After surgical exposure of the right radial artery, a ureteral catheter was passed into the vertebral artery for cerebral angiography. After the procedure, the artery was ligated without causing any harm to the circulation of the hand. In his attempts to pass the catheter to the vertebral artery, Radner often slipped into the ascending part of the thoracic aorta and supravalvular aortography was obtained. But not even this technique produced acceptable information, despite the use of iodopyracet as contrast medium. The reason was the small-bore catheter with inherent low injection rate when contrast medium

was injected by hand and the documentation with one film only. An adequate technique for documentation was not yet available. Radner was also the first to use a steering device to direct the tip of the catheter into the vertebral artery or the thoracic aorta (Fig. III, 57) [26].

The supravalvular technique for thoracic aortography via the radial artery according to Radner was taken up almost directly by the radiologists working in collaboration with Crafoord, one of the leading cardiovascular surgeons of the time (the first to perform a resection of the ste-

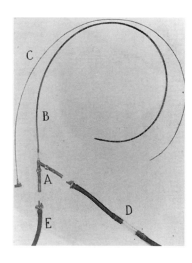

Fig. III, 57. Radner's technical resources to pass the catheter to the vertebral artery and sometimes to the ascending aorta. A steel wire increased the torque control of the catheter [26] (1949).

notic segment in coarctation of the aorta). The surgeons' need for exact documentation of the disease before exploration was imperative and forced the radiologists to improve their technique. Brodén et al. [27] and Joensson et al [16, 28] made remarkable contributions to improve the diagnostic information in cardiovascular radiology. By increasing the catheter diameter (they used a heart catheter) and applying counterpressure to reduce flow to other regions, they decreased the effect of dilution of the contrast medium. They soon found that injection by hand was not effective enough and therefore used an injector (Fig. III, 58) that could inject 50–80 ml of 70% iodopyracet in 3–5 s. With their selective angiocardiography technique, they studied mainly the right heart and the pulmonary arteries, and included pressure recordings since *'changes of the left side of the heart are not yet accessible to radical therapy'* [28]. Consequently, they felt no need to push for selective studies of the left atrium or ventricle, or the coronary arteries.

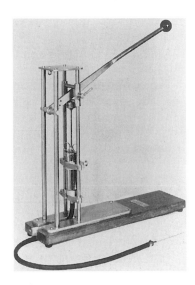

Fig. III, 58. The manual pressure injector used by Joensson for selective angiocardiography in the late forties.

They were, however, prepared to examine coronary arteries since they gave good examples of the vessels at thoracic aortography. They also found it quite possible to catheterize the coronary arteries: by accident, they entered the right coronary artery and deposited contrast medium,

which was not realized until the angiographic films became available for review [27]. They noted that no ECG changes were observed during the injection and that the patient felt no discomfort. They warned others, however, to place the tip of the catheter low in the ascending aorta to avoid the 'mishap'. Thus, radiology was ready for coronary angiography long before clinicians were interested in documenting coronary artery disease or surgeons prepared to perform bypass operations.

Joensson [28], not being completely satisfied with the Radner catheter technique, punctured the carotid artery percutaneously in caudal direction for thoracic aortography. He was the first to use a guide-wire (a 28-cm-long silver thread) to bring the needle down to the upper part of the ascending aorta (Fig. III, 59). 'The thread is very soft and has a rounded tip and it can do no damage if it is pushed down slowly and gently.' To prevent clotting, he used saline for flushing and, probably also for the first time, a guide-wire soaked in heparin.

Documentation

For optimum information, contrast medium has to be injected at a rate close to that of the blood flow in the region being studied. This was realized early and also that injection by hand was not always sufficient for an adequate study. Therefore, Dos Santos used a device that forced the contrast medium in by means of compressed air. A similar technique was used by Doss [29] for translumbar aortography. During the war, Fariñas [30] had problems obtaining rubber catheters and therefore punctured the femoral artery with a 1.5-mm trocar after blunt dissection. After compression of the femoral arteries, he injected 50 ml 70% Diodrast for 2.5–3.5 s, using a pump with a piston operated by an air compressor with a regulator and a manometer. The piston acted directly *'on the embolus of the syringe'*. In this way, he obtained retrograde abdominal aortograms of good quality. As mentioned above, Joensson obtained a similar flow rate through catheters using a manually operated injector. Similar techniques were used by others.

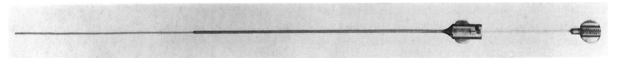

Fig. III, 59. A silver-wire needle used by Joensson (1949) to place the needle into the ascending aorta from the right carotid artery [28].

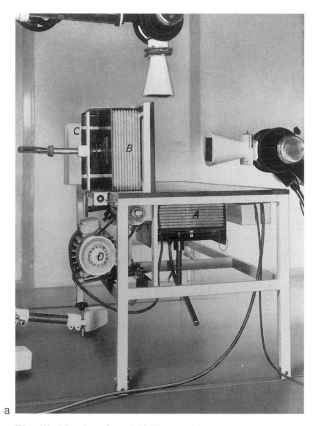

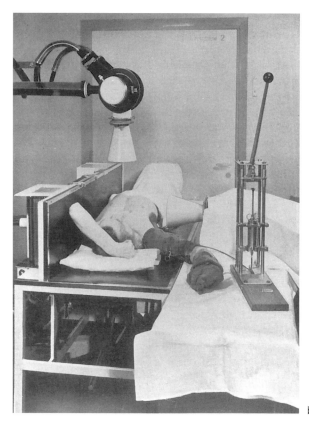

a   b

Fig. III, 60a, b. a) and **b)** The rapid cassette changer used for angiocardiography by Joensson (1951)

The documentation of the injected contrast medium was made with rather primitive injectors and in most places by one or two radiographs in only one projection at a time.

Castellanos et al. [13] used two X-ray tubes for simultaneous recording of one anteroposterior and one lateral angiogram. Robb and Steinberg [14] obtained two sequential films in the same projection. A number of cinefluorographic (i.e. filming of the fluorescent image) studies were made [31, 32]. The information was, however, not adequate and the radiation dose was high, and the technique was therefore not used for angiographic documentation in man.

One of the best known cassette changers is Caldas' 'radio-carousel', which gave Moniz the opportunity to do physiologic studies of the cerebral circulation [33, 34] using one frame per second in one projection. Barclay [35] developed an experimental cineradiographic unit in 1934 with which he studied, among other things, the renal circulation.

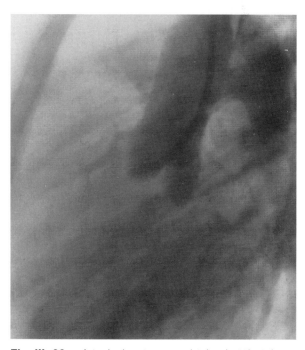

Fig. III, 60c. A typical aortogram obtained at that time.

The most common cassette changer employed for cerebral angiography was the manually operated box containing 2–4 cassettes (24 x 30 cm). One of the best known devices was made by Sanchez-Perez, later modified to a motor-driven unit in 1943 [36]. The cassette changer used later in the forties by Joensson and his group was put forward by Axén and Lind in 1948 [37]. It could perform cardiography in two simultaneous planes at 1–2 films per second (Fig. III, 60). In 1949, Gidlund [38] demonstrated his roll-film changer, a forerunner of the Elema roll-film unit with 12 exposures per second. Fredzell (s. Fig. V, 139) et al. [39] also put forward a biplane rapid cassette changer that could operate 12.5 radiographs per second with a cassette size of 18 x 24 cm. In addition a number of various types of machines were tested because of the great need for swift documentation, particularly in angiocardiography because of the rapid and large excursions of the heart from systole to diastole.

At the end of the forties, angiographers were well supplied with new technology for documentation of their efforts with new catheterization methods and with less toxic contrast media. The ground was now prepared for the giant step forward in angiographic technique that took place in the following decade.

The fifties

By the end of the forties, the number of angiographic procedures had markedly increased. New methods for improved visualization, particularly of the heart, the thoracic aorta, and the cerebral vessels, had become accepted procedures. Some of these new methods were called 'selective' when the tip of the catheter was placed so that injection of contrast medium gave information about a specific area such as selective angiocardiography [16]. There appeared other selective studies, but they were not named so. For instance, vertebral, subclavian, and carotid angiography are highly selective studies.

Radner in Lund and Joensson in Stockholm are those most often referred to, having formed the ground for catheter angiography. They were certainly pioneers in selective angiography. Why was Swedish radiology in the lead during this period in the same way as the Portuguese school was in the twenties? There is no straightforward answer to this, and probably many events add up for a new paradigm to occur. One fact is that the borders of the country are to a certain extent a limit for fast spread outside the country. At the same time, there is a need for a fast catching up with a new technique inside a country once it has appeared there. It is called competition. Another reason was that Sweden had escaped the destructive effects of the Second World War and that the technical advances in surgery occurring in the postwar period required preoperative mapping of the lesions. For instance, new advances in other areas of medicine improved cardiovascular radiology. A repetition of this will be found at the end of this decade when the surgeons wanted to perform coronary bypass surgeries. Another reason for the fast development in cardiovascular radiology in Sweden was the strong position of the radiologists in the clinical team, which was laid down already in the twenties by Goesta Forssell (s. Fig. I, 26).

The referring clinicians never questioned the radiologists' role in angiography. Of course, there was a limit set for the radiologists to act. Surgical exposure and suture of the femoral artery were reserved for the surgeon, and the same was the case with the radial artery. Teamwork was established by the surgeon and the radiologist but if the radiologist had some experience in surgery, he was permitted to explore the radial artery, which was ligated following completion of the angiogram.

During my first 2 years as a resident in radiology in Lund, 1949–1951, I had many opportunities to follow Radner in his catheterizations (Fig. III, 61). He was trained in medicine, radiology, and psychiatry before he entered neurosurgery. While there, he convinced his older colleagues that vertebral angiography would be worthwhile to perform in patients with posterior fossa lesions. He performed the entire procedure himself, from exploration of the radial artery, catheterization, and documentation. Considering the rather primitive situation in radiology at that time, it was a complicated procedure to keep the surgical wound sterile during fluoroscopy in complete darkness. He had to use his feet to move the small X-ray tube on the floor (Fig. III, 61) to follow the tip of the catheter to its position. When in place, anteroposterior and lateral views were obtained, each with three cassettes manually shifted by a resident. Radner had his dissertation in 1951 on vertebral angiography, and left thereafter to be become professor in internal medicine.

From what is said above, it can be understood that radiologists were not interested in performing angiography with a catheter passing into an open wound, pushing the catheter in darkness while extreme attention had to be paid to the

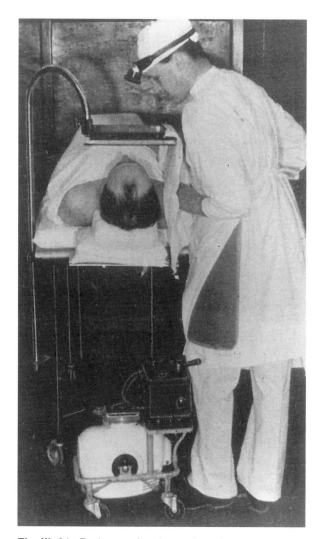

Fig. III, 61. Radner performing catheterization of the vertebral artery (approximately 1950). Note the primitive arrangements with the X-ray tube on a trolley and the small fluorescent screen.

fluoroscopy screen to follow the poorly visible catheter. The percutaneous introduction of catheters was therefore a giant step forward in diagnostic radiology. There were other factors of importance that made angiography to prosper in the fifties. New contrast media with higher contrasting effects and lower toxicity appeared. New types of catheters, and new types of documentation were other reasons for the fast change during this decade.

Contrast media

In 1950, acetrizoate sodium (Urokon) and diprotrizoate (Miokon) became available, replacing Diodrast. Both contrast media had three iodine

atoms in the molecule, giving a higher contrasting effect than any other previously used media. They also had a lower toxicity and lower irritating effect than before. Urokon and Miokon were almost completely replaced in the mid-fifties by the sodium and meglumine salts of diatrizoate (Urografin, Renografin, Hypaque), which are still used in many centres.

Vascular approach

Percutaneous puncture and contrast medium injection directly into vessels were performed in the early fifties for carotid angiography as well as for extremity angiography and venography.

Veins

The slow flow and easy access to the extremity veins and the iliac and caval veins gave opportunities during this decade to document thrombosis and to establish technical standards for the procedure. The cerebral veins were studied at cerebral angiography, thanks to new techniques for documentation by rapid serial angiography following carotid artery injection.

Moreover, the abdominal veins became available for venography during this decade. At attempts to catheterize the right heart, the Cournand catheter had often slipped into the hepatic veins, so radiologists knew how to reach these veins.

Rappaport [40] paved the way for more systematic analysis of the hepatic and renal veins in experiments on dogs. He used a steering device so that the catheter could be pushed into these veins from the femoral vein. Furthermore, the pelvic veins were observed by injection of contrast medium into the pelvic bones or into the wall of the uterus. Epidural phlebography was obtained in a similar way by injection of contrast material into the vertebrae.

The portal system was explored in many different ways. One was percutaneous splenoportal venography, first in dogs by Abeatici and Campi [41], soon to be followed by studies in man. Another method, used in man, was percutaneous hepatic puncture of the portal vein system introduced by Bierman et al. [42]. The first portal venogram had been performed in the forties during operation [43]. Splenoportal venography caused some complications. Therefore, Oedman [44] demonstrated the splenoportal venous system by celiac angiography, which was later improved by pharmacoangiography.

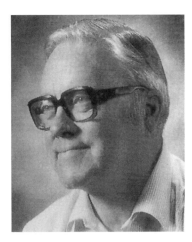

Fig. III, 62. S.I. Seldinger, the man who invented the technique of percutaneous catheterization and as a consequence opened up a new era in diagnostic radiology. Swedish radiologist, worked at Karolinska Institute in Stockholm and later in Mora.

Arteries

The year 1953 belongs to angiographic history. With the publication of Seldinger's [45] (Fig. III, 62) discovery of the ideal way to introduce a catheter into the body, the status of radiology changed in many countries. The reason for this was the fact that in most places angiography with catheters was a surgical procedure. From now on, radiologists could be in charge of the entire angiographic procedure.

A number of important developments formed the basis for Seldinger's successful innovation. The polyethylene catheter (PE catheter) was used in surgery late in the forties, and in 1950, Helmsworth et al. [46] used it for arteriography. Following this, Peirce [47] introduced the PE catheter percutaneously. The catheter passed through the needle into the femoral artery and then into the lumbar aorta. Although thin-walled, the PE catheter's lumen could not be too wide as it had to pass through the needle. As a consequence, the flow rate through the catheter was low, which limited the potential of this technique.

Seldinger, as a resident in radiology, assisted older colleagues in aortofemoral angiography and realized that the best way to improve the quality of the studies was to increase the flow rate by increasing the lumen of the catheter. He considered using a 30-cm-long needle with the PE catheter as a sheath on the needle so the catheter tip could reach the lumbar aorta. He rejected the idea as being too difficult to work with. Another way he considered was placing the needle through the distal part of the catheter via a side hole, but the PE catheter had a tendency not to follow the needle into the artery.

Then suddenly, Seldinger got a 'severe attack of common sense': puncture the artery, introduce a wire through the needle, remove the needle, push the catheter over the wire, advance them together, and then remove the wire [48] (Fig. III, 63).

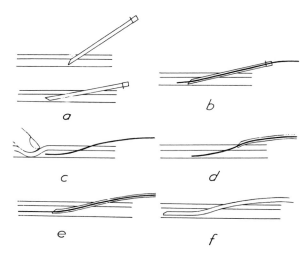

Fig. III, 63. Seldinger's original schematic presentation of percutaneous catheterization in 1953 [45].

Seldinger's method was known by all radiologists in Scandinavia interested in angiography by 1952. The cheap PE tubes were available to all and easy to shape for percutaneous use. Lumbar aortography with this technique began in most of the larger hospitals in Scandinavia that year. The primary consequences for radiology were:

- Catheterization of the lumbar aorta could be performed with the aid of fluoroscopy (in complete darkness) with no open wound.
- The patient could be moved for different projections without risking the sterility of a wound.
- The surgeon did not have to participate in the procedure.
- Angiography could be performed on wider indications with a limited number of complications.

The radiologist now had a method that enabled him to become a specialist not only for documentation of angiography procedures but also for the entire vascular investigation. This became even more important when it was realized that the catheter could be placed in ANY branch of the aorta for selective angiography. Thus, selective angiography, particularly of abdominal vessels, became the next important step in the history of angiography.

As previously mentioned, selective angiography had been performed, or attempts had been made in this direction, much earlier [4, 15, 22, 25]. Radner [49], for instance, showed, in addition to his other previously reported studies, that a metastasis could be demonstrated in the supraclavicular region at subclavian angiography. In 1951, Bierman and coworkers [50] proved that all main branches of the abdominal aorta could be catheterized from the brachiocephalic vessels with radiopaque 7F–9F catheters. Most often the carotid arteries were exposed for this procedure. These workers' main intentions were to demonstrate lesions by selective angiography and to treat lesions by regional arterial infusion of drugs. They also demonstrated that the subclavian, carotid, and internal mammary arteries could be reached with the same type of catheters from the femoral artery.

In the years following Seldinger's report on percutaneous catheterization, a great number of studies on lumbar aortography as well as on selective angiography of the branches from the lumbar aorta were published. Some difficulties were encountered because of the performance of the procedure in darkness, making it difficult to see the catheter as well as other details on the fluoroscopy screen. Various techniques were used to increase the visibility of the catheters. The most important was the image intensifier designed in 1948 by J.W. Coltman (s. Fig. V, 167) of Westinghouse [51]. The brightness gain of over 1000 meant that fluoroscopy could be performed in daylight, the image became sharper, and the catheters were easy to follow. It was not until the end of the fifties that image intensifiers became available for fluoroscopy, and not until the sixties that they were combined with TV systems.

Most radiologists during the fifties had to rely on indirect vision when following the catheters in the body. The new PE catheters for percutaneous introduction were not radiopaque and various techniques were used to render them visible on the screen. Contrast medium inside the catheter was usually difficult to see on the screen. The guide-wire was therefore usually kept in the catheter until it was in place, and some even placed a gold plate or heavy metal on the tip of the guide-wire.

When the catheter was to be directed into branches of the aorta, the problems with this fluoroscopy technique became even more obvious. It was therefore an important step forward when Oedman in 1955 [52] introduced the radiopaque PE catheter for percutaneous intro-

duction. Lead oxide was incorporated into the catheter material, making it thicker than the nonopaque PE catheter with the same lumen. However, the catheter was easily tapered so it could enter the femoral artery without difficulty. Furthermore, the catheter could be formed in hot water to any desired shape, depending on the actual vascular topography.

Other methods were also used to reach branches of the aorta. For instance, Rappaport [40] introduced for experimental work a steering device, and Gollman [53] a curved guide-wire for the same purpose in humans. Tillander [54] applied on the top of the catheter a few pieces of gold-plated soft iron so that an external strong magnet could bring the catheter to more peripheral branches of the coeliac artery.

The percutaneous femoral artery technique became the method of choice not only for the lumbar and thoracic aorta, but also for the brachiocephalic arteries. For example, the left vertebral artery was reached from below, replacing both Radner's technique and the direct percutaneous method introduced by Shimidzu in 1937 [18]. The first attempts from below were made during the fifties [55], but the method was not established until the next decade.

The coronary arteries were examined with increasing frequency due to the increasing awareness among the clinicians that documentation of coronary artery disease was necessary to provide adequate treatment. Di Guglielmo and Guttadauro [56] conducted a thorough analysis of the in vivo anatomy of the coronary arteries. Their material was based on the technique used in Joensson's department, such as supravalvular aortography. A number of reports appeared, describing various techniques for improved information because too often there was incomplete visualization of the coronary arteries. In man, the best information with the supravalvular technique was obtained when contrast medium was injected during cardiac arrest, provoked by acetylcholine [57]. In dogs, Dotter and Frische [58] used a balloon catheter with double lumen. The balloon was expanded, obstructing the aortic flow during injection of the contrast medium, and extraordinarily high-quality angiograms were obtained. Both methods were considered to be too risky and were not used as routine procedures. The main reason probably was the appearance of the selective technique for coronary angiography by the end of this decade. In 1959, Sones and Shirey [59] performed selective coronary angiography using catheters from the radial artery according to Radner.

Documentation

Contrast medium injection through catheters and needles for documentation is a crucial part of the angiographic procedure. This problem became particularly critical with the introduction of the PE catheters. Because of the way they were introduced into the vessels, they had an open end and were thus different from the previously used, surgically introduced, closed-end catheters. Since the percutaneous technique suddenly became available to all radiologists, the second half of this decade became a period of trial and error. Every angiographer came up with his own method of how to manipulate the catheter to obtain a safe and high-quality investigation.

The nonopaque catheters came in rolls of about 3 m with varying inner and outer diameters. For lumbar aortography, for instance, a 30-cm-long PE 205 catheter (OD/ID 2.08/1.35 mm) was used. The catheters were carefully tested for the required flow rates. It was soon realized that for the lumbar aortogram, a catheter with an end-hole was usually sufficient for the information needed. For the similar but wider catheter for thoracic (supravalvular), aortography one end-hole was not sufficient. During injection, the catheter recoiled, and at the end of the injection could often be found in the lumbar aorta or in one of the brachiocephalic arteries. Side-holes were therefore made close to the end-hole. For further improvement, the end-hole was occluded by various techniques. Gidlund [60] tested various models and also other types of catheters with closed ends. These were introduced differently, via a PE-sheath, a method later popular for exchange of catheters in angio-graphy (Fig. III, 64). They were also found to give more adequately selected information as needed, for example, in renal aortography.

The preparation of the radiopaque Oedman catheters for selective angiography was presented by the inventor [61]: tapering the tip over the guide-wire, shaping the catheter according to the vascular anatomy by heating in hot water, flaring the proximal end for Luer lock adaptation, and providing side-holes by a special puncturing instrument, all had to be prepared before the procedure could begin.

The amount and flow rate of contrast medium to be used depended on the local blood flow and the size of the vascular system to be examined. In the adult heart and the thoracic aorta, for instance, the deposition of the contrast medium had to be at a high rate (at least 25 ml/s), consist of a large amount (about 50 ml), and be ECG-triggered. In the renal artery of a normal kidney, 5–10 ml injected by hand was usually adequate.

Injection by hand was used for most selective studies where 10 ml or less of contrast medium was required. Otherwise, the injection was made with a high-pressure injector. Many types were already in use [29, 30] and new ones appeared. For larger amounts, particularly for cardioangiography and thoracic aortography, the Gidlund injector became very popular [60] (Fig. III, 65).

During the fifties, a number of new film changers appeared. The cassette changers for two planes [37] for cardioangiography were replaced. They caused a lot of vibration and noise. It was important to use high-speed radiography, particularly in angiocardiography. The only in-

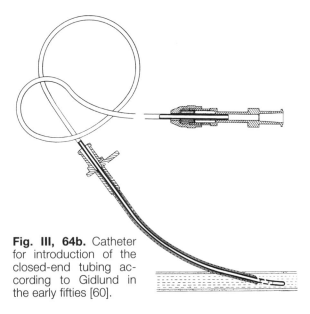

Fig. III, 64a. Puncture for introduction of the closed-end tubing according to Gidlund in the early fifties [60].

Fig. III, 64b. Catheter for introduction of the closed-end tubing according to Gidlund in the early fifties [60].

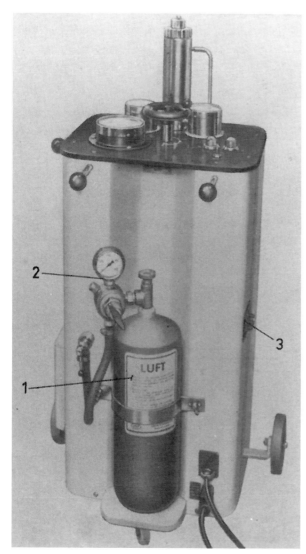

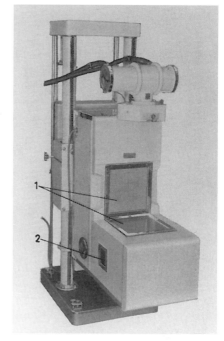

a

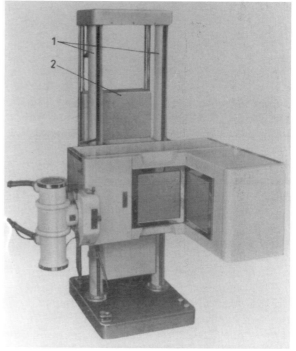

b

Fig. III, 65. The Gidlund high-pressure injector (1956) [60].

Fig. III, 66a, b. The Elema roll-film changer for examination in supine **a)** or upright **b)** positions with a maximum of 12 images per second [60].

strument that could produce 12 film per second in both planes was the Elema roll-film changer (Fig. III, 66). Direct cinefluorography of the regular fluorography screen was not adequate for this purpose because of its low resolution and the high radiation dose. It was, however, used with advantage for studying vascular physiology, e.g. circulation time of contrast medium through the heart and pulmonary vasculature (s. Fig. III, 100) [62]. Thus, during the fifties and for a great part of the next decade, the biplane roll-film changer was the best alternative to document congenital and acquired diseases of the heart [63].

With the development of the image intensifiers, which were ready to be utilized for cinecardiography in 1953, a completely new method for

documenting cardiovascular disease became available [64]. With the biplane cineangiocardiography [63, 65] utilizing a 5-inch or 11-inch image intensifier and 16-mm or 35-mm film cameras, new information of the heart was obtained (Fig. III, 67). The detail of the cinecardiogram

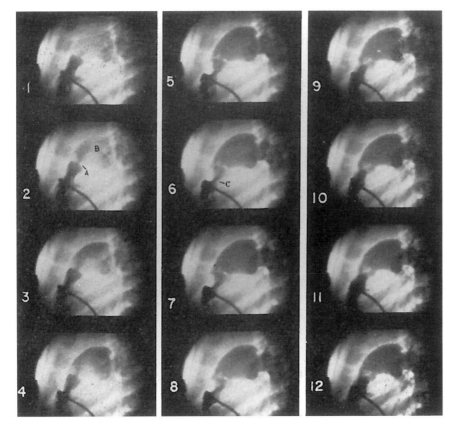

Fig. III, 67. Cine-angiocardiography with a five-inch image intensifier and a 16-mm camera by Sones in 1958 [64].

was not of the same quality as that observed on the conventional angiocardiogram. This was, however, well compensated for because *'studies of the moving film obviates the lack of clarity to some degree and permits more precise identification of valves, borders and outlines of vessels'* [65]. The enormous technical development during the fifties also included the improvement of generators and microelectronics so that the exposure time could be reduced to milliseconds and pulsed, with resultant lower radiation to the patient.

The Elema roll-film changer was also used for documentation at angiography in other parts of the body as was the Franklin unit [66]. At the same time (in 1953), the AOT Schoenander changer [67] appeared. In the Franklin changer, the roll-film was cut after exposure, while in the AOT the films were of regular 24 x 30 or 35 x 35 cm size. Both could operate at a maximum of 6 frames/s and be used for both vertical and horizontal documentation. To reduce scatter radiation, they were usually operated only in one plane at a time, and mostly for cerebral angiography. Another popular changer during the fifties was the modified Sanchez-Perez changer [36].

To estimate the flow pattern through the organ, the injection rate and the exposures were sometimes recorded with simultaneous ECG and pressure recordings. The pressure injectors were triggered with the exposures, both at full size and at cineangiography.

The sixties

When we entered the sixties, all the vessels in the body had been visualized by angiography. Various indications and techniques had been used to reach these goals. The angiographer's personal experience and devotion played an essential role in this development. Consequently, the success rate, the quality of the examinations, and the complications varied widely. The sixties became a period of consolidation of angiographic techniques but also marked improvement in diagnostic information and widening of the indications for angiography. The technical improvements, the complications, and the results of clinical and experimental research were recorded in numerous reports and textbooks. The most important of these was Abram's Angiography [68], which eventually became the 'Bible' for angiographers.

During this decade, angiography became a special procedure not only for diagnostic reasons. It became the radiologist's method with which he could demonstrate for the clinician the resectability of a lesion, for instance, by demonstrating the local and distant extent of a tumor or by revealing the severity of a cardiovascular lesion, particularly arteriosclerosis. In other words, angiography became essential for diagnosis and therapy, giving radiology an increasingly important position in clinical teamwork.

Angiographic anatomy was mainly defined during the previous decades. The improved technique of catheterization and documentation at superselective angiography revealed further anatomic and pathoanatomic vascular details. This led also to information about vascular physiology and pathophysiology. Pharmacoangiography became an important addition to this technique.

During the sixties, angiography took a completely new direction by being used not only for diagnostic purposes, but also for treatment in connection with the angiographic procedure. Interventional radiology had its beginning in 1964 when Dotter and Judkins [69] reported their first experience with transluminal treatment of arteriosclerotic obstruction. Their technique was soon adopted by other angiographers, but it was not until the next decade that percutaneous transluminal angioplasty (PTA) and other interventional radiological procedures became accepted and made a very important contribution to patient treatment. Interventional radiology is *the branch of radiology concerned with providing diagnosis and treatment of disease by a variety of percutaneous procedures performed under the guidance of radiological imaging* (coming issue of Dorland's Illustrated Medical Dictionary).

The necessary tool for angiography, the contrast medium, was with some modifications the same as during the second half of the fifties. It was high- osmolar and ionic, even though Almén in 1966 [70] had tested a dimer (6 iodine atoms per molecule) with lower osmolality and higher contrasting effect. The radiologists were aware of the toxic effects of the contrast media from the very beginning of angiography. It was, however, not until the classic experiments on neurotoxicity by Broman and Olsson in the late forties [71] that it became obvious that great care had to be taken with the increasing number of angiographic examinations performed. The general effects, including the hemodynamic and the local toxic effects of contrast media, became important, particularly when contrast medium was deposited in small branches partially occluded by the catheter tip. But the injected contrast medium can also have direct traumatic effects, caus-

ing subintimal dissection or even extraluminal deposits of contrast medium, depending on the jet.

The blood flow through vascular systems, or rather the flow of contrast medium, was evaluated early by serial angiography by Moniz [34] and in the thirties and by Greitz [72] and Gidlund [60] in the sixties. During the sixties, methods for blood flow measurements were performed by linear flow velocity [73], variation in contrast density [74], and a 'spillover' flowmeter technique [75].

Complications

Complications from angiographic procedures have not been previously discussed in detail but they were well known from the very first beginning of this technique, and deaths were reported. During the fifties, a number of comprehensive analyses of complications were made [76, 78]. During the sixties, further important contributions showed that complications may occur if specific precautions are not taken. Every aspect of the angiographic procedure had to be considered with great care, including the patient's condition, before the investigation could proceed. For instance, not only had the coagulation and bleeding time to be checked to prevent postangiographic hematoma formation, but the patient's general condition was also important, as was the presence of hypertension.

Baum et al. [79] (1966) showed that 'complications of no arteriography' were just as common as in those cases with arteriography. They studied the rate and character of reactions in consecutive vascular catheterizations in 1600 patients and found a similar rate of complication in those patients in whom angiography had been postponed as in those who had undergone the angiographic procedure. This does not mean that angiography is a harmless procedure, but shows that the complications are often unpredictable and that many of them are not due to unskilled operators. On the other hand, it is obvious that the important attributes of a successful angiographer are technical skill and sound clinical judgement.

The puncture site is one site where severe complications may occur. Hematoma formation, aneurysms, spasm, dissection, or occlusion, and nerve palsy may occur, but most are avoidable by proceeding with caution.

Catheter techniques

Needle puncture of a distal vessel or an organ followed by injection of contrast medium was common, among other purposes, for femoral arteriography, translumbar aortography, venography and splenoportography. This was eventually replaced during the sixties with the catheter needle technique [60] introduced for splenoportography by Seldinger [80]. Immediately after puncture, the needle was withdrawn and the softer catheter could be advanced, causing less trauma to the vessel wall or organ.

The catheter, no doubt, plays a substantial role since it is a foreign body introduced into the vascular system. Platelet adhesion to the catheter and clot formation are bound to occur. With special precautions (Macrodex, heparin), the clot formation can be reduced [81, 82, 83].

The mechanical local effects of the tip of the catheter, the jet of the contrast medium, and the traumatic effects of the guide-wires were additional important contributors to complications. The size (OD/ID), length, shape and make (brand) of the catheter were consequential. For instance, side holes close to the tip of the catheter were able to reduce the jet effect [60, 84, 85, 86]. The jet caused not only local trauma to the vessel but also recoil and whipping of the catheter. The percutaneous technique according to Seldinger required an open-end catheter. A closed-end heart catheter had to be introduced via a sheath [60] or created by occluding the tip after introduction [84, 87]. These methods were soon replaced by the hook-tail followed by the pigtail catheter. The catheter had a tapered distal part and when it passed up into the aorta, the reversed part could negotiate practically every aortic–arterial tortuousity or ulcer without trauma. It worked in the same way as flexible safety guide-wire [88, 89, 90] or the J-shaped catheter [91]. The pigtail catheter eventually became the preferred catheter for cardioangiography and aortography.

New catheter material was introduced during the sixties. The nonopaque PE catheters were still frequently used as were the Oedman radiopaque catheters. Woven Dacron, polyurethane, Teflon, and other plastics became available for clinical use [84, 92, 93]. They were tested for plastic memory and torque, details of importance in angiographic work. A number of different factors must be taken into account when selecting a catheter, such as length, thickness, calibre, resistance to mechanical stress, radio-opacity and elasticity.

The thrombogenicity of the catheters was also tested in vitro and in vivo in dogs [83, 94] and was found to be low with the nonopaque PE catheters and high with the radiopaque ones. That the catheters could cause severe complications during the angiographic procedure was well known to all angiographers, and therefore injections of heparin during the procedure became routine.

Guide-wires are of great concern for the angiographer. The original guide wire of Seldinger consisted of a long slender coil spring that was stiffened with a fixed wire core, except for its tip. Prioton et al. [88] modified it by using a movable core that facilitated transvalvular catheterization and superselective catheterization. It was also less liable to breakage. Since breakage nevertheless may occur, Dotter [89] constructed a safety spring that prevented a broken guide-wire from remaining in the vessel.

The guide-wires were also used to increase the torque control of catheters, particularly for superselective catheterizations. To prevent clot formation on the guide-wires, they were coated with a thin layer of Teflon to facilitate the catheterization procedure. The guide-wires could be preshaped to a certain extent [89, 90] which also accomplished some precaution against perforation of the vessel wall.

As expected, with the increasing numbers of studies performed, complications from the catheterization procedure became of increasing concern to angiographers during the sixties. Preventive means were recommended, some of which should be followed not only during the angiographic procedure but also afterwards [95].

During the sixties, coronary angiography became the most debated and, to radiologists, the most challenging subject. Various techniques were developed to obtain high-quality coronary angiograms without directly entering the coronary arteries. By depositing contrast medium in the coronary sinuses, a kind of semiselective technique was obtained with a single-loop or a double-loop technique [96, 97, 98]. It gave more information about the coronary vessels than the commonly used aortic root injection. The technique was developed mainly because of the risk of complications of selective coronary angiography, which were substantial in the early days. Despite the higher risks of complications, the Sones' technique was taken up by more and more centres following the clinical demands for more information about the coronary arteries.

Since the Sones' technique for entrance of the arterial system was essentially the same as the old Radner technique, angiographers looked for a percutaneous technique to replace the cutdown of the radial artery. The first attempts in this direction were presented by Ricketts and Abrams [99] by using preshaped catheters after percutaneous puncture of the femoral artery. The technique was, however, not established until 1967 by Judkins [100], and Amplatz et al. [92] (Fig. III, 68). After careful testing of a number of catheter material and shapes, they could show that a safe and reliable technique of percutaneous selective coronary angiography could be obtained from the femoral arteries. Particularly important in this respect was the Ducor catheter, designed by Viamonte and Stevens [93], made of polyurethane and stainless steel wires. Thanks to its excellent torque control, the Ducor catheter became the most commonly used catheter for coronary angiography.

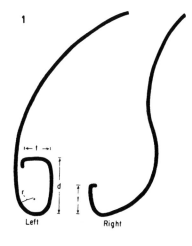

Fig. III, 68. Types of catheter according to Judkins (1967) for left and right coronary artery catheterization [100].

The brachiocephalic arteries were catheterized from the femoral arteries [101, 102] using a similar technique. The spinal arteries were explored in great detail by Dichiro et al. [103] and Djindjian [104]. A superselective technique from the axillary artery for visceral angiography was also developed, particularly for detailed information about hepatic and pancreatic lesions [105, 106]. Various techniques were used for small artery catheterization. One, the coaxial catheter [40, 84], was later used to a great extent while the many variations of steering devices constructed during the sixties [40, 70, 107, 108] were almost completely abandoned in the following decades.

Pharmacoangiography was introduced during this decade. Vasoconstricting and vasodilating drugs were injected intra-arterially before injection of contrast medium into the renal [109, 110,

111] and splanchnic circulation [112, 113] for improved diagnostic information. For therapeutic purposes, drugs had been infused intra-arterially in the hepatic artery in 1950 by Bierman et al. [114]. In the sixties, a few reports appeared on intra-arterial therapy with tholazoline for spasm in the superior mesenteric artery [115] and embolic material for angiomatous lesions [116, 117]. Other types of intravascular treatment beginning in the sixties and still in use today include the inferior cava filter to prevent thrombosis in the legs from reaching the pulmonary arteries [118] and the intra-aortic balloon pump for support in cardiogenic shock [119].

Documentation

Injectors

The technique for documentation of the angiographers' efforts varied and was mainly dependent on the aim of the procedure. The quality of the angiograms improved markedly with more commonly available remotely controlled injector–catheter systems and with technical improvements. Analyses were made of the factors that determine the delivery rates of the liquids through catheters. The contrast medium was delivered according to the type of lesion present, and flow charts were provided for each catheter and type of contrast medium used. All these factors contributed to high-quality angiographic studies and a reduced number of complications. A variety of injectors and film changers were already available at the beginning of the sixties. The Gidlund injector was still in use in many centres. A high-pressure portable injector was introduced by Amplatz in 1960 [120]. It was thermostatically controlled and powered by carbon dioxide. Two electrically powered injectors with mechanical drive were introduced during this decade. One was the Cordis injector, which became very popular and is still used in many places. The injection of contrast medium could be ECG-triggered and repeated several times, and the exact flow rates could be selected. The other was the Viamonte–Hobbs injector [121] with the same high reliability of injection as the Cordis injector and with an incorporated ground safe detector for improved safety. These two mechanical-drive electrically powered injectors eventually replaced the high-pressure gas-powered injectors.

Film changers

The film changers depended on the type of examination. The Elema roll-film changer was used in most places for cardiac and coronary angiography because of the cardiac contractions requiring a high rate of film exposure (12/s). In many centres, cardiac documentation was exclusively performed with cinefluorography and, eventually with increasing spatial resolution of the image intensifiers, with image intensifiers. The roll-film changers were replaced by cinefluorography or in combination with 100-mm photofluorography.

For documentation of vascular structures outside the heart, the Franklin and AOT changers were the most commonly employed film changers during the sixties. Amplatz' 'see-through changer' was also introduced during this period [122]. In comparison with other film changers, it had the advantage that the angiographic documentation on the 35-cm roll film could be checked simultaneously on a TV-monitor via the image intensifier.

For aortoiliac–femoral arteriography, the 35-cm cut-film or roll-film changers were most often utilized. To cover the entire arterial tree from the aorta, beginning at the level of the renal arteries, to the ankle-foot level, the patient had to be transported in increments of three or four steps with a movable table top. The quality of the examination was often not as good as desired and various measures were taken to improve the information. Single long films were utilized during the fifties but during the sixties long film changers were constructed to cover the entire field [123, 124]. Usually only two or three of these 1-m films were necessary to cover the entire vascular system.

From the seventies to today

By the end of the sixties, the thrombogenicity of catheters was being intensely investigated. This research continued during the seventies and is still going on. For many decades, heparin had been added to the solution used to flush the catheters during the catheterization procedure. Clot formation on the inside of the catheter could be prevented to a certain extent, but the amount of heparin injected in that way was not enough to protect clot formation on the outside. For that reason, the catheters and guide-wires were soaked in heparin and treated with benzalkonium heparin or with silicone grease [125,

126]. Wallace et al. [127] showed that systemic heparinization of the patient significantly reduced the complications due to thrombus formation, a technique that was soon adopted by most institutions. In those few instances of bleeding after catheter removal and despite compression after 10–15 min, protamine sulphate was given with good effect.

Other important investigations were made by light- and electron-microscopy of catheters and guide-wires. Surface defects, such as scratches, cracks, depressions and protrusions, could provoke thrombus formation [128, 129]. Particularly notable was the amount of fibrin harvested from between the coils of the guide-wires, and it appeared that cleansing of these was inefficient. Re-use of guide-wires was therefore not recommended. Teflon-coated guide-wires were found to have another problem. The Teflon covering, intended to reduce the coefficient of friction of the guide-wire, was partly shed from the wire during use and could cause microembolization [129].

Eventually, a number of factors were found to be the reason for the clot formation and embolization: the chemical composition of the catheter, the size (OD/ID), and the length of the catheter, various coating media, surface charge, and smoothness of the inner and outer sides of the catheter. Contrast media, particularly the ionic, and the flushing media act partly as anticoagulants [130, 131, 132] but they are effective only on the catheter's inner side.

Moderate or pronounced hematomas are seen in about 4% of patients after femoral catheterization. Delayed bleeding may also occur and the observed rate in a prospective series was 1.2% [133]. Bed rest for 24 h after the catheterization procedure and pressure dressings [134, 135] have been in use to reduce the hematoma formation, particularly, in patients who are uncooperative, on anticoagulant therapy, or hypertensive.

Also pseudoaneurysm and arteriovenous shunt may develop after a catheterization procedure. Their main cause is a faulty approach to the femoral artery precluding the application of effective compression when the catheter has been removed. The puncture site is too low and not in the common femoral artery, which is easily compressed over the femoral head [136].

The single most important factor of reducing complications due to clot formation and bleeding is a decrease in the OD of the catheter. With 4–5 F (OD 1.4–1.7 mm) new type 'high-flow' catheters, vascular complications can be avoided and angiography performed on an outpatient basis [135]. In those cases, the patients are observed for a few hours after the angiographic procedure and then sent home for a 24-h bed rest. Exceptions to this rule apply when the catheterization procedure was prolonged with repeated change of catheters, when interventional procedures have been performed, or when wider catheters have been used for specific reasons.

The transfemoral route of catheterization has always been the preferred technique because of the good size of the artery, the comfortable access to the vessel, and relatively easy control of the puncture site. The original Dos Santos technique of translumbar aortography for peripheral vascular disease was for a long period used in only a few places because of the serious complications that are sometimes observed. One reason was, of course, the inaccessibility of the puncture for compression, with risk of uncontrolled hemorrhage, and another the risk of puncture and contrast deposition in structures outside the aorta. With modern technique, exchanging the needle over guide-wire with a catheter, Amplatz and his coworkers showed that the translumbar catheterization was not followed by more complications than the transfemoral technique [137], which could be confirmed later in a large survey [138]. Further proof in this direction was the demonstration of only small para-aortic or psoas muscle hematomas by CT [139, 140, 141]. The utilization of high-flow, thinned-walled 4–5 F catheters further improved the percutaneous translumbar technique, which can be used to study the coronary as well as the brachiocephalic arteries.

The transaxillary technique for vascular approach is not as well tolerated mainly since a hematoma is more difficult to control, and trauma to the brachial plexus is not uncommon. A survey showed that significantly more complications occur with the transaxillary catheterization compared to the transfemoral or translumbar approach [138]. A miniaturization of instruments for angiography has been under way during the last two decades. Vessel dilators, catheter sheaths, coaxial catheters, balloon-tipped catheters, and flow-directed catheters are some of the various methods employed in modern angiography [142–150]. With these catheters, the angiographer can reach peripheral branches of the arterial tree for high-resolution diagnostic information as well as for various treatment purposes. The guide-wires have also become correspondingly smaller, some with torque control, others more rigid [149–153].

It is obvious that the high flow rate of contrast medium through a 4 F catheter cannot be achieved in the wide-lumen catheters, but about 20 ml/s can be given with low-viscosity contrast media with a 4 F high-flow nylon aortic flush catheter [146]. A combination with intra-arterial digital subtraction angiography will give high quality angiography.

The small catheter size modifies again the alternative for cerebral and coronary angiography, which can now be performed after percutaneous puncture of the brachial artery [154, 155].

Another approach to vessels in the body was transhepatic catheterization of the portal circulation. This had been performed, as previously mentioned, in 1952 by Bierman et al [42]. This technique was renewed in the seventies to reduce flow to esophageal or gastric varices by occlusion of the left gastric vein [156]. The pancreatic veins were also explored by this technique [157], which was later utilized for hormone assays in hormone-producing tumors of the pancreas.

The angiographic technique for diagnosing and treating gastrointestinal bleeding was introduced by Baum and Nusbaum in 1971 [158], and the infusion of vasopressin and later the addition of embolization became an important technique for a number of leaking vessels. Interventional angiography became an established method in the seventies for a variety of vascular conditions, of which hemorrhage, vascular aneurysms, angiomatous lesions, and tumor treatment are most important. Vascular dilatation with percutaneous techniques (PTA, PTCA, PTRA) was performed for treating stenosis of the femoral, coronary, and renal arteries.

The low osmolality, ionic and non-ionic contrast media became available during the seventies and were replacing the high osmolar, ionic contrast media because of less intense reactions, particularly in peripheral arteriography [159]. However, with intra-arterial digital subtraction angiography (DSA), the old ionic hyperosmolar contrast media may be used again but diluted to avoid any discomfort when injected.

Documentation

The documentation of the angiographic procedures changed during the last two decades but film changers for full-size serial radiography are still in use for specific purposes. The PUCK film changer became available. It could be connected directly to the U- or C-arm equipment, which became the modern angiography unit together with the carbon fiber table top.

Magnification angiography became a frequently used technique, particularly in Japan during the sixties [160]. The technique was found to be of value in cerebral, pulmonary, and renal angiography [161, 162]. The development of new diagnostic methods has reduced the importance of magnification angiography, which has been the topic in only a few reports during the last decade.

The most important technical improvements in angiographic documentation was initiated by Mistretta and his group in Madison, USA [163] and by Heintzen and his coworkers in Kiel, Germany [164]. It was the digital subtraction angiography technique, which meant a degradation of spatial resolution but achieved an enormous improvement in contrast resolution. A number of early reports documented that by intravenous injection of contrast medium, adequate information could be obtained of the cardiac chambers and arterial system, and flow measurements could be recorded [165, 166, 167]. However, it soon became obvious that intravenously injected contrast medium, because it was too diluted when reaching the arterial system, gave inadequate morphological arterial information. Therefore, soon after its introduction in clinical routine, contrast medium was again injected on the arterial side as before [168], but the contrast medium was given in a lower dose through smaller catheters than before.

The quality of the angiographic procedures using DSA has now increased to the extent that full-sized radiographic documentation is rarely necessary. This is particularly applicable to those vascular structures that are unaffected by cardiac, respiratory or gastrointestinal movements, such a as aorta, and brachiocephalic and iliofemoral arteries.

A limitation of the DSA technique for lower leg arteriography is the diameter of the image intensifier. Its maximum diameter of about 40 cm only can cover about a quarter of the body section for documentation. To overcome this limitation, the tube including the image intensifier, or the table top, has to be moved along the body for sequential documentation. Until recently, documentation was obtained by photofluorography, usually with incremental translation of the table top. These problems seem to be solved now with the PERIVISION system [169], which gives a high-quality DSA mapping of the peripheral vessels.

Another digital technique, the Fuji computed radiography system, has also been utilized for aortography and peripheral aortography [170]. A hexagonal large-format serial cassette changer with four imaging plates in a row and covering 100 cm of the body is used for this purpose. Six exposures are made after injection of 50 ml of contrast medium and adequate information of arteriosclerotic disease can be obtained.

The high resolution of the image intensifiers, thanks to the caesium-iodide input phosphor and other improvements over the years, has made photofluorography a competitor to full-size serial angiography in abdominal studies as well as in cardioangiography [171, 172]. For coronary angiography and cardioangiography, however, cineradiography is still most often used and in many places the only method for documentation. Digital videography is taking an increasing part and will eventually replace cineradiography except in areas where a very high recording rate is necessary.

Future of angiography

Today, we see a completely different role for angiography from that at the beginning of the seventies. With the advent of the gamma-camera in the sixties, radionuclide imaging became a competitor in documentation of diseases in organs (e.g. brain, liver, heart, kidney) but was often regarded complementary rather definitive. New radionuclides and new techniques, particularly SPECT (Single Photon Emission Computed Tomography) and PET (Positron Emission Tomography), have increased their roles in acquisition of information about organ function and disease. It is mainly in the localization of gastrointestinal bleeding that radionuclide imaging has replaced angiography [173].

Ultrasonography and CT have to a great extent replaced angiography (and radionuclide imaging) in the documentation of structural diseases of organs since the seventies, complemented by MR imaging during the eighties. The documentation of vascular disease, particularly arteriosclerosis and venous lesions, is still an important part of angiography. It is true that both duplex-Doppler and MR angiography eventually might take over most of the present indications for angiography, but the radiologist has over the years learned an extremely important lesson: he knows how to breach vessels with the smallest possible trauma, and how to treat vascular disease and organ lesions with percutaneous techniques.

It will take another decade or so before we see whether angiography can be replaced not only by MR technique but also by endoscopy [174] or intravascular ultrasound [175]. Perhaps, we will then also see intravascular treatment with these techniques and, perhaps, non-invasive medical treatment of arteriosclerotic disease.

References

1. Sicard, J.A., G. Forestier: Injections intravasculaires d'huile iodée sous contrôle radiologique. Compt. Rend. Soc. Biol. 88 (1923) 1200–1202
2. Berberich, J., S. Hirsch: Die röntgenographische Darstellung der Arterien und Venen am Lebenden. Klin. Wschr. 2 (1923) 2226–2228
3. Brooks, B.: Intraarterial injection of sodium iodide. Preliminary report. J. Am. Med. Ass. 82 (1924) 1016–1019
4. Moniz, E.: L'encéphalographie artérielle, son importance dans la localisation des tumeurs cérébrale. Rev. Neurol. 2 (1927) 72–89
5. Dos Santos, R., A. Lamas, J.P. Caldas: L'arteriographie des membres de l'aorte et de ses branches abdominales. Bull. et mém. Soc. Nat. Chir. 55 (1929) 587–601
6. Forssmann, W.: Über Kontrastdarstellung der Höhlen des lebenden rechten Herzens und der Lungenschlagader. Münchener Med. Wschr. 78 (1931) 489–492
7. Radt, P.: Eine Methode zur röntgenologischen Kontrastdarstellung von Miltz und Leber. Klin. Wschr. 8 (1929) 2128–2129
8. Moniz, E., A. Pinto, A. Lima: Die Vorzüge des Thorotrast bei arterieller Encephalographie. Röntgen-Praxis 4 (1932) 90
9. Swick, N.: Darstellung der Niere und Harnwege im Röntgenbild durch intravenöse Einbringung eines neuen Kontraststoffes, des Uroselectans. Klin. Wschr. 8 (1929) 2087–2089
10. Frey, S., H.G. Zwerg: Die röntgenologische Darstellung der Gefäße am lebenden Tiere und Menschen (Vasographie). Dtsche Zschr. Chir. 232 (1931) 173–186
11. Wohlleben, T.: Venographie. Klin. Wschr. 11 (1932) 1786–1789
12. Moniz, E., L. de Carvalho, A. Lima: Angiopneumographie. Presse Méd. 53 (1931) 996–999
13. Castellanos, A., R. Pereiras, A. Garcia: L'angiocardiographie chez l'enfant. Presse Med. 80 (1938) 1474–1477
14. Robb, G.P., I. Steinberg: Visualization of the chambers of the heart, the pulmonary circulation and the great blood vessels in man. A practical method. Am. J. Roentgenol. 41 (1939) 1–17
15. Chavez, I., N. Dorbecker, A. Celis: Direct intracardiac angiocardiography – its diagnostic value. Am. Heart J. 33 (1947) 560–593
16. Jönsson, G., B. Brodén, J. Karnell: Selective angiocardiography. Acta Radiol. 32 (1949) 486–497
17. Loman, J., A. Myerson: Visualization of the cerebral vessels by direct intracarotid injection of thorium dioxide (Thorotrast). Am. J. Roentgenol. 35 (1936) 188–193
18. Shimidzu, K.: Beiträge zur Arteriographie des Gehirnes – einfache perkutane Methode. Arch. Klin. Chir. 188 (1937) 295–316
19. Rousthöi, P.: Über Angiocardiographie. Vorläufige Mitteilung. Acta Radiol. 14 (1933) 419–424
20. Reboul, H., M. Racine: La ventriculographie cardiaque expérimentale. Presse Méd. 41 (1933) 763–767
21. Nuvoli, I.: Arteriografia dell'aorta toracica mediante puntura dell'aorta ascendente o del ventriculo S. Policlinico Sez. Prat. 43 (1936) 227–237
22. Radner, S.: An attempt at the roentgenologic visualization of coronary blood vessels in man. Acta Radiol. 26 (1945) 497–502
23. Ichikawa, T.: Schatten der Nierenarterie (I). Meine Methode zur röntgenologischen Darstellung der Nierenarterie. Zschr. Urol. 32 (1938) 563
24. Farinãs, P.L.: A new technique for arteriographic examination of the abdominal aorta and its branches. Am. J. Roentgenol. 46 (1941) 641–645
25. Radner, S.: Intracranial angiography via vertebral artery. Acta Radiol. 28 (1947) 838–842
26. Radner, S.: Technical equipment for vasal catheterization. Acta Radiol. 31 (1949) 152–154
27. Brodén, B., G. Jönsson, J. Karnell: Thoracic aortography. Observations on technical problems connected with the method and various risks involved in its use. Acta Radiol. 32 (1949) 498–508
28. Jönsson, G.: Thoracic aortography by means of a cannula inserted percutaneously into the common carotid artery. Acta Radiol. 31 (1949) 376–386
29. Doss, A.K.: Translumbar aortography – an apparatus for injecting the radiopaque media. Surgery 16 (1944) 422–424
30. Farinãs, P.L.: Retrograde abdominal aortography. Am. J. Roentgenol. 55 (1946) 448–451.
31. Ramsey, G.H.S., J.S. Watson Jr, T.B. Steinhausen, J.J. Thompson, F. Dreisinger, S. Weinberg: Cinefluorography. A progress report on technical problems, dosage factors and clinical impressions. Radiology 52 (1949) 684–690
32. Janker, R.: Roentgen cinematography. Am. J. Roentgenol. 36 (1936) 384–390
33. Caldas, J.P.: Artériographies en série avec l'appareil radio-carrousel. J. Radiol. Electr. 18 (1934) 34
34. Moniz, E., A. Lima, P. Caldas: Angiographies en série de la circulation de la tête. Rev. Neurol. 1 (1934) 489–510
35. Guy, J.M.: A.E. Barclay and angiographic research in Oxford. Br. J. Radiol. 61 (1988) 1110–1114
36. Sanchez-Perez, J.M.: The cranial seriograph and its utility in neurologic radiology for cerebral angiography. Surgery 13 (1943) 661–666
37. Axén, O., J. Lind: Om angiocardiografi på späda barn. Nord. Med. 38 (1948) 1143 (In Swedish)
38. Gidlund, A.S.: A new apparatus for direct cineroentgenolgy. Acta Radiol. 32 (1949) 81–88
39. Fredzell, G., J. Lind, E. Ohlson, C. Wegelius: Direct serial roentgenography in two planes simultaneously at 0.08 second intervals. Physical aspects of roentgen diagnosis, apparatus and its applications to angiocardiography. Am. J. Roentgenol. 63 (1950) 548–558
40. Rappaport, A.M.: The guided catheterization and radiography of the abdominal vessels. Can. Med. Ass. J. 67 (1952) 93–100
41. Abeatici, S., L. Campi: Sur les possibilités de l'angiographie hepatique. La visualisation du système portal. Acta Radiol. 36 (1951) 383–392

42. Bierman, H.R., H.L. Steinbach, L.P. White, K.H. Kelly: Portal venipuncture. A percutaneous, transhepatic approach. Proc. Soc. Exp. Biol. Med. 79 (1952) 550–552

43. Blakemore, A.H., J.W. Lord Jr.: The technique of using vitallium tubes in establishing porta-caval shunts for portal hypertension. Ann. Surg. 122 (1945) 476–489

44. Ödman, P.: Percutaneous selective angiography of the coeliac artery. Acta Radiol. (1958) Suppl. 159

45. Seldinger, S.I.: Catheter replacement of the needle in percutaneous arteriography. A new technique. Acta Radiol. 39 (1953) 368–376

46. Helmsworth, J.A., J. McGuire, B. Felson: Arteriography of the aorta and its branches by means of the polyethylene catheter. Am. J. Roentgenol. 64 (1950) 196–213

47. Peirce, E.C.: Percutaneous femoral artery catheterization in man with special reference to aortography. Surg. Gynec. Obstet. 93 (1951) 56–74

48. Seldinger, S.I.: A leaf out of the history of angiography. Radiology, edited by M.E. Silvester, F. Abecasis and J.A. Veiga-Pires. Elsevier Science Publishers BV, Excerpta Medica, Amsterdam 1987.

49. Radner, S.: Subclavian angiography by arterial catheterization. Acta Radiol. 32 (1949) 359–364

50. Bierman, H.R., E.R. Miller, R.L. Byron Jr, K.S. Dod, K.H. Kelly, D.H. Black: Intraarterial catheterization of viscera in man. Am. J. Roentgenol. 66 (1951) 555–567

51. Krohmer, J.S.: Radiography and fluoroscopy, 1920 to the present. Radiographics 9 (1989) 1129–1153

52. Ödman, P.: Percutaneous selective angiography of the main branches of the aorta (preliminary report). Acta Radiol. 45 (1956) 1–14

53. Gollman, G.: Eine Modifizierung der Seldingerischen Kathetermethode zur isolierten Kontrastfüllung der Aortenäste. Fortschr. Röntgenstr. 87 (1957) 211–214

54. Tillander, H.: Selective angiography of the abdominal aorta with a guided catheter. Acta Radiol 45 (1956) 21–26

55. Lindgren, E.: Another method of vertebral angiography. Acta Radiol. 46 (1956) 257–261

56. DiGuglielmo, I., M. Guttadauro: A roentgenologic study of the coronary arteries in the living. Acta Radiol. (1952) Suppl. 97

57. Lehman, J.S., R.A. Boyer, F.S. Winter: Coronary arteriography. Am. J. Roentgenol. 81 (1959) 749–763

58. Dotter, C.T., L.H. Frische: Visualization of the coronary circulation by occlusion aortography. A practical method. Radiology 71 (1958) 502–523

59. Sones, F.M. Jr., E.K. Shirey: Cine coronary arteriography. Mod. Concepts Cardiovasc. Dis. 31 (1962) 735

60. Gidlund, Å.: Development of apparatus and methods for roentgen studies in haemodynamics. Acta Radiol. (1956) Suppl. 130

61. Ödman, P.: The radiopaque polythen catheter. Acta Radiol. 52 (1959) 52–64

62. Janker, R., H. Hallerbach: Die Angiocardiokinematographie als Mittel zur Bestimmung der Lungenkreislaufzeit. Fortschr. Röntgenstr. 75 (1951) 290–291

63. Abrams, H.L.: An approach to biplane cineangiocardiography. 1. Background and objectives. Radiology 72 (1959) 735–740

64. Sones, F.M.: Cine-cardio-angiography. Pediatr. Clin. North Am. 5 (1958) 945–979

65. Abrams, H.L.: Biplane cinefluorography with eleven-inch image intensifiers. Cinefluorography: 191–212. Edited by G.H.S. Ramsey, J.S. Watson Jr, T.A. Tristan, S. Weinberg, W.S.Ch.C. Cornwell. Thomas Publishers, Springfield, IL 1960.

66. Rigler, L.G., J.C. Watson: A combination film changing device for general radiography. Radiology 61 (1953) 77–79

67. Sjögren, S.E., G. Fredzell: Apparatus for serial angiography. Acta Radiol. 40 (1953) 361–368

68. Abrams, H.L.: Angiography. Vol. I-II. Little, Brown and Co, Boston 1961.

69. Dotter, C.T., M.P. Judkins: Transluminal treatment of arteriosclerotic obstruction. Description of a new technic and a preliminary report of its application. Circulation 30 (1964) 654–670

70. Almén, T.: A steering device for selective angiography and some vascular and enzymatic reactions observed in its clinical application. Acta Radiol. (1966) Suppl. 260

71. Broman, T., O. Olsson: Experimental comparison of diodonum with sodium acetrizoate with reference to possible injurious effects on the blood-brain barrier. Acta Radiol. 46 (1956) 346–350

72. Greitz, T.: A radiologic study of the brain circulation by rapid serial angiography of the carotid artery. Acta Radiol. (1956) Suppl. 140

73. Büchner, H.: Angiokymographie und Stufenarteriographie. RÖFO 97 (1962) 345–352

74. Nordenström, B., S. Grim: A method for determination of blood flow with use of roentgen contrast medium. Radiology 84 (1965) 644–656

75. Olin, T., H. Redman: Spillover flowmeter. Acta Radiol. Diagnosis 4 (1966) 217–222

76. McAfee, J.G.: A survey of complications of abdominal aortography. Radiology 68 (1957) 812–824

78. Boblitt, D.E., M.M. Figley, E.F. Wolfman Jr.: Roentgen signs of contrast material dissection of aortic wall in direct aortography. Am. J. Roentgenol. 81 (1959) 826–834

79. Baum, S., G.N. Stein, K.K. Kuroda: Complications of "No arteriography". Radiology 86 (1966) 835–838

80. Seldinger, S.I.: A simple method of catheterization of the spleen and liver. Acta Radiol. 48 (1957) 93–96

81. Jacobsson, B., D. Schlossman: Thromboembolism of leg following percutaneous catheterization of femoral artery for angiography. Predisposing factors. Acta Radiol. 8 (1969) 109–118

82. Jacobsson, B.: Effect of pretreatment with Dextran 70 on platelet adhesiveness and thromboembolic complications following percutaneous arterial catheterization. Acta Radiol. 8 (1969) 289–295

83. Schlossman, D.: Thrombogenicity of vascular catheters. Thesis, University of Gothenburg, Orstadius Boktryckeri AB, Gothenburg 1972.

84. Olin, T.: Studies in angiographic technique. Thesis, Lund University, Sweden. Håkan Ohlssons Boktryckeri, Lund 1963.

85. Boijsen, E., M.P. Judkins: A hook-tail "closed-end" catheter for percutaneous selective cardioangiography. Radiology 87 (1966) 872–877

86. Rodriguez-Alvarez, A., G. Martinez de Rodriguez: Studies in angiocardiography. Am. Heart J. 53 (1957) 841–853

87. Hettler, M.: Angiographische Probleme und Möglichkeiten. II. Der perkutane Arterienkatheterismus mit an der Spitze verschlossenem Katheter als

Grundlage der Etagen-Aortographie. Fortschr. Röntgenstr. 92 (1960) 198–206

88. Prioton, J.B., A. Thévenet, M. Pelissier et al.: Cardiographie ventriculaire gauche par cathétérisme retrograde percutane fémoral. Presse Med. 65 (1957) 1948–1951

89. Dotter, C.T., M.P. Judkins, L.H. Frische: Safety guidespring for percutaneous cardiovascular catheterization. Am. J. Roentgenol. 98 (1966) 957–960

90. Judkins, M.P., H.J. Kidd, L.H. Frische, C.T. Dotter: Lumen-following safety J-guide for catheterization of tortuous vessels. Radiology 88 (1967) 1127–1130

91. Baum, S., H.L. Abrams: A J-shaped catheter for retrograde catheterization of tortuous vessels. Radiology 83 (1964) 436–437

92. Amplatz, K., G. Formanek, P. Stanger, W. Wilson: Mechanics of selective coronary artery catheterization via femoral approach. Radiology 89 (1967) 1040–1047

93. Viamonte, M. Jr., R.C. Stevens: Guided angiography. Am. J. Roentgenol. 94 (1965) 30–39

94. Zeitler, E., W. Schoop: Der Wandel in der Indikation zur Angiographie bei der arteriellen Verschlusskrankheiten. Fortschr. Röntgenstr. 112 (1970) 291–309

95. Lang, E.K.: Prevention and treatment of complications following arteriography. Radiology 88 (1967) 950–956

96. Paulin, S.: Coronary angiography. A technical, anatomic and clinical study. Acta Radiol. (1964) Suppl. 233

97. Bellman, S., H.A. Frank, P.B. Lambert et al.: Coronary arteriography. I. Differential opacification of the aortic stream by catheters of special design. N. Engl. J. Med. 262 (1960) 325–328

98. Hettler, M.G.: Die semiselektive, bilaterale Koronarangiographie. Eine neue klinische Untersuchungsmethode der Herzkranzarterien. Fortschr. Röntgenstr. 103 (1965) 249–261

99. Ricketts, H.J., H.L. Abrams: Percutaneous selective coronary cine arteriography. J. Am. Med. Ass. 181 (1962) 620–624

100. Judkins, M.P.: Selective coronary arteriography. Part I. A percutaneous transfemoral technic. Radiology 89 (1967) 815–824

101. Amundsen, P., P. Dietrichson, I. Enge, R. Williamson: Cerebral angiography by catheterization. Complications and side effects. Acta Radiol. Diagnosis 1 (1963) 164–172

102. Hinck, V.C., M.P. Judkins, H.D. Paxton: Simplified selective femorocerebral angiography. Radiology 89 (1967) 1048–1052

103. DiChiro, G., J. Doppman, A.K. Ommaya: Selective arteriography of arteriovenous aneurysms of spinal cord. Radiology 88 (1967) 1065–1077

104. Djindjian, R.: Technique de l'artériographie de la moelle epinière par aortographie selective. Presse Med. 76 (1968) 159–162

105. Boijsen, E.: Selective visceral angiography using a percutaneous axillary technique. Br. J. Radiol. 39 (1966) 414–421

106. Boijsen, E.: Selective pancreatic angiography. Br. J. Radiol. 39 (1966) 481–487

107. Cope, C.: A new maneuvreable guide for selective abdominal catheterization. J. Appl. Physiol. 16 (1961) 917–918

108. Wholey, M.H., V. Jackman: A new instrument. Controllable guide for angiography. Am. J. Roentgenol. 97 (1966) 500–503

109. Abrams, H.L., E. Boijsen, K.E. Borgström: Effect of epinephrine on the renal circulation. Angiographic observations. Radiology 79 (1962) 911–922

110. Abrams, H.L.: The response of neoplastic renal vessels to epinephrine in man. Radiology 82 (1964) 217–224

111. Olin, T., S. Reuter: A pharmacological method for improving nephrophlebography. Radiology 85 (1965) 1036–1042

112. Boijsen, E., H. Redman: Effect of bradykinin on celiac and superior mesenteric angiography. Invest. Radiol. 1 (1966) 422–430

113. Boijsen, E., H. Redman: Effect of epinephrine on celiac and superior mesenteric angiography. Invest. Radiol. 2 (1967) 184–199

114. Bierman, H.R., R.L. Byron Jr., E.R. Miller, M.B. Shimkin: Effects of intra-arterial administration of nitrogen mustard. Am. J. Med. 8 (1950) 535

115. Aakhus, T., G. Braband: Angiography in acute superior mesenteric arterial insufficiency. Acta Radiol. Diagnosis 6 (1967) 1–12

116. Luessenhoop, A.J., W.T. Spence: Artificial embolization of cerebral arteries. Report of use in a case of arteriovenous malformation. J. Am. Med. Ass. 172 (1960) 1153–1155

117. Doppman, J.L., G. DiChiro, A. Ommaya: Obliteration of spinal cord arteriovenous malformation by percutaneous embolization. Lancet I (1968) 477

118. Mobin-Uddin, K., R. McLean, J.R. Jude: A new catheter technique of interruption of inferior vena cava for prevention of pulmonary embolism. Ann. Surg. 35 (1969) 889–894

119. Kantrowitz, A., S. Tjönneland, P.S. Freed et al.: Initial clinical experience with intraaortic balloon pumping in cardiogenic shock. J. Am. Med. Ass. 203 (1968) 113–118

120. Amplatz, K.: A vascular injector with program selector. Radiology 75 (1960) 955–956

121. Viamonte, M. Jr., J. Hobbs: Automatic electric injector. Development to prevent electromechanical hazards of selective angiocardiography. Invest. Radiol. 2 (1967) 262–265

122. Amplatz, K.: New rapid roll film changer. Radiology 90 (1968) 130–134

123. Roy, P., A. Jutras, M. Longtin: Extra large field angiography. Technique and results. J. Can. Ass. Radiol. 12 (1961) 27

124. Amplatz, K.: Rapid long film changers. Angiography, 2nd edn., p. 75. Edited by H.L. Abrams. Little, Brown and Co., Boston 1971

125. Amplatz, K.: A simple non-thrombogenic coating. Invest. Radiol. 6 (1971) 280–289

126. Glancy, J.J., G. Fishbone, E.R. Heinz: Non-thrombogenic arterial catheters. Am. J. Roentgenol. 108 (1970) 716–723

127. Wallace, S., H. Medellin, D. de Jong, C. Gianturco: Systemic heparinization for angiography. Am. J. Roentgenol. 116 (1972) 204–209

128. G.H. Nachnani, L.S. Lessin, T. Motomiya, W.N. Jensen: Scanning electron microscopy of thrombogenesis on vascular catheter surfaces. N. Engl. J. Med. 286 (1972) 139–140

129. Anderson, J.H., C. Gianturco, S. Wallace, G.D. Dodd: A scanning electron microscopic study of angiographic catheters and guide wires. Radiology 111 (1974) 567–571

130. Raininko, R., M. Riihelä: Blood clot formation in angiographic catheters. In vitro tests with various contrast media. Acta Radiol. 31 (1990) 217–220
131. Dawson, P., P. Hewitt, I.J. Mackie et al.: Contrast, coagulation, and fibrinolysis. Invest. Radiol. 21 (1986) 248–252
132. Stormorken, H., I.O. Skalpe, M.C. Testat: Effect of various contrast media on coagulation, fibrinolysis, and platelet function. An in vitro and in vivo study. Invest. Radiol. 21 (1986) 348–354
133. Sigstedt, B., A. Lunderquist: Complications of angiographic examinations. Am. J. Roentgenol. 130 (1978) 455–460
134. Christenson, R., E.V. Staab, H. Burko, J. Foster: Pressure dressings and postarteriographic care of the femoral puncture site. Radiology 119 (1976) 97–99
135. Colapinto, R.F., P.W. Harty: Femoral artery compression device for outpatient angiography. Radiology 166 (1988) 890–891
136. Rapoport, S., K.W. Sniderman, S.S. Morse, M.H. Proto, G.R. Ross: Pseudoaneurysm. A complication of faulty technique in femoral arterial puncture. Radiology 154 (1985) 529–530
137. Haut, G., K. Amplatz: Complication rates of transfemoral and transaortic catheterization. Surgery 63 (1968) 594–596
138. Hessel, S.J., D.F. Adams, H.L. Abrams: Complications of angiography. Radiology 138 (1981) 273–281
139. Hagen, B., M. Vowinckel: Computertomographische Dokumentation retroperitonealer Hämatome nach translumbaler Aortographie. Fortschr. Röntgenstr. 133 (1980) 496–501
140. Amendola, M.A., J. Tisnado, W.R. Fields et al.: Evaluation of retroperitoneal hemorrhage by computed tomography after translumbar aortography. Radiology 133 (1979) 401–404
141. Gmelin, E., E. Rinast: Translumbar catheter angiography with a needle-sheath system. Radiology 166 (1988) 888–889
142. Smith, T.P., Z. Vlodaver, M.D. Darcy et al.: Improved vessel dilator for percutaneous catheterization. Radiology 163 (1987) 271–272
143. Rosen, R.J.: A new catheter for selective and superselective angiography. Cardiovasc. Intervent. Radiol. 9 (1986) 49–51
144. Wright, K.C., S. Wallace, C. Charnsangavej, Y.Y. Lee, C.H. Carrasco, C. Gianturco: Flow-directed catheter for superselective arterial catheterization. An experimental evaluation. Cardiovasc. Intervent. Radiol. 9 (1986) 54–56
145. Castaneda-Zuniga, W.R., J.L. Bass, J.E. Lock: Selective opacification of arteries with balloon-occlusion angiography. Radiology 138 (1981) 727–729
146. Becker, G.J., M.E. Hicks, R.W. Holden et al.: Screening for occlusive vascular disease with intraarterial DSA. Preliminary experience with a high flow 4-F catheter. Radiology 153 (1984) 823
147. Sawada, S.: Selective hepatic angiography using a balloon catheter guide. Radiology 156 (1985) 545–546
148. Bynum, L.J., J.E. Wilson III, E.E. Christensen, C. Sorensen: Radiographic techniques for ballon-occlusion pulmonary angiography. Radiology 133 (1979) 518–520
149. Chuang, V.P.: Superselective hepatic tumor embolization with Tracker-18. J. Intervent. Radiol. 3 (1988) 69
150. Okazaki, M., H. Higashihara, F. Koganemaru et al.: Emergent embolization for control of massive hemorrhage from a splanchnic artery with a new coaxial catheter system. Acta Radiol. 33 (1992) 57–62
151. Robinson, J.D., D.W. Hunter, W.R. Castaneda-Zuniga, K. Amplatz. A new torque guide wire. Radiology 165 (1987) 572–573
152. Sacks, B.A., J.C. Sequeira: Use of the 1 mm "J"-guidewire for selective catheterization. Radiology 132 (1979) 754–755
153. Lunderquist, A., M. Lunderquist, T. Owman: Guide wire for percutaneous transhepatic cholangiography. Radiology 132 (1979) 228
154. Morin, M.E., B.A. Willens, P.A. Kuss: Carotid artery. Percutaneous transbrachial selective arteriography with a 4-F catheter. Radiology 171 (1989) 868–870
155. Kamiya, H., S. Ohsugi, M. Ohno, M. Horiba, H. Hayashi: Coronary angiography by means of the percutaneous transbrachial approach. Radiology 179 (1991) 863–866
156. Lunderquist, A., J. Vang: Transhepatic catheterization and obliteration of the coronary vein in patients with portal hypertension and esophageal varices. N. Engl. J. Med. 291 (1974) 646–649
157. Göthlin, J., A. Lunderquist, U. Tylén: Selective phlebography in the pancreas. Acta Radiol. Diagnosis 15 (1974) 474–480
158. Baum, S., M. Nusbaum: The control of gastrointestinal hemorrhage by selective mesenteric arterial infusion of Vasopressin. Radiology 98 (1971) 497–505
159. Almén, T., E. Boijsen, S.E. Lindell: Metrizamide in angiography. I. Femoral angiography. Acta Radiol. 18 (1977) 33–38
160. Takahashi, S., S. Sakuma: Magnification radiography. Springer Verlag, Berlin 1975.
161. Takaro, T., S.M. Scott: Angiography using direct roentgenographic magnification in man. Am. J. Roentgenol. 91 (1964) 448–452
162. Greenspan, R.H., A.L. Simon, H.J. Ricketts, R.H. Rojas, J.C. Watson: In vivo magnification angiography. Invest. Radiol. 2 (1967) 419–431
163. Mistretta, Ch.A., M.G. Ort, J.R. Cameron et al.: A multiple images subtraction technique for enhancing low contrast, periodic objects. Invest. Radiol. 8 (1973) 43–49
164. Heintzen, P.H., R. Brenneke, J.H. Bürsch et al.: Automated videoangiocardiographic image analysis. Computer (IEEE) 8 (1975) 55–64
165. Meaney, T.F., M.A. Weinstein, E. Buonocore et al: Digital subtraction angiography of the human cardiovascular system. Am. J. Roentgenol. 135 (1980) 1153–1160
166. Bürsch, J.H., H.J. Hahne, R. Brennecke, D. Grönemeier, H. Heintzen: Assessment of arterial blood flow measurements by digital angiography. Radiology 141 (1981) 39–47
167. Crummy, A.B., Ch.M. Strother, J.P. Sacket et al.: Computerized fluoroscopy. Digital subtraction for intravenous angiocardiography and arteriography. Am. J. Roentgenol. 135 (1980) 1131–1140
168. Brandt-Zawadski, M., R. Gould et al.: Digital subtraction cerebral angiography by intraarterial injection. Comparison with conventional angiography. AJNR 3 (1982) 593–599
169. Hilbertz, Th., U. Fink, P. Kohz, U. Eberwein, W. Buchsteiner, E. Jenner: Perivision – a new standard in peripheral angiography. Electromedica 60 (1992) 2–5

170. Nitatori, T., J. Hachiya, T. Korenaga, Y. Furuya: Whole body intravenous digital subtraction angiography. Radiology 156 (1985) 829–830

171. Aakhus, T., L. Lantto, F. Kolmannskog, A. Winter: Comparison of image intensifier photofluorography and full-size radiography in abdominal angiography. Acta Radiol. 22 (1981) 39–47

172. Judkins, M.P.: Angiographic equipment. Abrams Angiography, Vascular and interventional radiology, 3rd edn., vol I, pp. 125–175. Edited by H.L. Abrams. Little, Brown and Co., Boston 1983.

173. Alavi, A., E.J. Ring: Localization of gastrointestinal bleeding. Superiority of 99mTc sulfur colloid compared with angiography. Am. J. Roentgenol. 137 (1981) 741–748

174. Ferris, E.J., K. Ledor, D.D. Ben-Avi et al.: Percutaneous angioscopy. Radiology 157 (1985) 319–322

175. Nishimura, R.A., T.J. Welch, A.W. Stanson, P.F. Sheedy II, D.R. Holmes Jr.: Intravascular US of the distal aorta and iliac vessels. Initial feasibility studies. Radiology 176 (1990) 523–525

Abdominal vessels

E. Boijsen

Radiography of the abdomen is an important part of diagnostic radiology and has been so since the X-rays came into use in clinical work. Plain radiography, i.e. radiography without the use of contrast media, has always been used both in cases where the clinical diagnosis is obvious and in cases where the symptoms are uncharacteristic and the diagnosis not known. In the former case the localization and extent of disease can be shown, and in the latter the radiographs can often establish a diagnosis in conjunction with the clinical findings and case history.

With the addition of contrast media to the gastrointestinal tract, further information is obtained about the abdominal organs. Eventually, contrast media were administered for information about the gallbladder, kidneys and biliary tree. Further improvement in diagnostic accuracy was obtained when contrast media were injected into the vessels.

Abdominal angiography is a radiographic method used for documentation of the vascular systems of the abdomen and retroperitoneum. Not only are the lumbar aorta, the inferior vena cava, and their large branches documented, but all vessels down to the capillary level can be recorded, the smallest ones as parenchymal accumulations of contrast medium. Information about the parenchymal organs and gastrointestinal tract is thus also obtained.

Contrast medium injected into the lumbar aorta is called lumbar aortography, into its branches selective angiography, and into the vena cava or its branches cavography or selective venography, respectively. Although these angiographic procedures still are very important both for diagnosis and for regional therapy, their numbers have reduced markedly during the last 20 years because of the development of non-invasive imaging methods.

Abdominal angiography is a relative latecomer in the history of radiology. By the year after Roentgen's discovery, arteries and veins were demonstrated in cadavers or amputated specimens. Heavy metal compositions were injected into the vessels, but the solutions were too toxic to be used in humans. It took more than 30 years before the lumbar aorta and its branches were documented radiographically *in vivo* in humans. The main reason was that because of toxicity no contrast medium was considered acceptable for intravenous or intra-arterial injection.

Percutaneous translumbar aortography

The first and most remarkable contribution to abdominal angiography came from Portuguese clinicians in the late twenties. In 1929, two years after Moniz' report on cerebral angiography, Dos Santos, Lamas and Caldas reported their first experience with percutaneous lumbar aortography [1]. After testing a number of radiopaque substances experimentally and clinically, Moniz had found that solutions of sodium iodide were most suitable for cerebral angiography. Consequently, Dos Santos used this agent but in a higher concentration (100%). Initially, he did not have any complications, but the procedure was difficult to accept for the patients since it had to be performed under lumbar anesthesia to avoid severe pain from the injection of sodium iodide. Extravasation was reported, but the pain was considered acceptable and not so severe as experienced with extravasation of Neo-salvarsan.

Dos Santos (Fig. III, 69) was well aware of the easy access to the lumbar aorta from the back, because he had often accidentally, without complications, punctured the lumbar aorta when injecting anesthetics into the para-aortic sympathicus

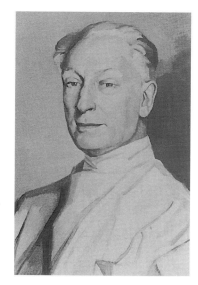

Fig. III, 69. Reynaldo dos Santos (oil painting) performed the first abdominal angiography in 1929 [1]. Surgeon in Lisbon. Also known as expert in art history.

chain. With this experience and with the well-known studies of Moniz at hand, Dos Santos was predestined to be the pioneer in abdominal angiography. In his first reports, he also discussed the potentialities of regional therapy by intra-aortic or intra-arterial injection of drugs.

The technique to puncture the lumbar aorta is today the same as that described by Dos Santos, but otherwise there is no resemblance to the present method of percutaneous lumbar aortography. A catheter of about the same diameter as the needle used by Dos Santos is introduced and the position of the catheter is carefully checked with an image intensifier–TV system before a contrast agent of low toxicity is injected. No lumbar spinal anesthesia is required and the patient will hardly feel the injection of the contrast agent.

Even if Dos Santos originally considered his method safe and harmless, he nevertheless had severe complications and even fatalities. One problem, later often referred to, was the risk associated with the blind puncture of the aorta. For instance, the tip of the needle could be positioned in one of the branches of the aorta and sodium iodide deposited directly into the celiac, mesenteric or renal arteries, with secondary thrombosis and organ necrosis, as later reported [2, 3]. In his first report, Dos Santos presented a case in which the celiac trunk was punctured, and thus he was the first to perform selective celiac angiography. No complications were observed in this particular case. Later on, with less toxic contrast media, selective celiac, superior and inferior mesenteric, and renal angiograms were performed inadvertently at percutaneous lumbar aortography without any complications in

most cases [3]. It became obvious that deposition of contrast medium in a branch of the aorta, selective angiography, gave far better information about the abdominal organs than translumbar aortography could. This technique could, however, not be performed routinely until 20 years after the first demonstration of a selective celiac angiogram by Dos Santos.

The method of percutaneous translumbar aortography was soon well known but did not receive immediate acceptance because of reluctance to puncture the aorta blindly. Also reports of serious complications dampened the radiologists' and clinicians' interest in the method. Furthermore, Henline and Moore [4] showed in 1936 in an experimental study that five of 19 dogs undergoing percutaneous translumbar aortography died because of bleeding shortly after the procedure, and another three died because of the toxicity of the contrast agent. The method was considered too dangerous and was therefore not taken up widely until after World War II, when new contrast media with lower toxicity were used [5, 6].

In a questionnaire to 450 radiologists and urologists in the United States in 1956, McAfee [3] found that 97% of all abdominal aortograms were performed as percutaneous transabdominal studies and that at that time very few angiograms were performed even in large hospitals. The fatalities reported in his enquiry were mainly due to renal damage caused by inadvertent direct injection of contrast agent into the renal artery. Also neurological and gastrointestinal complications were observed, mainly due to inadvertent injection of contrast agent into lumbar or mesenteric arteries. Intramural injections were frequent and were observed in 10% of the cases in one series [7].

Lumbar aortography – other techniques

In 1939, Robb and Steinberg [8] demonstrated an alternative to the translumbar method by injecting contrast medium intravenously and recording the diluted agent on the arterial side. However, they focused their interest on lesions in the heart and thoracic aorta, and therefore lumbar aorta and the renal arteries were observed in only a few of their cases. Later, this intravenous lumbar aortography became a practical method when the lumbar aorta could not be reached by any other modality. Subtraction methods were used and these became particularly popular in the beginning of the eighties as intravenous digital subtraction angiography.

Catheterization of the aorta for lumbar aortography from the femoral artery after surgical exploration of the vessel was performed in 1941 by Fariñas [9], who 5 years later also demonstrated the aorta by retrograde injection of contrast medium from the femoral artery. The femoral arteries distal to the puncture were compressed with the patient in Trendelenburg position, and the agent injected with a pressure injector.

The translumbar percutaneous technique was dominating until 1953 when Seldinger [10] published his method of percutaneous transfemoral lumbar aortography. The low complication rate as compared with the translumbar technique soon became obvious. Until this time, lumbar aortography was performed mainly by surgeons. With the Seldinger technique, it immediately turned into a method performable by radiologists.

When I entered radiology in 1949 at the Department of Radiology in Lund, very few abdominal angiographic procedures were performed. Olle Olsson, my chief and tutor, had visited Dos Santos in 1946 because he was convinced that the best way at that time to improve the diagnosis of renal disease was to perform angiography. And Dos Santos was the only man to learn from in Europe, because just after World War II abdominal aortography was hardly used in any other place (Fig. III, 70). He returned convinced of the impact renal angiography would have in the future. For several reasons previously mentioned, radiologists were not very interested in the translumbar method and even though this technique was to a certain extent used in our department, we preferred the transradial catheterization method introduced by Radner for vertebral and thoracic angiography, by bringing down a radiopaque ureteral catheter to the lumbar aorta from a cut down of one of the radial arteries.

This technique was not ideal. It was an awkward and difficult fluoroscopic procedure to advance the catheter to the lumbar aorta in complete darkness with an open wound in the elbow region. Furthermore, with the thin and narrow ureteral catheter, contrast medium could only be injected at a slow rate and the information of the renal arteries was often not optimal. Most important, however, was the risk of arm ischemia when the radial artery was ligated following the angiographic procedure. This happened in at least one patient who had lumbar aortography performed from the radial artery. Therefore, when the Seldinger method became available, we immediately turned to this technique. In a review of renal complications from lumbar aorto-

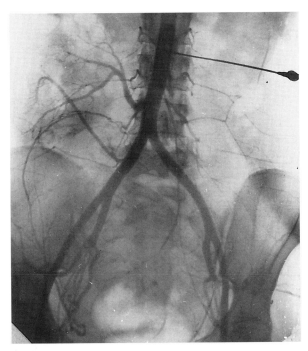

Fig. III, 70. Percutaneous translumbar aortography performed by dos Santos in a pregnant woman with a malpositioned and malrotated right kidney. The two right renal arteries have a low origin from the aorta and the right iliac artery. Gift from Prof. dos Santos to Prof. Olsson in 1946 when the latter visited Lisbon.

graphy at our department by Idbohrn in 1956, few complications were found with 54 transradial and 132 percutaneous transfemoral lumbar aortograms in comparison with previously reported translumbar aortography studies [11].

The history of abdominal angiography had a long period of trial and error, with a number of serious and even fatal complications. To a large extent, the problems emanated from inexperience, toxic contrast media given in too high concentrations and amounts, and technical mishaps. All these complications were markedly reduced when the Seldinger technique became available and new less toxic contrast agents were used. Over the years, continuous improvements in technique and increased experience among radiologists, including careful observation of the patients after the angiographic procedure, have definitely improved the safety, but complications can never be completely eliminated. Quality control in radiology has changed our attitude towards angiography. It means that patients' safety and comfort should be given priority and that, for this reason, the highest achievable information cannot always be obtained. Informing the patient before the examination and providing a careful follow-up are important responsibilities of the radiologists.

Selective abdominal angiography

During the early fifties, lumbar aortography performed as percutaneous transabdominal method or as a catheter method from the femoral arteries was mostly used for diagnosis and localization of intrinsic disease of the aorta and its main branches. To an increasing extent, aortography was also used for demonstrating lesions in the kidneys, liver and spleen [3, 12, 13, 14]. It was found by some that translumbar aortography was an adequate method in the diagnosis of renal cancer. For instance, Evans [14] correctly diagnosed 95% of all renal cancers operated on, but stressed that the diagnosis should only be based on high-quality angiograms. In other series, however, it was found that percutaneous translumbar aortography was not an acceptable method to distinguish renal cysts from cancer [15, 16].

As previously mentioned, inadvertent injection of contrast agent directly into the renal, celiac, and mesenteric arteries had markedly im-

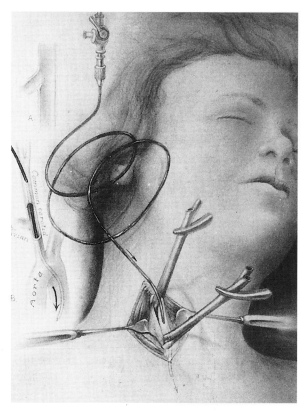

Fig. III, 71a, b. Catheterization technique of abdominal arteries (1951) according to Bierman et al. [17]. **a)** Cut down of the carotid artery for catheter introduction.

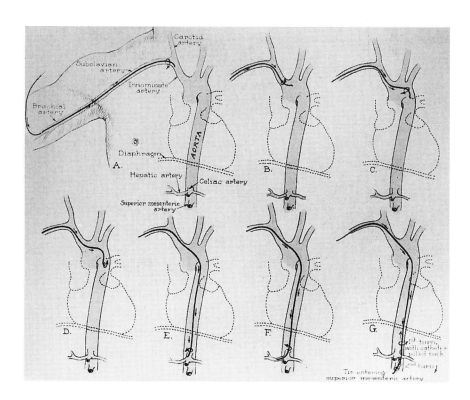

Fig. III, 71b. Introduction and passage of catheter from the brachial artery.

proved the diagnostic information [1, 12]. In most cases, this injection did not cause any harm, but in some severe complications were observed because too large an amount of hypertonic contrast media had been injected, or the vessels had become occluded following a subintimal injection. The logical consequence was the performance of selective angiography with lower concentrations and doses compared with those for aortic midstream injection.

The first truly intentional selective angiograms of branches of the lumbar aorta in humans were reported in 1951 by Bierman et al [17]. They stated: '. . . *if the major artery leading to a specific organ could be isolated to the exclusion of other viscera, not only could that specific organ be visualized roentgenographically, but also various chemotherapeutic agents could be administered in high concentration directly to neoplastic lesions involving this organ*'.

They were also aware of the fact that such catheterizations could give new pharmacological and physiological information about the abdominal organs. These statements are as relevant today as they were more than 40 years ago. After surgical exposure, usually of the right carotid artery, they could pass the catheter into the celiac artery in 23 of 24 patients. They also gave direct recommendations on how to perform the procedure and the first selective hepatic angiogram was presented (Fig. III, 71 and 72). Unfortunately, this technique of surgical exploration of

the carotid artery and of catheterization under fluoroscopy in complete darkness caused several cerebral complications and therefore never came into routine use.

Tillander [18] tested another method in 1951 with the same intentions as those of Bierman et al. In dogs and corpses he used magnetic guidance of a catheter with articulated steel tip and '. . . *under favorable conditions the catheter could be guided (from the left radial artery) into any of the arterial branches*' (of the lumbar aorta).

In 1952, Rappaport [19] showed that in dogs it was possible to bring the catheter from the femoral artery into the abdominal vessels with the aid of a guiding instrument. Later, modifications of this steering device were used in cases difficult to catheterize. The modern catheterization technique, supported by high-resolution image intensifiers and TV, flexible guide-wires and steerable catheters, has eliminated the use of guiding instruments.

The radiologists were well prepared for improved information of the abdominal vessels and organs when the percutaneous femoral catheterization method became available. A few years later, in 1956, a number of reports on selective abdominal angiography in humans appeared, with insertion of the catheter from the femoral arteries [20, 21], from the exposed radial artery [22, 23], and from a surgically exposed mesenteric artery [24]. Of particular interest was the

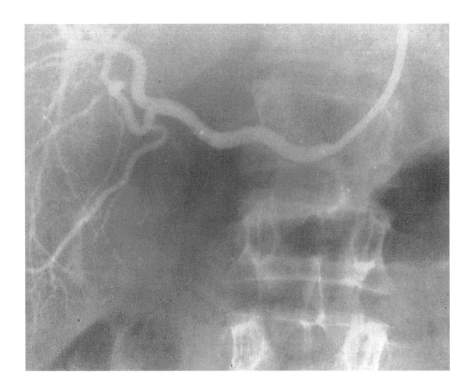

Fig. III, 72. The first selective catheterization of the hepatic artery and angiogram by Bierman et al. [17].

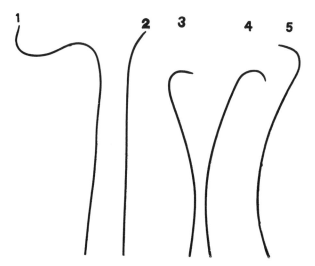

Fig. III, 73. Radiopaque catheters for catheterization of abdominal vessels according to Oedman [20]. Different shapes obtained by shaping the catheter in hot water just before catheterization. The catheter was shaped according to the expected anatomy of the vessel of interest.

report in 1956 by Ödman [20], who presented the radiopaque polythene catheter, which, depending on the vascular anatomy, could be shaped for selective angiography of branches of the aorta (Fig. III, 73). Tillander [22] used magnetic guidance of the catheter in humans and passed the catheter into the gastroduodenal artery. Injecting contrast medium in this position, he could for the first time show all the pancreatic arteries and accumulation of contrast medium in the entire pancreas (Fig. III, 74).

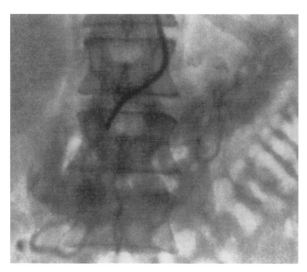

Fig. III, 74. Angiography of the gastroduodenal artery according to Tillander [22]. Accumulation of contrast medium observed, presumably in the gastric wall and probably also in a normal pancreas (1956).

Morino [23] used the Radner technique to perform selective abdominal angiography from the exposed radial artery. With further development in catheters and with modern fluoroscopy, percutaneous catheterization from the brachial and axillary arteries was later worked out both for selective angiography of abdominal vessels and for lumbar aortography [25–30].

Although neither Bierman's nor Tillander's technique was used further, their work paved the way for the selective and superselective angiography that became such important methods for the following two decades in the radiological diagnosis of vascular and parenchymatous lesions of the abdomen and retroperitoneum. The techniques established by Seldinger [10, 21] and Ödman [20] were soon accepted as standard methods in abdominal angiography, and readily adopted by radiologists because, as mentioned, the radiologist could now perform lumbar aortography or selective angiography without active participation of the surgeon.

Percutaneous translumbar aortography still prevailed but the numbers decreased. It was mostly used for the diagnosis of ischemic leg disease. In our radiology department, this method disappeared almost completely after 1953, since catheterization was performed from the left axillary artery when the catheter for some reason could not reach the lumbar aorta from the femoral arteries [27]. The complication rates with axillary artery catheterization was, however, higher than with the transfemoral method [31], and therefore intravenous lumbar aortography with subtraction technique was an alternative. This became very popular with the availability of digital subtraction angiography.

During the sixties and most part of the seventies, abdominal angiography, particularly as selective angiography, became the most commonly used procedure in our angiography rooms. They were regarded by the clinicians as highly important diagnostic procedures in parenchymal diseases of the upper abdominal and retroperitoneal organs, in traumatic lesions, and in vascular disorders. During the first years after the selective technique became available in 1956, the catheterization was performed in complete darkness because image amplification was not yet available. To be able to see the catheters during conventional fluoroscopy, the angiographer had to be well adapted to the darkness, and use thick-walled Ödman-Ledin catheters. Identifying the level where the arteries arose from the aorta was difficult in these circumstances. Therefore, a lead marker was placed on the abdominal wall at the level of L1 and its position documented with a radiograph. Since most of the upper abdominal vessels originate from the aorta at this level, it was a simple and wise step before the catheterization procedure. The catheters also had to be preshaped in hot water before the procedure. They were formed according to the anatomy, which was approximated and based on age, sex, degree of atherosclerosis, size and weight.

When the catheter was considered to be in the desired position, i.e. in the vessel to be catheterized, a test injection was made with radiographic documentation using a small amount of contrast medium. Because of the varying anatomy, too small a vessel could have been catheterized, the catheter could have blocked the artery with risk of parenchymal damage by the contrast agent, or a subintimal injection could ensue. Since the poor resolution at conventional screening could not exclude these and other complications, such a test injection was necessary. It was, however, time consuming and could also increase the risk of complications. To reduce these complications, at least in part, a mapping aortography was often performed before proceeding to selective catheterization.

During the first years, the final radiographic documentation at selective angiography was made with a homemade cassette changer, consisting of three cassettes that were shifted manually. Injection of contrast agent was made by hand or with an injector, depending on the vessels undergoing examination. Already in the late fifties, cassette changers and injectors driven by compressed air were available for more sophisticated documentation of the abdominal organs. In the early sixties, image intensifiers and TV became available for catheterization, in addition to simplifications of the catheterization procedure, thus reducing the complications. The consequences were that more manipulations could be performed for superselective technique and for improved diagnostic information. Later on, in the seventies, further advances were made when the interventional procedures were introduced for treatment of various abdominal lesions.

Indications and angiography methods

The number of indications for abdominal angiography increased continuously during the sixties. With increasing experience, the incidence of complications decreased and the referring clinicians became more interested in sending their patients for abdominal angiography, increasing the number of examinations. The reports in the radiological journals soon related the value of selective angiography in abdominal and retroperitoneal lesions and the radiologists made their clinical colleagues aware of the new indications and the improved information obtained with this technique. Obviously, the referring clinicians had to be motivated to use these investigations since they had the ultimate control of sending patients for angiography. Eventually, they accepted this new technique and appreciated the information obtained.

Lumbar aortography was used for the study of primary lesions of the lumbar aorta (atherosclerosis, aortitis, aneurysms) and of the origins of its branches (stenosis, occlusion). As a consequence of these changes, abnormal collateral circulations were defined as well as their importance for hypertension, intestinal angina, and malabsorption. Lumbar aortography was also used for arterial mapping before selective procedures, which followed if the midstream injection of contrast medium did not entirely disclose the expected lesion. In the mid seventies and thereafter, with improving resolution of ultrasonography, computed tomography, and magnetic resonance imaging, the indications for lumbar aortography diminished but is still of importance to verify findings made by the non-invasive methods or to evaluate findings further that are inconclusive.

Selective angiography of the celiac, mesenteric and renal arteries gave so much more information about the abdominal organs when compared to the conventional radiographic methods that there was no reason to perform prospective randomized studies to prove their superiority. With selective abdominal angiography, radiologists were for the first time in a position not only to show lesions in the liver, pancreas, spleen, bowel, kidneys or adrenals but also to show the altered vascular supply in the organs, and in cases of tumors, the abnormal vessels in the tumors. They were also able to define the normal blood flow and show changes in blood flow of the abdominal organs due to primary vascular lesions (atherosclerosis, angiomatous lesions, AV malformations, arteritis) or secondary vascular lesions (tumor infiltration or shunting, inflammatory lesions with aneurysm formation or rupture, traumatic lesions with vessel rupture or occlusion, or degenerative disease with dysplasia and varices). In addition, and most important, was the possibility to define preoperatively the exact site, local and distant extension, and resectability of a lesion.

Superselective angiography

As in all biological material, it was soon observed that the radiological diagnosis was not always correct and in fact sometimes misleading. For instance, a solid tumor could be completely overlooked because an extremely diminished blood supply and the displaced adjacent vessels gave a false impression of a cystic lesion. One reason was the relative limited spatial resolution of the system, which was partly due to the fact that the contrast medium was diluted by the high blood flow through the abdominal blood vessels. This could partly be compensated for by increasing the rate of the injection of contrast medium. There was, however, a limit to this injection technique. Too high an injection rate would cause the catheter to recoil with the tip ending up in the aorta or could deposit the contrast medium subintimally or could even perforated the vessel. To increase the contrast medium concentration in the arteries, the catheter tip could be positioned closer to the organ or lesion to be studied. The catheter was therefore brought further distally into the artery supplying a lesion, thereby reducing the dilution of the contrast medium. Superselective angiography of the hepatic, splenic, gastric, pancreatic, and mesenteric arteries eventually became routine procedures that were particularly important in the diagnosis of hepatic and pancreatic lesions, in accordance with the intentions of Bierman and Tillander in the early fifties [27, 28, 32, 33].

Magnification angiography was another method that became important, particularly in pancreatic and renal disease [34, 35]. Combined with superselective technique, even very small infiltrated arteries could be identified in the otherwise difficult diagnosis of pancreatic carcinoma (Fig. III, 75).

Balloon occlusion angiography was also tested as a method for increased information at angiography but was met with reluctance among angiographers because the hypertonicity and chemo-

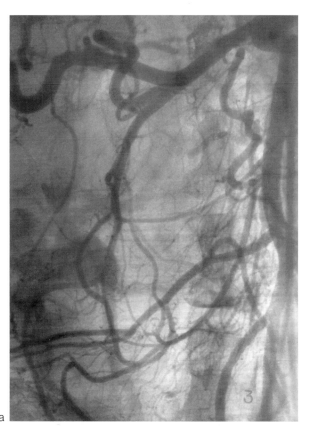
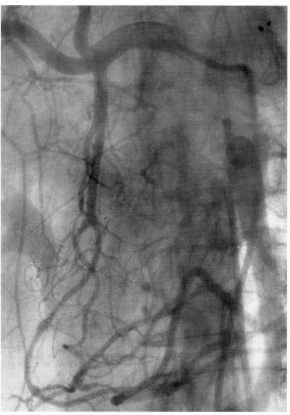

a   b

Fig. III, 75a, b. Magnification angiography (2,5 x) in two patients with small (2–3 cm) carcinoma in the head of the pancreas. **a)** Selective celiac and superior mesenteric angiography with two catheters. **b)** Selective hepatic and superior mesenteric angiography also with two catheters. An abundance of small arteries can be observed in the head of the pancreas and infiltration of some of these small arteries. No tumor vessels were found.

toxicity of the contrast media could cause severe organ destruction if injected into an occluded artery.

Pharmacoangiography with vasoconstrictive substances was another important method used to increase the information about the abdominal arteries. By slowing down the circulation, the contrast medium became less diluted. We performed our first examinations in dogs in 1962 to confirm the effect of adrenaline on the renal circulation [36]. The main intention at that time was to use it later in clinical renal angiography for improved demonstration of the abnormal vasculature in renal tumors. Later on, Abrams [37] confirmed that adrenaline gave better information about renal tumors than angiography without this drug. A number of other investigators followed, showing that also other vasoconstrictors (noradrenaline, angiotensin, vasopressin) had this effect, which sometimes improved the information about renal and renal pelvic tumors. Most important for this information was the fact that the vasoconstriction precluded the accumulation of contrast agent in the renal parenchyma, and therefore the renal arteries as well as the tumor vessels could be better defined. Thus, the fact that the tumor vessels reacted less to vasoconstrictive substances than the normal renal arteries was of less importance for this improvement in contrast resolution.

The vasoconstrictive effect of drugs was also used in the mesenteric and celiac arteries [38]. The various vascular beds all responded with vasoconstriction but in varying degree. The vasoconstrictive drugs were used extensively but how important they were for the final diagnosis has never been fully defined. No doubt, as a complementary to conventional angiography, the technique was in selected cases of great value.

Pharmacoangiography with vasodilating substances injected intra-arterially was also used extensively, but mainly for improved information of the splanchnic veins (see below). Due to the increased blood flow, particularly through the superior mesenteric artery, good arteriographic information was rarely obtained despite the increased rate and amount of injected contrast medium. Nevertheless, the technique could be used to show intestinal extravasation from an intermittently bleeding artery [39].

Abdominal veno- or phlebography

Venography of the inferior vena cava, hepatic and renal veins have always been relatively rare examinations because of the limited indications for their use and for the often incomplete information obtained of the entire hepatic and renal veins. Injection of contrast medium against the blood flow and the varying venous anatomy are the main problems in this respect.

Dos Santos [40] in 1935 was the first to report on inferior cavography performed after the saphenous vein was exposed. The technique, still often used today, was reported in 1947 by O'Loughlin [41]: Needle puncture of the femoral veins, compression of the femoral arteries, and Valsalva maneuver to reduce the flow of blood through the vena cava, and then injection of contrast agent. After the introduction of the Seldinger technique, catheterization of the lower inferior vena cava is often used instead.

For the introduction of catheters into the hepatic and renal veins, Rappaport [19] used in the early fifties the technique from the femoral veins, but later on the percutaneous method with preshaped catheters had become the method of choice. To improve the information, balloon catheters have been used in the inferior vena cava or they have been placed in the hepatic or renal veins. This was found to be rather effective for the hepatic veins, less so for the renal veins. Therefore, renal venography was performed after first blocking the flow in the renal artery by 10 mg adrenaline [42] or by a balloon catheter [43]. For evaluation of renal blood flow in hypertensive patients with renal artery stenosis, renal venography was performed without flow retardation [44].

Venography and cavography were performed mainly in patients who were expected to have thrombus formation, spontaneously or due to tumor invasion, but also in renal and hepatic disease processes that could involve the veins. Today, cavography and venography of the hepatic and renal veins are rarely used for diagnostic purposes since they have been almost completely replaced by the non-invasive methods, particularly duplex Doppler ultrasonography and magnetic resonance imaging.

Venography of the portal system

The portal vein and its tributaries were first examined radiographically by injecting contrast into the surgically exposed mesenteric vein. Then, in the early fifties, both percutaneous splenoportography and transhepatic portography were introduced. Of these, splenoportography became the method of choice for a long period. At that time, the transhepatic technique with a needle and wedge hepatic phlebography with a catheter, usually only gave information of the intrahepatic portal veins, and the mesenteric vein injection required an operation.

Despite the fact that the portal vein and its tributaries could be demonstrated at celiac and superior mesenteric angiography, this information often failed or was incomplete, particularly in patients with portal hypertension where a good venous demonstration was essential. Therefore, splenoportography prevailed for about a decade despite the 1% risk that the patient could have a severe intrahepatic hemorrhage following the procedure. When the superselective technique became available and splenic angiography performed with large amounts of contrast agent gave adequate information about the splenic and portal veins, the number of patients undergoing splenoportography diminished and this technique is rarely used today. For demonstration of the superior mesenteric and portal veins, pharmacoangiography of the superior mesenteric artery with vasodilating drugs became a routine procedure, while these drugs were of little aid at splenic angiography to show the splenic vein. The most commonly used drugs were bradykinin, tolazoline and prostaglandin [45, 46, 47]. Superior mesenteric pharmacoangiography and splenic angiography in combination usually gave adequate information in cirrhosis, portal hypertension and splenic thrombosis.

Twenty years after the first percutaneous portography was performed, the method was reintroduced by Wiechel [48], now with catheters. During the seventies, intense experimental and clinical research was performed not only on transhepatic but also on transumbilical catheterization of the portal venous system. For instance, not only the main stems of the portal vein were catheterized and visualized radiographically, but also the pancreatic veins could be analyzed in detail [49, 50]. Venous sampling became important for hormone assays in patients with endocrine tumors of the pancreas [51] and intestine [52, 53], in the same way as sampling of renin had been performed since 1969.

As a consequence of the transhepatic portal vein technique, the coronary vein was catheterized and occluded in patients with bleeding varices from portal hypertension, a method introduced by Lunderquist [54] in our department. A new approach to treat esophageal and gastric varices with coronary vein occlusion became available. A few years later, it did not turn out to be as effective as expected and trans-esophageal endoscopic obliteration gave better results.

Another completely different technique, transjugular intrahepatic portosystemic shunting, eventually became, in the eighties, an alternative to the operative portocaval shunts, which both in the acute and elective situations were considered to have high cost/benefit value. In 1967, Hanafee [55] had proposed another approach to the portal system, namely via transjugular catheterization. He and Rösch [56] showed experimentally two years later that an intrahepatic shunt could be created between an intrahepatic vein and a portal vein branch. Various techniques to keep the shunts open were tested but it was not until a metallic expandable stent was placed between the two systems that a practical, nonsurgical portocaval shunt had the potential of remaining patent [57]. This method has now been taken up as the primary method to create a portocaval shunt in patients with severe portal hypertension.

Interventional abdominal angiography

A new era in abdominal angiography has come with the so-called interventional technique. Angiography is in itself interventional, but the word stands for something more than just angiography. It is usually a therapeutic procedure with angiographic technique. No doubt the number of indications for angiographic studies have decreased markedly during the last 15–20 years but the interventional technique has given the radiologists new incitements to abdominal angiography. Thanks to the long experience the angiographer has in catheterization of abdominal vessels and due to the new material invented by angiographers in close cooperation with the industry, the radiologists are now in a position to treat patients with new methods. Thus, interventional abdominal angiography is now extensively used for treatment of a number of lesions, which previously needed surgical therapy, with better cost/benefit for both the patient and society.

The scope of this article is not to analyze all the various methods and indications for abdominal interventional angiography. The development has been fairly slow for several reasons. One is the fact that the referring physician with his responsibility for his patient has hesitated to have the radiologist perform a therapeutic procedure that was not scientifically proven to be better than conventional treatment. Since it is almost impossible to prove the superiority of interventional angiography by prospective randomized comparative studies, this slow development has to be accepted. Other reasons for the slow pace in the development of this new technology are the clinicians' reluctance to accept treatment methods he does not fully control, and economic considerations.

Some examples of interventional angiography in the portal circulation have been discussed. Also tumors of the liver and kidneys have been explored with interventional angiography, but so far there is no final answer as to whether or not this method will be used in the future. More successful is the treatment of vascular lesions. For instance, angioplasty of stenosis in the main branches of the lumbar aorta, and occlusion of arteriovenous fistulas, malformations, aneurysms, or vessel ruptures are important therapeutic measures that today are largely accepted by the medical profession. Particularly the difficult diagnosis and poor prognosis of gastrointestinal hemorrhage has been markedly improved thanks to the efforts by angiographers, of which Baum and his collaborators [58, 59] are the most important contributors. Subsequent technical developments, mainly endoscopic therapy, have reduced the importance of vasopressin-induced occlusion of a bleeding site in the bowel. The interventional procedure still prevails even if the original vasopressin method has been replaced with various methods of embolization [60].

Non-invasive abdominal angiography

Abdominal angiography is considered an invasive diagnostic method that causes discomfort and a certain risk even though it is relatively small compared to cerebral and coronary angiography. When intravenous digital subtraction angiography was introduced at the beginning of the eighties, it was hoped that this technique could take over some of the roles of conventional abdominal angiography. However, it was soon realized that intravenous digital subtraction angiography could only be used to visualize large vessels, such as the lumbar aorta and its largest branches. The spatial resolution was inferior and the highly diluted contrast medium, when injected intravenously, could not be enhanced enough despite the higher contrast resolution with digital subtraction. It was realized that intra-arterial digital subtraction angiography was required for adequate information. This means the return to an invasive procedure, but not to the same extent

as previously because smaller catheters as well as lower doses of contrast medium could be used.

When ultrasonography and computed tomography became available in the seventies, these non-invasive techniques replaced a number of angiographic procedures. Magnetic resonance imaging was introduced in the eighties and further reduced the indications for abdominal angiography. Digital subtraction angiography did not reverse this tendency and the number of diagnostic angiographic procedures decreased markedly. The advantage of not using catheters and the result of randomized prospective comparative studies proving that superior information can be obtained with non-invasive techniques paved the way for this new type of imaging of the abdominal organs.

During the last decade, we have seen marked technical improvements in all three non-invasive methods, which can visualize the vessels not only morphologically: they will also provide information of the flow dynamics to the organs. Despite this enormous development in radiology during the last decade, selective abdominal angiography still has an important role to play. No method can compete with the spatial resolution and the comprehensive vascular display achieved with conventional angiography. There is even a certain risk that the radiologist and the clinician rely too much on the information obtained with non-invasive imaging and forget the high information content obtained for small vascular lesions with abdominal angiography. Documentation with conventional angiography or digital subtraction angiography is often required to confirm findings observed with non-invasive imaging, before as well as after interventional angiography.

References

1. Dos Santos, R., A. Lamas, J. Caldas: L'arteriographie des membres, de l'aorte et de ses branches abdominales. Bull. Mem. Soc. Nath. Chir. 55 (1929) 587–601
2. Wagner, F.B. Jr, A.H. Price: Fatality after abdominal arteriography: prevention by now modification of technique. Surgery 27 (1950) 621–626
3. McAfee, J.G.: A survey of complications of abdominal angiography. Radiology 68 (1957) 825–838
4. Henline, R.B., S.W. Moore: Renal arteriography: preliminary report of experimental study. Am. J. Surg. 32 (1936) 222–229
5. Nelson, O.A.: Arteriography of abdominal organs by aortic injection: a preliminary report. Surg. Gynecol. Obstet. 74 (1942) 655–662
6. Wagner, F.B. Jr: Arteriography in renal diagnosis: preliminary report and critical evaluation. J. Urol. 56 (1946) 625

7. Boblitt, D.E., M.M. Figley, E.F. Wolfman Jr: Roentgen signs of contrast material dissection of aortic wall in direct aortography. Am. J. Roentgenol. 81 (1959) 826–834

8. Robb, G.P., I. Steinberg: Visualization of the chambers of the heart, the pulmonary circulation, and the great blood vessels in man. A practical method. Am. J. Roentgenol. 41 (1939) 1–17

9. Farinas, P.L.: A new technique for the arteriographic examination of the abdominal aorta and its branches. Am. J. Roentgenol. 46 (1941) 641–645

10. Seldinger, S.I.: Catheter replacement of the needle in percutaneous arteriography. A new technique. Acta Radiol. 39 (1953) 368–376

11. Idbohm, H.: Tolerance to contrast media in renal angiography. Acta Radiol. 45 (1956) 141–154

12. Rigler, L.G., P.C. Olfelt: Abdominal aortography for the roentgen demonstration of the liver and spleen. Am. J. Roentgenol. 72 (1954) 586

13. Edsman, G.: Malign tumour of the spleen diagnosed by lienal arteriography. Acta Radiol. 42 (1954) 461–464

14. Evans, A.T.: Renal cancer: translumbar arteriography for its recognition. Radiology 69 (1957) 657–662

15. Creevy, C.D., W.E. Price: Differentiation of renal cysts from neoplasms by abdominal aortography. Radiology 64 (1955) 831–839

16. Uson, A.C., M.M. Melicow, J.K. Lattimer: Is renal arteriography (aortography) a reliable test in the differential diagnosis between kidney cysts and neoplasms? J. Urol. 89 (1963) 554–559

17. Bierman, H.R., E.R. Miller, R.L. Byron Jr. et al: Intraarterial catheterization of viscera in man. Am. J. Roentgenol. 66 (1951) 555–568

18. Tillander, H.: Magnetic guidance of a catheter with articulated steel tip. Acta Radiol. 35 (1951) 62–64

19. Rappaport, A.M.: The guided catheterization and radiography of the abdominal vessels. Canad. Med. Ass. J. 67 (1952) 93–100

20. Ödman, P.: Percutaneous selective angiography of the main branches of the aorta (preliminary report). Acta Radiol. 45 (1956) 1–14

21. Edholm, P., S.I. Seldinger: Percutaneous catheterization of the renal artery. Acta Radiol. 45 (1956) 15–20

22. Tillander, H.: Selective angiography of the abdominal aorta with a guided catheter. Acta Radiol. 45 (1956) 21–26

23. Morino, F., A. Tarquini: Cateterismo attraverso l'arteria homerale per l'arteriografia dei rami collaterali dell'aorta addominale. Minerva Med. 47 (1956) 935

24. Schobinger, R., G. Blackman, R.K. Lin: Operative intestinal arteriography. Acta Radiol. 48 (1957) 330–336

25. Boijsen, E., G.L. Feinstein: Arteriographic catheterization techniques. Am. J. Roentgenol. 85 (1961) 1037–1052

26. Hanafee, W.: Axillary artery approach to carotid, vertebral, abdominal aorta, and coronary angiography. Radiology 81 (1963) 559

27. Boijsen, E.: Selective visceral angiography using a percutaneous axillary technique. Br. J. Radiol. 39 (1966) 414–421

28. Boijsen, E.: Selective pancreatic angiography. Br. J. Radiol. 39 (1966) 481–487

29. Becker, G.J., M.E. Hicks, R.W. Holden et al: Screening for occlusive vascular disease with intraarterial DSA. Preliminary experience with a high-flow 4-F catheter. Radiology 153 (1984) 823

30. Lederer, W., W.H. Dingler, J. Gaa et al: Die Wertigkeit des transbrachialen Zugangswegs für die arterielle Gefäßdarstellung unter Verwendung von 4-F-Kathetern. Fortschr. Röntgenstr. 151 (1989) 674

31. Hessel, S.J., D.F. Adams, H.L. Abrams: Complications of angiography. Radiology 138 (1981) 273–281

32. Reuter, S.R.: Superselective pancreatic angiography. Radiology 92 (1969) 74–85

33. Ariyama, J., H. Shirakabe, H. Ikenobe et al: The diagnosis of the small resectable pancreatic carcinoma. Clin. Radiol. 28 (1977) 437–444

34. Takaro, T., S.M. Scott: Angiography using direct roentgenographic magnification in man. Am. J. Roentgenol. 91 (1964) 448–452

35. Boijsen, E., P. Maly: Vergrößerungstechnik in der abdominellen Angiographie. Radiologe 18 (1978) 167–171

36. Abrams, H.L., E. Boijsen, K.E. Borgström: Effect of epinephrine on the renal circulation. Angiographic observations. Radiology 79 (1962) 911–922

37. Abrams, H.L.: The response of neoplastic renal vessels to epinephrine in man. Radiology 82 (1964) 217–224

38. Boijsen, E., H. Redman: Effect of epinephrine on celiac and superior mesenteric angiography. Invest. Radiol. 2 (1967) 184–199

39. Rösch, J., F.S. Keller, A.S. Wawrukiewicz et al: Pharmacoangiography in the diagnosis of recurrent massive lower gastrointestinal bleeding. Radiology 145 (1982) 615–619

40. Dos Santos, R.: Phlebographie d'une veine cave inférieur suture. J. Urol. Med. Chir. 39 (1935) 586

41. O'Loughlin, B.J.H.: Roentgen visualization of the inferior vena cava. Am. J. Roentgenol. 58 (1947) 617

42. Olin, T.B., S.R. Reuter: A pharmacoangiographic method for improving nephrophlebography. Radiology 85 (1965) 1036–1042

43. Georgi, M., M. Marberger, R. Günther et al: Retrograde Nierenphlebographie bei Ballonverschluß der Nierenarterie. Fortschr. Röntgenstr. 123 (1975) 341–347

44. Abrams, H.L., S. Baum, T. Stamey: Renal venous washout time in renovascular hypertension. Radiology 83 (1964) 597–609

45. Boijsen, E., H.C. Redman: Effect of bradykinin on celiac and superior mesenteric angiography. Invest. Radiol. 1 (1966) 422–430

46. Redman, H.C., S.R. Reuter, W.J. Miller: Improvement of superior mesenteric and portal vein visualization with tolazoline. Invest. Radiol. 4 (1969) 24–27

47. Davis, L.J., J.H. Anderson, S. Wallace et al: The use of prostaglandin E1 to enhance the angiographic visualization of the splanchnic circulation. Radiology 114 (1975) 281–286

48. Wiechel, K.L.: Tekniken vid perkutan transhepatisk portapunktion (PTP). Nord. Med. 86 (1971) 912 (in Swedish)

49. Göthlin, J., A. Lunderquist, U. Tylén: Selective phlebography of the pancreas. Acta Radiol. Diagn. 15 (1974) 474–480

50. Hoevels, J., A. Lunderquist, U. Tylén: Percutaneous transhepatic portography. Acta Radiol. Diagn. 19 (1978) 643–655

51. Lunderquist, A., M. Eriksson, S. Ingemansson et al: Selective pancreatic vein catheterization for hormone assay in endocrine tumors of the pancreas. Cardiovasc. Radiol. 1 (1978) 117–124

52. Reichardt, W., S. Ingemansson, A. Lunderquist, A. Nobin: Selective mesenteric phlebography in patients with carcinoid tumors. Gastrointest. Radiol. 4 (1979) 179–189

53. Haber, E., T. Koerner, L.B. Page et al: Application of a radioimmunoassay for angiotensin I to the physiologic measurement of plasma renin activity in normal human subjects. J. Clin. Endocrin. Metab. 29 (1969) 1349

54. Lunderquist, A., J. Vang: Transhepatic catheterization and obliteration of the coronary vein in patients with portal hypertension and esophageal varices. N. Engl. J. Med. 291 (1974) 646

55. Hanafee, W., M. Weiner: Transjugular percutaneous cholangiography. Radiology 88 (1967) 35–39

56. Rösch, J., W.N. Hanafee, H. Snow: Transjugular portal venography and radiologic portocaval shunt: an experimental study. Radiology 92 (1969) 1112–1114

57. Palmaz, J.C., R.R. Sibbit, S.R. Reuter et al: Expandable intrahepatic portacaval shunt stents: early experience in the dogs. Am. J. Roentgenol. 145 (1985) 821–825

58. Nusbaum, M., S. Baum: Radiographic demonstration of unknown sites of gastrointestinal bleeding. Surg. Forum 13 (1963) 374–375

59. Baum, S., M. Nusbaum: The control of gastrointestinal hemorrhage by selective mesenteric arterial infusion of vasopressin. Radiology 98 (1971) 497–505

60. Encarnacion, C.E., S.#Kadir, C.A. Beam, C.S. Payne: Gastrointestinal bleeding: treatment with gastrointestinal arterial embolization. Radiology 183 (1992) 505–508

Heart and coronaries - the pioneering age

J.W. Ludwig

The radiographic examination of the heart with contrast media

Only a few weeks after Roentgen's discovery in 1895, Haschek and Lindenthal [30] applied these new rays to visualize blood vessels. They injected a radiopaque substance into the blood vessels of an amputated hand and published their findings in the *Wiener Klinische Wochenschrift*. This was the first attempt to investigate the vascular system roentgenologically (see fig. III, 96).

It was not until 1910 that a similar report was published. Franck and Alwens [24] described in this year experiments on dogs and rabbits to obtain radiographic images of the heart cavities and major vessels. They injected a suspension of bismuth and oil into a large arm vein and saw this contrast medium travel through the heart and lungs. These experiments did not amount to further development. The next step was not until 1923 when Sicard and Forestier [64] injected 5 ml Lipiodol into the femoral vein of a dog. Under fluoroscopy they witnessed this contrast medium in the right ventricle, where it disintegrated into small droplets that were rapidly transported into the pulmonary arteries, causing multiple small emboli. After 10 min, the droplets of contrast medium could not be seen any more. The animals did not show any symptoms during these investigations. A similar experiment was performed on patients. They injected lipiodol into an arm vein and again saw multiple lung emboli due to the oil-containing contrast medium. Apart from severe coughing, no other symptoms were noted. In 1928, the Italian physician Montanari [44] probed the right side of the heart in an animal; this was followed by an attempt on a human cadaver.

A year later, in 1929, Forssmann (Fig. III, 76) introduced a catheter into a blood vessel, at first in a cadaver and then on himself until he observed, in a mirror placed before the fluoroscopic screen, that the catheter tip was in the right atrium. He took a radiographs of this finding. During this attempt on his own body he did not feel anything unusual. Forssmann's self-experiment had become the beginning of a revolutionary development in medicine, from which many new diagnostic and therapeutic possibilities originated.

In 1931, Forssmann [23] used the catheterization method on dogs to visualize the chambers of the heart. At first, he used a solution of 20% sodium iodide and later 50% Uroselectan. He injected the contrast medium into the right atrium of dogs and produced beautiful images of the contrast-filled right heart and pulmonary vessels. Attempts to take an angiocardiogram of himself, however, failed.

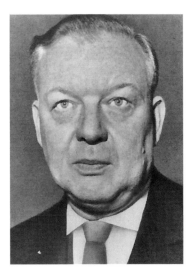

Fig. III, 76. Werner Forssmann (1904–1979). During his medical training, he conceived the idea of self-catheterization of the heart. The significance of his investigation was not immediately (1929) recognized. He turned to surgery. Nobel prize awarded only in 1956. Numerous awards, but none from the German Roentgen Society.

Heart catheterization and angiocardiography hardly developed at all in the years between 1929 and 1932, due to lack of necessary equipment.

In 1931, the Portuguese Moniz and his colleagues injected sodium iodide into rabbits via direct puncture into the right cardiac ventricle and produced an image of the right ventricle and pulmonary vessels. They called this technique angiopneumography [43] and it was used to visualize pulmonary vessels for various anomalies. Subsequently, they changed to a method in which they injected the contrast medium into the jugular veins of animals, and provided satisfactory images of the pulmonary arteries. Finally, they used the catheterization technique according to Forssmann on patients and obtained good images of the central pulmonary vessels. The sodium iodide used was too toxic, but with the organic contrast medium synthesized by Binz and Raeth (Fig. III, 3) [7], the Uroselectan, they could perform less risky experiments.

Diodrast, which was developed later and less toxic, increased the possibilities. This was a breakthrough for the further development of angiocardiography.

In 1933, Rousthöi [57] published his experiences demonstrating the cardiac cavities in animals (Fig. III, 56a). This publication 'Über Angiokardiographie' preceded Ameuille's publication [1] of 1936 in which he described success in demonstrating the right side of the heart in patients by means of Forssmann's method.

In 1937, the Cuban paediatricians Castellanos and coworkers published their work 'La angiocardiographie radio opaca' [14], the first report of a successful angiocardiography, performed on children up to age of six years. Numerous publications on congenital heart diseases followed, primarily describing congenital anomalies of right heart and septal defects. Changes in the pulmonary arteries were also successfully visualized.

Contiades, Ungar and Naulleu [17] showed in a large number of experiments that relatively large amounts of 50% Uroselectan injected intravenously into children only induced minor and quickly passing reactions on breathing and circulation. They injected 10–20 ml in 2 s into a vein of the arms or legs. Apart from children with a ventricular septal defect, they did not succeed in filling the left side of the heart.

In 1938, Robb and Steinberg [56] succeeded in demonstrating the left side of the heart and aorta for the first time, when they injected 20–40 ml of 70% Diodrast intravenously in 2 s.

In 1939, Castellanos and Pereiras [13] introduced retrograde aortography by antegrade injection of a contrast medium into the peripheral arteries of the arm and thus succeeding in filling the aorta. In 1940, Farinas advanced the tip of a radiopaque catheter from the femoral artery to the thoracic aorta and produced beautiful radiographs of the aorta after injecting a contrast medium.

Cournand, Ranges and Richards published in 1941 their first examinations of the circulation using catheterization of the heart and introduced this method for clinical investigations.

In 1947, Chávez, Dorbecker and Celis [16] described guided angiography in which they advanced a catheter through a vein into the right heart and pulmonary artery. A few years later, they advanced a catheter from an artery into the left ventricle to inject a contrast medium. Joensson and coworkers [32] applied the method of selective angiography more often in the following years.

In 1951, Ponsdomenec and Nunez [51] recommended the percutaneous selective technique by percutaneous puncture of the left ventricle. They obtained excellent images with this technique. Other entries to the left ventricle, such as transbronchial and transthoracic punctures, had also been tried by Morrow and Bjoerk. But with the introduction of the percutaneous transfemoral catheterization technique, described by Seldinger in 1953 (Fig. III, 62) [62], the catheterization via the femoral artery was clearly the superior technique for angiocardiography, from its technical aspect as well as from its low complications rate. The catheterization method via a peripheral vein or artery to reach the right or left side of the heart had finally become the favored method of visualizing the heart radiographically. Since then, the number of investigations and publications on angiocardiography of both congenital and acquired changes has become extraordinarily large.

In context with the congenital conditions, the names of Helen B. Taussig [70], Shinebourne [63], Elliot [21], Keith [35], Edward, Schad and Amplatz should be mentioned, and in context with the acquired conditions, such as valvular deformities, the name of Chaillet [15] among others. As to coronary artery diseases, the names of Sones, Proudfit and Bruschke deserve mention.

The development of modern imaging techniques, such as echography, computed tomography and magnetic resonance imaging, has rendered the application of angiocardiography superfluous in certain fields. Nevertheless, angiography still holds its place in diagnosing pathological changes.

The radiographic investigation of pulmonary vessels with contrast medium

The first investigations of the pulmonary artery by injecting radiographic contrast media, either via veins or into the right atrium, have already been mentioned.

It was not until 1951 that Bolt and coworkers [9] described selective pulmonary angiography with visualization of the vessels in the pulmonary periphery. A satisfactory assessment of the peripheral pulmonary vessels was not possible by angiocardiography because of dilution of the contrast medium. Furthermore, the simultaneous filling of all pulmonary arteries resulted in a superimposition of vessels, interfering with their assessment. In selective catheterization, the catheter is advanced through the right atrium and the right ventricle into the right or left pulmonary artery or smaller branches, achieving a good visualization of the corresponding vascular region with a relatively small amount of contrast medium. The most important indications for pulmonary angiography are the diagnosis of vascular anomalies, both congenital and acquired, and the confirmation of lung emboli, as well as the evaluation of pulmonary changes in pathological processes, when surgery is contemplated.

At first, angiography of the pulmonary artery and its branches had been performed with very simple equipment. A major improvement was the introduction of the fully automatic cut-film changer. Later, this radiographic technique was supplemented by cineangiography for the diagnosis of lung emboli and other conditions. This technique combined with the selective injection into a branch of the pulmonary artery through a balloon catheter, as described by Ferris and coworkers [22], became a very effective method of obtaining an accurate diagnosis.

Digital subtraction angiography combined with ECG-triggered radiographs, developed during the last few years, contributed to further refinement of the technique used for diagnosing pulmonary emboli. With intravenous injection of contrast medium (Fig. III, 77) into an arm vein or the right atrium, good results, compared to the cut-film changer, can be obtained, as described by Pond and coworkers [50] and Piers and coworkers [49]. Emboli in smaller than third-order pulmonary branches could, however,

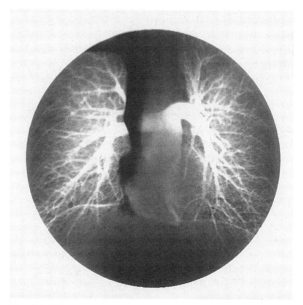

Fig. III, 77. Intravenous injection of contrast medium and ECG-triggered image to visualize the pulmonary arteries. No changes on either side.

remain undetected. Digital subtraction angiography was also performed by selective injection through catheters in the pulmonary artery or in one of its branches, among others by Goodman and coworkers [25] and Snijder. While adequate image quality was achieved, no definite conclusion about the optimal method of visualizing pulmonary emboli can presently be given. Further evaluation is needed here.

With intra-arterial digital subtraction angiography (DSA), the images are immediately at one's disposal and less contrast medium needs to be injected because of the system's high contrast resolution. The use of DSA has great advantages in the recently developed treatments for vascular anomalies of the lungs such as arteriovenous fistula. Using this new radiographic technique for the catheter embolization of these vascular changes offers a higher degree of safety and can achieve better results.

Radiographic investigation of the coronary arteries with contrast media

In 1928, Moniz described the technique of carotid angiography and its use in determining cerebral changes. Cerebral angiography, like angiography of other vascular regions, had made considerable progress, but visualization of the coronary arteries lagged behind and remained less developed in the early phases of angiography since good, nontoxic contrast media were not available. Furthermore, surgical treatment of angina pectoris was still unknown.

In 1933, Rousthöi [57] had made the first attempt to visualize the coronary arteries (Fig. III, 56). He did this on rabbits by introducing a catheter via the right common carotid artery until the tip was in the ascending aorta. The coronary arteries became partially and faintly recognizable after the injection of the contrast medium Thorotrast. Reboul and Racine [54] made similar animal experiments in the same year, but with only mediocre results.

In 1942, Castellanos and Pereiras were able to demonstrate the left coronary artery via the femoral artery in a nearly mature sheep embryo by means of retrograde angiography.

In 1945, Radner [53] could radiographically visualize the human coronary arteries *in vivo* for the first time. This was performed on five patients with an injection of contrast-medium into the aorta via a transsternal puncture, applying a technique used first in 1936 by Nuvoli [46] in a patient with an aneurysm of the thoracic aorta.

Hoyes and del Campo [31] obtained vague images of the coronary arteries in three of seven patients given contrast medium into the ascending aorta via an intercostal puncture. All of these attempts to visualize the coronaries were, however, not very successful. In 1950, Gordon [26] performed a follow-up examination on 1200 angiograms in which the contrast medium had been injected intravenously into a cubital vein, with very slight contrast visible in one or both coronary arteries in only 10 patients. In 48 patients, Di Guglielmo and Guttadauro injected the contrast medium intravenously into an arm vein but were not able to visualize a single coronary artery. Visualization of the coronary arteries seemed to have adequate results only when the contrast medium concentration was high in the aortic bulbus.

In 1952, Di Guglielmo and Guttadauro [18] published the results of coronary investigations on 159 patients after administering the contrast medium through a catheter via the brachial artery into the aorta. The best results were obtained when the catheter tip was in the middle third of the ascending aorta. In 70% of the cases, an image of partially filled coronary arteries had been obtained.

Sloman and Jefferson [65] obtained good images of the coronary arteries in 1960 in dogs by injecting rather high doses of contrast medium into the left ventricle. Lehman [37] per-

formed transthoracic ventriculography on 230 patients and in most cases mitral valve defects were identified. In 202 successful examinations, only 7% showed both coronaries. In most cases these poor results were caused by reflux into the left atrium, leaving a markedly diluted contrast medium for the coronary arteries.

In 1960, Joensson and Helstrom [33] injected the contrast medium into the left ventricle of a few patients. They used a catheter via the brachial artery, producing a satisfactory filling of the coronary arteries. However, a good assessment of the quality of these vessels was not possible, in part due to the superimposed left ventricle, which was also filled with contrast medium. Lehmann and coworkers [38] surmounted this superimposition by a suprasternal puncture of the aorta and an injection of contrast medium above the aortic valves. The coronary arteries were well visualized in approximately 10% of the cases.

Many other methods were tried to increase filling of the coronary arteries to enhance their visualization, ultimately to improve their diagnostic evaluation. The most important were:

- Methods to increase inflow of blood into the coronary arteries. According to Gregg and coworkers [27], this could be accomplished by decreasing cardiac output, increasing aortic pressure and reducing the heart rate, resulting in a relatively longer diastole and increasing the coronary filling which mainly takes place during diastole.
  - Unschel and Roth [74] injected the contrast medium during the diastole into the aortic root. Schad and coworkers [36, 58, 59, 60] developed a high-pressure injector, allowing phase-triggered injections into the aortic root. During two or three consecutive diastolic periods, the contrast medium was injected, visualizing all coronary arteries. Contrast medium was injected during diastole at 20 ml per cardiac cycle. This remarkably improved the results in comparison with the continuous injection.
  - Other methods for better coronary filling were developed by Brofman [10] and Elder, Haight and coworkers [29] and Templeton and coworkers [71]. They all resulted in usable images but were too complicated. The Dotter and Frische [19] method, which reduced the left ventricular output and induced a short asystole by acetylcholine injections, was too elaborate and risky.
- Methods of increased intrabronchial pressure, based on Boerema and Blickman's [8] experiments of inducing better coronary filling.

Nordenstroem [45] used this technique of increased intrabronchial pressure under total anesthesia. Here the aortic root was injected with 1 ml contrast medium (Urografin 76%) per kg body weight. This gave reasonable results in 430 patients but this technique was abandoned because of its inconvenience (anesthesia!) and future developments.

– Gregg and Sabiston [28] discovered that the coronary arteries could fill better during a short asystole. They attained this by injecting acetylcholine. A minor dilution occurred when the contrast medium was injected during this period, producing an enhanced visualization of the coronary arteries.

Arnuff and Buffaard [3] applied this method and injected 50 ml contrast medium (Vasurise 76%) via a catheter into the aortic root over 3–4 s. The coronary arteries of 24 patients were examined without serious adverse reaction, but the individual reaction to acetylcholine varied greatly and normal sinus rhythm did not always return spontaneously. Using the same method, Sloman and Jefferson administered atropine immediately after the contrast-medium injection, while Bilgutay and Lillehei [6] attached a pacemaker before the acetylcholine injection. Other disadvantages of the method were that radiographs of the vessels could not be obtained in various stages of the cardiac cycle, which is a requisite for an adequate assessment. Furthermore, since the radiographs could not be repeated in different projections, this method was entirely abandoned.

– Methods in which the contrast medium was injected, where possible, before the coronary orifices:

• Injection via a special catheter: the rate of blood flow is lower along the wall of a vessel than in the centre. Ohlsson [47] found that the flow rate in the distal part of the ascending aorta was less, and during some phase in the cycle even retrograde. Bellman [5] designed a catheter, later improved by Paulin [48], with a distal end that was ring-shaped and had side holes. Through this catheter 40–50 ml contrast medium (Urografin 76%) was administered. The radiographs produced were excellent. The investigation was successful in 228 of 234 patients. Duex [20], and Tsuzuki [73] also applied this technique to their patients successfully. Later developments have completely superseded this method too.

• Injection of contrast medium into the coronary sinus of the ascending aorta by means of a catheter, with the catheter tip placed exactly in front of the orifice of the coronary artery. Miller and coworkers [42] used this method on dogs, and Sones [67] on 137 patients in 1958. Contrast medium (20–30 ml Hypaque 76% per injection) was administered over approximately 5 s. The coronary arteries were well visualized in 90% of cases. Even this technique was later abandoned in favor of selective injection into the coronary arteries.

– Contrast-medium injections by means of a catheter selectively introduced into the right or left coronary artery. In 1958, Sones [66, 67] injected a contrast bolus into the right coronary artery by accident and produced an excellent image. He had injected 20 ml of contrast medium with the high pressure injector. The patient did not suffer any complications. Afterwards, Sones developed coronary angiography. As early as 1966, he had reported his examinations on 4200 patient with 35 000 angiograms of the coronary arteries. He used a specially designed catheter that was introduced through the brachial artery into the origin of the right or left coronary artery. Shortly afterwards, this method was introduced in a number of radiology departments throughout the USA, (by Lehman [37, 38], Judkins and Amplatz [2] among others) and was copied in Europe by Bruschke [11] and Lichtlen [39]. Judkins (Fig. III, 78) [34] had developed two different catheters to probe the left or the right coronary artery separately. In the meantime, catheters were inserted using the Seldin-

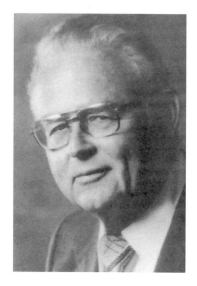

Fig. III, 78. Melvin P. Judkins (1922–1985). General practitioner until 1960, then interest in radiology. Under the influence of Charles Dotter and Mason Sones, he developed a method to catheterize the coronary arteries with special catheters.

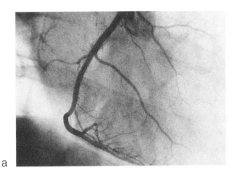
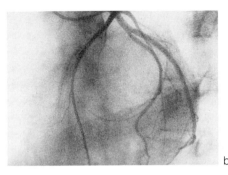

a

b

Fig. III, 79a, b. a) Normal right coronary artery in right oblique projection. **b)** Normal left coronary artery in left oblique projection (1976).

ger technique (into the femoral artery in the groin; Fig. III, 62) and not via the brachial artery. Subsequently, the catheters went through a series of slight modifications (Fig. III, 68), but selective coronary angiography as described and improved by Sones, Lichtlen [40], Bruschke and Ludwig [12] (Fig. III, 79) became the coronary imaging method, and is now used throughout the world in the examination of cardiac patients.

In the beginning, no adequate equipment was available to document angiographic radiographs and much development was necessary before today's image quality could be obtained.

In 1938, Robb and Steinberg [56] measured the mean circulation time before the injection of contrast medium, to determine the optimum time interval for taking the radiographs. This was limited to two or three radiographs with each injection with the equipment of those days. The equipment consisted of a Bucky table, holding the radiographic film that had to be changed

quickly. The ability to take more radiographs over a shorter period was paramount, to visualize both anatomical structures and functional changes.

In the course of time, two main imaging systems, the direct and indirect methods, were developed. The radiographs in the direct method were projected onto film by direct exposure. Its high resolution was its greatest advantage, revealing many details. The degree of contrast resolution was relatively low, and large amounts of contrast medium had to be injected to obtain a good image. One of the great merits of Ziedses des Plantes was his introduction of the photographic subtraction technique. Its higher contrast resolution results in more recognizable details and requires a smaller amount of contrast medium.

The development of X-ray tubes with rotation anode (Bouwers, 1929) was necessary for the exposure of a film-screen combination, which was rather insensitive at the time and produced a relatively grainy image. Radiation output had in-

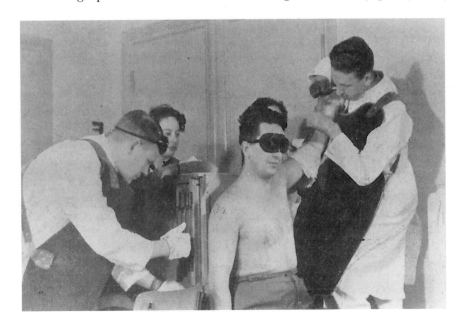

Fig. III, 80. Angiocardiography to demonstrate pulmonary arteries by means of a manual cassette changer (Koch).

creased by a factor of 10 and the thermic properties had also improved. This resulted in shorter exposure times and more exposures in quick succession. A great number of systems were developed to change radiographic films rapidly.

In 1934, Pezieras and Caldas designed their cassette-changing mechanism (Radiocarousel) and subsequently many other investigators, working in the field of experimental angiography, developed other rapid film changers, with frequencies of two to 12 films per second. In 1943, Schwarzschild [61] built a cassette changer for cassettes in the size of 35 x 35 cm, which could take a radiograph every one second. This changer was manually operated and the principle was later improved by the Dutch roentgenologist Oefner and described thoroughly in Swieringa's thesis [69]. Until 1960 (Fig. III, 80), this changer was used for pulmonary angiography. In 1951, Rethmeier [55] built a fully automatic system, that also recorded the exposure time and concurrent electrocardiogram.

Thomson, Figley and Hodges [72] designed in 1949 an automatic roll-film apparatus for the size 25 x 35 cm, achieving a frequency of five exposures per second. This size was not suitable for pulmonary vessels because of its small field size. In 1948, Axén and Lind [4] of the Swedish Elema-Schoenander company had the initiative to develop this system into a proper operating automatic apparatus, which took two films per second in two projections. Its use in angiocardiography facilitated not only examination of the anatomy and dynamics of the heart, but also of individual cardiac segments. After a series of improvements, six radiographs could be taken per second simultaneously in two projections (Fig. III, 66). This system was used for the diagnostic evaluation of the entire heart and pulmonary vascularity, but less for coronary angiography, and then only by Judkins [34] and Nordenstroem. Almost from the beginning, the radiographic documentation of these vessels was by the indirect method.

In the indirect method, the X-ray image on a fluorescent screen is photographed via a lens or reflex camera, producing an image that is much reduced in size. The initially built systems required magnifying projection of the individual images for interpretation. The advantage of the indirect method was the higher image frequency.

In 1937, Stewart, Hoffman and Ghiselin [68] took cinematographic images during an experiment with a fast-flowing liquid contrast medium. The result was bad, the image details limited. In the early fifties, the next development was documentation with very sensitive cameras such as the Bouwer's 'Odelca' reflex camera (see fig. V, 14), which took four photographs per second with an image size of 7 x 7 cm in two projections simultaneously. The spatial resolution was approximately 30 lines per millimeter. The contrast resolution, however, was not high, but could be improved with the aid of the subtraction method. This recording technique was used for angiography in a few clinics and had been described by Vlassenroot [75] among others (Fig. III, 81).

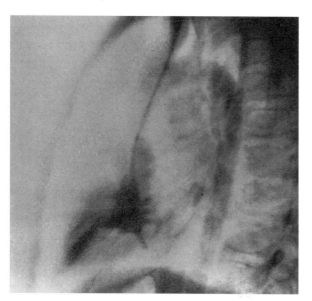 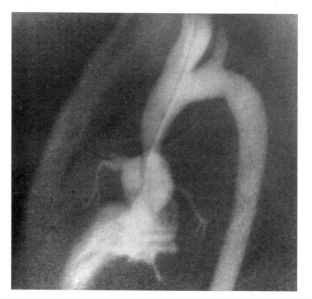

Fig. III, 81a, b. Lateral view in angiocardiography with "Odelka" camera. **a)** Barely visible supravalvular aorta stenosis in an eleven-year-old patient (injection of 20 ml 80% Diagnost via a catheter in the left ventricle). **b)** Photographic subtraction of photograph a). The supravalvular aorta stenosis is obvious, as well as slight filling of the coronary arteries.

The optical image intensifier, introduced in the early fifties, was of great importance for the practical application of coronary angiography, both for the fluoroscopic and radiographic techniques (Fig. III, 67). Without image intensifier, the position of the catheter, particularly in selective methods, would have been almost impossible. The first radiographic image intensifiers had to be operated with mirror systems, which restricted the examiner to a particular area.

Adding a television system to the image intensifier gave the examiner more freedom of movement, which was of particular importance for projections other than the anteroposterior projection. Recording images by cinematography was realized in practice only after the image intensifier had become available. In the sixties, the possibility of pulsed exposure was developed, which reduced the exposure time per image independently of the shutter speed of the camera. As a result of the pulse technique, the patients's radiation exposure time and the necessary radiation of the X-ray tube were almost halved. Up to 200 images per second could be taken with a 16-mm camera. A frequency of 50 photographs per second is considered very good for the clinical investigation of the heart and coronary vessels.

Electronic subtraction of images had already begun in the late fifties. A 'memory reel' on magnetic tape with several tracks had been developed. On each track, one-half of a television image could be recorded. Image 1 was subtracted from image 10, image 2 from 11, etc. The system could be applied for cerebral angiography since the immobilization of the patient's head avoided motion artifacts. The arterial phase was imaged in red, the venous phase in blue. The subtraction was analogous and was displayed during international radiological congresses in Munich (1959) and Montreal (1963). This system did not last long, however, because of unsatisfactory image quality.

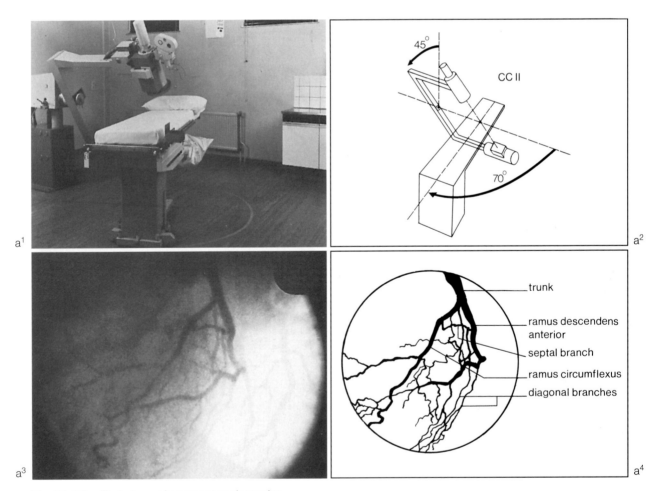

Fig. III, 82a. Technique of coronary angiography.
a¹) and a²) Position of table and U-arm with X-ray tube and image intensifier in craniocaudal projection. a³) Left coronary artery in craniocaudal projection. a⁴) Schematic drawing of c.

A few years previously, attempts had been made to improve the image details of cinematographic images by means of a 'harmonizer'. This required taking a contact print from an original 35-mm film on a fine-grained film with high gradation, which was accomplished by a 'flying spot scanner'. The result was an edge-enhancement that made the image look like a pen-and-ink drawing. Chaillet (1954) initiated the investigations, but the development was not continued because of an increase in image artifacts. The spatial and contrast resolution had been increased in the seventies and eighties due to optimization of the systems, and relatively small amounts of contrast medium were needed to visualize the cardiac chambers and valves well. The small amount of contrast medium required for selective coronary angiography made it possible to take successive radiographs in multiple different projections.

The development of equipment capable of producing not only frontal, lateral and in-between projections, but also caudocranial and craniocaudal projections was decisive to obtain optimal radiographic images of the coronary arteries in their entire length parallel to image plane (Fig. III, 82). Finally, anatomical changes could be established upon reviewing images both in static and dynamic view. Powerful computers gave a new impetus to image processing. The DSA is a new step in noise reduction and image manipulation, and also improves coronary arteriography.

But there were other options. In addition to the determination of ventricular volume, displacement of the ventricular wall was better detectable. Moreover, radiographs in two planes provide three-dimensional information. In this manner, the cross-section at the site of a stenosis of the artery could be detected and its proportional narrowing assessed. This digital processing has also been applied for coronary angiography, and has led to further improvement of diagnostic radiology (Fig. III, 83).

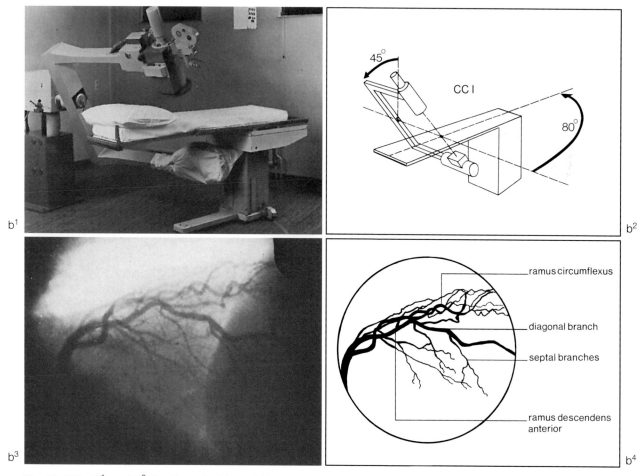

Fig. III, 82b. b^1) and b^2) Position of table and U-arm with X-ray tube and image intensifier in caudocranial projection. b^3) Left coronary artery in caudocranial projection. b^4) Schematic drawing of c.

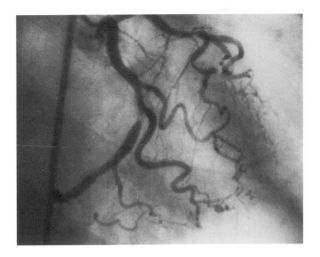

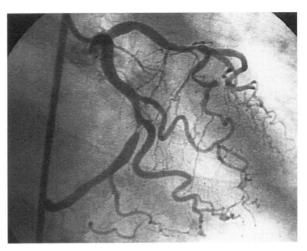

Fig. III, 83a, b. Cinematographic visualization of left coronary artery, conventional and digital processing. **a)** Conventional processing. Stenosis of circumflex and anterior descending arteries.

Fig. III, 83b. The same as in figure a. but after digital processing. Degree of stenosis can be assessed more accurately.

The modern treatment methods of angina pectoris or cardiac infarction, by means of coronary surgery or angioplasty, could not have developed without modern angiocinematography.

References

1. Ameuille, P., G. Ronneaux, V. Hinault, Desgrez, J.M. Lemoine: Remarques sur quelques cas d'artériographie pulmonaire chez l'homme vivant. Bull. Mem. Soc. Med. Hop. Paris 52 (1936) 729

2. Amplatz, K., G. Formanek, P. Stanger, W. Wilson: Mechanics of selective coronary artery catheterization via femoral approach. Radiology 89 (1967) 1040

3. Arnulf, G., P. Buffard: Die Arteriographie der Koronarien mittels Azetylcholin. Fortschr. Röntgenstr. 92 (1960) 115

4. Axén, O., J. Lind: A table for routine angiocardiography. Synchronous serial röntgenography in two planes at right angles. J. Am. Med. Ass. 143 (1950) 540

5. Bellman, S., H.A. Frank, P.B. Lambert, S. Littmann, J.A. Williams: Coronary arteriography. Differential opacification of the aortic stream by catheters of special design, experimental development. N. Engl. J. Med. 262 (1960) 325

6. Bilgutay, A.M., C.W. Lillehei: A new method for coronary arteriography. Acethylcholine with controlled return of heart rate using a cardiac pacemaker. J. Am. Med. Ass. 180 (1962) 1095

7. Binz, A., C. Raeth: Über biochemische Eigenschaften von Derivaten des Pyridins und Chinolins. Biochem. Z. 203 (1928) 218

8. Boerema, J., J.R. Blickman: Reduced intrathoracic circulation as an aid in angiography. The Journal of Thoracic Surgery 30 (1955) 129

9. Bolt, W., W. Forssmann, H. Rink: Selektive Lungenangiographie in der praeoperativen Diagnostik und in der inneren Klinik. Ed. G. Thieme Verlag, 1957

10. Brofman, B.L., J.C. Elder: Cardioaortic fistula. Temporary circulatory occlusion as an aid in diagnosis. Circulation 16 (1957) 77

11. Bruscke, A.V.G.: The diagnostic significance of the coronary arteriogram. Thesis, Groningen 1970

12. Bruschke, A.V.G., J.W. Ludwig: Craniocaudal projections in coronary arteriography. In: coronary angiography and angina pectoris by P.R. Lichtlen. Ed.: Thieme Publishers, Stuttgart 1976

13. Castellanos, A., R. Pereiras: Counter-current aortography. Rev. Cuba. Cardiol. 2 (1939) 187

14. Castellanos, A., R. Pereiras, A. García: La angiocardiografia radio-opaca. Arch. Soc, Estud. Clin. (Habana) 31 (1937) 523

15. Chaillet, J.L.: Cineradiography of cardiac valves in man. Thesis, Utrecht 1965.

16. Chávez, I., N. Dorbecker, A. Celis: Direct intracardiac angiocardiography: Its diagnostic value. Am. Heart J. 33 (1947) 560

17. Contiades, Ungar et Nauleau J.: Recherches expérimentales sur l'action vasculaire des produits de contraste en artériographie. Presse méd. 14 octobre 1935

18. Di Gluglielmo, L., M. Guttadauro: A roentgenologic study of the coronary arteries in the living. Acta Radiol. (1952) Suppl. 97

19. Dotter, C.T., L.H. Frische, W.S. Hoskinson, E. Kawashima, R.W. Phillips: Coronary arteriography during induced cardiac arrest and aortic occlusion. Arch. of Int. Med. 104 (1959) 720

20. Düx A.: Koronarographie. Methodik, Indikation und Ergebnisse. G. Thieme Verlag, Stuttgart 1967

21. Elliot, L.P., L.M. Bargeron, P.R. Bream, B. Soro, G.C. Curry: Axial cineangiography in congenital heart disease. Section II: Special lesions. Circulation 56: 1084–1093

22. Ferris, E.J., P.L. Smith, W.N. Lim, J.L. Whittle, C.B. Bice, T. Angtuaco: Radionuclide-guided balloon occlusion pulmonary cineangiography: An adjunct to pulmonary arteriography. 1978–1980

23. Forssmann, W.: Über Kontrastdarstellung der Höhlen des lebenden rechten Herzens und der Lungenschlagader. München. Med. Wschr. 78 (1934) 489

24. Franck, O., W. Alwens: Kreislaufstudien am Röntgenschirm. Münch. med. Wschr. 51 (1910) 950

25. Goodman, P.C., M. Brant-Zawadszki: Digital substraction pulmonary angiography. Am. J. Roentgenol. 139 (1982) 305–309

26. Gordon, A.J., S.A. Brahms, M.L. Sussman: Visualization of the coronary circulation during angiocardiography. Am. Heart J. 39 (1950) 114

27. Gregg, D.E.: Coronary circulation in health and disease. Lea and Febiger. Philadelphia, 1950.

28. Gregg, D.E., D.C. Sabiston: Current research and problems of the coronary circulation. Circulation 13 (1956) 916

29. Haight, C., M.M. Figley, W.J. Ellsworth, H. Sloan, J.A. Meyer, M.S. Bert, D.E. Boblitt: Experimental coronary arteriography. The effects of some modifications of the circulation. The Journal of surgical research 2 (1962) 7

30. Haschek, E., O.T. Lindenthal: A contribution to the practical use of the photography according to Röntgen. Wien. Klin. Wschr. 9 (1896) 63

31. Hoyos, J.M., C.G. del Campo: Angiography of the thoracic aorta and coronary vessels. Radiology 50 (1950) 211

32. Jönsson, G., B. Brodén, J. Karnell: Selective angiography. Acta Radiol. (Stockh) 32 (1948) 186

33. Jönsson, G., L. Hellstrom: Roentgenographic demonstration of the coronary arteries. Acta Radiol. 53 (1960) 273

34. Judkins, M.P.: Selective coronary arteriography. Radiology 89 (1967) 815

35. Keith, J.D., R.D. Rowe, P. Vlad: Heart disease in infancy and childhood. Ed.: MacMillar, New York.

36. Künzler, R., N. Schad: Atlas der Angiokardiographie: angeborener Herzfehler. Ed.: G. Thieme Verlag, Stuttgart.

37. Lehman, J.S.: Coronary arteriography. Practical considerations. Progress Cardiovascular diseases 2 (1960) 36

38. Lehman, J.S., R.A. Boyer, F.S. Winter: Coronary arteriography. Am. J. Roentgenol. 81 (1959) 749

39. Lichteln, P.: Zur Indikation des selektiven Koronarographie. Schweiz. Med. Wschr. 97 (1967) 195

40. Lichteln, P.: Coronary angiography and angina pectoris. Ed.: Thieme Publishers, Stuttgart 1976

41. Ludwig, J.W.: Coronariografie. Thesis, Amsterdam 1969

42. Miller, E.W., W.J. Kolff, C.R. Hughes: Angiography of the coronary arteries in dogs. During perfusion with a heart lung machine in combination with cardiac arrest in coronary artery surgery. Cleveland Clinic Quarterly 24 (1957) 123

43. Moniz, E., L. de Carvalho, A. Lima: Angiopneumographie. Presse Med. 53 (1931) 996

44. Montanari, A.: Zur Sondierung des Gefäszsystems. Bemerkungen zu den Arbeiten von Forssmann. Klin. Wschr. 9 (1930) 501

45. Nordenström, B.: Contrast examination of the cardiovascular system during increased intrabronchial pressure. Acta Radiol. Suppl. 200

46. Nuvoli, I.: Arteriografia dell'aorta toracica mediante punctura dell'aorta ascendente o del ventricolos. Policlinico (Prat.) 43 (1936) 227

47. Ohlsson, N.M.: Left heart and aortic blood flow in the dog. Precision motion analysis of high speed cinefluorographic recordings. Acta Radiol. (1962) Suppl. 213

48. Paulin, S.: Coronary angiography, technical, anatomic and clinical study. Acta Radiol. (1964) Suppl. 233

49. Piers, B.P., F. Verzijlbergen, C.J.J. Westermann, J.W. Ludwig: A comparitive study of intravenous digital substraction angiography and ventilation perfusionscan in suspected pulmonary embolisms. Chest 91 (1987) 837–843

50. Pond, G.D., T.W. Ovitt, M.B. Capp: Comparison of conventional pulmonary angiography with intravenous digital subtraction angiography for pulmonary embolic disease. Radiology 147 (1983) 345

51. Ponsdomeneck, E.R., V.B. Nunez: Heartpuncture. Am. Heart J. 41 (1951) 643

52. Proudfit, W.L., E.K. Shirey, W.C. Shelton, F.M. Sones: Certain clinical characteristics correlated with extent of obstructive lesions demonstrated by selective coronary arteriography. Circulation 38 (1968) 947

53. Radner, S.: An attempt at the rontgenologic visualization of coronary blood vessels in man. Acta Radiol. 26 (1945) 497

54. Reboul, H., M. Racine: La ventriculographie cardiaque expirimentale. Presse Méd. 1 (1933) 763

55. Rethmeier, B.L.: Een toestel voor angiocardiographie. Nederlands Tijdschrift voor Geneeskunde 47 (1951) 3493

56. Robb, G.P., I. Steinberg: A practical method of visualization of chambers of the heart, the pulmonary circulation, and the great blood vessels in man. J. Clin. Invest. 17 (1938) 507

57. Rousthöi, P.: Über Angiokardiographie. Vorläufige Mitteilung. Acta Radiol. 14 (1933) 419

58. Schad, N., R. Künzler, T. Onat: Differential diagnosis of congenital heart disease. Georg Thieme Verlag, Stuttgart 1958

59. Schad, N., J.P. Stuck, J. Wellauer: Die Angiokardiographie durch intermittierende Kontrastmittelinjektion. Dtsch. Röntgenkongr., Teil A (1966) 216

60. Schad, N., J.P. Stuck, J. Wellauer: Die intermittierende Phasengesteuerte Kontrastmittelinjektion in das Herz. Fortschr. Röntgenstr. 102 (1965) 619

61. Scharzschild, M.M.: Multiple cassette-changer for angiocardiography. Radiology 40 (1943) 72

62. Seldinger, S.I.: Catheter replacement of needle in percutaneous arteriography: New technique. Acta Radiol. (Stockholm) 39 (1953) 368

63. Shinebourne, E.A., F.J. Macartney, R.H. Anderson: Sequential chamber localisations logical approach to diagnosis in congenital heart disease. Br. Heart J. 38; 327–340

64. Sicard, J.A., G. Forestier: Injections intravasculaires d'huile iodée sous controle radiologique. C.R. Soc. Biol. (Paris) 88 (1923) 1200

65. Sloman, G., K. Jefferson: Cine-angiography of the coronary circulation in living dogs. Br. Heart J. 22 (1960) 54

66. Sones, F.M. Jr., E.K. Shirey: Cine coronary arteriography. Mod. Conc. Cardiovasc. Dis. 31 (1962) 735

67. Sones F.M., E.K. Shirey, W.L. Proudfit, R.N. Westcott: Cine coronary arteriography. Circulation 20 (1959) 773

68. Stewart, W.H., W.J. Hoffman, F.H. Ghiselin: Cinefluorography. Am. J. Roentgenol. 38 (1937) 465

69. Swieringa, J.: Intrapulmonale bronchuscysten. Academisch proefschrift, Utrecht 1952. Scheltema en Holkema, Amsterdam.

70. Taussig, H.B.: Congenital malformations of the heart. Ed.: Harvard University Press, Cambridge 1960.

71. Templeton, J.Y., R.R. Greening, C. Fineberg, P.G. Peter, J.R. Griffith, C.L. Reese, D.L. Clark, S. Wallace: Inflow occlusion for coronary arteriography: experimental comparison with other methods. Journal of thoracic and cardiovascular surgery 46 (1963) 818

72. Thompson, W., M. Figley, F.J. Hodges: Full cycle angiocardiography. Radiology 53 (1949) 729

73. Tsuzuki, M., H. Kiefer, H. Reindell: Erfahrungen mit der Koronararteriographie nach der Paulinschen Methode. Med. Klin. 62 (1967) 1118

74. Urschel, H.C., E.J. Roth: Coronary arteriography. A new electronically controlled method. IXth. International Congress of Radiology, 1959, München.

75. Vlassenroot, G.E.: Toepassing van de subtractie methode bij de kleinbeeld-angiocardiografie. Thesis, Amsterdam, 1961

Heart and coronaries - evolution of digital angiocardiography

P.H. Heintzen

Motivation

The tremendous progress in cardiovascular surgery that has taken place over the last few decades has increased the requirements for preoperative and postoperative diagnosis to such a degree that even highly sophisticated X-ray cinematography with its excellent spatial, temporal and contrast resolution is unable to answer satisfactorily all questions arising in clinical practice.

Today, it is mandatory not only to 'display' the correct anatomical structure of complex, congenital cardiac defects, even in newborns, but also to clarify the functional consequences of congenital defects, valvular heart diseases or vascular diseases in various organ systems (especially in the coronary circulation) with regard to their prognosis and indications for surgery.

Subjective criteria of evaluation are therefore in many cases no longer adequate for either the diagnosis or the control of success or quality. Angiocardiography consequently had to be further expanded to include angiocardiometry.

In tune with the development of computed tomography, cardiovascular radiology has for this reason become the 'pacemaker' of medical digital image processing.

Volumetry and densitometry

Quantitative evaluations of contrast images of the heart go back to the late fifties and early sixties. Based on various models, Swedish authors (Arvidson [11, 12] and Gribbe et al [13]) as well as American authors (Dodge et al [14, 15], Chapman et al [16]) developed procedures to determine cardiac volumes, especially those in the left ventricle by means of cut films or cineangio-

cardiograms. Initially, these were manual time-consuming evaluation methods which, in spite of their great pathophysiological importance, could not be applied extensively in clinical practice.

The search for quantitative evaluation of the image information was not only limited to the recognition of contours of the cardiac ventricles, but also attempted quantitative analysis of the entire optical density and grey-value information, i.e. a radiodensitometric image analysis. The potential possibilities of the densitometric evalua-

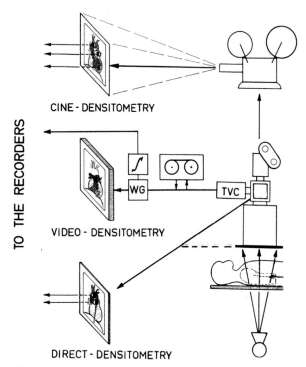

Fig. III, 84. Diagram of three methods for the recording of radiographic contrast densitograms: cinedensitometry, videodensitometry and direct image-intensifier-fluorescent-screen densitometry [22].

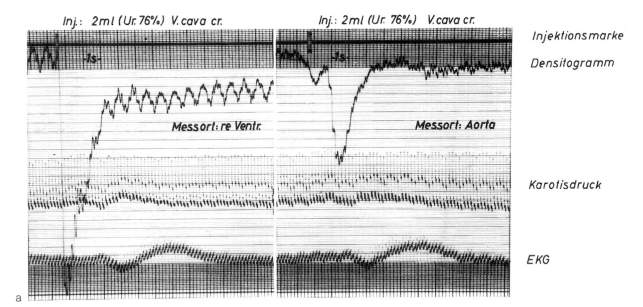

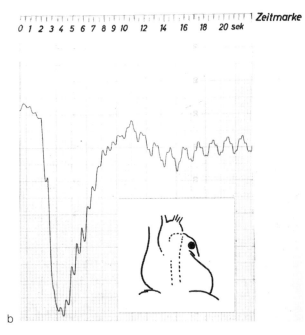

Fig. III, 85a, b. Two examples of experimentally **(a)** and clinically **(b)** obtained "contrast-medium dilution curves" at different measurement sites by means of fluorescent-screen densitometry **(a)** and cinedensitometry **(b)**, of the pulmonary artery after injection of contrast-medium into the cubital vein [20].

tion of angiocardiograms using various methods have been described by Wood et al [17], Heintzen [18] and Heintzen et al [19, 20, 21, 22] (Fig. III, 84). Examples of the first cine- and fluoroscopic densitograms from the central cardiovascular structures are illustrated in fig. III, 85.

However, the prerequisites for quantitative density measurements with conventional radiologic techniques had to be developed first,

namely: (a) methods to stabilize X-ray beams (Heintzen et al [1, 23, 24]), and (b) conditions under which Lambert-Beer's law was valid with regard to X-ray attenuation caused by contrast media (Buersch et al [25]; Heintzen et al [26]).

After this had been accomplished, it became feasible to use the contrast medium injected during angiocardiography as a quantitatively measurable 'indicator' of the blood distribution and blood flow in the projected image without necessitating insertion of a probe into the heart. The first 'contrast-medium dilution curves' obtained from experimental and clinical studies with direct densitometry and cinedensitometry met the expectations of the respective procedures (Heintzen et al [22]; Rutishauser [27]).

Physiologically tested concepts of this contrast-indicator technique provided totally new quantitative evaluation capabilities of the dynamic image information that previously could only be evaluated subjectively. But this process required electronic methods for measurements and evaluation.

Videodensitometry and videometry as preliminary stages to digital angiocardiography

In the sixties, image intensifier television systems signified the beginning of electronic image processing and prepared the way for rapid and versatile image processing (Gebauer et al [28]).

The transformation of angiocardiographic image information into electronic 'video signals' led to the development of videodensitometry by Sturm and Wood at the Mayo Clinic [29]. Osypka designed the first videodensitometer in our electronic laboratories in 1966. Over the following years, videodensitometry with pulsed X-ray exposures and regions-of-interest has become a quantitative method that could be clinically applied (Heintzen, [30]; Heintzen and Pilarczyk [31]; Buersch [32]; Buersch et al [33]).

Digital processing of video angiocardiograms was first performed for automated determination of ventricular volumes as part of videometry, both in the USA (Wiscomb [34]; Robb [35]; Ritman et al [36]) and by our group. Volumetry of the ventricles was based on the synchronous evaluation of biplanar angiocardiograms that were displayed on a monitor operating in the 'split screen' mode (Osypka and Heintzen [37]) and temporarily stored on a magnetic tape or disk together with physiologic (ECG, pressure) and alphanumeric reference data (Fig. III, 86).

The ventricular contours were manually, semiautomatically or fully automatically outlined, then digitized image-by-image, and sent to an on-line digital computer (CDC 1700) that was programmed to calculate the ventricular volumes automatically (Heintzen et al [1, 38, 39]). Using synchronous integration of intracardiac pressure values contained in the image information (Fig. III, 86), the computer could generate pressure-volume diagrams of the ventricles that characterized the mechanical work and working conditions of the ventricles (Heintzen et al [40]). Thus, videodensitometry and videometry were the first steps into the era of 'computer angiocardiography'.

Modalities of digital angiocardiography

Partial digitalization of X-ray television signals with temporary storage in a digital matrix rapidly led to the realization that, *'since the advantages of electronic image transfer (modulation, subtraction, harmonization, storage and reproduction) and the electronic data processing of functional and morphological parameters cannot be denied, a development has begun which, via a further improvement in television image quality, will logically result in a replacement of the cine technique'* (Heintzen [42]; paper given at the 51st German Roentgen Congress, Munich, May 1970).

The rapid development of modular electronic techniques made it possible to build digital image memories with real-time recording on magnetic disks, initially, of individual television images and, finally, of entire angiocardiographic image series (Heintzen et al [43]).

In the course of this development, the work groups of Wood at the Mayo Clinic, USA [44], of Mistretta at the University of Wisconsin, USA [45], of Nudelman et al at the University of Arizona, USA [46], and of Hoehne and colleagues in Hamburg, Germany [4, 47], as well as of

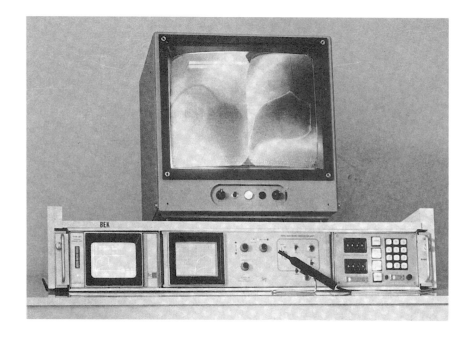

Fig. III, 86. First volumetric unit with automated, digital evaluation by biplane and/or cineangiocardiograms. Biplane levocardiogram with an adaptable videodensitometric measurement window for the left ventricle. ECG and pressure-proportional horizontal "bars" are stored in the biplane image information so that pressure-volume diagrams can be obtained from the integrated image information [38,39] (1970).

our own interdisciplinary team in Kiel have made substantial contribution before the introduction of commercial image processors by the industry (Heintzen and Buersch [2]; Heintzen and Brennecke [5]; Mistretta et al [3]).

The industry began to show interest after the presentation and publication of the contrast-en-

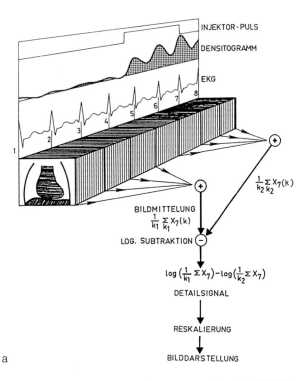

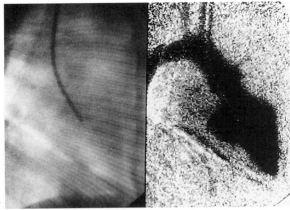

b

Fig. III, 87a, b. First digital subtraction angiocardiogram of the left ventricle obtained after the method shown as diagram **a)**. Four corresponding heart phase images were integrated before and after injection of contrast medium and then electronically subtracted. On the left in Fig. **b**, the conventional angiocardiogram with its image of best contrast is shown, with the left ventricle hardly recognizable. On the right, the levocardiogram from the same angiogram is shown after digital subtraction and electronic contrast enhancement [48] (1976).

hancement of a left cardiac ventricle achieved by digital subtraction revealed the importance for the entire angiographic and angiocardiographic radiology (Fig. III, 87) (Brennecke et al [48, 49, 50]; Heintzen et al [51]). Other groups primarily concentrating on applications in general radiology, such as Mistretta et al [3], who were already involved in dual-energy subtraction techniques, and Nudelmann et al [46] who worked on photoelectric procedures to digitize X-ray images, also stimulated the interest of the industry by their participation and promoted the field of digital subtraction angiocardiography.

After the first commercial systems had become available in 1980/1981, digital subtraction angiocardiography (DSA) spread swiftly. A complete survey of the literature would go beyond the scope of this review. To display vascular and cardiac anomalies following the only minimally invasive intravenous injection of contrast medium seemed to be a particularly attractive aspect of DSA. As it is often the case with new developments, the initial scepticism towards intravenous DSA was followed by an overestimation until its true diagnostic indications could be defined through experience and after improvements of the commercial systems. DSA proved to be advantageous for selective vascular injection of contrast medium, primarily arterially, but also for intracardiac administration of contrast medium (Ovitt et al [52]; Crummy et al [53]). Moreover, the accuracy of geometric measurements could be improved (Lange et al [54].

With regard to the technical developments of the equipment, the simple "mask-mode" subtraction, a postprocessing mode preceding the computer processing, has evolved into bus-oriented systems with rapid processors, functional modules and instant access storage devices (Fig. III, 88) [55].

Cost-benefit analyses have shown that twice as many patients can be examined at lower costs with a DSA system than with conventional equipment (Koster et al, [56]). The following commercial installations should be mentioned: DCI from Philips, DIVAS from CGR, and ANGIOTRON, DIGITRON and, lastly, HICOR from Siemens.

The knowledge gained from additional experimental and clinical studies showed that digital subtraction angiocardiography, though important, was only the beginning of the more universal and relevant applications of digital image processing in radiology and, particularly, in cardiovascular radiology.

The digitizing, storing and on-line processing of complete angiocardiographic image series

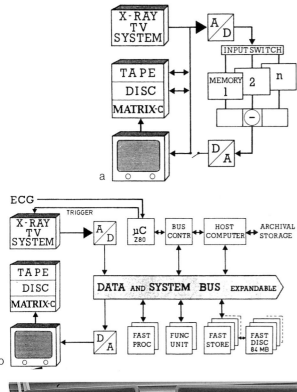

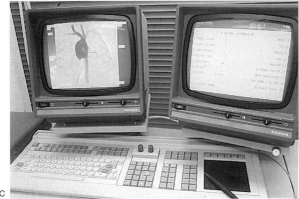

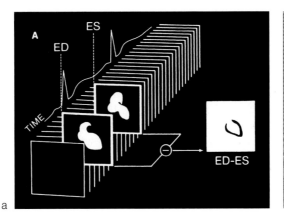

makes digital subtraction angiocardiography the most simple case of digital angiocardiography, which can process (in principle with the full array of generally available image processing programs applied to any arbitrarily selected images sequence) various combinations of images from an image series in many different ways, thereby increasing information by more than just eliminating background and enhancing contrast. Variable combinations of summation and subtraction procedures applied to ECG-triggered selected images or groups of images enable the quantitative acquisition of physiologically important, functional cardiac states. For instance, end-diastolic/end-systolic difference images can reveal abnormalities of the contraction process, wall motion, and ejection fraction (Fig. III, 89), and summation images can display myocardial volume and abnormal myocardial perfusion (Fig. III, 90) (Heintzen et al [51]; Radtke et al [57]; Buersch et al [58, 59, 60]). The up to this time analogue technique of videodensitometric determination of the regurgitation fraction in valvular insufficiency has recently been included into the program of a digital angiography system (DIGITRON 2) (Onnasch et al [61]).

Digital functional angiocardiography

In 1979, Brennecke [62, 63], a member of our bioengineering staff, developed, with the support of the 'Deutsche Forschungsgemeinschaft' (German Research Foundation), a microprocessor-guided image processor ('ISAAC', Image Sequence Acquisition and Analysis Computer), which achieved a rapid digitalization and flexible processing of entire image series with the aid of special functional units, thus providing the technical requirements for an efficient functional angiocardiography.

Fig. III, 88a-c. Architecture of various digital image processing systems. Simple commercial, first-generation subtraction unit (1981) **(a)**, bus-oriented **(b)**, modern image workstation (i.e. DIGITRON) **(c)**, (Heintzen, 1984 [7]).

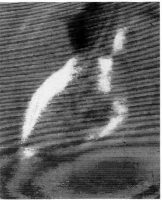

Fig. III, 89a, b. Enddiastolic-endsystolic differential images of the left ventricle **(b)** by selective ECG-triggered images according to the diagram **(a)** to illustrate the contractions and movements of the endocardial contour.

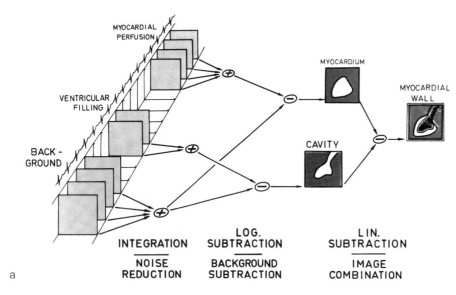

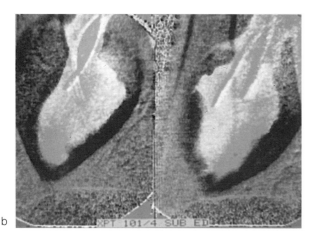

a

b

Fig. III, 90a, b. Diagram of the procedure to display the perfused myocardium by selective ECG-triggered image groups of an angiocardiographic image series **(a)**. Contrast display of the "capillary phase" of myocardial perfusion during systole and diastole **(b)** [51,58].

A digitally stored image series, displayed as a three-dimensional data block (Fig. III, 91), can be conceptually seen as the sum of separately digitized images or as a matrix of pixel densitograms.

The flexible, program-controlled access to such a data block permits both the simple subtraction processes, possibly as a preliminary step in processing, and the generation of functional or parametric images. New image qualities and physiologically relevant information could be derived from the sum of the separate images: the spatial distribution of temporal criteria; the arrival time of contrast medium; the time of maximum concentration of contrast medium; or the area under the pixel densitograms, reflecting the thickness of the contrast medium in a vessel and therefore representing a 'volumetric-parametric image'.

Through a physiologically meaningful combination of such functional parameters obtained from angiocardiograms, it was possible to gain new insights into the function of the cardiac and circulatory systems. Time parameter images can illustrate the temporal dissemination and distribution of the contrast medium, which takes the place of an 'indicator', in the vessels and organs. By virtue of these features, they are suitable for comparative, semiquantitative circulatory and perfusion studies, particularly in the evaluation of such symmetrical organs as lungs (Buersch et al [64]) and kidneys (Hoehne et al [65]; Buersch et al [66, 67]). Nevertheless, they have been applied in analyzing changes in myocardial perfusion after experimental infarction (Fig. III, 92) (Buersch et al [69, 70]) as well as in determining the coronary flow reserve (Vogel et al [71, 72]; van der Werf et al [73]; Nissen et al [74]).

Combining time and volumetric parameters, as developed by Buersch et al in our laboratories [66, 67, 68, 69, 70], opens entirely new methods to display and analyze blood-flow images. By varying the temporal segmentation, the progression of the contrast medium bolus can be assessed at defined time intervals. If volumetric parameters are included, angiographic flow measurements in arterial vessels (Fig. III, 93 and 94) as well as shunt calculations are possible (Fig. III, 95).

The development of digital functional angiocardiography is still at its beginning. As with digital subtraction angiocardiography, it can be expected to have a great impact on the diagnosis of cardiovascular diseases as soon as commercial radiographic systems are developed for easy application of these methods.

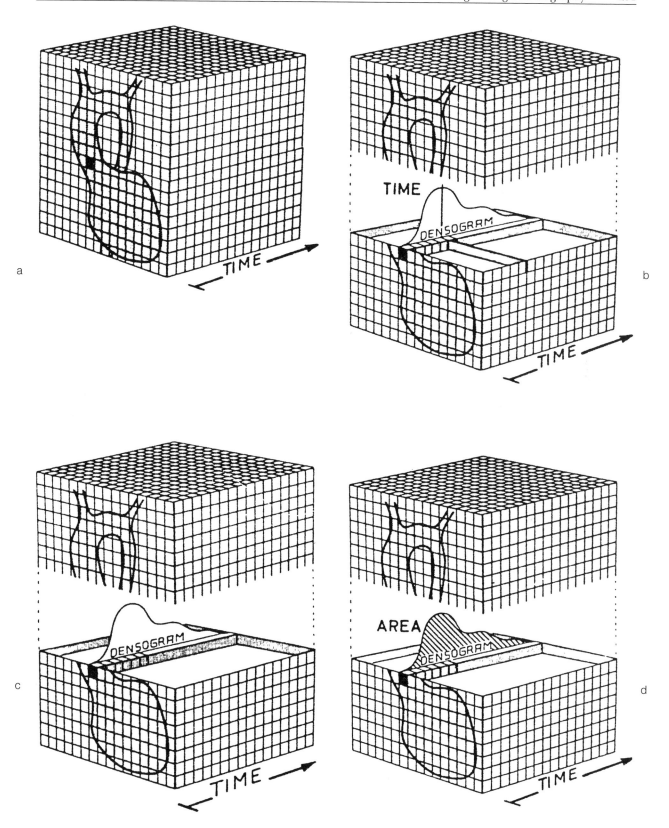

Fig. III, 91a-d. Schematic display of the data block from a digitized image series **(a)** illustrating the information stored can be viewed as a matrix of "pixel densitograms" **(b)**. Each densitogram allows the extraction of characteristic time parameters (e.g. arrival time or maximal value of the contrast medium bolus **(c)**, allows the collection of volumetric parameters from the area of the entire densitogram **(d)**.

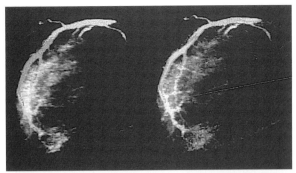

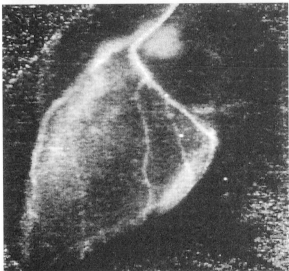

Fig. III, 92. Functional angiocardiogram (time-parameter images) of coronary perfusion following experimental closure of the circumflex branch or the anterior descending branch of the left coronary artery. The amount of myocardium of reduced or absent perfusion is seen in the time-parameter images [9] (1986).

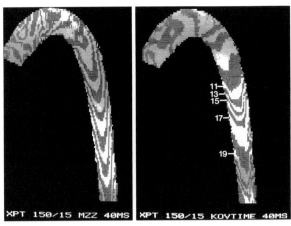

Fig. III, 93. Illustration of the procedure of temporal segmentation of the contrast-medium bolus progressing through the aorta. The mean circulation time (MZZ) in the left image and the covariance time in the right image were selected as time parameters. The advancement of these "parameters" is recognized via the black-and white lines marking each segment every 40 milliseconds. Whereas the mean circulation time is equal to the mean flow, the covariance time (kovtime) of the concentration of the bolus permits recognition of a pulsatile flow pattern. The sum of the areas under each pixel densitogram of the respective segments allows the automatic evaluation of the volume of this segment. The blood flow can be derived from the volume changes during these 40 milliseconds [69] (1986).

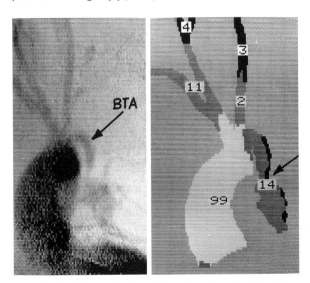

Fig. III, 95. Determination of the size of the shunt in a Blalock-Taussig anastomosis (14% in relation to the ejected volume of the left ventricle = 99%) using the described principles of the quantitative, digital densitometric functional angiocardiography [5] (1993).

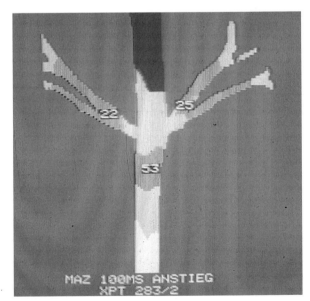

Fig. III, 94. Application of the concept outlined in Fig. III,93 to determine the flow in the renal artery. Temporal segmentation and parallel densitometric computation of the segmental volume allow the calculation of the relative blood flow distribution in the renal artery and descending aorta (see figures). The relative values can be converted to absolute flow values through geometric calibration of the aortic diameter [66] (1991).

In the meantime, procedures of digital electronic image processing in angiocardiography have begun to replace cinematography, solely on the basis of their rapid, flexible, easily controllable and reliably reproducible processing of information, although improvements are still imperative as to the storage of relevant clinical and forensic information. The technology is already there but, as the history of radiology has shown, the complex process of the clinical implementation of a medicotechnical innovation depends on many unpredictable factors and generally takes longer than expected.

References

1. Heintzen, P.H.: Roentgen-, Cine- and Videodensitometry. Fundamentals and Applications for Blood Flow and Heart Volumne Determination. Internat. Workshop Conf.Kiel, March 1969 Thieme, Stuttgart 1971
2. Heintzen, P.H., J.H. Bürsch: Roentgen-Video-Techniques for Dynamic Studies of Structure and Function of the Heart and Circulation. Internat Workshop Conf. Kiel, April 1976. Thieme, Stuttgart 1978
3. Mistretta, C.A., A.B. Crummy, C.M. Strother, J.F. Sackett: Digital Subtraction Arteriography. An Application of Computerized Fluoroscopy. Internat. Symposium, Madison, May 1981, Year Book Medical Publishers, Chicago 1982
4. Höhne, K.H.: Digital Image Processing in Medicine. Internat. Symposium, Hamburg, October 1981. Lecture Notes in Medicaln Informatics, Vol. 15, Springer, Berlin Heidelberg New York 1982
5. Heintzen, P.H., R. Brennecke: Digital Imaging in Cardiovascular Radiology. Internat. Workshop Conf. Kiel, Mai 1982. Thieme, Stuttgart 1983
6. Sigwart, U., P.H. Heintzen: Ventricular Wall Motion. Internat. Symposium, Lausanne, April 1982. Thieme, Stuttgart 1984
7. Riemann, H.E., J. Kollath: Digitale Radiographie; 1. Frankfurter Gespräch über Digitale Radiographie. Bad Nauheim, Sept. 1984. Schnetztor, Konstanz 1985
8. Just, H., P.H. Heintzen: Angiokardiographie. Current Status and Future Developments. Internat. Symposium, Titisee 1982. Springer, Berlin Heidelberg New York 1986
9. Heintzen, P.H., J.H. Bürsch: Progress in Digital Angiocardiography. Proc. Internat. Symposium Kiel, October 1986. Kluwer Academic Publishers, Boston Dordrecht Lancaster 1988
10. Mancini, G.B.J.: Clinical Applications of Cardiac Digital Angiography. Raven Press, New York 1988
11. Arvidsson, H.: Angiocardiographic observations in mitral disease, with special reference to volume variations in the left atrium. Acta Radiol. (1958) Suppl. 158
12. Arvidsson, H.: Angiocardiographic determination of the left ventricular volume. Acta Radiol. 56 (1961) 321
13. Gribbe, P., L. Hirvonen, J. Lind, C. Wegelius: Cineangiographic recordings of the cyclic changes in volume of the left ventricle. Cardiologia 34 (1959) 348
14. Dodge, H.T., H.L. Tannenbaum: Left ventricular volume in normal man and alterations with disease. Circulation 14 (1956) 927)
15. Dodge, H.T., H. Sandler, D.W. Ballew, J.D. Lord: The use of biplane cinefluorography for measurement of left ventricular volume in man. Am. Heart J. 60 (1960) 762
16. Chapman, C.B. O. Baker, F.J. Reynolds, F.J. Bonte: Use of biplane cinefluorography for measurement of left ventricular volume in man. Circulation 18 (1958) 1105
17. Wood, E.H., R.E. Sturm, J.J. Sanders: Data processing in cardiovascular physiology with particular reference to roentgenvideodensitometry. Mayo Clin. Proc. 39 (1964) 849
18. Heintzen, P.H.: Kontrastmittelverdünnungskurven. Wiss. Kolloquium der Hamb. und Kieler Univ. Kinderklinik, Kiel. 7. Juli 1964
19. Heintzen, P.: A simple method for the recording of radiopaque dilution curves during angiocardiography. Am. Heart J. 69 (1965) 720
20. Heintzen, P., J. Bürsch: Kontrastmittelverdünnungsverfahren. Kreislaufmessungen, Band V, 149 (1965)
21. Heintzen, P., J. Bürsch: Methods for angiocardiodensitography: a new indicatortechnique. Circulation 32 Suppl. II (1965) 110
22. Heintzen, P., J. Bürsch, P. Osypka, K. Modenhauer: Röntgenologische Kontrastmitteldichtemessungen zur Untersuchung der Herz- und Kreislauffunktion. Z. Elektr. Med. 12 (1967) 82 und 145
23. Heintzen, P.: Usefulness and limitations of conventional x-ray equipments for densitometric measurements. In: Heintzen, P.: Roentgen-, Cine- and Videodensitometry. Thieme Stuttgart 1971
24. Heintzen, P., P. Osypka: Quantitative Analyse der Leuchtdichte- und Strahlungsimpulse an Röntgen-Bildverstärker-Cinepulsanlagen. I. Verhalten bei Serienimpulsen und Verfahren zur Strahlenstabilisierung für die Cinedensitometrie. Fortschr. Röntgenstr. 111 (1969) 115
25. Bürsch, J., R. Johs, P. Heintzen: Untersuchungen zur Gültigkeit des Lambert-Beer'schen Gesetzes bei der röntgenologischen Kontrastmitteldichtemessungen. Fortschr. Röntgenstr. 112 (1970) 259
26. Heintzen, P., K. Moldenhauer: The x-ray absorption by contrast material. In: Heintzen, P.: siehe [1] S. 73
27. Rutishauser, W.: Kreislaufanalyse mittels Röntgendensitometrie. Huber, Bern-Stuttgart-Wien 1969
28. Gebauer, A., J. Lissner, O. Schott: Das Röntgenfernsehen. Technische Grundlagen und klinisch-röntgenologische Anwendung. Thieme, Stuttgart 1965
29. Sturm, R.E., J.J. Sanders, E.H. Wood: A Roentgen videodensitometer for circulatory studies. Fed. Proc. 23 (1964) 303
30. Heintzen, P., J. Pilarczyk: Videodensitometry with contoured and controlled windows. In: Heintzen: siehe [1] S. 56
31. Heintzen, P.: Videodensitometry with pulsed radiation. In: Heintzen: siehe [1], S 46
32. Bürsch, J.H.: Quantitative Videodensitometrie. Grundlagen und Ergebnisse einer röntgenologischen Indikatormethode. Habilitationsschrift. Christian-Albrechts-Universität Kiel 1973
33. Bürsch, J.H., P.H. Heintzen, R. Simon: Videodensitometric studies by a new method of quantitating the amount of contrast medium. Eur. J. Cardiol. 1 (1974) 437

34. Robb, R.A.: Computer aided contour determination and dynamic display of individual cardiac chambers from digitized serial angiocardiographic film. In: Heintzen: siehe [1] S. 170
35. Wiscomb, W.K.: A hardware system for man-machine interaction in the study of left ventricular dynamics. In: Heintzen: siehe [1] S. 165
36. Ritman, E.L., R.E. Sturm, E.H. Wood: A biplane videometry system for dynamic (60/second) studies of the shape and size of ventricular structures, particularly the left ventricle. In: Heintzen: siehe [1] S. 179
37. Osypka, P., P. Heintzen: Neue elektronische Verfahren zur Verbesserung der Herzkatheterisierungstechnik und Angiokardiographie. Verh. Dtsch. Ges. Kreislaufforschung 34 (1968) 234
38. Heintzen, P., V. Malerczyk, J. Pilarczyk, K.W. Scheel: A new method for the determination of left ventricular volume by use of automatic video data processing. Circulation 42, Suppl. III (1970) 100
39. Heintzen, P., V. Malerczyk, J. Pilarczyk, K.W. Scheel: On-line processing of the video-image for left ventricular volume determination. Comp. Biomed. Res. 4 (1971) 474
40. Heintzen, P., V. Malerczyk, J. Pilarczyk: A videometric technique for automated processing of pressure volume diagrams. Comp. Biomed. Res. 4 (1971) 486
41. Heintzen, P.H., R. Brennecke, J.H. Bürsch, H.J. Hahne, P.E. Lange, K. Moldenhauer, D. Onnasch, W. Radtke: Quantitative analysis of structure and function of the cardiovascular system by roentgen-video-computer techniques. Mayo Clin. Proc. 5 (1982) 78
42. Heintzen, P.: Technische Fortschritte in der Röntgenfernsehkinematographie mit gepulster Strahlung. Röntgen-Bl. 24 (1971) 604
43. Heintzen, P.H., R. Brennecke, J.H. Bürsch, P. Lange, V. Malerczyk, K. Moldenhauer, D. Onnasch: Automated videoangiocardiographic image analysis. Computer IEEE 8 (1975) 55
44. Robb, R.A., E.H. Wood, E.L. Ritman, et al: Three dimensional reconstruction and display of the working canine heart and lungs by multiplanar x-ray videometry. Computer IEEE 8 (1975) 151
45. Mistretta, C.A., R.A. Kruger, T.L. Houk, et al: Computerized fluoroscopy techniques for non invasiv cardiovascular imaging. Proc. SPIE 152 (1978) 65
46. Nudelman, S.: Photoelectronic Digital Radiology. Past, present and future. In: Heintzen, P.H., R. Brennecke: Digital imaging in cardiovascular radiology. Thieme, Stuttgart 1983
47. Höhne, K.H., M. Böhm, W. Erbe, G.C. Nicolae, G. Pfeiffer, B. Sonne: Computer angiography: a new tool for x-ray functional diagnostics. Med. Orogr. Technol. 6 (1978) 23
48. Brennecke, R., T.K. Brown, J.H. Bürsch, P.H. Heintzen: Digital processing of videoangiographic image series using a minicomputer. Proc. Comp. Cardiol. IEEE Computer Society, Long Beach (1976) 225
49. Brennecke, R., T.K. Brown, J.H. Bürsch, P.H. Heintzen: A system for computerized video-image preprocessing with application to angiocardiographic roentgen-image series. In: Nagel, H.H.: Digitale Bildverarbeitung. Springer, Berling-Heidelberg-New York (1977) 244
50. Brennecke, R., T.K. Brown, J.H. Bürsch, P.H. Heintzen: In: Heintzen, P.H., J.H. Bürsch: Roentgen-Video-Techniques. Thieme (1978) 150

51. Heintzen, P.H., R. Brennecke, J.H. Bürsch: Computerized videoangiocardiography. In: Kaltenbach, M., P. Lichtlen: Proc. 3rd Symposium on coronary heart disease. Thieme, Stuttgart (1978) 116
52. Ovitt, T.W., P.C. Christenson, H.D. Fisher, et al: Intravenous angiography using digital video subtraction: x-ray imaging system. Am. J. Roentgenol. 135 (1980) 1141
53. Crummy, A.B., C.M. Strother, J.F. Sackett, et al: Computerized fluoroscopy: digital subtraction for intravenous angiocardiography and arteriography. Am. J. Roentgenol. 135 (1980) 1131
54. Lange, P.E., B. Ewert, W. Radtke, H.J. Hahne, D.G.W. Onnasch, P.H. Heintzen: Angiocardiographic volume determination of the left ventricle in children. Value of digital subtraction techniques after selective injection. In: Doyle, E.F., M.A. Engle, W.M. Gersony, W.J. Rashkind, N.S. Talner: Pediatric Cardiology, Springer, New York, (1985) 313
55. Pfeiler, M., P. Marhoff: Zur Technik der digitalen Röntgenbildverarbeitung insbesondere der digitalen Subtraktionsangiographie. Electromedica 51 (1983) 20
56. Koster, W.G., Van der Put: Kosten-Nutzen-Analyse der digitalen Subtraktionsangiographie. In: Riemann, H.E., J. Kollath: Digitale Radiographie. Schnetztor, Konstanz, (1985) 40
57. Radtke, W., J.H. Bürsch, R. Brennecke, H.J. Hahne, P.H. Heintzen: Bestimmung der linksventrikulären Muskelmasse mittels digitaler Angiokardiographie. Z. Kardiol. 70 (1981) 302
58. Bürsch, J.H., W. Radtke, T. Rünger, K. Moldenhauer, B. Hoffmann, P.H. Heintzen: Endocardial and epicardial contour detection of the left ventricle by digital angiocardiography. In: Sigwart, U., P.H. Heintzen: Ventricular wall motion. Thieme, Stuttgart (1984) 49
59. Bürsch, J.H., H.J. Hahne, C. Beyer, S. Seemann, L. Meissner, R. Brennecke, P.H. Heintzen: Myocardial perfusion studies by digital angiography. Proc. Comp. Cardiol. IEEE Computer Society, Long Beach (1983) 343
60. Bürsch, J.H., W. Radtke, R. Brennecke, H.J. Hahne, P.H. Heintzen: Assessment of myocardial perfusion by digital angiocardiography. In: Just, H., P.H. Heintzen (eds) (1986) 365
61. Onnasch, D.G.W., U. Jarrens, P.H. Heintzen: Determination of ejection and valvular regurgitant fraction by on-line digital densitometry – methodology, validation, and application. Intern. J. Cardiol. Imag. 7 (1991) 113
62. Brennecke, R., H.J. Hahne, K. Moldenhauer, J.H. Bürsch, P.H. Heintzen: A special purpose processor for digital angiocardiography. Design and applications. Proc. Comp. Cardiol, IEEE Computer Society, Long Beach (1979) 343
63. Brennecke, R., H.J. Hahne, P.H. Heintzen: A multiprocessor system for the acquisition and analysis of video image sequences. In: Pöppl, S.J., H. Platzer: Erzeugung und Analyse von Bildern und Strukturen, Springer Berlin-Heidelberg-New York (1980) 113
64. Bürsch, J.H.: Densitometric studies in digital subtraction angiography: assessment of pulmonary and myocardial perfusion. Herz 10 (1985) 208
65. Höhne, K.H., M. Böhm, W. Erbe, et al: Die Messung und differenzierte bildliche Darstellung der Nierendurchblutung mit der Computerangiographie. Fortschr. Röntgenstr. 129 (1978) 667

66. Bürsch, J.H., H.J. Hahne, R. Brennecke, D. Gröne-meyer, P.H. Heintzen: Assessment of arterial blood flow measurements by digital angiography. Radiology 14 (1981) 39

67. Bürsch, J.H.: Use of digitized functional angiography to evaluate arterial blood flow. Cardiovasc. Intervent. Radiol. 6 (1983) 303

68. Bürsch, J.H., C. Ochs, H.J. Hahne, P.H. Heintzen: Experimentelle Nierendurchblutungsmessungen mit der digitalen Funktionsangiographie. Der Radiologe 25 (1985) 381

69. Bürsch, J.H., P.H. Heintzen: Parametric imaging. Radiologic Clinic of North America. W.B. Saunders Company, USA 23 (1985) 321

70. Bürsch, J.H.: Wall thickening, muscle mass and infarct size. In: Mancini, G.B.J.: Clinical cardiac applications of digital angiography. Ravens Press, New York 1988

71. Vogel, R.A. et al: Visualization of myocardial perfusion using application of digital radiographic technique to selective coronary arteriography. Am. Cardiol. 49 (1982) 935

72. Vogel, R.A., M. Lefree, E. Bates, et al: Application of digital techniques to selective arteriography: use of myocardial contrast appearance time to measure coronary flow reserve. Am. Heart J. 107

73. Van der Werf, T., R.M. Heethaar, H. Stegehuis, N.H.J. Pijls, F.L. Meijler: Comparison of time parameters derived from myocardial time-density curves in patients before and after percutaneous transluminal coronary angioplasty. In: Heintzen, P.H., J.H. Bürsch: Progress in digital angiocardiography. Kluwer Press, Dordrecht-Boston 1988

74. Nissen, S., J.L. Elion, A.N. de Maria: Methods for calculation of coronary flow reserve by computer processing of digital angiograms. In: Heintzen, P.H., J.H. Bürsch: siehe [9] S. 237

75. Heintzen, P.H.: Digital angiocardiography. In: Collins, S.M., D.J. Skorton: Cardiac imaging and image processing. McGraw-Hill Book Company, New York (1986) 239–279

Peripheral vessels

E. Zeitler

The history of radiological imaging of the peripheral vessels had already begun a month after Roentgen's famous address to the Physical Medical Association in Wuerzburg [1]. E. Haschek and O.T. Lindenthal had injected Teichmann's mixture into the arteries of an amputated hand and had taken a photograph applying Roentgen's technique [2]. The photograph, published in 1896 (Fig. III, 96), was an important step towards visualizing arteries in living human beings. Impressed by such photographs that were taken in the first few months after Roentgen's discovery, W.G. Morton [3], Professor at the New York Postgraduate Medical School, stated in 1896: *'The X-rays have opened a new era in anatomic education, where the arteries and veins of dead bodies can be filled with "opaque" substances. We will thus be able to recognize and understand them in more detail than with any other anatomic preparation technique.'*

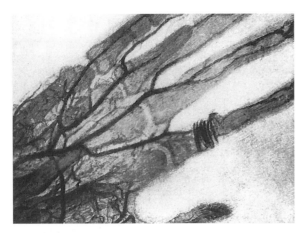

Fig. III, 96. Radiograph of an amputated hand after injection with "Teichmann's mixture" in the arteries by Haschek and Lindenthal in Vienna in January 1896.

The first X-ray atlas of the systemic arteries of the body [4] appeared in England 25 years after the discovery of X-rays, containing excellent reproductions of radiographs of the vascular system taken in cadavers.

The intravital visualization of vessels at first did not achieve the same precise information, due to
- the lack of nontoxic radiopaque media that can be injected in sufficient concentration and quantity, and
- the absence of technical capabilities to obtain radiographic images in rapid sequence.

Development of contrast media

The idea of studying the heart with contrast agents apparently first occurred to Franck and Alwens [5], who introduced a suspension of bismuth and oil into the hearts of dogs and rabbits directly through the large veins. They were able to observe the passage of opaque droplets from the heart into the lungs. J.A. Sicard and G. Forrestier [6] tried Lipiodol to visualize blood vessels. Injection of a few milliliters of Lipiodol into the vein of the forearm did not produce any adverse effects. These successful investigations encouraged Sicard and Forrestier to apply the injection of the femoral artery clinically. The artery was surgically exposed and after arteriotomy injected with Lipiodol under observation. In an elderly patient with a gangrenous foot, they were able to determine the site of the vascular obliteration. Unfortunately, Sicard interrupted his investigations on vessels for his greater interest in myelography with Lipiodol.

In 1923, J. Berberich, assistant at the Senckenberg Institute for Pathology, and S. Hirsch, senior physician of the medical department in Frankfurt am Main, also reported the first results of intravital visualization of vessels [7].

In Volume I of the series 'Radiological Practice' published by W. Alwens, F. Dessauer, R. Grashey et al., S. Hirsch [8] reported in detail on the characteristics of radiation absorption of 70 different solutions, such as sodium iodide, strontium bromide and sodium chloride, as well as on the contrast obtainable in the roentgen image under various tube voltages. The intravital demonstration of arm veins and hand arteries with a 20% strontium bromide were impressive. Venous valves and finger arteries could be differentiated (Fig. III, 97). The first successful visualization of leg arteries by B. Brooks [9] (Fig. III, 98) was obtained with sodium iodide. His first patient was a diabetic with a large ulcer on his right leg, and a vascular occlusion was suspected. At the moment of injection, he compressed the vein proximally from the exposed artery after he had clamped the femoral artery proximally, giving enough time to visualize the vessel in different projections. The radiographs delineated the arteries well, except for the anterior tibial artery, which supplied the gangrenous region of the foot. A sympathectomy consequently performed relieved the pain and healed the gangrene.

Brooks described his experiences on 25 arteriograms, and after that devoted himself to other fields. Ensuing investigators assessed the quality of arteriograms with sodium iodide solutions [10, 11] differently. In part, this could be due to the amount of contrast medium used as well as to the image contrast and the selected injection site. All tests with iodinated oils in arteriographies and venographies were soon abandoned because of the fragmentation and drop-like segregation of the contrast column, though adverse reactions had not occurred.

According to R. Barke [12], 1929 belongs to the most fruitful years in the history of the development of contrast media. After intensive experiments with halogen pyridine derivatives, A. Binz

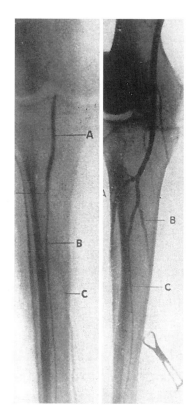

Fig. III, 98. Arteriography of the legs after injection with sodium iodide by Brooks in 1924.

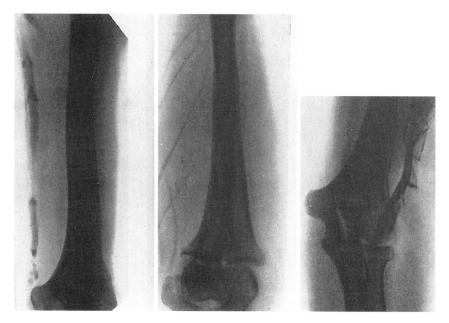

Fig. III, 97. Fluoroscopically guided radiographic visualization of arm veins and elbow arteries with 20% strontium bromide by Berberich and Hirsch (1923).

(see fig. III, 3) and C. Räth [13] had found a preparation suitable for radiographic opacification of the urinary tract and blood vessels and which was later called by von Lichtenberg 'Uroselectan'. M. Swick (see fig. III, 51a) [14] described the clinical experience with this contrast medium for excretory urography, and M. Ratschow [15] reported on vasography with particular consideration of the varicography.

In 1929, Dos Santos (Fig. III, 69) et al [16, 17] still used a 10% sodium-iodide solution for the first translumbar abdominal aortography to visualize the aorta, and the pelvic and leg arteries, while W. Forssmann (Fig. III, 76) [18] already employed a 40–50% solution of Uroselectan to visualize the heart and pulmonary vessels. Osborne et al [19] as well as Bronner, Hecht et al. had contributed substantially to the development of nephrotropic contrast media [20, 21].

Later, 'Perabrodil' proved to be tolerated well and was increasingly used to visualize veins and arteries until it was replaced by tri-iodinated contrast media 20 years later [22, 23, 24].

During the period between 1929 and the end of World War II, fundamental investigations on the radiological demonstration of the arteries and veins of the extremities were performed and the first epoch of reconstructive surgery of venous and arterial disorders evolved.

The interplay between the development of reconstructive operations and optimizing angiographic methods had begun. Retrograde catheterization of the abdominal aorta for angiography after incisional exposure of the superficial femoral artery by P.L. Fariñas [22] (Fig. III, 99) has largely been forgotten. It was the forerunner of Seldinger's decisive development of the percutaneous technique of catheterization of vessels over a wire (Fig. III, 62) [23].

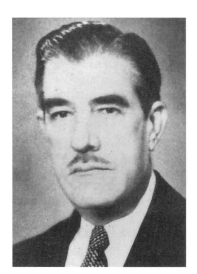

Fig. III, 99. Pedro Leandro Fariñas (1892–1951). Worked in Havanna, developed his own method for the arteriographic examination of the Aorta and its branches.

The synthesis of acetribenzoate ('Urografin') inaugurated the era of the tri-iodinated nephrotropic contrast media [25, 26]. These strong hydrophilic salts of tri-iodoxybenzoic acid derivatives carry an electric charge and dissociate in aqueous solution. This dissociation characterizes the physicochemical reaction and determines its osmolality [27]. The osmotic pressure with ionic contrast media was two to five times higher than that of blood. The high osmolality is partly responsible for the adverse reactions of ionic contrast media, particularly for the pain in arteriography of the extremities. Despite these reactions, arteriography was no longer carried out under general anesthesia, but under local anesthesia confined to the puncture site in the groin [28].

After contrast medium injection, several coagulation parameters can change, reducing the risk of thrombus formation. Also the blood osmolality can increase after repeated injections of contrast medium over a short period of time. Pauses had to be observed if large amounts of ionic contrast medium are used [29].

During this period of angiography, severe complications after peripheral arteriography [30] were only observed in 1–2% of the examinations, a complication rate similar to that with phlebography [31]. Analyzing angiographic examinations, it became increasingly difficult to differentiate the influence of the contrast medium from other influences, such as angiographic technique and examiner's expertise, as well as the patient's general attitude and perception of the disclosed risks (anxiety). In the following years several tri-iodinated contrast media were used: amidotrizoate, iotrizinate, iothalamate, ioxaklate and metrizoate [32, 33].

The introduction of non-ionic water-soluble contrast media was a considerable step forward with lasting impact on the reduction of adverse reactions, including the slight and moderately severe reactions [34, 35]. The non-ionic contrast media have no electric charge in an aqueous solution and have a very low, almost hemoisotonic osmotic pressure. This leads to less impairment of the biological membranes and to a low protein bond, which improves the general patient tolerance and has considerably reduced the risk for all indication, but especially for angiographies [36, 37]. As a result of this progress in contrast medium, tolerance and the introduction of digital techniques with reduced amounts of contrast medium, the arteriography of extremities could, like phlebography of the legs previously, develop into a routine method performed on an outpatient basis [38, 39].

Equipment

That arterial calcifications can be recognized on radiographs of the skeleton was already described in 1896 [5]. Due to the flowing blood in the arteries and veins, the intravital visualization of the vascular lumen was at first only possible under fluoroscopy or on individual radiographs that happened to exposed at the right time [7, 9].

The development of the radiographic technique of angiography of the extremities was based on two aspects: on the one hand, testing of fluoroscopically guided spot films obtained in modified positions and projections after various contrast medium applications, and on the other hand, designing of radiographic techniques in accordance with the hemodynamics of the blood flow in the entire length of the upper and lower extremities.

In this way, two principles could be continually improved:

– the use of cassettes for film-screen radiographs in fixed table positions, and
– the use of automatic film changers with movable table top.

In the latter technique, the patient is transported stepwise from one section to the next against the blood flow, either manually or automatically with variable programs.

Janker [39] (Fig. III, 100) wrote *'The drum for 96/20 cm cassettes and the cartridge for 96/20 cm images on roll-film are available for angiography of the legs.'* The drum could obtain six successive images, the roll-film changer enabled more. The interval between two exposures could be selected to be 2 s for the drum, 1 s for the cartridge, or at various lengths. As to recognizing detail,

it was undoubtedly a good method. For functional diagnoses, however, more radiographic images were necessary. As early as 1952, Janker, together with the vascular surgeon Paessler [40], performed a lumbar aortography (4 exposures/s) for the visualization of both leg arteries (12 exposures/s) and had a fairly good result by using a 35-mm film. To demonstrate all segments of both legs, the patient was moved into the 40 x 40 cm image field during the radiographic procedure.

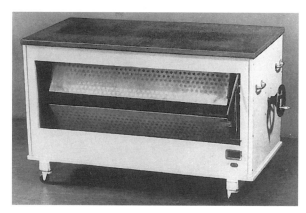

Fig. III, 101. Cassette drum for arteriography of the legs according to Janker (1954).

Janker's cassette drum (Fig. III, 101) and the cassette changer after Paessler and Wentzlik for serial angiography of the abdomen and the extremities (Fig. III, 102) were successfully used for many years [24, 30]. Operated with a manual cassette transport for three exposures in the aortic and pelvic region and for four exposures for each leg, the latter system was used by many clinics up to the seventies. This equipment could be employed both for translumbar aortography (Fig. III, 102) and for retrograde counter-current aortography from both femoral arteries [40]. Arteriography of the legs (Fig. III, 103) could, however, be carried out after a single retrograde puncture of the femoral artery with manual or pressure injection [23b].

The angiography table after Hasse and Ziplack (Fig. III, 104) used several full-size film cassettes, placed serially adjacent to each other. With the patient remaining unchanged in position, X-ray tube and long cassette transporter could be independently moved stepwise. Skin marks determined the stops for the next position. A well coordinated team of technicians or nurses was essential for this radiographic technique. Using this technique, the coworker of the founder of

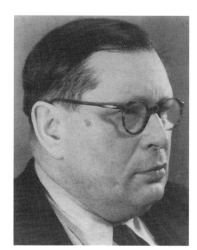

Fig. III, 100. Robert Janker (1894–1964). Worked in Bonn, where he established a private institute. Fluoroscopy and Cinematography were his main interest. Also many other developments, such as the cassette drum. Well-known books on radiographic technique.

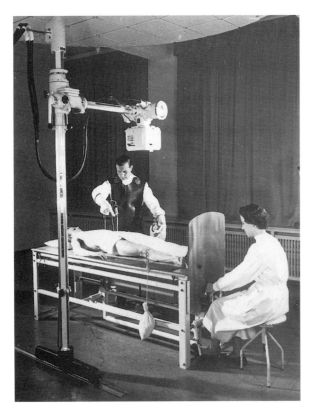

Fig. III, 102. Cassette changer for serial angiography of the abdomen and extremities, after Paessler and Wentzlik (1955).

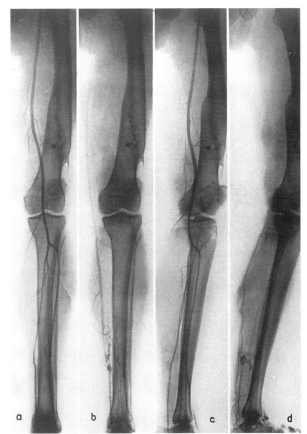

Fig. III, 103. Serial angiography of femoral arteries taken with the 96 x 20 cm cassette drum after Janker, a) and b) sagittal and c) and d) oblique projection (1954).

angiology in Germany, Max Ratschow, worked out all essential parameters for angio-organopathies and angioneuropathies, first in Halle/Saale and later in Darmstadt [30]. An angiographic differentiation between inflammatory and noninflammatory vascular diseases could not be achieved since the angiographic pattern of 'arterial obliteration' is the same for the different vascular diseases. Based on these angiographic examinations and patient's history and clinical data, M. Ratschow summarized peripheral vascular diseases under one term, 'peripheral occlusive vascular disease' (POVD) [30].

Using cinematography, R. Janker developed an angiographic unit with a sliding table to image the arteries in the extremities with a single contrast medium injection (Fig. III, 105). This was the predecessor of the automatic table-transport technique that was to be developed later. With this equipment, he could document the different contrast filling of both legs, depending on the degree of occlusion or obliteration (Fig. III, 106). He pointed out that arteriography of the legs via the femoral artery often had to be supplemented by lumbar aortography to demonstrate the

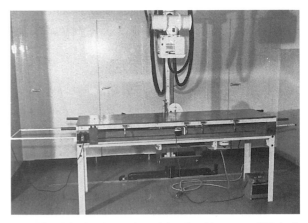

Fig. III, 104. Angiography table after Hasse and Ziplack with sliding table top and X-ray tube. (From: Ratschow, M.: Angiology, Thieme-Verlag, Stuttgart 1959).

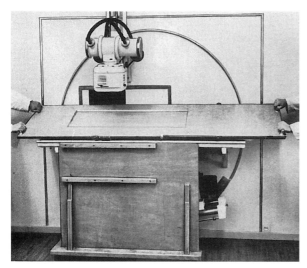

Fig. III, 105. Sliding table top to visualize the arteries of the extremities with cine-equipment after Janker (1954).

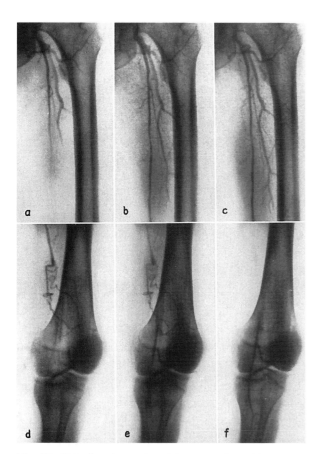

Fig. III, 106. Arteriography of the upper leg with a distal occlusion of the superficial femoral artery. Serial radiographs with the 70-mm film camera after Janker (1954).

pelvic arteries. In his institute, oscillography and rheography were used as very efficient means in selecting the appropriate imaging technique and exposure time [42]. The later development of controlled exercise oscillography [43] and stress tests with the Doppler ultrasound technique [44] had a lasting impact on the indications for arteriography of the lower extremities.

The advances in modern vascular surgery, such as surgical and percutaneous thromboendarterectomy (TEA) with the ring stripper [45] and, more importantly, the femoropopliteal bypass techniques by Kunlin [46] using the autologous saphenous vein or a Dacron prosthesis, required a precise knowledge of the individual manifestation of the chronic peripheral arterial occlusive disease. Employing a three-point indication [45] that included the clinical stage according to Fontaine, the operability, and the angiographic findings, together with the feasibility and technique of the surgical vascular reconstruction, made a consequent mapping of the incoming and outgoing vessels indispensable [47]. As a result, the visualization of the arteries of the lower leg and foot became increasingly more important [48] in acute and chronic arterial obliterations.

With the increasing clinical acceptance of Seldinger's retrograde catheterization technique [23a] or Hettler's closed-end catheter technique [41a,b], the translumbar puncture was performed less and less for aortoarteriography [47, 49, 50]. Thus, puncture and catheterization techniques and the use of ever more appropriate catheter materials gained in importance. In addition to Seldinger's technique, Hettler's technique provided the first opportunity to use closed-end catheters and for the first time incorporated the principle of a sheath for the exchange of catheters [41a,b]. Due to differences in the vascular occlusion pattern between both sides related to length of the obliteration and extent of the collateral circulation, the resultant asymmetric flow of contrast medium occasionally precluded a simultaneous visualization of both sides and required a repeat examination. This applied to each type of movable table used with a cut-film changers. Typical cut-film changers with broad applications are the AOT cut-film changer, the PUCK changer, and the Franklin changer.

A three-phase technique for arteriography of the pelvis and lower extremity was designed by Viehweger [51] in 1963 (Fig. III, 107). The X-ray tube was tilted in four radiographic positions without moving patient or cassette system. The arteries from the level of the kidneys to the

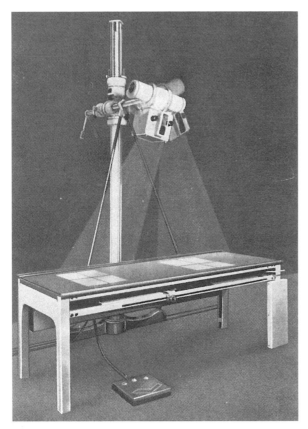

Fig. III, 107. Angiographic work place with three-phase technique after Viehweger. X-ray tube and collimator light field are placed for exposure positions one and four. (From: Heberer, Rau, Schoop, 1974).

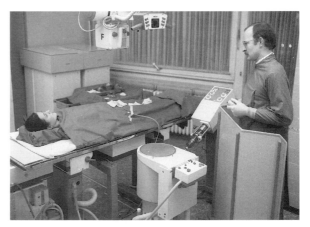

Fig. III, 108. Angiography table with automatic tabletop transport with an adjustable PUCK changer and ratchet switch.

feet were documented on a 35 x 120 cm film cassette loaded with four full-size films. Viehweger and Buechner [52] had shown that substantial distortions did not occur with this type of tube-tilting techniques [52] as long as the midline remained exactly focused. Unfortunately, the system was not further developed.

This technique may have become more widespread if digital subtraction angiography (DSA) had not been developed and angiography of the extremities with automatic table transport over an AOT or PUCK changer had not found such broad acceptance (Fig. III, 108).

Digital subtraction angiography

On the basis of experiments with computerized video–television systems [53, 54, 55, 56] the first digital subtraction angiographies after administration of contrast medium in vascular disorders was published in the early eighties.

Although the high expectations of a noninvasive intravenous angiography technique have only been partly realized, DSA (Fig. III, 109) and other digital angiographic methods have increasingly been applied throughout the world in addition to conventional angiography with automatic transport of the table or imaging system. Intravenous DSA [61], 10 years after its introduction and even after proposed placement of a thin catheter in the caval veins or right atrium, is used only in special circumstances, namely for the perioperative evaluation of vascular surgery, in interventional radiology, and for the diagnosis of abdominal aortic aneurysms (Fig. III, 110) or central occlusions in the pelvic or femoral arteries [57, 58, 59, 60], as a semi-invasive alternative to ultrasound and arterial DSA.

Arterial catheterization from the inguinal or antecubital regions [62, 63] has increasingly been accepted after introduction of 4 and 5 French catheters. Together with the use of very soft atraumatic guidewires (Terumo guidewire among others) the risk associated with arterial catheterization could be substantially reduced. Neither plaque detachment in the abdominal and pelvic region, nor serious complications at the puncture site have been observed. The arterial application of contrast media had enabled a more precise diagnosis (Fig. III, 109 and 113). In addition, the amount of contrast medium could be reduced. The adverse reactions and subjective complaints have become very low with the now almost exclusively used non-ionic contrast media [37, 38] in examinations performed without general anesthesia.

With a post-procedural observation period of 2–4 h, angiography of the pelvis and legs as

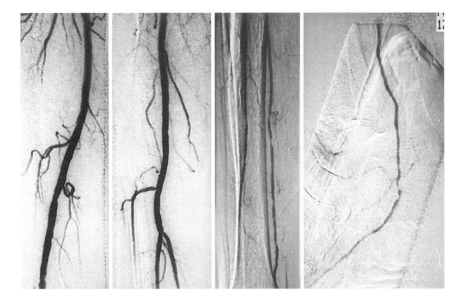

Fig. III, 109. Stepwise digital subtraction angiography (DSA) of the arteries of the lower extremities, virtually eliminating any interference from superimposed skeletal structures. Stenoses can be seen in femoral and pedal arteries as well as occlusions of the anterior tibial artery and dorsal pedal artery.

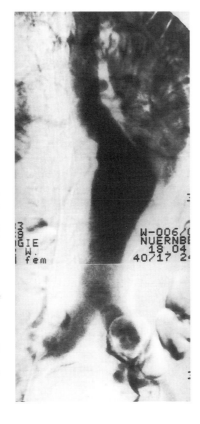

Fig. III, 110. Intravenous digital subtraction angiography in an infrarenal aorta aneurysm. The extent of the aneurysmal dilatation can be recognized as well as the absent lumbar arteries, its infrarenal location and the opacification of the left kidney after preceding administration of contrast medium.

DSA began as a video-subtraction technique and became a fully digitalized examination technique. Universal radiographic systems, primarily utilizing a C-arm arrangement with a large radius for lateral and oblique imaging, were available not only for the extremities, but also for the torso as well as for the extra- and intracranial vessels. These units have a wide range of applications for angiography of the extremities and for interventional radiology, including the options to treat arterial occlusions with percutaneous transluminal angioplasty (PTA) or to use intra-arterial embolization, thrombolysis and local infusion, as well as to perform fluoroscopically controlled biopsy and drainage. The angiographic units have been designed for multiplanar projections and for pelvic and femoral angiographies (Fig. III, 111) with only one injection of contrast medium into the abdominal aorta, just as in the early days of the first conventional angiographies with AOT changers (Fig. III, 112). The difference is that today the patient and the table remain fixed, while the imaging system consisting of X-ray tube, image intensifier, television circuit, and digital radiographic system moves in programmable steps [66, 67].

The digital systems provide advantages by enabling the exact measurements of vessels and stenoses as to length and diameter. The relative degree of a stenosis, expressed in percentages, can be determined objectively by diameter or density differences. This allows immediate quantification of the results of therapeutic interventions, and a objective measure for progression or regression of the disease.

well as shoulders and arms is increasingly performed on an outpatient basis [64, 65]. It is now possible to shorten the hospital stay of patients requiring active intervention and to avoid hospitalization of patients with vascular occlusive disease not suitable for active therapeutic intervention. Moreover, patients can be screened for complaints unrelated to vascular disease.

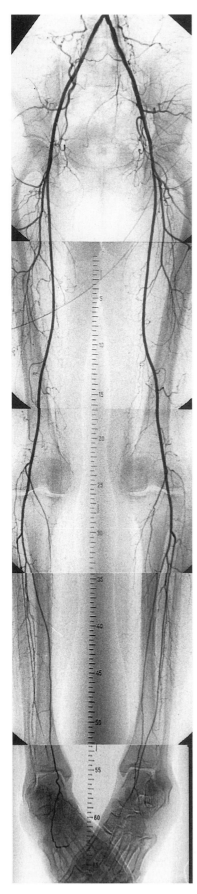

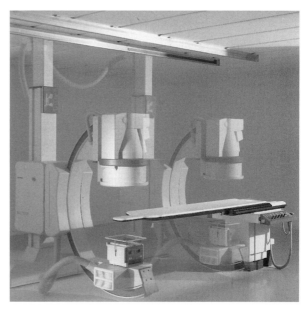

Fig. III, 112. Technical installation of a Multiscop with electronically controlled, movable C-arm unit relative to the fixed examination table.

Fig. III, 111. Intra-arterial DSA with visualization of the pelvic and femoral arteries from the aorta down to the pedal arteries in a patient in supine position and automatic transport of the X-ray tube (MULTISCOP with PERIVISION).

Of the image intensifiers developed as part of the imaging systems, the large-diameter intensifier has proven most valuable for angiography of the extremities. Depending on the need, it is mounted either above or below the angiographic table. It requires, however, specific collimator systems between the legs as well as filters to compensate for the different thickness of the various sections of the extremities. The use of full-size film changers is becoming superfluous since, in addition to digital image recording, the high resolution 100-mm image (Fluorospot) can be integrated into this system. The latter is particularly beneficial for instant documentation of changes occurring in the course of therapeutic interventions.

Digital subtraction angiography of peripheral vessels can also be performed after direct puncture of the femoral or cubital artery for the injection of a very small amount of contrast medium. Using a matrix of 1024 x 1024 in digital subtraction angiograms, a satisfactory visualization of digital arteries in the hands and feet (Fig. III, 113) is possible [48, 63].

Despite the high standard of spatial resolution with conventional radiological techniques and 100-mm image-intensifier fluorography, it becomes increasingly apparent that spatial resolution in the peripheral vessels is not the only criterion for diagnostic examinations. Increasingly, noninvasive examinations are demanded and are available.

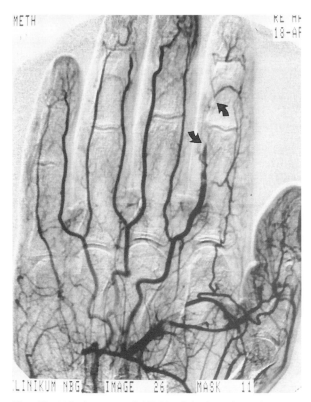

Fig. III, 113. Intra-arterial DSA of the hand arteries.

Noninvasive angiography of peripheral vessels

Today, color-coded duplex sonography [68, 69] and, increasingly, MR angiography [70, 71] are used as noninvasive methods to diagnose arterial or venous diseases of the arms and legs.

At present, neither method is capable of visualizing the peripheral vascular system from the aorta down to the pedal arteries or from the pedal veins up to the vena cava. Nevertheless, the functional flow analysis of arteries and veins provides essential diagnostic parameters. Typical examples include the demonstration of femoral and pelvic obliterations or the detection of pelvic or femoral venous thrombi. Duplex sonography, if carried out by experienced examiners with reliable modern equipment, not only complements angiography, but can also resolve clinically unclear cases and make angiography superfluous. In all cases considered for therapy by surgery or interventional radiology, an angiogram is still imperative. With an improved preliminary diagnosis, angiography can be better targeted and possibly performed immediately prior to a necessary therapeutic intervention. The number of di-

agnostic arteriograms and phlebograms [32, 72] can undoubtedly be reduced by duplex sonography. On the other hand, interventional angiographic methods are increasingly used in certain pathological conditions.

Thus, the discovery of X-rays has resulted not only in a diagnostic, but also in a therapeutic benefit. The patient can often be spared the risk of surgery and an extended hospital stay.

Up to now, MR angiography as well as duplex sonography can only cover sections of a certain range. Pelvis, knee or shoulder can be visualized with special techniques, such as 'phase imaging' or 'time-of-flight-technique' without the use of contrast media and without puncture or catheterization (Fig. III, 114) [73, 74]. Quantitative objective assessment of vascular pathology cannot only be established by changes of the vascular cross-section, but also, and even more so, by changes of the intraluminal blood flow. Further developments will likely mean a better analysis of the peripheral vessels by magnetic resonance angiography. It is uncertain, however, whether magnetic resonance imaging will have its place in the morphologic or functional diagnostic evaluation.

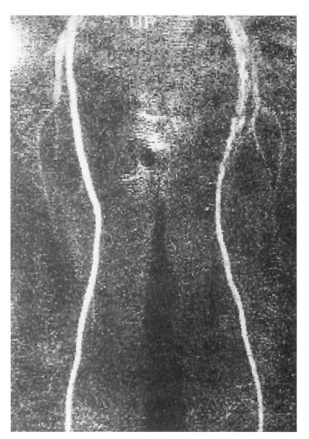

Fig. III, 114. MR angiography of femoral arteries.

Today, 100 years after the discovery of X-rays, there is no doubt that angiographic radiology provides the best objective morphological diagnosis of vascular diseases. It serves as the reference method for all other new imaging systems that do not use X-rays. It has also contributed to the development of vascular surgery and minimally invasive therapies, such as interventional radiology. It will continue to be of great value for interventional radiological and surgical treatments of many vascular diseases.

References

1. Roentgen, W.C.: Über eine neue Art von Strahlen. Erste Mitteilung. Sitzungsbericht der physikalisch-medizini\schen Gesellschaft. Würzburg 137, 1895

2. Haschek, E., Lindenthal D.Th.: Ein Beitrag zur prakti\schen Verwertung der Photographie nach Roentgen. Wiener Klin. Wschr. 9 (1896) 63

3. Morton, W.G., Hammer, E.W.: The X-ray, or Photography of the Invisible and its Value in Surgery. New York, Ameri\can Technical Book Co. 1896

4. Orrin, H.C.: The X-ray Atlas of the Systemic Arteries of the Body. Baillière, Tindall and Cox, London, 1920

5. Franck, O., Alwens, W.: Kreislaufstudien am Röntgen\schirm. Münch. med. Wschr. 57 (1910) 950

6. Sicard, J.A., Forestier, G.: Injections intravasculaires d'huile iodée sous controle radiologique. Compt. rend. Soc. Biol. 88 (1923) 1200

7. Berberich, J., Hirsch, S.: Die röntgenographische Dar\stellung der Arterien und Venen am Lebenden. Münch. med. Wschr. 49 (1923) 2226

8. Zeitler, E.: Aspekte der Extremitätenangiographie. Verlag Hans Huber, Bern, 1976

9. Brooks, B.: Intraarterial injection of sodium iodid. J. Am. Med. Ass. 82 (1924) 1016

10. Charbonnel, Massé: Artériographie des membres avec l'iodure de sodium, spécialement dans les artérites. Brill. mem. Soc. natl. chir. 55 (1929) 735

11. Dos Santos, R., Lamas, A.C., Pereira-Caldas, J.: Arteriografia da aorta e dos vasa abdominais. Med. contemp. 47 (1929) 93

12. Barke, R.: Röntgenkontrastmittel. VEB Georg Thieme, Leipzig, 1970

13. Binz, A., Räth, G.: Die Chemie des Uroselectans. Klin. Wschr. 9 (1930) 2297

14. Swick, M.: Darstellung der Niere und Harnwege im Röntgenbild durch intravenöse Einbringung eines neuen Kontraststoffes, des Uroselektans. Klin. Wschr. 8 (1929) 2087

15. Ratschow, M.: Uroselektan in der Vasographie unter besonderer Berücksichtigung der Varicographie. Fortschr. Röntgenstr. 42 (1930) 37–45

16. Dos Santos, R., Lamas, A., Caldas, J.P.: Arteriografia des membros. Med. Contemp. 47 (1929) 1

17. Dos Santos, R., Lamas, A., Caldas, J.P.: Artériographie des membres et de l'aorte abdominales. Masson et Cie, Paris, 1931

18. Forssmann, W.: Über Kontrastdarstellung der Höhlen des lebenden rechten Herzens und der Lungenschlagader. Münch. med. Wschr. 78 (1931) 489

19. Osborne, E.D., Sutherland, C.G., Schell, A.J., Rowntree, L.G.:
Roentgenography of the urinary tract during excretion of sodium iodid. J. Am. Med. Ass. 80 (1923) 368

20. Bronner, H., Hecht, G., Schüller, J.: Ausscheidungs-Pyelographie mit "Abrodil". Fortschr. Röntgenstr. 42 (1930) 206

21. Bronner, H., Kleinofen, P.: Einfluss der Diurese auf die Darstellung der Harnwege mit Perabrodil. Klin. Wschr. 16 (1937) 1056

22. Fariñas, P.L.: New technique for angiographic examination of the abdominal aorta and its branches. Am. J. Roentgenol. 46 (1941) 641

23a. Seldinger, S.J.: Catheter replacement of the needle in percutaneous arteriography. A new technique. Acta radiol. 39 (1953) 368

23b. Seldinger, S.J.: Arteries of the Extremities. In: Hdb. der Medizinischen Radiologie, Bd. X/3. Ed. Diethelm, L., Olsson, O., Strnad, P., Vieten, H., Zuppinger, A., Springer Verlag Berlin 1964, 400–472

24. Bruwer, A.J. (Editor): Classic Descriptions in Diagnostic Roentgenography. Charles Thomas Publisher, Springfield, Fig. 1964
– Glaser, O.: Wilhelm Conrad Roentgen. S. 23–46
– Abrams, H.L.: Card-Angiography and Thoracic Aortography. S.492
– Lessmann, F.P.: Phlebography. S. 653

25. Wallingford, V.H.: 3-Carboxylic-acylamino- 2,4,6-trijodbenzoic acids and the ethylester and nontoxic salts. US Patent 2 (1952) 611, 786

26. Langecker H., Harwart, A., Junkmann, K.: 3,5-Diacetylamino-2,4,6-trijodbenzoesäure als Röntgenkontrastmittel. Naunyn-Schmiedebergs Arch. Exp. Pathol. 222 (1954) 584–590

27. Sovak, M. ed: Radiocontrast agents. Springer Verlag Berlin, Heidelberg, New York, Tokyo (1984)

28a. Zeitler, E.: Kontrastmittelrisiko arterieller Angiographie. In: Kontrastmittelzwischenfälle, Symposium 1977, Schering AG, Berlin, S 117–121

28b. Zeitler, E.: Risks of arteriography under local anaesthesia. Ann. Radiol. 21 (1978) 491–492

29. Mann, S., Zeitler, E.: Verhalten der Serumosmolalität bei hohen Kontrastmitteldosen im Rahmen der Angiographie. Fortschr. Röntgenstr. 122 (1975) 135

30. Heberer, G., Rau, G., Schoop, W.: Angiologie, Begr. v. M. Ratschow. G. Thieme Verlag, Stuttgart, 1974

31. Zeitler, E.: Röntgenologische und nuklearmedizinische Diagnostik. S. 297–460 in Ehringer, H., Fischer, H., Netzer, C.O., Schmutzler, R., Zeitler, E.: Venöse Abflußströmungen, Enke Verlag Stuttgart 1979

32. Weber, J., May, R.: Funktionelle Phlebographie. G. Thieme Verlag Stuttgart 1990

33. Schmiedel, E.: Pharmakodynamik und Verträglichkeit von Röntgenkontrastmitteln. Röntgen-Bl. 40 (1987) 1–8

34. Speck, U., Siefert, H.M., Klink, G.: Contrast media and pain in peripheral arteriography. Invest. Radiol. 15 (1980) 335–389

35. Almén, T.: Effects of Metrizamide and other contrast media on the isolated rabbit heart. Acta radiol. Suppl. 335 (1973) 216

36. Björk, L., Erikson, U., Ingelman, B.: Clinical experience with a new type of contrast medium in selective coronary arteriography. Fortschr. Röntgenstr. 114 (1971) 816

37. Taenzer, V., Zeitler, E.: Contrast Media in Urography, Angiography and CT. G. Thieme Verlag Stuttgart 1983

38. Peters, D.E., Zeitler, E.: Röntgenkontrastmittel. Springer Verlag, Berlin, Heidelberg, 1991
39. Janker, R.: Röntgenologische Funktionsdiagnostik. Verlag W. Girardet, Wuppertal-Elbersfeld 1954
40. Pässler, H.W.: Abdominale Aortographie mit besonderer Berücksichtigung der bilateralen retrograden Serienaortographie ohne Katheter. Fortschr. Röntgenstr. 98 (1963) 279
41a. Hettler, M.: Die sichere Arterienpunktion als Grundlage der Extremitätenangiographie und des Arterienkatheterismus. Fortschr. Röntgenstr. 92 (1960) 97
41b. Hettler, M.: Der perkutane Arterien-Katheterismus mit an der Spitze verschlossenem Katheter als Grundlage der Etagenaortographie. Fortschr. Röntgenstr. 92 (1960) 198
42. Friedmann, G.: Oscillographie und Rheographie als Voruntersuchungen bei der Extremitätenarteriographie. Röntgen-Bl. 7 (1954) 99
43. Schoop, W.: Praktische Angiologie. 4. Aufl. (Belastgs-Oscillogr.) G. Thieme Verlag Stuttgart 1987
44. Bollinger, A.: Funktionelle Angiologie. Lehrbuch und Atlas, Thieme Verlag Stuttgart, 1979
45. Vollmar, J.: Rekonstruktive Chirurgie der Arterien. G. Thieme Verlag Stuttgart 1975
46. Kunlin, J.: Le traitement de l'artérite oblitérante par la greffe veineuse. Arch. Mol. Coeur 42 (1949) 371
47. Kappert, A.: Lehrbuch und Atlas der Angiologie. 12. Aufl. Verlag Huber, Bern, 1984
48. Zeitler, E.: Die selektive Katheterangiographie der A. femoralis superficialis. Electromedica 5 (1975) 167–178
49. Wenz, W.: Abdominale Angiographie. Springer Verlag, Berlin, 1972
50. Zeitler, E.: Aorto-Arteriographie. In: Angiologie, Begr. v. M. Ratschow, Heberer, G., Rau, G., Schoop, W.
51. Viehweger, G.: Die Drehphasentechnik. Deutscher Röntgenkongress. Thieme Verlag, Stuttgart, 1963, S. 236
52. Büchner, H.: Der Zentralstrahl ist für die Röntgenprojektion völlig bedeutungslos. Fortschr. Röntgenstr. 107 (1967) 540
53. Mistretta, C.A., Crummy, A.B., Strother, C.M.: Digital angiography: A prospective study. Radiology 139, 273 (1981)
54. Brennecke, R., Brown, T.K., Bursch, J., Heintzen, D.M.: Computerized video-image processing with application to cardioangiographic Roentgen image series. In: Nagel, H.H. (Ed.): Digital Image Processing. Springer Verlag, New York 1978, 244
55. Ovitt, T.W., Nudelmann, S.N., Fisher, D. et al.: Computerassisted video subtraction for intravenous angiography. Presented at work in progress at RSNA Chicago, Fig. Nov. 27 – Dec. 2, 1977
56. Christenson, P.C., Ovitt, Th.W., Fisher III, H.D., et al.: Intravenous angiography using digital video subtraction: Intravenous cervico-cerebrovascular angiography. Amer. J. Roentgenol. 135 (1980), 1145–1152
57. Crummy, A.B., Strother, Ch.M., Sackett, J.P. et al.: Computerized fluoroscopy: Digital subtraction for intravenous angiocardiography and arteriography. Amer. J. Roentgenol. 135 (1980), 1131–1141
58. Meany, T.F., Weinstein, M.A., Buonocore, E., et al.: Digital subtraction angiography of the human cardiovascular system. Am. J. Roentgenol. 135 (1980), 1153–1160
59. Seyferth, W., Marhoff, P., Zeitler, E.: Digital Subtraction Angiography (DSA); electromedica 2/82, S. 60–68
60. Seyferth, W., Marhoff, P., Zeitler, E.: Transvenöse und arterielle digitale Videosubtraktionsangiographie (DVSA). Fortschr. Röntgenstr. Heft 3, Band 136 (1982) 237–358
61. Zeitler, E.: Zehn Jahre digitale Subtraktionsangiographie am Klinikum Nürnberg. Electromedica 59 (1991) 102–104
62. Thurn, P., Felix, R. (Hrsg.) Standortbestimmung der digitalen Subtraktionsangiographie (DSA). Schering, Berlin, 1984
63. Zeitler, E.: Angiographie bei peripheren Durchblutungsstörungen. Internist 30 (1989) 406–410
64. Langer, M.: Ambulante digitale Subtraktionsangiographie. Schering, Berlin, 1986
65. Zeitler, E.: DSA unter stationären und ambulanten Bedingungen. Jahrbuch der Radiologie 1987, 27 – 47 Verlag Regensberg und Biermann, Münster
66. Fink, U.: Peripheral DSA with automated stepping. Eur. Rad. 13 (1991) 50
67. Darcy, M.D.: Lower-extremity arteriography: current approach and techniques. Radiology 178 (1991) 615
68. Jäger, K.: Duplex-Sonographie peripherer Arterien, Grundlagen und klinische Anwendung. Basel, Habilschrft. 1990
69. Fobbe, F., Koennecke , H.C., el Bedew, M., Heidt, P., Buese-Landgraf, J., Wolf, K.J.: Diagnostik der tiefen Beinvenenthrombose mit der farbkodierten Duplexsonographie. Fortschr. Röntgenstr. 151 (1989) 569–573
70. Dumoulin, C.L., Hart, H.R.: Magnetic Resonance Angiography. Radiology 161 (1986) 717–720
71. Marchal, G., Bosmans, H., van Hecke, P.: Magnetic Resonance Angiography. Review in MR: State of the Art. European Radiology Syllabus (1991) 166–178
72. Hach, W.: Phlebographie der Bein- und Beckenvenen. Schnetztor-Verlag GmbH, Konstanz, 1985
73. Laub G.A., Kaiser, W.A.: Angiography with Gradient Motion Refocussing. J. Comp. Ass. Tomogr. 12 (1988) 377–382
74. Peters, P.E., Bongartz, G., Drews, C.: Magnetresonanzangiographie der hirnversorgende Arterien. Fortschr. Röntgenstr. 152 (1989) 528–533

Lymphatic system

L. Beltz

Historical overview

The existence of lymphatic vessels has been known since antiquity. Hippocrates considered them as vessels transporting white blood, and Aristotle as containing colorless liquid. It was not before 1622 that Gaspare Asellius recognized the lymphatic vessels as a system separate from arteries and veins. In a dog, Pecquet described the cisterna chyli and thoracic duct which passed the liver, naming it ductus chyliferous in 1651. In 1653, the Swede Rudbeck discovered the lymphatic valves, and the same year the anatomist Bartholinus from Copenhagen gave the milky vessels their present name 'vasa lymphatica' (English: lymphatic vessels or lymphatics).

In this historical overview, we will pass over the early discoverers of the lymphatic system, their observations, speculations, and sometimes very personal priority battles, and will instead refer to the early publications by Asellius, 1627; Pecquet, 1651; Bartholinus, 1651 and 1653; Rudbeck, 1653; Barthels, 1909; Jossifow, 1930; and Rouviere, 1932. The fundamental work on the pathophysiology of the lymphatic circulation primarily came from Rusznyak et al, 1969.

Already in the early days, it has been tried to visualize the lymphatic vessels in the living. In detailed investigations, Mascagni studied the human lymphatic vessels and published his results in copperplate engravings in his work 'Vasorum Lymphaticorum Corporis Humani Historia et Ichnographia' (1787), which depicts the lymphatic vessels in detail that rivals present-day radiographic images.

After mentioning the history of classic anatomical and physiological investigations, our interest should focus on the feasibility of radiographic visualization. The first radiographs of lymphatic vessels were taken by Shdanov (1932) in cadavers and animals, with visualization of the lymphatic vessels following injection of mercury, lead, and silver compounds. The first direct injection of contrast medium into a lymph node was reported by Carvalho and coworkers in 1931.

In 1952, the English surgeon J.B. Kinmonth opened the lymphatic system to diagnostic radiology. He discovered a suitable vital dye (patent blue) to visualize the vessels, developed a meticulous technique of direct puncture of the lymphatic vessels and injected a water-soluble contrast medium to study lymphedema. The disadvantage of a water-soluble contrast medium was its fast diffusion across the wall of the lymphatic vessels. Not until iodinated oily contrast media, such as the iodinated ethyl ester of a mixture of mono- and di-iodinated saturated and unsaturated fatty acids mixed with poppy seed oil as carrier (Lipiodol UF, Ethiodol), was used, the visualization of the lymphatic system succeeded. Due to storage of contrast medium in the nodal sinusoids, the lymph nodes remain opacified over a long period of time.

In the sixties, the radiological evaluation of the lymphatic system advanced rapidly (Tjernberg, 1962; Servelle, 1962; Abbes, 1963; Arvay and Picard, 1963; Koehler et al, 1964; Ruettimann and Del Buono, 1964; Fuchs, 1965; Weissleder, 1965; Wiljasalo, 1965; Gerteis, 1966):
- The knowledge of the anatomy of the lymphatic vessels and lymph nodes increased (Jacobsson and Johansson, 1959; Gerteis, 1966; Wirth, 1966).
- The various forms of lymphedema of the extremities could be radiographically visualized and further defined (Jacobsson and Johansson, 1959; Kaindl et al, 1960; Servelle, 1962; Godart et al, 1964; de Roo, 1966; Gruwez

and Goldstein, 1968; Foeldi, 1969 and 1971; Clodius, 1977).

– The extent and localization of lymphomas could be shown, above all in the torso and here particularly in the retroperitoneum, and, with some limitation, further differentiated (Ruettimann and Del Buono, 1964; Fuchs, 1965; Weissleder, 1965; Luening et al, 1976; Elke and Beltz, 1984).

– This method gained great importance in the search for metastases in patients with urogenital tumors. The characteristic findings of impaired lymph drainage secondary to tumorous obstruction and the development of collateral lymphatic pathways provided new knowledge about the pattern of metastatic spread (Beltz, 1970 and 1980).

One limitation of the described method has remained until today. The lymphatic vessels can only be stained, dissected and injected with the oily contrast medium at a few anatomic sites. The pedal lymphography has remained the preferred approach to visualize the lymphatic vessels in the legs, the lymphatic vessels and lymph nodes in the groins and in the retroperitoneum, and the thoracic duct as well as some of the lymph nodes in its drainage area.

Lymphographic technique

Before presenting the radiographic anatomy of the lymphatic system, the technical aspects of lymphography should be reviewed here. The technique of lymphography was developed by the English surgeon Kinmonth (Fig. III, 115) in 1952 and is still in general use today, though with many suggested modifications not to be included in this presentation. Staining the lymphatic vessels with dye for the dissection has remained unchanged and is still valuable today, independent of the injection site. In pedal lymphography, the lymphatic vessels are stained following subcutaneous injection of 1 ml patent blue dye into the dorsum of the first interdigital clefts. The best site for the surgical preparation of the lymphatic vessels proved to be the level of the first and second cuneiform bones or navicular bone where the lymphatic vessels are of wider caliber than further distally. Numerous needles and sets of surgical instruments for cannulating the lymphatic vessels are on the market. Most commonly used is Ruettimann's and Del Buono's (1964) special cannula, but various other customized sets of surgical instruments with catheters are

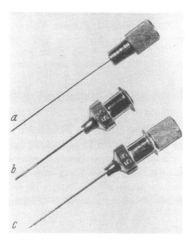

Fig. III, 115a–c. Lymphatic cannulation technique (1964).

Fig. III, 115a. Needle.

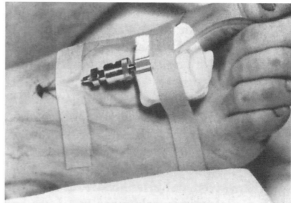

Fig. III, 115b. Puncture.

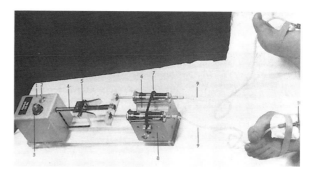

Fig. III, 115c. Foot after puncture and connected to the infusion pump.

on the market (Altaras, 1969, Luening et al, 1976). Water-soluble iodine contrast media are undoubtedly best tolerated, but are only suitable for diagnosing disorders of the lymphatic vessels due to rapid diffusion and only transient storage in the lymph nodes, precluding an adequate morphologic assessment of nodal structures. Thus, lymphography still depends on the use of iodinated oily contrast media (Lipiodol UF, Ethiodol).

Adverse reactions and complications

Some adverse reactions and complications that could occur in the use of iodinated oily contrast media should be mentioned:

– The oily contrast medium enters the venous system from the thoracic duct and moves into the lungs where it becomes lodged in the pulmonary capillaries as oil emboli, potentially causing pulmonary infarcts, pulmonary edema and lipoid pneumonia. Using correct technique (not too much contrast medium), the incident of these complications is approximately 1:2500 examinations performed.

– Allergic reactions to the oily contrast medium have not occurred, as far as we know, but have been observed to the dye used for staining of the lymphatics, particularly to patent blue dye. The allergic reaction develops soon after the injection of the dye (immediate type) and usually is easily reversible. A severe allergic shock is rare.

– The oily contrast medium causes a dilatation of all sinuses within the lymph nodes during the first day after the injection. The contrast medium is only stored and not actively incorporated into the cells, compressing the intervening reticular tissues. Already after a few days, the phase of accelerated resorption and phagocytosis develops. Foreign-body giant cells and occasionally plasma cells appear, and a sclerosis of the supportive tissue framework develops and, eventually, nodal fibrosis, which remains recognizable for years. It is important to note that neither lymphatic vessels nor lymph nodes lose their function. The lymphatic vessels remain patent, as proven by follow-up lymphograms, and the lymph nodes maintain their filtering and storage functions. Nevertheless, three possible disadvantages or contraindications have been repeatedly mentioned:

  • Through damage of the cannulated lymphatic vessels, lymphedema can progress, particularly when secondary to hypoplasia of the lymphatic system;
  • There is the risk of the propagation of tumor cells and metastatic spread to the next higher regional group of lymph nodes;
  • The histologically observed changes in the lymph nodes may induce a malignant conversion of the lymphatic tissue (Guetgemann, 1968).

In summary, it can be stated that by using the correct technique, such as careful preparation of the vessels, and individual selection of the total amount of contrast-medium injected (radiological control of the disturbed or undisturbed contrast-medium drainage), the most frequently occurring complications could be avoided. The increase in lymphedema as a result of lymphography is usually transient. Up to now, lymphographic dissemination of tumor cells leading to metastatic spread has not been proven, and carcinomatous nodal transformation induced by lymphography with oily contrast medium has not been observed. The initially reported complications have almost exclusively resulted from a faulty technique.

Anatomy

Extremities

A superficial or prefascial (subcutaneous) system is distinguished from a deep (subfascial) lymphatic system. The pedal lymphography will predominantly opacify the lymphatic vessels of the superficial system of the lower extremities (Fig. III, 116a).

The lymphatic vessels are classified according to caliber and localization: the vessels of the first

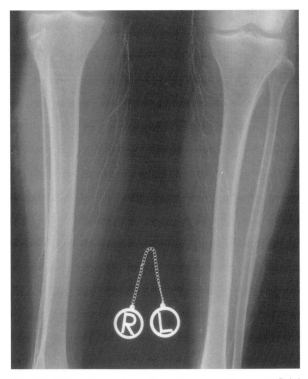

Fig. III, 116a. Normal lymphangiogram of the superficial or prefascial ventromedial lymphatic chain of the legs. The lymphatic vessels run medially and increase in number cranially.

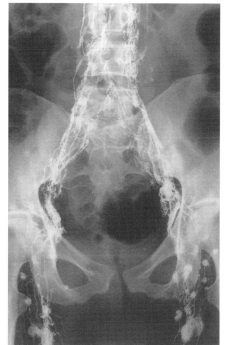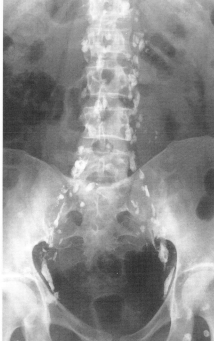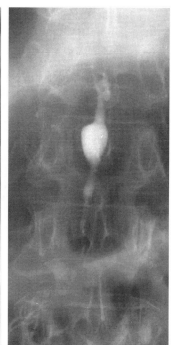

Fig. III, 116b. Normal lymphangiogram or filling image of the subinguinal and retroperitoneal (iliac and lumbar) lymphatic vessels. In all sections interganglionic anastomoses are present. **c)** Normal lymphadenogram or storage image of the inguinal and retroperitoneal lymph nodes. Three to four hours after injection, the contrast medium has left the vessels and is stored in the lymph nodes.

Fig. III, 116d. Cisterna chyli: contrast medium that is not stored in the lymph nodes reaches the subphrenic cisterna chyli via the lumbar trunci.

order are the collectors (lymphographically demonstrable), the vessels of the second order are the precollectors, and the vessels of the third order are the lymphatic capillaries. In the lower extremities, the anteromedial prefascial lymphatic trunk drains the cutaneous capillaries and accompany the greater saphenous vein. The interpretation of the pathologic lymphogram is based on the analysis of the number, caliber and course of the lymphatic vessels. The evaluation of lymphangiopathies also requires the histological examination of the wall of the lymphatic vessel (Jacobsson and Johansson, 1959; Kaindl et al, 1960; Kinmonth, 1972).

Inguinal region and retroperitoneum

The lymphatic vessels of the anteromedial trunk drain into the subinguinal lymph nodes and thereafter into the inguinal (groin) lymph nodes. From there, efferent lymphatic vessels pass under the inguinal ligamentum into the pelvis and continue along the external iliac artery and vein. They form three chains and are called

external iliac lymphatic vessels because of their location.

In the common iliac vein region, these three chains continue and drain into the lumbar lymphatic plexus, which accompanies the abdominal aorta and inferior vena cava (Fig. III, 116b). At the level of the second lumbar vertebra, the lymphatic vessels form two lumbar trunks, which drain into the cisterna chyli (Fig. III, 116d).

Thoracic duct

The inferior end of the thoracic duct is the cisterna chyli, which is intra-abdominal in location, and from there it ascends in front of the thoracic spine. The thoracic duct is initially to the right side of the aorta, inclines to the left at the level of the thoracic aperture, to drain with several ducts and trunks into the junction of the left subclavian and internal jugular vein (angulus venosus). The termination can also be on the right or bilateral. The thoracic duct's normal caliber ranges between 1 and 4 mm (Fig. III, 116e).

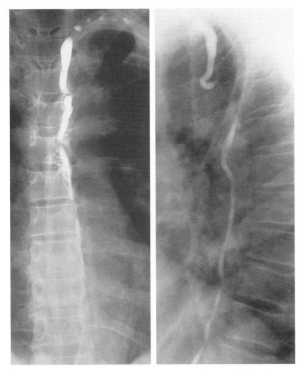

Fig. III, 116e. Thoracic duct in two planes. The ductus runs in front of the spinal column to the upper thoracic aperture and opens into the left angulus venosus with several branches. With increased lymph volume (liver cirrhosis), the ductus is dilated as shown in this case.

There is a distinction between lymphangiogram (visualization of the lymphatic vessels) or filling phase (Fig. III, 116b) and lymphadenogram (visualization of the lymph nodes) or storage phase (Fig. III, 116c). With the currently injected total amounts of Ethiodol, a nodal opacification adequate for diagnostic evaluation can persist for up to 12 months (Fig. III, 117 a–c). Thus, the therapeutic response of nodal pathology can be followed without reinjecting contrast medium (Fig. III, 124 a, b; Fig. III, 125 a–c).

Diseases of the lymphatic vessels

Lymphedema

A classification of the peripheral lymphedema is found in table III, 3. Heredity, age of onset and precipitating factors are primarily considered in this classification, less so morphological changes in the lymphatic vessels and corresponding lymphographic criteria, such as aplasia, hypoplasia or hyperplasia of lymphatic vessels and their histologic findings.

In patients referred for radiologic evaluation, three conditions predominate:
– Acquired primary lymphedema with hypoplasia. Congenital primary lymphedema with hyperplasia of the lymphatic vessels is rather rare.
– Secondary lymphedema in tumors, after trauma, during inflammation or after surgical intervention.
– Post-traumatic or postsurgical decompensated lymphedema (Brunner, 1969), or secondary lymphedema in primary dysplasia of lymphatic vessels (Beltz, 1981).

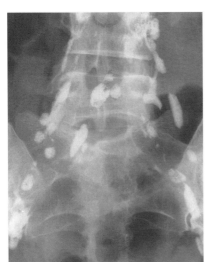
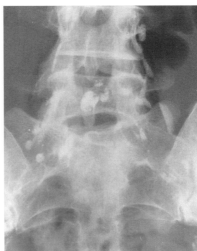
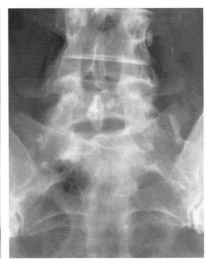

Fig. III, 117a-c. Follow-up lymphadenograms: duration of the visible stored contrast medium in normal retroperitoneal lymph nodes. **a)** Lymphadenogram, 24 hours after the injection, **b)** after two months, **c)** after ten months.

Table III, 3. Classification of peripheral lymphedema

I. Primary lymphedema
   a) hereditary, congenital lymphedema (Nonne 1891, Milroy 1892)
   b) hereditary, noncongenital lymphedema (Meige 1898)
   c) congenital, nonhereditary lymphedema
   d) acquired lymphedema
      – hypoplasia
      – aplasia
      – lymphangiectasia

II. Secondary lymphedema
   a) tumorous lymphedema
   b) traumatic lymphedema
   c) postsurgical lymphedema
   d) inflammatory lymphedema
   e) parasitic lymphedema

III. Combined phlebolymphedema
   1. lymphedema in primary venous disorders
      a) varicosis
      b) postphlebitic syndrome
      c) thrombophlebitis
      d) venous ulcer
      e) venous insufficiency
   2. Tumorous phlebolymphedema

IV. Differential diagnosis
   a) primary lymphedema in mixed congenital angio-dysplasias
   b) primary lymphedema together with other diseases (Turner-syndrome, hereditary recurrent intrahepatic cholestasis)
   c) Lipoedema (tree-trunk or fatty leg)

Primary lymphedema

Lymphangiectatic edema (Fig. III, 118a) is usually a unilateral lymphedema of the foot, the ankle or the entire leg accompanied by anomalous lymphatic vessel of the torso (Fig. III, 118b). This type is usually congenital but not hereditary (Malan and Puglionisi, 1964).

Hypoplasia of the lymphatic vessels is a more frequently acquired primary lymphedema with a decrease in lymphatic vessels in the prefascial vascular tracts. Lymphographically, a reduction in number and frequently also a narrowed lumen can be recognized (Fig. III, 119). In 1960, Kaindl et al have described a disease of the intima as lymphangiopathia obliterans.

Secondary lymphedema

It is the role of lymphography to localize and analyze the damage of the lymphatic vessels causing the secondary lymphedema. Secondary lymphedema is characterized by the following lymphographic findings:
– Total or partial blockage of the level of the damaged lymphatic vessels, with local distension (edema) distally and backflow of contrast medium into lymphatic vessels of the second and third order.
– Drainage through collateral vessels to bypass the local damage (Jacobsson and Johansson, 1962; Picard and Gallet, 1966; Gruwez and Goldstein, 1968; Brunner et al, 1970; Clodius, 1977).

Fig. III, 118a, b. Primary congenital lymphedema; six-year-old boy. **a)** Hyperplastic, lymphangiectatic lymphedema of the right leg in primary congenital lymphedema. **b)** A concomitant retroperitoneal lymphatic disease is present: systemic angiomatous dysplasia with ectatic lymphatic vessels, valvular insufficiency, reflux into pubic and scrotal lymphatic vessels, scrotal lymphedema, osteolymphangiomatosis (1984).

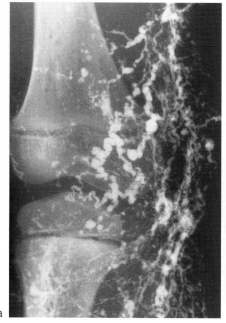
a

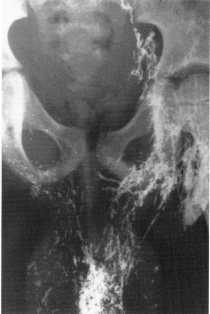
b

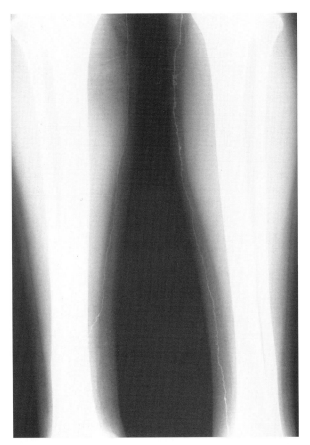

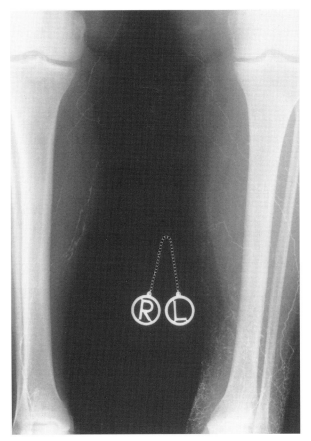

Fig. III, 119. Primary acquired lymphedema in hypoplasia. A 24-year-old female patient, hypoplastic lymphatic vessels showing a decreased caliber and fewer valves. Cutaneous and subcutaneous fibrosis are present (1984).

Fig. III, 120. Secondary tumorous lymphedema, 60-year-old female patient, cervix carcinoma, stage III. Mainly left-sided lymphedema with partly dilated and tortuous lymphatic vessels, retrograde filling of the precollectors and lymphatic capillaries (dermal backflow) (1984).

The most frequent causes of secondary lymphedema are tumors (Fig. III, 120), trauma, infection and postsurgical changes in lymph circulation, particularly following surgical interventions in the inguinal region or axilla.

Even today lymphography is always indicated to clarify edemas of unclear etiology, to recognize mixed forms (e.g. combined lymph–phlebo–edema) or to distinguish lymphedema from lipidemia (so-called trunk leg or regional adiposity). In our experience, approximately 50% of the patients with lipidemia are found to have dysplasia of the lymphatic vessels (usually hypoplasia).

Lymphatic and venous systems

Embryology can explain the close relationship between lymphatic vessels and veins. However, the lymphatic system is not only ontogenetically but also functionally related to the venous system.

Almost all venous diseases alter the lymph circulation. Combined phlebo–lymph–oedema can be observed in varicosity of the legs, in the post-thrombotic syndrome, in thrombophlebitis, and also in ulcers of the lower leg due to stasis. In cases with such a compound damage, only lymphography together with simultaneous venography can lead to the correct diagnosis.

In the mixed forms of angiodysplasia, the arterial, venous and lymphatic circulation must be examined to assure exact classification (Malan and Puglionisi, 1964, 1965).

Central lymphangiopathies

In accordance with the pathological findings of the lymphatic system of the extremities, central angiopathies can also be broadly classified into aplasia, hypoplasia, and hyperplasia of the lymphatic system, whereby this classification primarily applies to the main lymphatic vessels below the diaphragm less so to the thoracic duct. The hyperplastic form is the most frequent disease affecting the retroperitoneal lymphatic system, and is lymphographically characterized by varicose or angiomatous abnormalities, chylous reflux and chylous effusion (Fig. III, 118b).

Lymphatic cysts

Primary lymphatic cysts arise from the walls of dysplastic vessels (Fig. III, 121). The disposition for the cyst formation is congenital. Lymphatic congestion alone does not lead to cyst formation.

Secondary lymphatic cysts or lymphoceles can nearly always be traced back to previous surgical interventions, particularly to lymphadenectomies. The lymphatic vessels are dissected during surgery, and the lymph extravasates from the damaged vessel into the surrounding tissues to form a localized accumulation of chyle. Lymphoceles are created cavities without epithelial lining. Nowadays, lymphoceles are no longer assessed lymphographically, but, if necessary, with ultrasound or computed tomography.

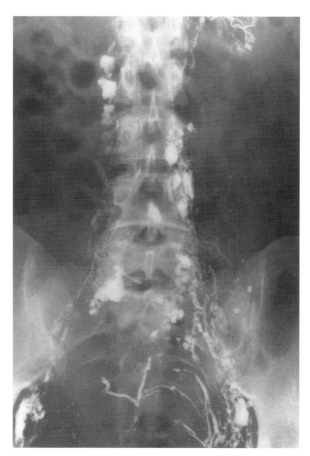

Fig. III, 122a, b. Chylascites in retroperitoneal dysplasia of lymphatic vessels. A 26-year-old female patient. **a)** Dysplastic lymphatic vessels with numerous retroperitoneal fistulous communications.

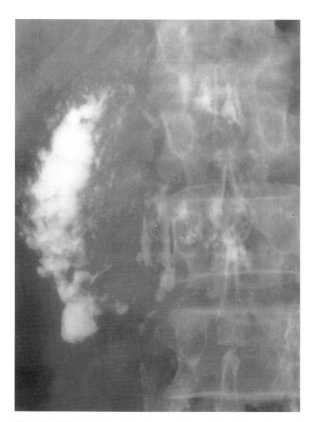

Fig. III, 121. Multicystic retroperitoneal lymphangioma. A 59-year-old male patient. A lymphangioma with large cysts mainly localized in the right retroperitoneum (1984).

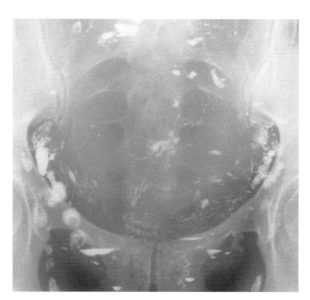

Fig. III, 122b. A delayed film obtained upright shows free leakage of contrast medium into the pelvic cavity (1984).

Chylous effusion

Chylous effusion is caused by a disorder of the lymphatic system with chylous reflux and leakage of chyle into one of the body cavities (chylothorax, chylous ascites and chylopericardium), as well as into an organ (e.g. chyluria), but rarely into the skin (cutaneous chylous blisters or chylous cysts) (Picard, 1967; Beltz, 1980).

There are either primary lymphatic dysplasias (Fig. III, 122 a, b), primary lymphatic tumors (Fig. III, 123 a, b) or, rarely, secondary abnormalities of the lymphatic vessels in tumors, after trauma or surgical intervention, in infections, or in parasitic infestations (Table III, 4). Since the chylous genesis of the effusion is generally known, lymphography should elucidate its underlying cause and possibly locate the site of the lymph fistula. Localizing a fistula is easy in

Table III, 4. Causes of chylous effusions

– Congenital malformation or dysplasia of lymphatic system with
  • congenital chylous effusion
  • acquired chylous effusion
– Chylous effusion in primary tumors of the lymphatic system (lymphangiomas and lymphangiomyomas) and in lymphoceles
– Chylous effusion in malignant and benign tumors
– Posttraumatic chylous effusion
– Postsurgical or iatrogenic chylous effusion
– Inflammatory and parasitic chylous effusion
– Chylous effusion in venous disorders (thrombosis or increases venous pressure)

cases with local vascular damage but can be difficult in a systemic disease of the lymphatic vessels.

Filariasis, which only occurs in tropical countries, is by far the most frequent cause of chyluria. It is produced by a mechanical obstruction of the lymphatic vessels infested with parasites (Picard, 1967).

Tumors of the lymphatic system

Lymphangiomas and lymphangiomyomas are rare benign tumors of the lymphatic system. While lymphangioma simplex (i.e. capillary lymphangioma, usually a superficial lymphangioma), lymphangioma cavernosum or cysticum, and the large-cyst lymphangioma in the neck are no indications for a lymphographic examination, the retroperitoneal and mediastinal lymphangiomas (Fig. III, 121) can be visualized lymphographically; this is also true of the rare lymphangiomyomatosis that only affects females (Fig. III, 123a).

Lymph node diseases

Lymphography is not indicated for benign lymph node diseases, but cognizance of benign changes (nodal phase) is important, primarily to interpret early lymphadenographic features of malignant lymph node processes correctly.

Defects of fibrolipomatous degeneration in the lymph nodes are most frequent, and are secondary to age-related degeneration of the lym-

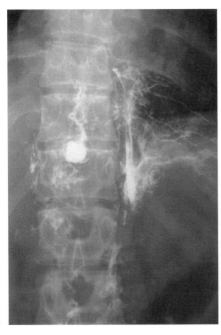

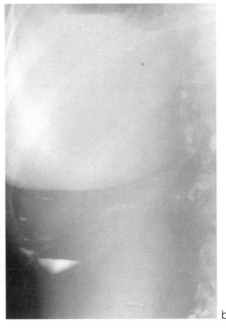

Fig. III, 123a, b. Retroperitoneal and mediastinal lymphangiomyoma and chylothorax. **a)** In the retroperitoneum and posterior mediastinum, angiomatous tumor of the lymphatic vessels with numerous fistulous communications. **b)** Thorax in an upright position: free leakage of contrast medium into the sinus in chylothorax.

a

b

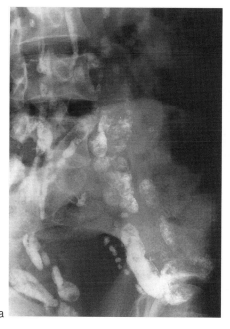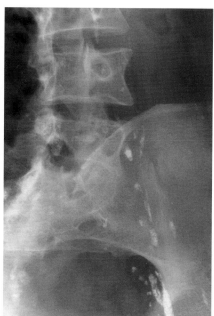

Fig. III, 124a, b. Hodgkin lymphoma. A 36-year-old male patient. **a)** Clearly enlarged retroperitoneal lymph nodes with a partly cystic, partly indistinct storage structure. The periphery of the lymph nodes is preserved. **b)** Follow-up five months later, after radiation therapy: tumor completely regressed, unremarkable lymph nodes.   a   b

phatic tissues with thinning of the nodal tissue. They are also called benign fibrolipomatous storage defects. Reactive lymph node hyperplasia, often a nonspecific finding in inflammatory and also noninflammatory diseases, also belongs to the benign lymph node diseases. Follicular hyperplasia, lymph-node tuberculosis, often accompanied with calcifications, and sarcoidosis are other benign lymph node diseases. Finally, rheumatic diseases accompanied by inflammatory nodal reactions should be mentioned. The characteristic lymphadenogram of these benign and often chronic inflammatory lymph-node processes have been described by many authors (Tjernberg, 1962; Ruettimann and Del Buono, 1964; Wiljasalo, 1965; Viamonte and Ruettimann, 1980; Elke, 1984).

Malignant lymph node diseases

The malignant lymph node diseases, of course, represent the most prominent indications for lymphography. It is important to evaluate
– the extent of the primary malignant lymphoma,
– and the lymphogenic metastatic spread of other primary tumors.

Primary malignant lymphomas

Only through lymphography it became apparent how often the lymph nodes within the retroper-

itoneum are involved in malignant lymphatic diseases. In the sixties, it was discovered that primary lymph node neoplasias could be confined to the retroperitoneum. One would have expected some insight from autopsies, but the postmortem findings usually came from patients who had died in the late or disseminated phase. Until the introduction of computed tomography, lymphography was routinely used to stage malignant lymphomas and was also always used on patients with suspected retroperitoneal nodal metastases.

The early histologic classification dividing Hodgkin's disease or lymphogranulomatosis and the old classification of non-Hodgkin lymphoma with diseases entities of reticulosarcoma, lymphosarcoma, and Brill–Symmers disease have now been abandoned in favor of the modern classification for Hodgkin and non-Hodgkin lymphomas.

Systematically analyzing lymphadenograms for many years, lymphologists have endeavored to find a more exact differentiation of the various malignant lymph node diseases (Fig. III, 124 a, b). In 40–50% of primary malignant lymphomas, lymphography shows involvement of retroperitoneal lymph nodes with a sensitivity of approximately 95% (Arvay and Picard, 1963; Wiljasalo, 1965; Fuchs et al, 1969; Ruettimann, 1974; Luening et al, 1976; Elke and Beltz, 1984).

Computed tomography has replaced lymphography to a large extent in the visualization of primary malignant lymphomas but lymphography is still indicated when the findings of computed tomography are indeterminate or contradict the

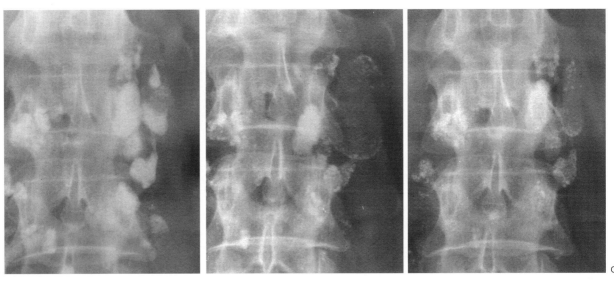

a   c

Fig. III, 125a-c. Nodal metastasis in a cervix carcinoma, stage III, in a 53-year-old female patient. **a)** Left para-aortic, a somewhat irregularly shaped storage defect in a not enlarged lymph node. At first, this region was not irradiated. **b)** Follow-up lymphadenogram after five months: marked enlargement of the lymph node, larger central defect, periphery largely spared. **c)** Follow-up two months later, after telecobalt therapy: complete regression.

clinical results (Strijk et al, 1987). While ultrasound and computed tomography only recognize nodal enlargement, the lymphadenogram has the advantage of structural analysis, providing more precise differentiation between benign and malignant lymph-node diseases. But even today, a definitive diagnosis cannot be expected from lymphadenograms, and lymphography has not replaced the histological result. In the early stages, without obvious enlargement of the lymph nodes, lymphography with its fine structural parameters is of more help in the diagnosis than the cross-sectional methods. The interpretation of these delicate nodal parameters is only meaningful when the lymphography is performed before medical therapy or surgery (Elke, 1984).

Lymph node metastases

Metastases from urogenital tumors are particularly suitable for the lymphographic diagnosis since the metastatic spread of these tumors follows the lymphatic drainage to the retroperitoneal and inguinal lymph nodes. These tumors include renal cell carcinoma and bladder carcinoma as well as tumors of the male genital organs, such as prostate carcinoma, testicular carcinoma and penile carcinoma, and tumors of the female genital organs, such as cervix carcinoma, corpus carcinoma, and ovarian carcinoma, as well as carcinomas of the vagina and vulva.

The lymphographic diagnosis of metastatic deposits in the lymph nodes is based on the synopsis of several criteria found in the filling and storage phase. During the filling phase, displacement of the lymphatic vessels, partial or complete lymph blockage with stasis of contrast medium, and evidence of collateral vessels are of high diagnostic value. In the storage phase, nodal enlargement and defects caused by tumor deposits are analyzed (Fig. III, 125).

Lymphography contributes greatly to the diagnosis and therapy of the above-mentioned tumors, summarized as follows:
– Determination of the extent of nodal spread for staging of urogenital carcinomas.
– Consideration of surgical options, particularly for planning a lymphadenectomy in addition to the resection of the primary tumor. Postsurgically, the extent of the radical surgery can be assessed by means of plain radiographs of the abdomen.
– The opacified nodes harboring metastases can be included in the radiation treatment field.
– The effect of the therapy can be monitored by obtaining follow-up plain radiographs of the abdomen for the evaluation of the opacified lymph nodes (lymphadenograms) (Fig. III, 125).

The lymphographic accuracy is between 85 and 90%, but these numbers have been (and still are) challenged. Using the cervix carcinoma as example of an urogenital tumor, the difficulties of correlating lymphographic and histological findings will be illustrated.

At autopsy, the incidence of metastases was found to be between 60 and 70%, which can be considered advanced metastatic disease. In the clinical context, the stage is determined by the lymphographically demonstrated incidence of metastases, which for the cervix carcinoma was found as follows:

Stage I   15–20%
Stage II   35–40%
Stage III   over 50%

For the cervix carcinoma, it is a particularly demanding task to determine the lymphographic accuracy by correlating the lymphographic findings with the histologic findings. The metastatic lymph nodes may not be enlarged, making it very difficult to distinguish nodal metastases from benign nodal changes such as fibrolipomatosis. Furthermore, the lymph nodes are numerous, and an exact correlation can only be achieved if all excised lymph nodes are examined for subtle histological changes, as done by Gerteis (1969) on up to 80 separate histological sections. Gerteis could attain an accuracy of more than 90%, which could only be equalled by very few authors (Arvay and Picard, 1963; Gerteis, 1966 and 1972; Reiffenstuhl, 1967; Fuchs et al, 1969).

False-negative findings can be attributed to small metastases that can only be detected microscopically.

If the lymphographic results are compared with other imaging methods, computed tomography reveals an almost similar accuracy for para-aortic nodal metastases. Lymphography remains by far superior in the search for pelvic nodal metastases. Consequently, lymphography has retained its role, particularly for the cervix carcinoma, where its accuracy in diagnosing nodal metastases amounts to 90–95% while computed tomography only yields a 65–70% overall accuracy.

References

Abbes, M.: Aspects actuels de la lipiodo-lymphographie. A propos de 200 explorations. Ann. Chir. (Paris) 17 (1963) 689

Altaras, J.: Verbesserte Technik der Lymphographie und ihre Ergebnisse. In: Deutsche Röntgengesellschaft. Deutscher Röntgenkongreß 1968. Hrsg. F. Gauwerky, Thieme Stuttgart 1969

Arvay, N., J.D. Picard: La lymphographie. Masson, Paris 1963

Asellius, P.: De lactibus, sive lacteis venis, quarto vasorum mesaraicorum genere, novo invento. Diss. Lugd. Bat. et off J. Maire 1627

Barthels, P.: Das Lymphgefäßsystem. In: Handbuch der Anatomie des Menschen. Hrsg. von Bardeleben, Fischer, Jena 1909

Bartholinus, T.H.: Vasa lymphatica nuper Hafniae in Animantbus inventa, et Hepatis exsequiae. G. Holst, Hafniae 1653

Bartholinus, T.H.: Anatomica, ex Caspari Bartholini parentis Institutionibus, omnium recentiorum, et proprries observationibus tertium ad sanguinis circulationem reformata. F. Hack, Leyden 1651

Beltz, L.: Lymphgefäße. In: Schinz, H.R., W.E. Baensch, W. Frommhold, R. Glauner, E. Uehlinger, J. Wellauer: Lehrbuch der Röntgendiagnostik. 6. Auflage. Thieme Stuttgart 1981

Beltz, L., J.D. Picard: Lymphangiopathies. In: Viamonte, M., A. Rüttimann: Atlas of lymphography. Thieme Stuttgart 1980

Beltz, L.: Lymphblock und Kollateralkreislauf. Habil. Bonn 1970

Brunner, U.: Das Lymphödem der unteren Extremitäten. Aktuelle Probleme in der Angiologie, Bd. 5, Huber, Bern 1969

Brunner, U., R. May, W. Schoop, E. Witzleb: Das dicke Bein. Aktuelle Probleme in der Angiologie, Bd. 9, Huber, Bern 1970

Carvalho, R., A. Rodriguez, S. Pereira: Sur une nouvelle méthode de mise en évidence des lymphatiques chez le vivant. Bull. Ass. Anat. (Nancy) 25 (1931) 101

Clodius, L.: Lymphedema. Supplement to lymphology. Thieme, Stuttgart 1977

Elke, M., L. Beltz: Lymphsystem. In: Schinz: Radiologische Diagnostik, 7. Auflage. Hrsg. von W. Frommhold, H. Stender, P. Thurn. Thieme Stuttgart 1984

Földi, M.: Disease of lymphatics and lymph circulation. Akademiai Kiado, Budapest 1969

Földi, M.: Erkrankungen des Lymphsystems. Witzstrock, Baden-Baden 1971

Fuchs, W.A.: Lymphographie und Tumordiagnostik. Springer, Berlin 1965

Gerteis, W.: Persönliche Mitteilung 1969

Gerteis, W.: Darstellungsmethoden des Lymphgefäßsystems und praktische Lymphographie. In: Lymphgefäßsystem, Handbuch der allgemeinen Pathologie. Bd. III/6, Springer, Berlin 1972

Gerteis, W.: Lymphographie und topographische Anatomie des Beckenlymphsystems. Enke, Stuttgart 1966

Godart, S., J. Collette, J. Dalem: Pathologie chirurgicale des vaisseaux lymphatiques. Acta chir. Belg. Suppl. 1 (1964) 1

Grau, H.: Vergleichende Anatomie des Lymphgefäßsystems. In: Lymphgefäßsystems, Handbuch der allgemeinen Pathologie. Bd. III/6, Springer, Berlin 1972

Gruwez, J., M. Goldstein: Les methodes d'exploration en pathologie vasculaire peripherique. Acta chir. Belg. Suppl. 2 (1968) 1

Gütgemann, A.: Persönliche Mitteilung 1968

Huth, F.: Allgemeine Pathologie des Lymphgefäßsystems. In: Lymphgefäßsystem, Handbuch der allgemeinen Pathologie. Bd. III/6, Springer Berlin 1972

Jacobsson, S., S. Johansson: Lymphangiography in lymphedema. Acta Radiol. (Stockh.) 57 (1962) 81

Jacobsson, S., S. Johansson: Lymphographic changes in lower limbs with varikose veins. Acta chir. Scand. 117 (1959) 334

Jacobsson, S., S. Johansson: Normal roentgen anatomy of the lymph vessels of upper and lower extremities. Acta radiol. (Stockh.) 51 (1959) 321

Jossifow, G.M.: Das Lymphgefäßsystem des Menschen. Fischer, Jena 1930

Kaindl, F., E. Mannheimer, L. Pfleger-Schwarz, B. Thurnher: Lymphangiographie und Lymphadenographie der Extremitäten. Thieme, Stuttgart 1960

Kappert, A.: Lehrbuch und Atlas der Angiologie. Erkrankungen der Arterien, Venen, Kapillaren und Lymphgefäße. 8. Auflage Huber, Bern 1976

Kinmonth, J.B.: Lymphangiography in man. Clin. Sci. II (1952) 13

Kinmonth, J.B.: The Lymphatics, diseases, lymphography and surgery. Arnold, London 1972

Koehler, P.R., G.T. Wohl, B. Schaffer: Lymphangiography, a survey of its current status. Am. J. Roentgenol. 91 (1964) 1216

Kubik, S.: Klinische Anatomie. Bd. III: Thorax. Thieme Stuttgart 1969

Kubik, S., G. Töndury, A. Rüttimann, W. Wirth: Nomenclature of the lymph nodes of the retroperitoneum, the pelvis and the lower extremity. In: A. Rüttimann: Progress in Lymphology. Thieme Stuttgart 1967

Kubik, S.: Die normale Anatomie des Lymphgefäßsystems unter besonderer Berücksichtigung der Sammelgebiete der Lymphknoten der unteren Körperhälfte. In: J. Becker, F. Gauwerky: Maligne Lymphome. Urban and Schwarzenberg, München, Berlin, Wien 1969

Lüning, M., M. Wiljasalo, H. Weissleder: Lymphographie bei malignen Tumoren. Thieme Stuttgart 1976

Malan, E., A. Puglionisi: Congenital angiodysplasias of the extremities. J. cardiovasc. Surg. (Tornio) (1964/65) 5, 87 and 6, 255

Malek, P., J. Kolc, A. Belan: Lymphography of the deep lymphatic system of the thigh. Acta Radiol. (Stockh.) 51 (1959) 422

Mascagni, P.: Vasorum lymphaticorum corporis humani historia et ischnographia. Carli, Senis 1787

Pecquet, J.: Experimenta nova anatomica, quibus incognitum hactenus chyli receptaculum et ab eo per thoracem in ramos usque subclavious vasa lactea deteguntur. Janssonium, Amstelaedami 1661

Picard, J.D., J.P. Gallet: Étude radioclinique des lymphoedemes de l'enfant. Presse méd. 74 (1966) 29

Picard, J.D.: La lymphographie au cours des chyluries (à propos de 30 observations). J. Urol. Néphrol. 73 (1967) 671

Reiffenstuhl, G.: Das Lymphknotenproblem beim Carcinoma colli uteri und die Lymphirradiatio pelvis. Urban and Schwarzenberg, Berlin, München, Wien 1967

Roo, T. de: Atlas of Lymphography. Stenfert Kroese, Leiden 1975

Roo, T. de: Lymfografie bij lymfoedeem van de extremiteiten. Ned. T. Geneesk. 110 (1966) 523

Rouviere, H.: Anatomie des lymphatiques de l'homme. Masson, Paris 1932

Rudbeck, O.: Nova exercitatio anatomica, exhibens Ductus Hepaticos Aquosos et Vasa Glandularum Serosa, nunc prinum inventa, aeneisque fguris delineata. Euchar. Lauringerus, Arosiae 1653

Rusznyak, I., M. Földi, G. Szabo: Lymphologie, Physiologie und Pathologie der Lymphgefäße und des Lymphkreislaufes. Fischer, Stuttgart 1969

Rüttimann, A.: Progress in Lymphology I. Thieme Stuttgart 1967

Rüttimann, A.: Erkrankungen des retroperitonealen Lymphsystems. In: Lehrbuch der Röntgendiagnostik, 6. Auflage. Hrsg. H.R. Schinz, W.E. Baensch, W. Frommhold, R. Glauner, E. Uehlinger, J. Wellauer. Thieme Stuttgart

Rüttimann, A., M.S. del Buono: Die Lymphographie. In: Ergebnisse der medizinischen Strahlenforschung, Bd. I. Hrsg von H.R. Schinz, R. Glauner, A. Rüttimann. Thieme Stuttgart 1964

Servelle, M.: Oedemes chroniques des membres. Masson, Paris 1962

Shdanov, D.A.: Röntgenologische Untersuchungsmethoden des Lymphgefäßsystems des Menschen und der Tiere. Fortschr. Röntgenstr. 46 (1932) 680

Strijk, S.P.: Lymphography and abdominal computed tomography in staging non-Hodgkin Lymphoma. Acta Radiol. (Diagn) 28 (1987) 263–269

Strijk, S.P., C. Boetes, G. Rosenbusch, J.H.S. Ruijs: Lymphography and abdominal computed tomography in staging Hodgkin disease. Fortschr. Röntgenstr. 146 (1987) 312–318

Tjernberg, B.: Lymphography. Acta radiol. (Stockh.) 1962 Suppl 214

Viamonte, M., A. Rüttimann: Atlas of lymphography. Thieme Stuttgart 1980

Viamonte, M., P.R. Koehler, M. Witte, Ch. Witte: Progress in lymphology II. Thieme Stuttgart 1970

Weissleder, H., V. Bartos, L. Clodius, P. Malek: Progress in lymphology. Avicenum, Czechoslovak Med. Press, Prague 1981

Weissleder, H.: Die Lymphographie. Ergebn. inn. Med. Kinderheilk. N.F. 23 (1965) 297

Welin, S., S. Johansson: Lymphography. In: Handbuch der medizinischen Radiologie, Bd. VIII. hrsg. von L. Diethelm, O. Olsson, F. Strnad, H. Vieten, A. Zuppinger. Springer, Berlin 1968

Wiljasalo, M.: Lymphographic differential diagnosis of neoplastic disease. Helsinki, Helsingfors 1965

Wirth, W.: Zur Röntgenanatomie des Lymphsystems der inguinalen, pelvinen und aortalen Region. Fortschr. Röntgenstr. 105 (1966) 441 u. 636

Chapter 4

Invisible light sliced

Improved diagnostics by new representation of anatomy

Introduction

G. Rosenbusch, M. Oudkerk, E. Ammann

'We are, as far as we know, able to bring the separate parts of the body on the screen or photographic plate from any point of view.... We will not discuss all the possibilities here, but will provide a general outline of the individual parts of the body on two main levels, in which the most differentiable will be visible without diminishing the high value of oblique views in any way.... One should not only be cognizant of the anatomical relationships, but should learn to recognize the three-dimensional anatomical relationships correctly from the given projections of the roentgen images. One should not be satisfied with the surface view but should attain a sensibly reconstructed transparency.'

Gocht's description (1898) is still valid today. Although the difficulties of assessing three-dimensional characteristics from ordinary photographs were well known, it was nevertheless often possible to say something about the structure of a lesion.

Three-dimensional vision is possible because each eye sees a slightly different image, and the combination of these two images provides the three-dimensional picture. To observe objects, various stereoscopic instruments have been developed, as early as the late nineteenth century, which looked like binoculars. The American Elihu Thomson, who worked as an adviser to General Electric and who had 700 patents to his name in the field of electricity, wrote as early as 1896 that normal radiographs display simple shadows in a single plane and that it was difficult to say if an object or part of an object was lying above or below it. Thomson's stereoscopic method was to take one photograph in the usual way and then a second one in which the Crookes' tube was moved while the object remained in the same place. The negatives of the two photographs were mounted in the stereoscope and viewed. Thomson described the effect as remarkable.

In 1903, Albers-Schoenberg mentioned the stereoscopic investigation as *'one of the more modern achievements of roentgenography. The wish to have stereoscopic images of individual parts of the human skeleton is an extraordinary claim, because the depth dimensions as well as the interrelated position of the single bones is not revealed by the nature of the roentgen plates. Particularly in evaluating the congenital hip dislocation, it is important to learn more about the position of the femoral head in relation to the acetabulum since the method of operation is based on the knowledge of this relationship. Furthermore, the determination of foreign bodies appears to benefit from a good stereoscopic technique because the measuring methods generally proved to be too ponderous and too cumbersome.'* The interest in stereoscopy was such that more than one method was developed (Figs. IV, 1–3). Albers-Schoenberg, however, dedicated no more than 12 pages on stereoscopy in his book 'Röntgentechnik' (1903) of 260 pages.

A 'stereo X-ray tube' was developed with two anodes at a distance of 6-10 cm and the cathodes laterally - two tubes acting as one – with no need to move the device. The two tubes were used sequentially in stereograms, often after a change of film. Until approximately 25 years ago, stereograms were employed to localize calcifications in the interior of the skull and to diagnose space-occupying masses in the brain. Today stereoradiography is only used occasionally for therapeutic intervention.

Various ideas have been developed for imaging structures in layers to permit characterization of organs and their lesions, facilitating a more accurate diagnosis and resulting in better directed therapy. The considerable progress in the development of tomography was performed by indivi-

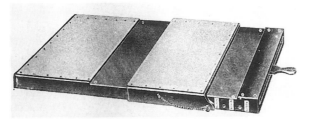

Fig. IV, 1. Sliding cassette for stereoscopic radiographs (R.G.S. 1912).

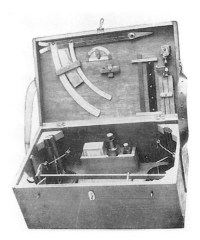

Fig. IV, 3. Instruments for localization after Fuerstenau-Weski (Sommer, 1919).

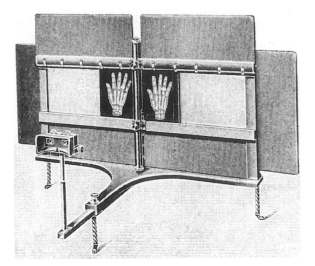

Fig. IV, 2. Film viewer for stereoscopy (Siemens-Archive).

duals who were not satisfied with the existing means.

They often worked independently, and applied for patents that were only occasionally awarded. As early as 1915/1916, C. Baese in Italy and Karel Mayer in Poland presented designs. The list of pioneers includes A.M.E. Bocage, F. Portes, and M. Chaussé in France, A. Vallebona in Italy, B. G. Ziedses des Plantes and D.L. Bartelink in The Netherlands, and E. Pohl and G. Grossmann in Germany.

Although many of these investigators had applied for patents before Ziedses des Plantes, he is considered to be the real developer of modern tomography because he worked out the theoretical physical foundations.

Industry did not always adopt these new ideas willingly and colleagues also were not always open to new ideas. Thus, Ziedses des Plantes reported that during his studies (1921/1922) in the course on microscopic histology he was under the impression that the microscopic image was actually a cross-sectional image.

'In those days, I thought that it would be nice when this could be attained in roentgenology. One had to take radiographs that often presented one plane or plane section in detail so that overlapping images could be avoided.... In a microscope the rays are first focused and then deviated, therefore providing a detailed image in the plane of focus. The same should also be possible with roentgen rays without questions of lenses or mirrors, namely by passing all rays through the same focus. When you move the roentgen tube and roentgen film so that all rays do exactly the same thing, like in the microscope, the tube and the film move in such a circle, or better even in a spiral, that you will attain the roentgenologic image of a cross-section.' (Interview).

The professor of roentgenology at the University of Utrecht thought that the ideas of Ziedses des Plantes were interesting, but without practical value. At Christmas 1928, when Ziedses des Plantes was on call as an assistant in the neurology department, he had radiographs of the skull taken of a neurologic patient with persistent psychiatric symptoms, with no abnormality demonstrated. Autopsy a few days later revealed a tumour at the base of the skull with erosion of the sella turcica. Ziedses des Plantes then reintroduced his idea that in tomographic images these changes might have been visible.

He consulted his chief assistants, set-up a scale model, and went to a Dutch roentgen equipment factory in Delft. They were willing to construct such an instrument, but after inquiry it appeared that Bocage, Portes, and Chausse had already obtained a similar patent in France. (These devices, however, were never used, probably because, as Ziedses implied, they were not successful.) The instrument-maker of the neurology clinic then constructed the apparatus for Ziedses des

Plantes. He also went to Philips with his model and showed them the results. The roentgenology adviser for Philips, Dr. G. J. van der Plaats, thought initially that the method was of little value, but changed his mind after reconsideration. He was of the opinion that a roentgen image should be detailed, whereas the tomographic method is actually based on blurring of structures that should not be visualized. The full development of tomography, as this technique is generally referred today, took three to four decades; other terms applied to this technique are stratigraphy, planigraphy, and laminagraphy.

Tomography was also combined with other techniques, for example, pneumoencephalography, retroperitoneography, intravenous urography, kymography, and later angiography. Other developments produced stereolaminagraphy and cinetomography. Many of these techniques were interesting from an experimental point of view, but were not adopted in everyday practice. A long battle for supremacy ensued between the many independent designs.

So far tomography could take longitudinal sections. The requirement for transverse axial slices was particularly strong in radiotherapy for the targeted radiation of tumours, and also in diagnostic radiology to gain insight into pathoanatomical relationships. As early as 1936, H. Vieten conceived a design to obtain transverse tomographic images by combining old, classical and modern tomography. The prototype saw further development, but did not attain its full potential.

In the seventies, the computer was introduced into diagnostic radiology. Hardly any other field of clinical medicine was influenced by the computer as profoundly as radiology, where its properties are particularly suitable. New imaging methods feasible through new methods of measurements added new dimensions, which created radiology as we know it today. Imaging was not only performed by X-rays but also by non-ionizing rays as ultrasound, and radio waves as in magnetic resonance imaging.

While the transverse tomograph with its synchronous movement between patient and film-cassette rotation via an electric shaft had not succeeded, computed tomography (CT) made its triumphant appearance in 1973. X-ray tube, generator, table and, to a certain extent, detector were familiar principles. New were the computer and a software program that computed a tomogram from many thousands individual values to produce an image on the monitor. Also new were the precision requirements for movement of the gantry and for the tube voltage, which

had to be extremely constant during the entire scan, initially for a period of 5 min.

For this reason, only the head could be initially imaged by neuroradiologists: the patient's head was placed in an elastic support, the water bag, which conformed to the skull and eliminated air as cause of image artifacts.

As a result of CT, neuroradiology and general radiology saw a stormy development, although in the seventies the spatial resolution was ten times lower, the exposure time 30–300 times longer, and the cost about five times higher in comparison with conventional radiographic imaging. CT, however, offered a higher contrast resolution than any film-screen system, and produced an image of anatomical details without superimposed structures. High-voltage slip rings allowed continuous rotation, and the X-ray tube output could be increased to 40 kW with a continuous output of 4–5 kW. The cathode was given a so-called spring focal spot, allowing the measurement of twice the number of image projections. Also the concept of the single-tank generator was rediscovered, and tube and generator rotate continuously around the patient. The continuous rotation of the X-ray source together with new ideas in the reconstruction algorithm brought the spiral, and with it the visualization of volume.

Using electromagnetic deflection of the electron beam, scan times of 50 ms have been attained. For volume scans with the spiral technique, the tube output exceeds 100 kW and its continuous output 10 kW. Here, the development of new hardware operated with newly written software for postprocessing algorithms was the key to the success. This technique can also be used for interventional procedures and biopsies as well as for quantitative image processing. Furthermore, improved connectivity via networking of the images allows correlation with other imaging modalities.

A general cure for cancer may not be available for a long time, possibly never, in view of the different causes of cancers and their diverse biology. Despite this, therapeutic advances have been made in recent decades, based on better understanding of tumour biology, the introduction of cytostatics, more refined surgical techniques, and new developments in radiation therapy that permit higher radiation doses without increasing the damage to the surrounding healthy tissues.

Conventional transverse tomography was already established in radiation planning to localize tumours, but computed tomography allows a far better localization and can exactly compute and determine the radiation fields and radiation doses for single- and multiple-field techniques as well as for rotational techniques.

Studies comparing conventional with CT-supported therapy planning revealed that the planning had to be changed in approximately one half of the patients because of inadequately assessed tumor volume by the conventional method. In abdominal tumors, a change of therapy was required in 86% of the cases.

In addition to intrinsic tumour parameters, the basic requirements for good therapeutic results include the assessment of regional or distant metastases, for which CT and ultrasonography are well suited. The tumour stage has also to be taken into consideration in planning the therapeutic approach. Moreover, the reactions of the tumour and its metastases should be monitored during therapy, particularly when cytostatics are used. The size of the tumour and its metastases should be measured before therapy and on follow-up scans to assess changes in size, with further treatment depending upon the found therapeutic response. CT is of particular value in monitoring the therapeutic effect, but ultrasonography and increasingly also MRI are important.

Finally, in neuroradiology many earlier important examination methods have become obso-

lete. Only through old textbooks would a 45-year-old radiologist have heard of pneumoencephalography, and it is doubtful if he would know how such an examination was performed or its results interpreted. The mechanically so impressive and precise apparatuses used to perform pneomoencephalograms can now be found exclusively in museums.

The precision expected form radiologists increases in line with neurosurgical progress. The type of process and its exact location, size and vascularity must be known before surgical intervention. With older methods, such as pneumoencephalography and angiography, sufficient information could often be obtained, but only CT allowed a noninvasive entry into the cranial cavity that is also faster and provides a more reliable diagnosis. More intracranial information is also important for treating head injuries, which have become more frequent as a result of traffic accidents and life in the modern industrial world. The prognosis has improved considerably for this type of patient because the diagnosis of an intracranial haematoma can often be made while the patient is still conscious, that is, in the period where surgical removal of the haematoma has the best chance of success.

Conventional tomography

F.E. Stieve

Introduction

Body section radiography is a procedure by means of which objects at depth are represented, avoiding the summation effects of normal projection radiographs. The properties of the radiograph obtained depend above all upon the body section to be imaged, but also upon eliminating superimposed structures.

Imaging of selected body sections is possible because two of the three components of the system X-ray source, object and receiving medium, are moved during exposure under constant geometric conditions in a coordinated manner so as to ensure that all points of the selected object layer are projected to the same point of the receiving medium, while those outside that layer are subject to continuous variations on the imaging system and thereby 'blurred', i.e. represented by inadequate contrast.

Vieten (1936) gave the following definition of tomography [35]:

'The principle of preferential imaging of a given body section by elimination of all details outside this layer consists of coordinated motions of two components of the recording system, i.e. focus, object and film, conducted during exposure of the film such that the relationship of the distances between focus and object layer on the one hand and between focus and film (or between object layer and film) on the other hand remains constant. All X-rays passing through points of a layer for which this condition is fulfilled will then coincide with equal points on the film in any phase of the motions, and a sharp image of the relevant body section will be obtained. For all points outside this layer, however, the relationship of the distances varies during movement; they are therefore continuously projected to different positions of the film, and will be blurred and underexposed.'

This description is valid even today, although the receiving medium or imaging system is no longer film. Fig. IV, 6 shows the principle of preferential imaging of body sections according to Vieten.

Historical review

Karol Mayer's observations [17] must be regarded as precursors of classical tomography. As early as 1914 he described a procedure in which the X-ray tube was moved in order to keep images of the heart free of superimposed structures, while the object to be recorded and the film or X-ray screen remained stationary [8, 18]. Mayer described this principle in detail in 1935 on the occasion of a dispute concerning the claims for priority referring to a publication by Grossmann [10, 11]. A procedure which served a similar purpose was that described by Carlo Baese [1] in a patent granted in 1915 which was entitled 'Method of, and apparatus for, the localization of foreign objects in, and the radiotherapeutic treatment of, the human body by X-rays'. This procedure is based upon the principle of moving the X-ray source and film and was the basis of moving-field therapy and tomography which were further developed later.

The practice of body-section imaging using X-rays and the theory of planographic imaging were developed independently of each other and almost simultaneously by Andre Bocage (Fig. IV, 4) and B.G.A. Ziedses des Plantes (Fig. IV, 5) [41]. Bocage [4] was the first to describe the basic principles in a patent specification in 1921. It was patented in 1922 as a method and device for radiographic reproduction of a body section under conditions excluding structures

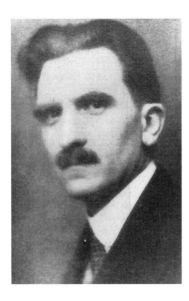

Fig. IV, 4. André Edmund Marie Bocage (1892-1953). French Dermatologist and pioneer in Tomography. His "direct analytic radiography" of 1921 found no interest and was not realized until 1938.

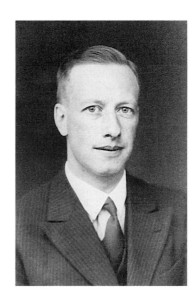

Fig. IV, 5. Bernard Georg Ziedses des Plantes (1902-1993). Dutch neurologist, who already worked on technical problems of roentgenology in Utrecht. He developed or discovered planigraphy and subtraction. For many years neurologist in Rotterdam and later professor of Radiodiagnostics in Amsterdam.

in front and back. It is based upon findings Bocage made when examining wounded soldiers during the First World War.

It was almost at the same time that B.G.A. Ziedses des Plantes began to conduct research into planigraphy that he published in his doctoral thesis entitled 'Planigraphie en Subtractie' in 1934 [42].

Further studies and contributions referring to planigraphy, most of which were made independently of each other and with no knowledge of the other publications or patents, were furnished by Portes and Chaussé [22], Pohl [21], Kieffer [14], Bartelink [2, 3], Vallebona [31], and others, to name only the most important authors. They were reflected in numerous constructional realizations, with a first practicable apparatus developed by J. Massiot in 1935 [15]. The most important publications and patents concerning tomography of the early years are summarized in Table IV, 1.

The knowledge that the position of the image recording system would permit imaging of layers perpendicular to the body axis goes back to Bocage as well. In 1922, he had pointed out that the object layer to be recorded depends upon the form and position of the image recording system. Moreover, Ziedses des Plantes reported that planigraphic images might also be obtained with the imaging system in any desired oblique position. The relevant geometric derivation was another contribution made by Vieten. It led to the method of transverse axial tomography specified in a patent application by Vieten in 1936 [34], and was independently described by Watson in 1937 [36]. Practical designs were developed, again without most of the authors knowing of

the publications by others, in 1947 by Ch. Frain and F. Lacroix in France [6], A. Vallebona in Italy [32], in 1948 by S. Takahashi in Japan [29], in 1949 by A. Gebauer and F. Wachsmann in Germany [7] and by J. J. Stevenson (1950) [25] and W. Watson (1951) [37] in England. It was, above all, S. Takahashi [28, 29, 30] who furnished extensive experimental evidence and basic knowledge to this technique which must be regarded as a precursor of computed tomography.

The constructional principle of body-section imaging using X-rays

Form of movement

As the description of the basic principles of tomography suggests, there are essentially three approaches to the construction of tomographic equipment. All have been realized technically and some are available today:

– *Movements of the X-ray tube and imaging system*

Movements may be one-dimensional or multidimensional following a circular arc or a straight line. Circular movements were realized by, among others, G. Grossmann [10, 11] in the tomographic apparatus and in the POLYTOME [24] developed by Massiot/Philips [15, 16]. Some tomographic equipment also provide for movement at plane–parallel levels, e.g. the PLANIGRAPH by Siemens, a technical solution employed in most of the available tomographic attachments.

Table IV, 1. Time table of the development of tomography.

1915	C. Baese [1]	Method of, and apparatus for, the localisation of foreign objects in, and the radiotherapeutic treatment of, the human body by the X-rays. Eng. und Ital. Patent.
1921	A.E.M. Bocage [4]	Procédé et dispositifs de radiographie sur plaque en mouvement. Franz. Patent.
1921	F. Portes et M. Chaussé [22]	Procédé pour la mise au point radiologique sur un plan sécant d'un solide, ainsi que pour la concentration sur une zone déterminée d'une action radiotherapeutique maximum et dispositifs permettant la réalisation. Franz. Patentschrift 1922.
1927	E. Pohl [21]	Verfahren und Vorrichtung zur röntgenographischen Wiedergabe eines Körperschnittes und Ausschluß der davor und dahinter liegenden Teile. Deutsche Patentschrift.
1929	J. Kieffer [14]	X-ray device and method of technic. US Patent.
1930	A. Vallebona [31]	Una modalità de technica per la dissociazione delle ombre applicata allo studio del cranio. Radiol. med (Torino) 27: 1090
1931	B.G.A. Ziedses des Plantes	Een bijzondere methode voor het maken van röntgenphotos van schedel en wervelkolom. Ned. T. Geneesk. 75: 5218–5222 [41]
1931	D.L. Bartelink	Einrichtung zur Bildherstellung mittels Röntgenstrahlen. Schweizer Patent 155930
1935	G. Grossmann	Tomographie I. Fortschr. Röntgenstr. 51: 61–80 [8] Tomographie II. Fortschr. Röntgenstr. 51: 191–208 [10]
1935	H. Chaoul	Ein neues Röntgenuntersuchungsverfahren zur Darstellung von Körperschichten und seine Anwendung in der Lungendiagnostik. Fortschr. Röntgenstr. 52; Kongr.H. 43: 46–50.
1935	J. Massiot [15]	Essais d'une aparail pour radiographie analytique. Bull. Soc. Radiol. méd. France 23: 395–398.
1936	W. Watson	Improvements in or relating to X-ray apparatus. Engl. Patent 480459
1936	H. Vieten [35]	Verfahren zur röntgenographischen Darstellung eines Körperschnittes. Deutsches Patent 672518.
1941	M. de Abreu	Roentgen geometry in formation of roentgenographic image (applications of tomography). Rev. méd. bras 11: 181–232.
1941	S. Takahashi [28]	Study of the technique of the radiographic delineation of the cross section of the body (Study on Rotatography and Crossgraphy). 4th Report Tohoku. J. exp. Med 54: 1.
1947	Ch. Frain et F. Lacroix [6]	Courbe-enveloppe et coupes horizontales. J. Radiol. Electrol. 28: 142–143.
1948	A. Vallebona	Prime ricerche su di un nouvo metodo radiographico: Stratigraphia assiale con radiuazioni perpendicolari all'asse. Ann. Radiol. diagn. (Bologna) 20: 57–64.
1949	A. Gebauer	Körperschichtaufnahmen in transversalen (horizontalen) Ebenen. Fortschr. Röntgenstr. 71: 669–696.
1949	W. Watson	Simultaneous multisection radiography. Radiology 5: 669.
1950	Y.V. Paatero [20]	A new tomographical method for radiographing curved outer surfaces. Acta Radiol. (Stockh.) 32: 117–184.
1950	J. Stevenson [25]	Horizontal body section radiography. Br. J. Radiol. 23: 319.
1950	S. Takahashi	A method to take radiograms of the transsection of the body at any inclination and curvature. Tohoku J. exp. Med. 52: 38

– Movement of the patient and image recording system

Here again, the movement is either one-dimensional, utilized in the system proposed by Vallebona-Bozetti [32, 33], or multidimensional, corresponding to the constructional principle of most systems for transaxial tomography.

– Movement of the X-ray tube and patient

This form of movement has several disadvantages not only in the construction of the system but also in the potential for error in section imaging. It has seldom been realized in praxis.

Position and form of the image recording system

As shown in Fig. IV, 6 position and form of the body section to be recorded depend upon the form and position of the image recording system. In classical tomography, the image is obtained at a level that is plane-parallel to the table top since the image recording system is also at a plane-par-

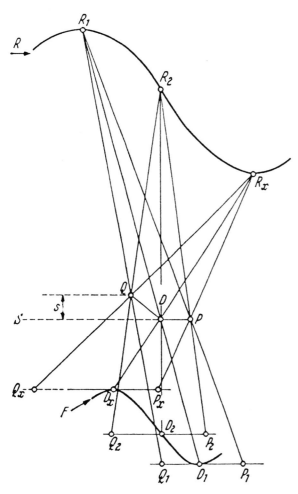

Fig. IV, 6. Principle of preferential visualization of body sections after Vieten [27].

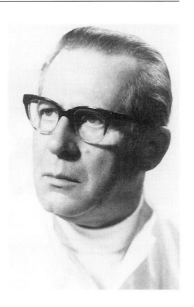

Fig. IV, 7.
Heinz Vieten (1915-1985). radiologist at the University Clinic in Düsseldorf. In addition to general diagnostic problems, he made important contribution to the development of transverse tomography.

within the range of the primary beam, of which any desired straight or curved area may be selected for imaging, depending upon the position of the image recording system (Fig. IV, 8). This is possible since any point of a three-dimensional structure is related to a point within the space where, due to the movement, the requirement for constant image ratios remains fulfilled, and where no change occurs in any relative projection during the movement.

In fact, the virtual three-dimensional image is generated infinitely frequently in an infinite number of magnification scales, corresponding to the infinite number of theoretical possibilities for reproducing an image at a wider or shorter distance to the object, i.e. more or less magnified.

From a great number of theoretical possibilities, the reproduction in straight plane sections, i.e. so-called transverse sections, has been realized, whereby either X-ray source and image recording system perform circular movements on transverse paths, as described by Vieten and Watson and realized in computed tomography today, or patient and image recording system are moved relative to the X-ray source, which is fixed, as applied in the case of classical transverse axial tomography and realized by Vallebona, Gebauer and Wachsmann, Watson and others.

Imaging of objects with a curved image recording system was used by Paatero [20] for obtaining radiographs of the jaws in 1949. The procedure, called Pantomography, is still of basic importance for orthodontics and dental medicine today [12]. This technique moves either the X-ray source and image recording system that corresponds

allel level. Deviations from this principle have been rare.

The conditions for a tomographic image, however, are neither bound to a plane that is plane-parallel to the table top and thereby horizontal to the table top with the focal spot following a parallel path or a path along a spheric arc, nor bound to the position of the fulcrum about which the system moves.

In this respect, projections in tomography are basically different from those of conventional radiographs: while the latter always represent only a two-dimensional object, the image of which may be somewhat distorted depending upon the position of the image registering system, every tomographic image will produce a complete three-dimensional 'virtual' radiograph (Vieten, Fig. IV, 7) of the total recording object

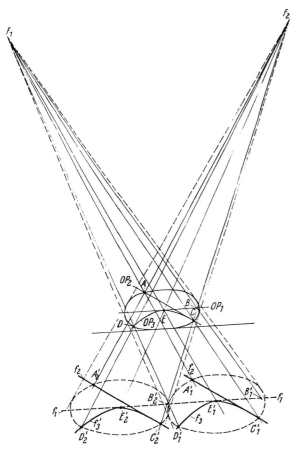

Fig. IV, 8. Projection of a "virtual" three-dimensional radiograph of the space outside the object at an arbitrary distance. Depending on position and type of imaging system (f_1, f_2, f_3) certain sections (OP$_1$, OP$_2$, OP$_3$) of the object can be imaged from this projectional system [27].

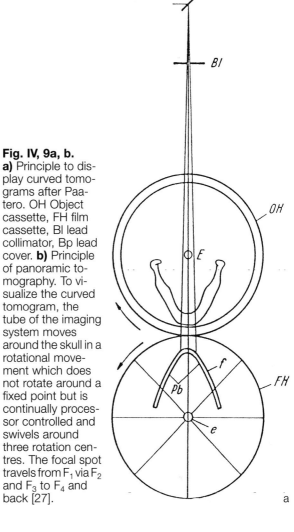

Fig. IV, 9a, b.
a) Principle to display curved tomograms after Paatero. OH Object cassette, FH film cassette, Bl lead collimator, Bp lead cover. **b)** Principle of panoramic tomography. To visualize the curved tomogram, the tube of the imaging system moves around the skull in a rotational movement which does not rotate around a fixed point but is continually processor controlled and swivels around three rotation centres. The focal spot travels from F_1 via F_2 and F_3 to F_4 and back [27].

a

in form to the position of the jaws or the patient and curved image registering system (i.e. the film-screen combination) with the X-ray tube remaining stationary.

In the systems most frequently used today, X-ray source and cassette rotate around the skull, but the fulcrum is not fixed but, under processor control during the tomographic procedure, changes continuously around three rotation centres along a parabola. In addition, the X-ray beam is collimated by a slit diaphragm fitted to the tube and by a second diaphragm, a few millimeters wide and about 15 cm long, placed in front of the cassette. These diaphragms create a very narrow effective radiation beam and reduce the proportion of scattered radiation (Fig. IV, 9).

Another principle to be mentioned consists of multiple layer imaging. In systems using this principle, the position of the fulcrum has a limited influence on the position of the layer to be im-

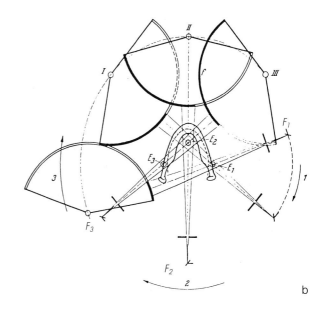

b

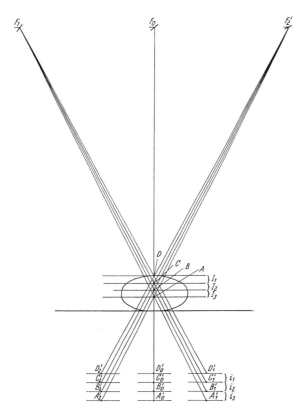

Fig. IV, 10. Principle of multiple tomography (simultaneous multisection). More than one tomogram can be obtained by exposing several films separated by small gap [27].

aged. The level of the image plane will only correspond to the fulcrum plane when the object points in the fulcrum plane are continuously projected to the same point during the movement, i.e. when the two parts have the same range of motion. For an image recording system situated closer to or farther away from the tube in relation to the fulcrum plane, the motion speed changes for this position and another plane is imaged. This principle has been realized in the case of simultaneous multilayer imaging (Fig. IV, 10)

Nomenclature

The various forms of body section imaging were given different names by the authors who developed or invented them. For instance, Vallebona called the procedure he developed stratigraphy, Ziedses des Plantes referred to his procedure as planigraphy, Bartelink and Kieffer used the term body-section radiography, Grossmann tomography, Moore laminography, Kieffer vertigraphy and Tailland radiotomy.

In 1962, the International Commission on Radiation Units and Measurements (ICRU) [13] recommended in Handbook 89 that the term 'tomography' should be generally used for all procedures, even though other terms might have historical claims. This term has been used in the meantime and is generally accepted, with increased recognition after the introduction of computed tomography.

Additional ICRU recommendations containing definitions of terms are given here as excerpts:

Object plane. The plane of the object that is shown in the image, whether it is a plane or curved surface. Its level is preselected by the position and form of the recording system and the geometric relationship of the recording system to the object and focal spot.

Section thickness. The sum of the planes that the eye cannot distinguish by differences in sharpness, i.e. planes that have not been subject to detectable blurring, even if they are not at the level of the mathematical fulcrum. These planes lose the motion unsharpness in the general unsharpness. The effective thickness of a section is determined by an absolute or arbitrary factor.

The proposals by the ICRU are intended to introduce on an international level only terms that can be exactly defined and experimentally verified. The ICRU therefore do not consider 'section thickness' a suitable term and recommend 'selectivity', 'section interval' and 'efficiency coefficient' as better terms.

Section interval. This proposal is based on the fact that it is of no practical relevance to state whether the tomographic image shows a section thickness of 1 cm, for instance. This would only mean that details of smaller diameter are contained in the section, but not whether they are detectable. The section interval refers to the detail size, i.e. the distance between one object plane and the next.

Selectivity. Selectivity refers to the degree of elimination of redundant shadows.

Efficiency coefficient. The efficiency coefficient refers to the excursion of 1 cm above the object plane and determines the section interval.

Blurring. It refers to the track traveled by a structural density outside the object plane due to motion. The recorded density is called blurring. The geometrical degree of blurring indicates the magnification factor necessary to be applied to an area in the object plane to produce the blurred shadow.

Exposure angle. The exposure angle is the angle through which the central beam moves during exposure. In pluridirectional movements, the effective exposure angle is the mean value of all exposure angles.

Level. The level indicates the site of a plane within the object or relative to the height of the fulcrum in relation to the object support.

Section interval. The section interval is the distance between one layer and the next, mostly expressed in millimeters or centimeters.

Movements.

Unidirectional (linear): the system moves in a single plane.

Pluridirectional: the system moves in more than one plane. Simple pluridirectional movements include the basic forms of circle, spiral and ellipse. The compound pluridirectional movements are combinations of simple movements and include spiral, hypocycloidal and cloverleaf.

All these forms of movement have been realized in tomographic devices. For details see Handbuch der Medizinischen Radiologie: 'Bevorzugte Darstellung einzelner Koerperschichten' or Golden's Diagnostic Radiology, Section 17: Tomography: Physical Principles and Clinical Applications.

Image generation

Tomographic image and projection image share the same basic principle: an image is created by X-rays that have passed through the patient. The emerging radiologic image is then transformed into a visible image.

To use X-rays in diagnostic radiology, it is important to know that radiographic images partly follow laws that are quite different from those of photographic images:

- The radiograph is a 'transmission image' of differences in attenuation converted to differences in optical density by the image recording system, and has no direct relationship to light reflection from a visible object, as in photography.
- Radiographic imaging follows the laws of central projection, i.e. objects are magnified in relation to their position, with the magnification increasing with the distance from the image recording system.
- The perceptible minimum difference of an object depends on the thickness and density of the tissue traversed by the X-ray beam in relation to adjacent structures. For an image contrast of approximately 10% compared to air, the minimum difference is about 4–5 mm for tissue, 0.2 mm for bone, and 0.004 mm for io-

dine contrast medium with a concentration of 2 mg/cm^2. These values depend upon the radiation energy.

- In addition, the radiograph is the result of the summation of individual superimposed shadows, which might produce structures that do not really exist. This summation effect is partially offset in the tomographic image.
- The recorded radiologic image as well as the reviewed image is further degraded by scattered radiation produced within the body and contained in the radiologic image. Scattered radiation reduces contrast and, in addition, changes the contrast of an object relative to its position within the scattering body. Furthermore, scattered radiation increases unsharpness since it acts as radiation arising from a large area.
- Superposition and summation give rise to structures not corresponding to actual object structures. They produce interference effects, referred to as object noise, which may affect the perceptibility of objects with low contrast. The noise effect also is partially offset in tomography.
- Finally, the sharpness of the recorded image is influenced by the finite extension of the X-ray source (focal spot size) in relation to the location of the object to be imaged as well as to the image recording system. The sharpness also depends on the object contour and on object motion during exposure.

Several authors have addressed the question how far the mentioned laws operate on tomography. The first and fundamental investigations are from Ziedses des Plantes. In his Doctoral Thesis of 1934, he studied the influence of tomographic imaging on the radiologic image and the resulting radiograph.

He concluded from his experiments:

- The unsharpness of the tomographic image border increases with the exposure angle, in part due to a wider tangent zone (increased obliquity) of the X-ray beam.
- Composite pluridirectional movements (i.e. a spiral movement in his experiments), due to more homogenous blurring of components outside the object plane, provided better results with regard to homogeneity of the object and its contours than unidirectional linear blurring or simple circular blurring.
- Object components with high contrast may produce sharply defined contours, even when they are located outside the layer, thus appearing to belong to it (so-called core shadows).

In the 1960s, P. Edholm [5] studied the formation of tomographic images and how the image formation is influenced by different forms of motion. He studied experimentally and calculated mathematically the factors determining the density and border of the tomographic images, and furnished the following conclusions, which supported and supplemented my own observations and calculations:

– In comparison with the projection image, the density of an object is reduced in the tomographic image. This is related, in part, to the imaged layer and, in part, to the distribution of the density over a wider area.

– Differences in density may occur between the center of the object and its border, especially for spherical objects with a border consisting of concave and convex components. The interior convex component of the shadow will be perceived by the viewer as the contour of the object. The concave component corresponds to the accompanying blurring and is either perceived as free zone or not seen at all. The viewer will interpret the region of the maximum gradient as the object contour.

– Contours can only be perceived as such when the differences in density produced in the tomographic image have a steep gradient in relation to the surroundings.

– The tomogram always represents a section, i.e. the differences in dose or density values are recorded as the sum of the depth-related object sections.

– These structures can be superposed by object shadows from particles located outside the object plane. They are referred to as redundant shadows. Their presence depends on the degree of blurring of the system and they are therefore more apparent with linear blurring than with pluridirectional blurring. Nevertheless, eliminating shadows outside the layer reduces the visualized structures. As a result, it is possible to perceive even particles of weak contrast that are not perceptible in conventional radiographs due to poor signal–noise ratio.

– Small particles of low contrast, however, are only recordable in the tomogram if the unsharpness is less than the particle size and if the blurring is free of contrast from attenuating structures in the adjacent layers that exceed the contrast in the particles within the layer. The changes of the image contour and the gradient caused by blurring are most homogenous with pluridirectional movements of the system, thus producing an impression of sharpness that largely is directionally independent.

– The unidirectional movement produces non-uniform blurring of the image border, with maximal blurring of structures perpendicular to the obscuring movement, i.e. steep gradient, and no blurring of structures parallel to it. The latter structures are sharply delineated and add the impression of increased sharpness to the image. As structures from outside the focal plane, they are detrimental and create a false image of the object plane.

These and other factors that affect the tomographic image presentation are responsible for the differences between tomography and projection radiography as well as for the differences between the various tomographic systems as to formation and content of the tomographic image.

Radiation exposure

Surface dose

Comparison of radiation exposures should be based on equal exposure conditions to reduce interfering factors as much as possible. Using equal exposure conditions (radiation energy, distances and film dose for film–screen combinations of equal sensitivity), the surface dose is greater for linear tomography than for conventional radiography. For the layers near the film, the entrance dose is the highest, the maximum dose the lowest and the peripheral dose decrease the most shallow. For the layers near the tube, the conditions approximate those in conventional radiography. The dose at the edge decreases to about 1%, reaching values of 0.5% or less outside the field.

With circular, hypocycloidal and spiral movement, the dose is distributed over a greater area than with linear blurring for the same exposure angle. The surface dose is more heterogeneous and the values at the margin are only 20–30% of the mean value. With a field size of 20 x 20 cm, the 10% value of the surface dose is reached within the object layer at about 16 cm from the centre in layers near the film and about 2 cm closer in layers near the tube. The entrance dose in the centre does not essentially differ from the values measured with linear tube movement. The values are, however, generally up to 30% higher than those of stationary imaging with equal projections. Fig. IV, 11 shows the dose distribution on the surface, as measured from the midline of a water phantom of 20 cm thickness using linear tube movement. The dif-

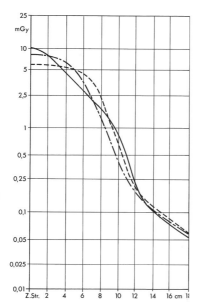

Fig. IV, 11. Surface dose [27] on the side towards the X-ray tube measured in the midline of a 20-cm water phantom at various section levels. Linear blurring, FFA 140 cm, field size 20 x 20 cm on the film. 80 kV, 2 mm Al, section thickness 3 cm -; 9.5 cm -.-.-.; 16 cm ——. Reference value S = 100 at the cassette [27].

tant from the tube, was especially found in layers near the tube. The closer the object plane is to the radiation exit side, the lower the dose in the layer. Furthermore, there is a flatter dose decrease along the periphery. Fig. IV, 12 shows the dose distribution in a 20-cm water phantom for stationary recording compared to tomographic images in 3-cm layer height, measured as distance from the object support.

Similar conditions are also found when assessing the integral dose. It is lowest in layers distant from the tube, reaching values equal to those in stationary recording when layers in the body centre are considered, and exceeds the values of stationary recordings by almost 10% in layers close to the tube, when all other conditions are equal.

Except for the somewhat different conditions at the field margins, the dose conditions in tomography correspond fairly well to those in conventional radiography. There is no dose increase within the layer.

ferences might be due to different obliquity of the radiation and different field sizes on the surface. This is supported by the observation that surface dose and exposed field increase with the exposure angle [26].

Distribution of dose within the body

These studies were conducted to find out whether in tomography the maximum dose within the layer is greater than the surface dose at the tube side. The measurements mentioned above show that the relative increase in the dose observed in the center of the radiation entrance field, which was most pronounced in layers dis-

Dose required at the image recording system

The dose required for a given optical density for the same film–screen combinations changes since some of the radiation enters the cassette surface and film-screen combination obliquely during tomography. As a result, the dose required with the employed film-screen combinations is higher than with perpendicular incidence of the radiation. The increase depends on the effective exposure angle, with the most frequently used exposure angles of 30–40° having an average dose increase of 10% in comparison with a perpendicular incidence.

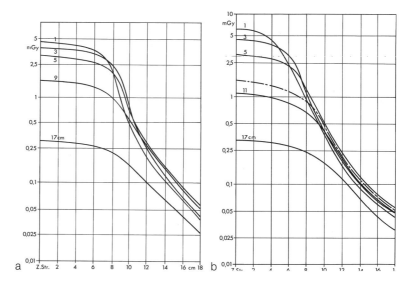

Fig. IV, 12a, b. Distribution of the dose in a 20-cm water phantom in upright position **(a)** compared with tomograms of 9.5 cm section thickness **(b)**, technical data as in Fig. IV,11. Section plane -.-.- [27].

Dose values at the exit side of the phantom measured for each individual projection are found to increase by about 15 and 30%, respectively, as a result of oblique irradiation of the body when the exposure conditions are almost unchanged and the tube voltage is about 70 kV. This means that, at constant dose rate of the tube, the oblique projections with oblique irradiation contribute considerably less to the image generated than the projection with perpendicular incidence of radiation.

To offset this shortcoming, an exposure system was developed that measured the dose rate above the cassette and kept it constant. The tomograms generated using automatic exposure control differ not only by more constant image quality but also by considerably enhanced homogeneity due to the greater effective exposure angle and the more uniform dose in all projection directions.

Quality assurance

Poor image quality is often more easily detected in tomography than in conventional radiography. It is for this reason that the question of quality control was addressed relatively early. The testing procedures are based on recommendations of the International Commission for Radiological Units and Measurements (ICRU) [13], prepared and published in 1962. These are still relevant today as can be seen from the recommendations by the expert commission of the World Health Organization (WHO, 1982) [38] and the National Council on Radiation Protection and Measurements (NCRP Report No 99, 1988) [19].

The following performance characteristics are essential for the testing of the equipment:

Exposure angle, including assessment of the symmetry of the movement path.

ICRU have indicated a procedure to assess both the exposure angle and constancy of motions. The motions are often not constant, especially in tomographic attachments. The precision of the pendulum angle should not vary by more than ±5% from the indicated value.

Selection of the level and graduated scale

The levels should be reproducible with a tolerance of ±2 mm.

Resolution

The resolution can be tested visually. It should approximate the conditions of stationary recordings, though it is clearly somewhat lower due to the oblique incidence. However, the visual resolution for high-contrast lead grids should not be worse than about 10% of the value with stationary recordings under equal conditions.

Assessment of section intervals, selectivity and the efficiency coefficient or the layer thickness.

These conditions should be tested using a lead grid with a bar thickness of 0.2–3 mm diameter. A similar phantom may be used to assess the selectivity and the efficiency coefficient. Details of the measuring procedure are contained in the ICRU recommendations.

Mechanical stability

Especially the tomographic attachments frequently in use today are unstable when used over prolonged periods of time and require regular periodic checkups. This applied to both the motions and the constancy of scale setting and object plane.

Radiation exposure

According to the data given in this section 6, the radiation exposure on the entrance surface of the phantom, depending upon the pendulum angle, shall not exceed the incident dose in stationary recordings by 30% with all other conditions equal.

The dose for the film-screen combination should not exceed 10% of stationary radiographs under equal exposure conditions. A film-screen combination with a speed of 200 or 400 may be used in general, except for tomograms requiring a higher resolution, such as tomograms of the inner ear, which must be performed using film-screen combinations with a speed of 100.

Indications, performance and limitations

General considerations

Tomography is an imaging procedure with its indications, apart from a few exceptions, derived from the clinical findings and from imaging findings of preceding radiological and nuclear medical examinations. Tomography should be confined to areas that require more detailed examination to answer specific clinical questions. The approach is guided by the findings of preceding radiographic studies, which determine the site to be examined as well as the appropriate projections and section intervals. In general, it is useful to examine the body region of interest in two planes perpendicular to each other. To optimize the information, the size of the selected films is often smaller than the size of the plain radiographs and has to be individualized for each case. Tomographic films in two projections provide topographic information that reveals the relationship to adjacent organs and structures and that facilitates the observation of pathologic conditions over the course of time.

Tomography complements the findings of conventional radiography by eliminating superimpositions inherent in projectional images. To compare the findings observed during the course of a disease and its therapy, it is generally necessary to select the same projections. Changing projections on subsequent examinations may lead to misinterpretations and wrong decisions.

The imaging parameters will generally be the same as used in the corresponding plain radiographs. Since the contrast is affected by the selected section thickness and the size of the examined organ or part of body in the preselected projection, the tube voltage should not be too high. It is generally advisable to use a grid with a not too high grid ratio. It should be a linear grid appropriate for the focus-film distance and the pluridirectional movement of the central beam.

'Rare earth' screens with a resolution of about six line pairs per millimeter and a speed of 200 (or 400 with about 5 LP/mm for the abdominal region) are proven film-screen combinations, with a few exceptions such as imaging of the skeleton.

The films used should have a high gamma since the relatively thin sections reduce contrast in comparison to plain radiographs.

Film processing is subject to the same requirements as conventional films.

Finally, it is important that the examining physician inspects the obtained films immediately after the tomographic examination to find out whether the area of interest if fully represented. With individualized specific instructions, the examination can also be performed by a qualified radiographer or other assistants.

Indications for tomography

The following considerations may serve as basic rules for indications for tomography:

– Tomography largely frees the plain radiograph from superimposed densities and lucencies, thus permitting imaging of processes or details in the organ of interest.

– It eliminates most summation and subtraction effects in the region of interest. Thus, section imaging also permits representation of contrast-poor circular foci in the lung as well as small defects in the skeleton. This effect is frequently called 'structural depletion' but is actually due to a changed signal–noise ratio with a reduced organ-dependent noise.

– Tomography only displays organ borders with contours of the imaged section that are perpendicular to the projection, i.e. parallel to the useful radiation beam. Therefore, it may be necessary to select other than standard projections. This requirement was pointed out by Ziedses des Plantes [42] in his 1934 monograph. A detailed description of this effect is given in a monograph by Edholm (1960) [5]. Because of the finite extension of the layer, the detail contrast is reduced. This reduction is partly offset by a decrease in scattered radiation that enters the area to be imaged since its field size is clearly smaller than that of the plain radiograph. Therefore, proper coning should be practiced.

– The plain radiographs or other image studies of the body region to be examined must be available for the tomographic examination, otherwise the examination cannot be properly conducted and the structures in question seen on the plain radiograph cannot be visualized and identified with certainty. In particular, pulmonary findings that are at different 'depths' may be overlooked. Therefore, care must be taken to include at least the organ of major clinical interest in its entirety. This may frequently require several projections.

– When tomograms of the organ are already available, they are necessary to obtain a comparable examination. Tomograms only display partial sections that are different from corresponding projections of the plain radiographs.

For the purpose of comparison, the same projections should be selected if possible.

The following sections describe the most important indications, subdivided according to organs. This description does not claim to be comprehensive. Every indication follows from the clinical problem and the observed findings, as well as from the knowledge and experience gained from radiographic imaging of normal and pathologically altered organs. Details are found in various monographs and are discussed here.

Tomography of the chest

Tomography of the chest is of great importance for diagnosing pathologic changes in the lungs. A detailed account of the achievement of this procedure and its limitations was already given in the early years of tomography, e.g. by H. Chaoul and his school (1934, 1935). K. Greineder [9] was the first to compare the tomographic findings with organ sections from autopsy specimens. B.R. Young [40] summarized the findings by proposing the performance of tomography in any case of a pulmonary finding inadequately explained by plain radiographs.

Chest tomography is still in the domain of diagnostic radiology. It may be considered equal to computed tomography in a number of instances, particularly, in the diagnosis of advanced tuberculous and other inflammatory processes in the lung, and in the delineation of cavities and loss of pulmonary tissue.

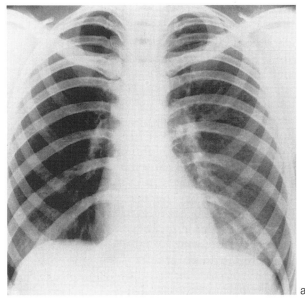

a

Fig. IV, 13a-c. Right bronchial adenoma. **a)** Chest radiograph. Right lung increased radiolucency. Right hilar density smaller than left.

Furthermore, tomographic sections of the lung can answer the question of the presence of more nodules in addition to nodules seen in plain radiographs, with these additive nodules

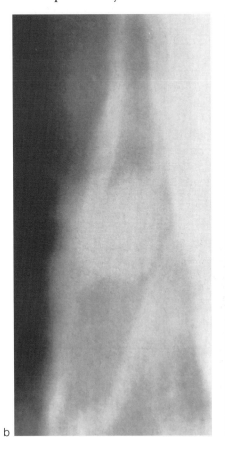

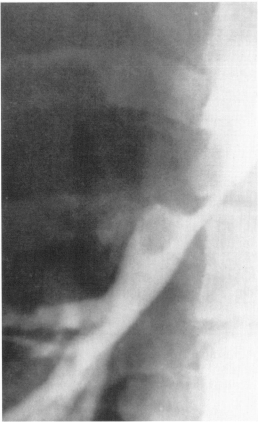

Fig. IV, 13b-c.
b) Frontal tomogram at a depth of 11.5 cm. Right main bronchus shows a pigeon-egg-sized density. **c)** Right bronchogram. Defect in the opacified bronchus (Gebauer et al, 1959).

b

c

possibly requiring further histological clarification. Tomography is also suited for the localization and evaluation of abscesses. However, the differential diagnosis between malignant and benign processes, especially if they arise in the bronchial tree, should now be reserved for endoscopy or percutaneous fine needle biopsy or other invasive procedures.

Section imaging of the hilus, including bronchial tree (Fig. IV, 13), hilar vessels and lymph nodes, still remains an indication for conventional tomography, especially when computed tomography is not available. For this purpose, two projections (AP and lateral) are generally necessary to demonstrate the findings. Occasionally, special oblique projections may be required to visualize the bronchial structures in question parallel to the image plane. Only such a projection might visualize outline and course of a bronchus.

When the findings are unclear, sonographic or endoscopic examinations of the hilus and tracheobronchial tree might be indicated.

Processes along the chest wall, including pleural space, are better visualized by computed tomography than by conventional tomography. If computed tomography is not available, conventional tomography should be performed by selecting a projection that has the margins of the process almost perpendicular to the projection plane and parallel to the central ray. The most appropriate projection should be determined by fluoroscopy if feasible.

Tomography of the mediastinum including heart and large vessels

The diagnosis of processes within the mediastinum, especially those not recognizable as mediastinal enlargements, is best achieved with endoscopic methods (e.g. mediastinoscopy), possibly with excisional biopsy. This approach is superior to tomography, which, however has been proved a suitable screening method for determining site and extension of mediastinal abnormalities.

In cardiac imaging, conventional tomography has been largely replaced by sonography and nuclear medicine. For the diagnosis of changes in the chambers of the heart and the coronary vessels, various cardiological examinations are available, such as Tl-201 scintigraphy, echocardiography and coronary angiography. Tomography can no longer be seen the method of choice. Sonography of the heart and its vessels was well established even before the introduction of computed tomography.

Indications for tomography of the skeletal system

In generalized diseases of the skeletal system, tomography only has a subordinate role. General metastatic spread within the skeletal system is primarily a domain of nuclear medicine. To assess general bone loss, osteodensitometric procedures have a greater impact than tomography, even in cases of more regional bone loss in the extremities. However, for localized osseous findings, tomography may still provide important in-

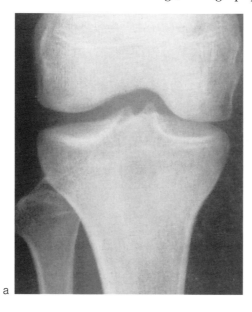
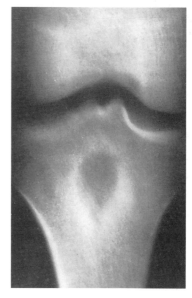

Fig. IV, 14a, b. Brodie's abscess in the proximal tibia metaphysis. **a)** Plain radiograph. Lucency hardly visible. **b)** Frontal tomogram. Lucency and surrounding sclerosis clearly visible (Gebauer et al, 1959).   a   b

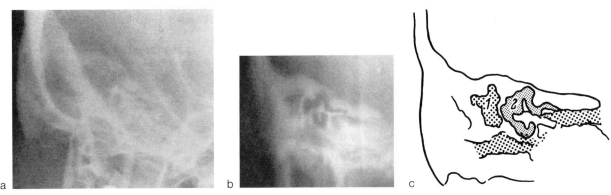

Fig. IV, 15a-c. Sequestered labyrinth. **a)** Plain radiograph in Stenvers projection. **b)** Tomogram of the petrous bone in Stenvers projection. **c)** Diagram: 1 = antrum; 2 = sequestered labyrinth (Gebauer et al, 1959).

formation, complementary to the information of plain radiographs obtained in two projections. This also applies to the diagnosis of fractures, degenerative processes, and destruction due to infection or inflammation (Fig. IV, 14). More recently, this has been successfully supplemented by magnetic resonance imaging, if available, e.g. in the diagnosis of osteomyelitis. Tomography can also aid in delineating localized metastases or localized manifestations of generalized bone diseases.

Tomography is still important for examinations of the facial bones, especially mandible and maxilla. In this context, orthopantomography, often without plain radiographs, is frequently the method of choice. Orthopantomography is indicated for the following conditions:
- Examinations of diseases that preclude opening of the mouth for intraoral diagnosis. This includes fractures and their sequelae, oral and dental tumors including maxillary and mandibular tumors, advanced infections and changes in the temporomandibular joints.
- Examinations where the film size for intraoral imaging is inadequate, as individual film or film series, for a radiographic survey.
- Imaging any sections of mandible and maxilla that cannot be represented on intraoral films. These include not only diagnosis in and around the teeth but also in the region of the ascending ramus of the mandible, the temporomandibular joints and adjacent paranasal sinuses, and the nasopharyngeal region.
- Periapical lesions with margins exceeding the size of an intraoral film.

Orthopantomography is generally accepted in dental medicine and is increasingly used in general radiology. Numerous designs are available.

This speaks for the suitability of this diagnostic procedure and is an indication of its steadily enlarging applications.

Another frequently used diagnostic procedure is the tomography of the facial bones, including the sinuses. Now and as before, tomography is generally used to discover mucosal changes, to diagnose inflammatory processes, and to detect destructive changes including fractures in the region of the facial bones (Fig. IV, 15). It is easier performed than computed tomography, less time consuming, and associated with a lower radiation exposure.

Tomography of skeletal parts oriented parallel to the longitudinal axis should be mentioned, as a mean of visualization without superimposed structures. This includes tomography of the sternum and long bones, to visualize inflammatory processes and advanced tumors as well as structures immediately adjacent to these bones.

Conventional tomography is also used to clarify processes involving the joints, if necessary combined with contrast-medium administration and performed as a double-contrast method, which so far has not yet entirely been replaced by magnetic resonance imaging.

Abdomen

Tomography of the kidneys and renal pelves is still justified as a method of providing images free of superimposed structures.

Imaging kidneys and intrarenal collecting system free of any intestinal air in pediatric cases, improved imaging of the renal and adrenal contours, especially in suspected mass lesions, and improved imaging of the intrarenal collecting system are all still used. Here again, however, tomography is largely being replaced by sonography. The same is true for imaging of the gall bladder and bile ducts, while imaging of the pancreas was never valid indication for tomography.

Conclusions

During the past decades, the progress in imaging technology and interventional radiology, including new diagnostic surgical procedures, has improved the efficiency of diagnostic radiology, providing the basis for the delivery of effective therapies. The multitude of diagnostic procedures now available worldwide allows a targeted diagnostic evaluation. The indications for conventional tomography have considerably changed and are more limited, but several areas remain where conventional tomography is still superior today, especially in view of its relatively uncomplicated technical equipment and simple performance.

Recently, experts have addressed the issue of diagnostic equipment needed for institutions where technical or financial reasons preclude the installation of highly technical equipment. In the Technical Report 795 [39] of the World Health Organization, these experts state that good basic patient care requires a universal stand for conventional radiography, an ultrasound unit and, if possible, a tomographic device and a fluoroscopic system. This emphasizes the necessity of having conventional tomography equipment installed and operative in every radiology department. The sequence of examinations recommended for the evaluation of most important diseases should be followed.

Future developments and trends

In the industrialized countries, body section imaging is an examination that is primarily performed by computed tomography and magnetic resonance imaging. Both methods have the advantage of superb image processing and high contrast resolution, but computed tomography is burdened by a higher radiation exposure in comparison to conventional tomography. This one is of the reasons that CT is generally used as a supplemental rather than a primary procedure, e.g. in intravenous pyelography to eliminate superimpositions.

Pantomography is advantageous and increasingly used for the evaluation of teeth and jaw. With film-screen systems containing rare-earth phosphors, the radiation exposure could be reduced by 50% to values that are clearly below those for usual dental radiographs with intraoral films (e.g. Rimkus et al. [23]). These applications should be encouraged in dentistry and orthodontics.

According to recommendations by a commission of experts of the World Health Organization, conventional tomography should continue to be a diagnostic procedure available in private practice and hospitals providing medical care at level I.

Improvements in image quality can certainly be achieved by applying digital methods, such as digital storage phosphor systems. However, this is still an investigational modality and not yet available in hospitals and practices.

Digital tomosynthesis, described recently, probably has little prospect of being introduced into diagnostic radiology to any large extent despite its clearly reduced radiation exposure.

Thus, conventional tomography, with the notable exception of pantomography, will be restricted to applications that provide the diagnostic information at lower cost and less radiation and to situations where more technical and expensive equipment is not available.

Summary

Tomography is a radiographic method based on principles conceived and practically applied in the early years of diagnostic radiology. It is a method that can eliminate interfering overlying densities, thus providing a better visualization of the body region in question, and that has the advantage of being performed with little additional effort.

The radiation exposure of a tomographic radiograph is similar to that of a conventional radiograph obtained under comparable conditions. Dedicated applications, such as pantomography, have an assured position in the diagnostic evaluation of the teeth and jaw. Other applications of conventional tomography also have established indications despite the introduction of new tomographic technologies.

References

1. Baese, C.: Method of apparatus for the localisation of foreign objects in and the radiotherapeutic treatment of the human body by X-rays. Italian Patent (1915)

2. Bartelink, D.L.: Nouveau procédé radiographique de mise en évidence d'une région osseuse déterminée. J. Belge. Radiol. 21 (1932) 447–450

3. Bartelink, D.L.: Röntgencoupes. Ned. T. Geneesk. 76 (1932) 23

4. Bocage, A.E.M.: Procédé et dispositif de radiographie sur plaque en mouvement. Franz. Patentschr. Nr. 534 464 (1922)

5. Edholm, P.: The Tomogram, Its Formation and Content. Acta Radiol. (1960) Suppl. 193 Stockholm

6. Frain, Ch., F. Lacroix: Courbe-enveloppe et couppes horizontales. J. Radiol. Electrol. 28 (1947) 142–143

7. Gebauer, A., F. Wachsmann: Geometrische Betrachtungen und technische Fragen zur Herstellung transversaler (horizontaler) Körperschichtaufnahmen. Röntgen-Bl. 2 (1949) 215–229

8. Grossmann, G.: Tomographie I. Fortschr. Röntgenstr. 51 (1935) 61–80

9. Greineder, K.: Das Schichtbild der Lunge, des Tracheobronchialbaums und des Kehlkopfes. Leipzig, G. Thieme 1941

10. Grossmann, G.: Tomographie II. Fortschr. Röntgenstr. 51 (1935) 191–208

11. Grossmann, G.: Praktische Voraussetzungen für die Tomographie. Fortschr. Röntgenstr. 52 (1935) Kongreßh. 44: 46–50

12. Höxter, E.A., A. Schenz: Röntgenaufnahmetechnik. Teil Panorama-Schichtaufnahmen. 14. Auflage, 28–29, Siemens AG, Berlin und München (1991)

13. International Commission on Radiological Units and Measurements (ICRU): Methods of Evaluating Radiological Equipment and Materials; Measurement of the caracteristics of body-section radiographic equipment. Handbook 89: 15–26. United States Department of Commerce. National Bureau of Standards, U.S.A. (1963)

14. Kieffer, J.: X-ray device and method of technic. U.S.A. Patent Nr. 195 4321 (1929/34)

15. Massiot, J.: Essai d'un appareil pour radiographie analytique. Bull. Soc. Radiol. méd. France 23 (1935) 395–398

16. Massiot, J.: Histoire de la Tomographie. Medica Mundi 19 (1974) 106–115

17. Mayer, K.: Radyologiczne Rözpozanie Roznizkowe Chorob Sera i Aorty. Krakow: Gebethner and Co (1916)

18. Mayer, K.: Zur Tomographie. Fortschr. Röntgenstr. 52 (1936) 622–623

19. National Council on Radiation Protection and Measurements: Quality Assurance for Diagnostic Imaging Equipment. NCRP Report No. 99. National Council on Radiation Protection and Measurements. Bethes da, MD. USA (1988)

20. Paatero, Y.A.V.: A new tomographical method for radiographing curved outer surfaces. Acta radiol. (Stockholm) 32 (1949) 117–184

21. Pohl, E.: Verfahren und Vorrichtung zur röntgenographischen Wiedergabe eines Körperschnittes und Ausschluß der davor und dahinter liegenden Teile. Dtsch. Patentschr. 544 4200 (1927)

22. Portes, E., M. Chaussé: Procédé pour la mise au point radiologique sur un plan sécant d'un solide, ainsi que pour la concentration sur une zone déterminée d'une action radiotherapeutique maximum et dispositifs permettant la réalisation. Franz. Patenschr. Nr. 541 941 (1922)

23. Rimkus, D.S., B.M. Gill, N.A. Baily, L.B. Talner, P.J. Friedman: Digital Tomosynthesis: Phantom and patient studies with a prototype unit. Comp. Med. Imag. Graph. 13 (1989) 307–318

24. Sans, R., J. Porcher: Le Polytome. J. Radiol. Electrol. 31 (1952) 300

25. Stevenson, J.J.: Horizontal body section radiography. Brit. J. Radiol. 23 (1950) 319–334

26. Stieve, F.E.: Radiation exposure to body section radiography. Acta Radiol. 55 (1961) 465–485

27. Stieve, F.E.: Bevorzugte Darstellung einzelner Körperschichten. In: Handbuch der Medizinischen Radiologie, Band III: 715–1041. H. Vieten et al., ed. Springer, Berlin, Heidelberg und New York (1973)

28. Takahashi, S.: Study of the technique of the radiographic delineation of the cross section of the body (Study on Rotatography and Crossgraphy). 4th Report, Tohoku J. exp. Med. 54 (1941) 1

29. Takahashi, S.: Rotation Kymography. Nippon Acta Radiol. 9 (1948) 1–14

30. Takahashi, S.: Theory of blurring of X-ray images and occurence of obstructive shadows in rotatory cross section radiography. Tohoku, J. exp. Med. 58 (1953) 63–68

31. Vallebona, A.: Una modalità di tecnica per la dissociazione della ombre applicata allo studio del cranio. Radiol. med. (Torino) 27 (1930) 1090

32. Vallebona, A.: Nouvelle méthode roentgenstratigraphique. Radiol. clin. (Basel) 16 (1947) 279–285

33. Vallebona, A.: New application of stratigraphy. Proc. 6th Int. Congr. Ron Radiology, London (1950) 89–92

34. Vieten, H.: Verfahren und Apparatur zur Anfertigung von Schichtaufnahmen in beliebig gestellten und beliebig gestalteten Schichten. Dtsch. Patentanmeldung 54949 IX/30a vom 8.5.1936

35. Vieten, H.: Verfahren zur röntgenographischen Darstellung eines Körperschnittes. Dtsch. Patentschr. 672 518 (1936)

36. Watson, W.: X-ray apparatus. Brit. Patent of 26.12.1937 (1937)

37. Watson, W.: Improvements in or to apparatus for radiography and X-ray fluoroscopy. Brit. Patent. 705 297 (1951)

38. World Health Organization (WHO). Quality Assurance in Diagnostic Radiology. World Health Organization, Geneva (1982)

39. World Health Organization (WHO). Effective choices for diagnostic imaging in clinical practice. Technical Report Series 795. World Health Organization, Geneva (1990)

40. Young, B.R.: The value of body section Roentgenography (Planigraphy) for the demonstration of tumors, non neoplastic disease and foreign bodies in the neck and chest. Am. J. Roentgenol. 47 (1942) 83–99

41. Ziedses des Plantes, B.G.A.: Enen bijzondre methode voor het maken van röntgenphotos van schedel en wervelkolom. Ned. T. Geneesk. 75 (1931) 5218–5222

42. Ziedses des Plantes, B.G.A.: Planigraphie en Subtractie. Röntgenographische differentiatie methoden. Thesis, Kemnik en Zoon NV, Utrecht (1934)

Computed tomography - technical development

W.A. Kalender

'If we give free rein to our fantasy and imagine perfecting the new photographic process with the aid of Crookes' tube until one part of the soft-tissue structures of the human body remains transparent and a layer located underneath can be imaged on the plate, this would be of invaluable assistance in diagnosing innumerable diseases not directly associated with bone structures.'

Translation of an excerpt from 'Frankfurter Zeitung', 7 January 1896.

Historical overview

As has been reported in the previous section, concepts of tomographic imaging using X-rays were developed at a very early date. The unknown author of the above article appearing in the feature supplement of the 'Frankfurter Zeitung' expressed truly prophetic ideas only a few days after the first reports were published on Roentgen's discovery of X-rays and prior to their first medical use. Although we do not know exactly what the author had in mind when he conceived the possibility of displaying *'a layer located underneath . . .'* the soft tissue structures of the human body, it was certainly not computed tomography as we know it today. Perhaps he wished to obtain a view similar to that with an anatomical preparation after superimposed layers of tissue have been removed. His assessment that *'. . . this would be of invaluable assistance in diagnosing innumerable diseases not directly associated with bone structures'* was in any case correct. One should, however, avoid overinterpretation of this quotation; the development of tomography, modern methods of reconstructing digital images, and today's powerful computers were all still undreamed of.

Computed tomography (CT) first became feasible with the development of modern computer technology in the sixties, but some of the ideas on which it is based can be traced back to the first half of this century. In 1917 the Bohemian mathematician J.H. Radon [1] proved in a fundamental research paper that the distribution of a material or material property in an object layer can be calculated if the integral values along any number of lines passing through the same layer are known. The first optical applications of this theory were developed for radioastronomy by Bracewell in 1956 [2], but they met with little response and were not exploited for medical purposes.

The first medical applications were by the physicist A.M. Cormack, who worked on improving radiotherapy planning at Groote Schuur Hospital, Cape Town, South Africa. Between 1957 and 1963, and without knowledge of previous studies, he developed a method of calculating radiation absorption distributions in the human body based on transmission measurements [3]. He postulated that it must be possible to display even the most minute absorption differences, i.e. different soft-tissue structures. However, he never had occasion to put his theory into practice, and first learned of Radon's work much later, a fact that he regretted by stating that earlier access to this knowledge would have saved him a lot of work [4]. While familiarizing himself with Radon's work, Cormack discovered that Radon had himself been unaware of still earlier work on the subject by the Dutch physicist H.A. Lorentz who had already proposed a solution of the mathematical problem in 1905 [5].

Successful practical implementation of this theory was first achieved in 1972 by the English engineer G.N. Hounsfield (Fig. IV, 16), who is

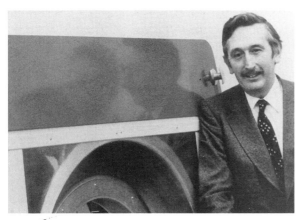

Fig. IV, 16.. Godfrey Hounsfield (born in 1919). English Engineer, who developed the first CT-Scanner at EMI. Together with the American physicist A.M. Cormack (born in 1924) he received the Nobel Prize for medicine in 1979.

now generally recognized as the inventor of computed tomography [6]. Like his predecessors, Hounsfield worked without knowledge of the above-mentioned earlier findings. His success took the entire medical world by surprise, and he achieved his remarkable breakthrough neither at a renowned university nor with a leading manufacturer of radiological equipment, but with the British firm EMI Ltd, which had never previously been involved in medical engineering. This invention gave EMI, which had until then manufactured only records and electronic components, a monopoly in the CT market that lasted for 2 years, and the terms 'EMI scanner' and 'CT scanner' became almost synonymous. In 1974 Siemens became the first traditional manufacturer of radiological equipment to market a head CT scanner, after which many other companies quickly followed suit. A boom followed, reaching its peak in the late seventies with 18 companies offering CT equipment. Subsequently, eleven of these, including EMI, had withdrawn from the market.

The first clinical CT images were produced at the Atkinson Morley Hospital in London in 1972. The very first patient examination performed with CT offered convincing proof of the effectiveness of the method by detecting a cystic frontal lobe tumor [7]. The first publications were by Hounsfield and by Ambrose, both in 1973 [6, 8]. This invention was immediately and enthusiastically welcomed by the medical community,

and has often been referred to as the most important radiological invention since the discovery of X-rays; its later development only confirmed these early expectations. Computed tomography has become a very important factor in diagnostic radiology. While only 60 EMI scanners had been installed by 1974, it is now estimated that approximately 25 000 clinical installations will exist by 1995. In 1979 Cormack and Hounsfield, a physicist and an engineer, were awarded the Nobel Prize for medicine in recognition of their outstanding achievements.

Table IV, 2. Historical overview: the development of CT

1895	W.C. Roentgen discovers 'a new kind of rays' later referred to as 'X-rays' or 'roentgen rays' in his honour.
1917	J.H. Radon develops the mathematical foundation for reconstructing cross-sectional images from transmission measurements [1].
1963	A.M. Cormack describes a technique for calculating the absorption distribution in the human body [3].
1972	G.N. Hounsfield and J. Ambrose conduct the first clinical CT examinations.
1973	First publications dealing with CT [6,8].
1974	60 clinical CT installations
1975	First whole-body CT scanner in clinical use [10].
1979	Hounsfield and Cormack awarded the Nobel Prize.
1983	First clinical examinations performed with electron beam CT [12].
1989	First clinical examinations with spiral CT [14–18]
1995	Approximately 25 000 clinical CT installations.

Perception in slices –
the principle of computed tomography

Computed tomography is a digital technique, i.e. the body is not seen as a unit but is subdivided into slices. These slices or layers are composed of discrete, square-shaped volume elements ('voxels') corresponding in height to the thickness of the slice (Fig. IV, 17a). The value of each of these volume elements is displayed in one picture element ('pixel') of the image matrix. The reconstruction of such images from measurements (or scans) can be performed by various methods. The simplest general concept is that a system comprising N independent equations obtained from the measured values exists, from which M unknowns, the pixels, should be calculated or reconstructed. This can be expressed very graphically for very small image matrices (Fig. IV, 17b). For practical applications, the number of measurements 'N' should be clearly greater than the number of pixels 'M'.

The required acquisition of values measured within the patient is achieved by scanning a transverse anatomical slice from as many different perspectives as possible. For this purpose, both the X-ray source and the detector system must rotate around the patient (Fig. IV, 17c). The beam is collimated to a pencil beam or narrow fan beam. In contrast to conventional tomography, only the slice actually displayed in the image is traversed by the X-ray beam. The measured signals are not influenced or falsified by structures located in adjacent slices.

Fig. IV, 17a-e. Diagram of scan and image reconstruction in CT.

Fig. IV, 17a. In CT, the slice under examination must be imagined as consisting of discrete volume elements, the contents of each being displayed in a corresponding pixel of the image matrix.

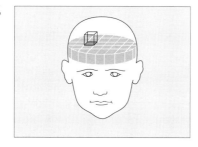

Fig. IV, 17b. In the simplest case of only four pixels, four transmission measurements (four equations in four unknowns) already suffice to reconstruct the corresponding 'image'.

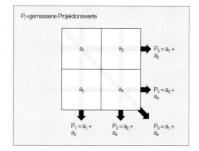

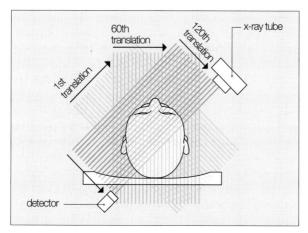

Fig. IV, 17c. The attenuation of X-rays by anatomic structures in the slice is measured from various perspectives. The image is reconstructed from these projections.

In a CT scan, the attenuation of the X-radiation is measured along the lines between the focal spot of the X-ray tube and the detector. These measurements are the 'line integrals' that Radon [1] and Cormack [3] had postulated in their research. Integration here means that the attenuation of the beam by every volume element is summed along the measuring beam. Together, all measurements or line integrals detected from the same direction form a projection.

For high image quality, particularly with fine image matrices, the largest possible number of projections and measurements per projection must be acquired. For the data quantities normally processed by today's CT systems, the algebraic reconstruction methods mentioned above (Fig. IV, 17b) and also used by Hounsfield in his first studies require too much processing time. Today the convolution and back projection technique is usually employed. The principles of image reconstruction have been described in numerous textbooks and articles. Although other techniques such as Fourier reconstruction should also be mentioned [9], they will not be discussed here in any great detail. It would seem both more important and more interesting to explain what tissue properties are displayed in a CT scan and why this technique exhibits such a high degree of contrast sensitivity.

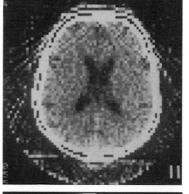

Fig. IV, 17d. 1974: display with an image matrix of 80 x 80 pixels and a 13-mm section thickness.

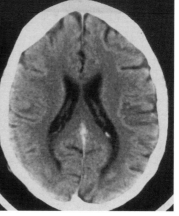

Fig. IV, 17e. 1983: Display with an image matrix of 1024 x 1024 pixels and a 5-mm section thickness.

A CT scanner measures the attenuation of X-rays in tissue. This depends on both the density and the atomic number of the tissue contained in the volume element under observation. The measured variable is physically designated as the linear attenuation coefficient μ. In the image, μ is displayed relative to the attenuation of water and specified in CT values commonly called Hounsfield units (HU) in honour of the inventor of computed tomography:

$$\text{CT value} = \frac{\mu - \mu\text{H}_2\text{O}}{\mu\text{H}_2\text{O}} \cdot 1000 \text{ HU}$$

This scale defines water as having a value of zero HU, and assigns a value of -1000 HU to air. Because of their low density, lung tissue and fat have negative CT values. Most other tissues lie within the positive range. For muscles, connective tissue and most organs this fact is chiefly attributable to the physical density of the organ's tissue. For bone and calcifications, however, the higher atomic number of calcium results in a higher attenuation value, and hence account for the high CT values typically ranging from 1000 to 2000 HU.

By its excellent soft-tissue contrast that had never been achieved before, CT convinced radiologists of its diagnostic value from the very beginning. This is not just due to the use of high doses and the resulting low pixel noise, since even conventional X-ray exposures can attain a low noise level. Rather, it is primarily the display without overlapping structures and with contrast enhancement that explains this capability. Soft tissues also display contrasts in conventional X-ray images. Unfortunately, they are concealed by superimposed bone structures and soft-tissue/air contrasts. The sections of CT depict the contrast in a volume element or a region in comparison with adjacent volume elements or regions without interfering superimpositions. As a result, even differences in density of only a few HU can be detected, which is a fascinating fact considering that 1 HU corresponds to a density difference of only 1/1000.

Technical development of CT

The development of CT hardware began on the basis of Hounsfield's experimental set-up (first generation: Fig. IV, 18a), which differed only slightly from the first clinical unit and the first commercial units (second generation, Fig. IV, 18b). Both operated according to the translate-rotate principle, i.e. the radiation source and

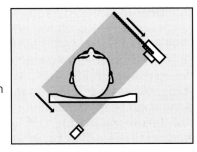

Fig. IV, 18a-f. Block diagram of different CT scanners (See text for explanation). **a)** Hounsfield's experimental set-up with only one detector element (pencil beam).

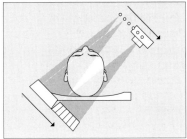

Fig. IV, 18b. Set-up of first commercial cranial CT scanner with small detector arrays (fan beam).

the detector scanned the object in a linear translation movement, rotated 1° and then repeated this procedure. Hounsfield thus acquired 180 projections, each with 160 measured values for a total of 28 800 data per scan [6]. This sufficed to reconstruct an image comprising 6400 pixels, i.e. with an 80 x 80 matrix. The scan took 5 min and the image reconstruction also required 5 min. Hounsfield specified an examination time of 35 min for scanning six sets of two images each with a section thickness of 13 mm. These were remarkable performance data. Hounsfield had already performed the first tests back in 1969 using an isotope source with a scan time of 9 days per phantom image [7].

Almost all commercial translate-rotate scanners offered only a scan field for cranial examinations. The first attempt to perform CT scans on all regions of the body again employed the translate-rotate principle [10]. In 1974, Ledley and coworkers commissioned their ACTA (Automatic Computerized Transverse Axial) scanner, which acquired a scan field of 48 cm in a 6-min scan. Although this could demonstrate the potential of CT for whole-body imaging, obvious problems occurred with respect to respiratory excursions and patient movements and with the long exposure times required to scan larger anatomical regions. The main goal of CT development in the mid-seventies was to reduce the scan times to only 20 s so that scans of the torso could be performed during a single breath-hold. The solution to this problem was the introduction of the fan-beam technique.

Instead of scanning a transmission profile with a pencil beam, in the fan-beam technique a large detector arc is exposed and a complete projection is acquired simultaneously. This results in much better utilization of the available output of the X-ray tube. The translation movement is not required, so that the system needs only a rotation movement (Fig. IV, 18c,d). The first whole-body tomographs equipped with a fan-beam system were launched in 1975. The 'unattainable 20-s barrier' had finally been broken. In the first scanners of this type, both the tube and the detector rotated around the patient. While this technique resulted in higher technical demands, it also brought advantages with regard to costs and image quality (third generation: Fig. IV, 18c). Shortly thereafter, scanners featuring a stationary, ring-shaped detector surrounding the patient in which only the tube had to be moved were introduced (fourth generation: Fig. IV, 18d). The purely rotation systems quickly prevailed, and the translate-rotate systems have almost completely disappeared. The discussion as to the best type of scanner is still going on, although the third generation has successfully established its predominance from a purely numerical standpoint.

Regardless of the given type of scanner, the image quality always depends greatly on the scan time, since deliberate and involuntary patient movements can impair image definition and cause artifacts. In conventional CT systems the electrical energy is fed to the X-ray tube through a cable. This prevents fast and continuous rotation and makes it necessary to accelerate the scanner in one direction, decelerate it following a 360° scan, and then accelerate it again for the next scan. 'Fast scanners' employing this technique attained scan times of only 2 s but fell short of the wishes voiced by clinicians and radiologists. The goal of providing the shortest possible scan times was therefore further pursued through many creative approaches. Three of these have taken shape: continuously rotating conventional systems, electron-beam scanners (Fig. IV, 18e), and volume CT scanners (Fig. IV, 18f).

In 1987, the introduction of continuously rotating CT systems (Siemens SOMATOM PLUS and Toshiba 900S) brought decisive new im-

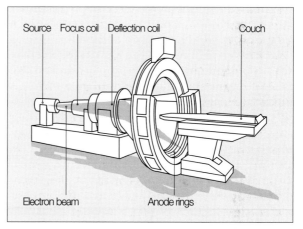

Fig. IV, 18e. C-100-electron-beam scanner to scan 8.8 mm slices in the millisecond range (Imatron Co., San Francisco, USA).

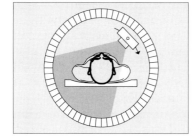

Fig. IV, 18c. Fan-beam scanner with moving detector arm to scan an entire anatomical region.

Fig. IV, 18d. Fan-beam scanner with fixed, ring-shaped detector surrounding the patient.

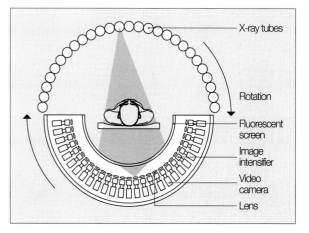

Fig. IV, 18f. Volume scanner with dynamic spatial reconstruction for simultaneous scan of 240 0.9 mm slices (Mayo Clinic, Rochester, USA).

pulses to computed tomography. This innovation not only reduced the scan time to 1 s, but also provided the basis for extended dynamic examinations and spiral CT. The vast majority of today's CT scanners are designed according to the continuous rotation principle.

A lot of consideration had, however, already been given at a much earlier date to the best way of reducing scan times and acquiring complete volumes [11]. Electron beam scanners with a ring-shaped anode surrounding the patient had already been proposed as early as 1977. The electron beam is electromagnetically guided over this target, and the scanning procedure is completed in only 50-100 ms without mechanical movement. The first CT scanner of this type was developed by D.P. Boyd [12]. Several dozen such scanners were subsequently sold and installed by the Imatron Co. (Fig. IV, 18e). Although this 'cine CT' is suitable for a wide range of applications, it will not enjoy widespread use before several technical improvements and a reduction in costs have been achieved.

An entirely different approach was followed by R.A. Robb and coworkers [13], who backed the use of conventional technology. In an enormous experimental set-up, they planned to install 28 X-ray tubes opposite 28 fluorescent screens in such a way that all of these components would continuously rotate around the patient (Fig. IV, 18f). This scanner was actually constructed only in a stripped-down version designed for physiological animal experiments and enabled simultaneous scanning of 240 slices with a section thickness of 0.9 mm at intervals of 1/60 s. Although this technical concept has been abandoned because of the costs involved and the poor image quality attained, its primary goal, i.e. to perform volume scanning employing thin slices in the shortest possible time, is still being sought.

Table IV, 3. Performance characteristics of CT: 1972 – 1995

	1972*	1995*
Min. scan time	300 s	0.1 – 1 s
Data per scan	57,6 KB	2 MB
Image matrix	80 x 80	1024 x 1024
Power	2 kW	60 kW
Section thickness	13 mm	1 – 10 mm
Spatial resolution	3 lp/cm	15 lp/cm
Contrast resolution	5 mm/	3 mm/
	5 HU/50 mGy	3 HU/30 mGy

* Typical values

Volume scans with spiral CT

With CT, the two-dimensional, slice-by-slice display of anatomical volumes gained full acceptance for the first time in the history of radiology. But the scanning of individual slices requires time to move the patient and give him a breathing pause between exposures. There is also a risk of organs being displaced by respiratory excursions or patient movement during interscan delays. This can cause problems especially when searching for lesions in the lung or liver. At any rate, a continuous scan cannot be guaranteed. The total scan time per organ is often longer than desirable, particularly in cases where a contrast medium has been injected.

The introduction of continuously rotating scanners opened up the possibility of continuous, i.e. contiguous sections, scanning of complete organs or body segments. This principle is based on continuous movement of the patient through the scan field during the scan, with the scan beam moving along a helical path in relation to the patient (Fig. IV, 19a). This requires a great deal of effort for image reconstruction since the data for the planar scans must be calculated from the data set of the volume scan. Still, this technique offers the advantage that image reconstruction can be performed for any table position within the scan volume (Fig. IV, 19b). It is also possible to define the levels retrospectively for calculating the sectional images, if necessary overlapping, to ensure a reliable diagnosis of small lesions with optimum contrast (Fig. IV, 19c). Volume scans employing this scan technique were first introduced by W.A. Kalender and coworkers in 1989.

Like the basic concept of computed tomography, theories about spiral CT were simultaneously and independently conceived at different locations. The earliest references to spiral CT were made in 1986, when I. Mori described the scanning technique and possible reconstruction algorithms, however, without reporting any results [19]. Independently of Mori's achievements, W.A. Kalender and P. Vock began their own work on spiral CT in 1988 and in cooperation with M. Oudkerk were able to present extensive and convincing clinical results by 1989 [14, 15, 16, 17, 18]. At the same time and without knowledge of the other research, Y. Bresler and C.J. Skrabacz conducted their investigations of spiral CT at the University of Illinois [20]. They emphasized the fact that these reflections were of a purely theoretical nature, and this opinion was upheld as late as 1990 by

Fig. IV, 19a, b. Working principle and results of spiral CT.

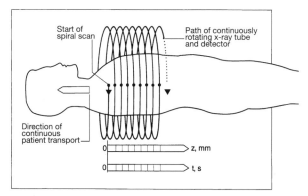

Fig. IV, 19a. During the scan, the patient is continuously moved through the scan field, thus enabling contiguous scanning of entire organs [14].

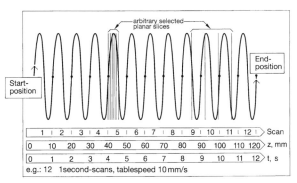

Fig. IV, 19b. Images can retrospectively be reconstructed in any position desired within the scanning volume, whereby the data for a planar image must be interpreted from the spiral data set.

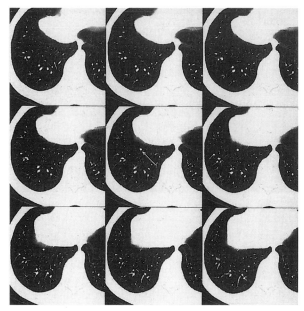

Fig. IV, 19c. By virtue of its continuous scanning of the volume of interest and optimized, retrospective selection of the image plane, the spiral CT yields increased contrast and diagnostic certainty when searching for small lesions.

an American CT manufacturer who assured them that such methods offered no prospect of success [21]. Despite this scepticism, spiral CT emerged within only a few years to become a most promising CT technique. Full acceptance was finally attained at the end of 1992, and this method is now regarded as the universal technique for CT.

The reasons are entirely practical. In comparison to single-slice scanning, the examination time has been considerably reduced. In many cases, e.g. in paediatrics, geriatrics and traumatology, this represents a considerable reduction in the patient's discomfort and the examiner's effort. Diagnostic certainty increases, especially in the detection of small, focal lesions [22, 23, 24, 25, 26]. In examinations requiring a contrast medium, an entire organ can be examined at a relatively high contrast level, using less contrast medium compared with prolonged examinations of individual slices [27, 28]. The possibility of performing an overlapping image reconstruction retrospectively provides an ideal basis for multiplanar and 3D displays (Fig. IV, 20) [29]. Single-slice exposure scanning would require additional scans and increased radiation exposure, but both of these drawbacks are generally eliminated in spiral CT. Instead of performing overlapping scans, overlapping images are simply reconstructed. The dose required for spiral CT is generally lower since repeat scans because of respiratory motion are almost entirely unnecessary and overlapping scans are no longer required for 3D displays. Furthermore, scans are frequently performed at reduced mA values as adjustment of the limiting output of X-ray tube to the longer exposure for spiral CT scans [30].

The total benefits offered by spiral CT have led to its being regarded as the universal CT scanning method of the future. It has not only replaced single-slice scanning but has also facilitated the development of completely new examination techniques including vascular imaging, also referred to as CT angiography [31, 32, 33, 34, 35]. Intravenous injection of contrast medium, in many cases already required as part of the CT examination, normally suffices. This keeps time requirement, patient discomfort and costs relatively low. Various possibilities are available for viewing and documentation. While the diagnosis is usually made on the basis of the original images or 2D reformatting, the findings are often also documented in 3D form (Fig. IV, 21). These 3D images offer the additional advantage that the vascular tree can be viewed from various, retrospectively selected view points.

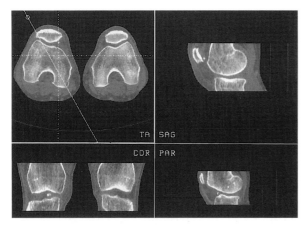

Fig. IV, 20a-c. Spiral CT enables contiguous, three-dimensional display of the human anatomy. **a.** High resolution in freely selected image planes.

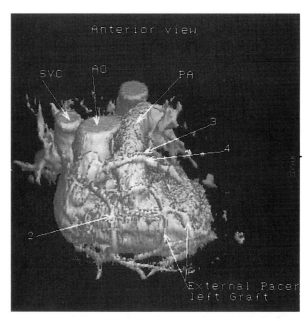

Fig. IV, 20b. Contiguous display - even with moving or pulsating structures.

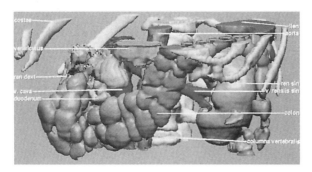

Fig. IV, 20c. Contiguous imaging even of organs subjected to respiratory movements (Source: K.H. Hoehne).

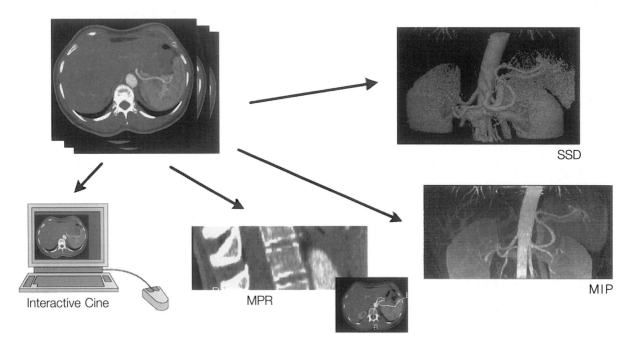

Interactive Cine   MPR   SSD   MIP

Fig. IV, 21. Angiography with spiral CT. Usually displayed in a interactive cine mode of 2D images.
In addition, reformations can be obtained in various orientations, along coronal and sagittal planes as well as along curved interfaces (MPR: multiplanar reconstruction). Documentation of the finding usually as 3D display, either as surface rendering (SSD) or as "maximum intensity projection" (MIP).

Special CT applications

Computed tomography is today a routine method of diagnostic radiology. The images it provides are predominantly used for qualitative assessment of anatomical and pathological details and seldom for quantitative information. A number of applications have, however, become established to support special techniques and indications or to provide quantitative information.

Although only briefly outlined in this section, such special applications constitute no small portion of all CT applications and also underscore the fact that CT has become a fully developed imaging technique. When the digital imaging modality CT was first introduced, the hope was expressed that it would eventually enable quantitative diagnosis of tissue or organs [36, 37, 38, 39, 40]. This expectation is reflected in the term still used in France, i.e. 'tomodensitométrie': tomographic or slice density measurement.

Fig. IV, 22a-d. Special CT examinations involving quantitative assessment of tissue properties.

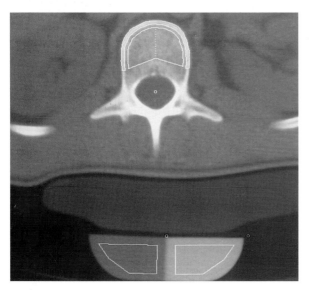

Fig. IV, 22a. Measurement of bone mineral content in the lumbar spine to diagnose and monitor osteoporosis.

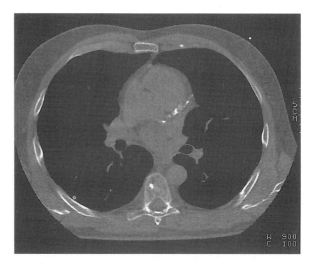

Fig. IV, 22c. Quantitative assessment of plaque volume and calcification in the coronary arteries with EBT.

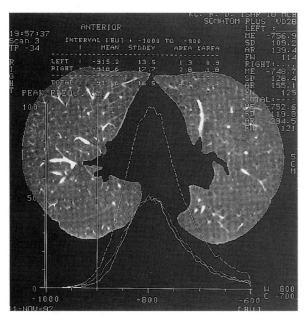

Fig. IV, 22b. Assessment of the lung density and structure under spirometric control.

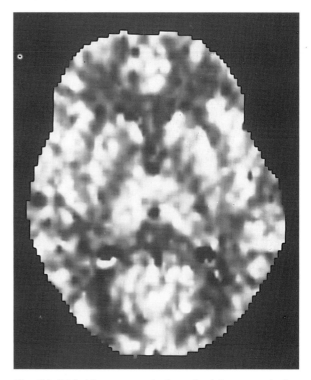

Fig. IV, 22d. Measurement of cerebral tissue perfusion with stable xenon.

Its basic applications consists of measuring geometric values, such as distances, areas, volumes or angles. This presents no particular problem since CT displays the anatomy three-dimensionally and without distortion. However, quantitative presentation of the density or other characteristics of tissue are of equal interest. Initial applications consisted of bone density measurements as part of the diagnostic evaluation of osteoporosis [36, 39]. In contrast to other transmission techniques, CT offers the advantage of excluding superimposition effects and distinguishing cortical and trabecular bone. This technique has been more or less perfected since. Dual-energy techniques and special calibration methods were used to optimize precision. Automatic evaluation techniques (Fig. IV, 22a) and exactly predefined examination protocols ensure high reproducibility of the measurements [41, 42].

Density measurements are also performed on numerous other tissues. They can be useful in characterizing tumors or in differentiating between cystic and solid lesions. One particularly important and well-established application is the measurement of the density and structure of lung tissue. Although quantitative CT (QCT) of the lung attracted a great deal of interest at the end of the seventies, adequate technical methods have only been available since 1990. These include spirometric control of the patient's respiratory condition and the resulting breath-controlled triggering of the CT scanner [43] plus automated evaluation techniques [44], to ensure a high level of reproducibility (Fig. IV, 22b).

Even greater demands are placed on the efficiency of a CT scanner by an application that has emerged only during the last few years: quantitative determination of the plaque volume and calcium content in the coronary arteries (Fig. IV, 22c). The most important prerequisite for this application was millisecond-range imaging. Its technological basis was provided by the principle of electron-beam tomography as noted above. Typically, 40 successive ECG-triggered 3-mm scans would then be acquired at 100-ms intervals, followed by evaluation based on a threshold technique [45, 46]. The chief aim of this method is to detect disorders of coronary arteries through early, non-invasive quantitative determination of calcifications, and provide an objective technique for follow-up examinations. The correlation between calcification, angiographically detected stenoses, and clinical findings is still under investigation. Nevertheless, this method can already be classi-

fied as a cost-effective examination technique that minimizes patient discomfort.

Functional examinations performed with CT scanners have also become established. Especially noteworthy are measurements of tissue perfusion, which can be performed either with intravenous bolus injection of an iodinated contrast-medium or under inhalation of xenon. For cerebral blow flow measurement with stable xenon, a mixture of xenon, oxygen and ambient air is inhaled by the patient for several minutes, scans are taken usually at 1-min intervals during the wash-in and wash-out phases. With special evaluation techniques chiefly derived from the Fick principle, tissue perfusion can be calculated in absolute values expressed in ml/min/100 g of tissue (Fig. IV, 22d).

These examples of quantitative CT hardly cover the entire range of special applications. From special examination techniques, such as functional heart scans with cine or interventional CT, to special evaluation techniques, such as surgical planning (computer aided surgery (CAS)) and radiotherapeutic planning or biomechanical calculations, a wide selection of diagnostic and therapeutic applications is supported. CT has the decisive benefits that the anatomy is displayed with a very high resolution, in three dimensions and without distortion, and that the displayed calculated values enable quantitative assessment of tissue characteristics.

'Quo vadis CT?' – A technical view

Computed tomography must, of course, always be compared with other imaging techniques. In addition to the diagnostic and clinical benefits, humane aspects, such as the length of examination, degree of invasiveness and cost-effectiveness must also be assessed. Imaging by means of magnetic resonance tomography (MR) and ultrasound, neither of which require ionizing radiation, made tremendous progress during the eighties. At that time it was even expected that CT would largely be replaced by these techniques. These expectations proved false: CT lived on, and rapidly resumed its development at the beginning of the nineties. Further advances included numerous special applications, in addition to spiral CT dealt with above. CT offers fast and simple performance of examinations coupled with a high degree of diagnostic certainty. Contiguous sections obtained with spiral CT is one important issue here, and another is the easy interpretation of CT images. The latter is possible because even though CT images often show less contrast than MR images, they remain largely unaffected by the examination parameters and are thus easier to compare.

From a technical standpoint CT is a fully developed imaging technique, which nevertheless still offers many prospects for further improvement. The trend away from single-slice scans and toward the acquisition of complete volumes will continue. Further increases in tube power and shorter scan times will always be on the agenda. While new technical approaches do exist, the breakneck speed of technical development witnessed in the early years of CT will be difficult to repeat.

More and faster advances can be expected in the areas of image reconstruction, processing and evaluation, since the general progress in the field of computer technology can be utilized here. Instantaneous image reconstruction and real-time 3D displays are certainly to be expected. Image segmentation with the aid of artificial intelligence and the presentation of findings in revolutionary new 3D display forms, such as virtual reality, are promises that still seem rather futuristic at this time. As part of the overall development taking place in our 'age of information', such technologies will both advance and sustain the clinical benefits offered by CT and other imaging techniques.

References

1. Radon, J.H.: Über die Bestimmung von Funktionen durch ihre Integralwerte längs gewisser Mannigfaltigkeiten. Ber. vor Sächs. Akad. Wiss. 69 (1917) 262
2. Bracewell, R.N.: Strip integration in radioastronomy. J. Phys. 9 (1956) 198–217
3. Cormack, A.M.: Representation of a function by its line integrals, with some radiological applications. J. Appl. Physics 34 (1963) 2722–2727
4. Cormack, A.M.: Early two-dimensional reconstruction (CT-Scanning) and recent topics stemming from it. Nobel Lecture, December 1979. J. Comput. Assist. Tomogr. 4 (1980) 658–664
5. Cormack, A.M.: 75 Years of Radon Transform. J. Comput. Assist. Tomogr. 16 (1992) 673
6. Hounsfield, G.N.: Computerized transverse axial scanning (tomography). Part I. Description of system. Br. J. Radiol. 46 (1973) 1016
7. Hounsfield, G.N.: Computed medical imaging. Nobel Lecture, December 1979. J. Comput. Assist. Tomogr. 4 (1980) 665–674
8. Ambrose, J.: Computerized transverse axial scanning (tomography). Part II. Clinical application. Br. J. Radiol. 46 (1973) 1023–1047
9. Brooks, R.A.: Principles of computer assisted tomography (CAT) in radiographic and radioisotopic imaging. Phys. Med. Biol. 21 (1976) 689–732
10. Ledley, R.S., G. di Chiro, A.J. Luessenhop, H.L. Twigg: Computerized transaxial x-ray tomography of the human body. Science 186 (1974) 207–212
11. Iimuma, I.A., Y. Tateno, Y. Umegaki, E. Watanabe: Proposed system for ultra fast computed tomography. J. Comput. Assist. Tomogr. 1 (1977) 494
12. Boyd, D.P., M.J. Lipton: Cardiac computed tomography. Proc. IEEE 71 (1983) 298
13. Robb, R.A., E. Hoffman, L.J. Sinak, L.D. Harris, E.L. Ritman: High-speed three-dimensional x-ray computed tomography: The dynamic spatial reconstructor. IEEE 71 (1983) 308–319
14. Kalender, W.A., W. Seißler, E. Klotz, P. Vock: Spiral volumetric CT with single-breathhold technique, continuous transport, and continuous scanner rotation. Radiology 176 (1990) 181–183
15. Vock, P., H. Jung, W.A. Kalender: Single-breathhold volumetric CT of the hepatobiliary system. Radiology 173 (1989) 377
16. Vock, P., H. Jung, W.A. Kalender: Single-breathhold spiral volumetric CT of the lung. Radiology 173 (1989) 400
17. Kalender, W.A., W. Seißler, P. Vock: Single-breathhold spiral volumetric CT by continuous patient translation and scanner rotation. Radiology 173 (1989) 414
18. Oudkerk, M., W.A. Kalender: CT of hilar adenopathy with 1-second and subsecond scan times. Radiology 173 (1989) 452
19. Mori, I.: Computerized tomographic apparatus utilizing a radiation source. United States Patent Number: 463 0202, Dec. 16, 1986
20. Bresler, Y., C.J. Skrabacz: Optimal interpolation in helical scan 3D computerized tomography. Proceedings IEEE Conf. Acoust. Speech and Sig. Proc. (1989) 1472–1475
21. Bresler, Y.: Persönliche Mitteilung. 1992
22. Vock, P., M. Soucek, M. Daepp, W.A. Kalender: Lung: Spiral volumetric CT with single-breathhold technique. Radiology 176 (1990) 864–867
23. Costello, P., W. Anderson, D. Blume: Pulmonary Nodule: Evaluation with spiral volumetric CT. Radiology 179 (1991) 875–876
24. Remy-Jardin, M., J. Remy, L. Wattinne, F. Giraud: Central pulmonary thromboembolism: Diagnosis with spiral volumetric CT with the single breath hold technique – comparison with pulmonary angiography. Radiology 185 (1992) 1–8
25. Costello, P., C.P. Ecker, R. Tello, G.G. Hartnell: Assessment of the thoracic aorta by spiral CT. Amer. J. Roentgenol. 158 (1992) 1127–1130
26. Kalender, W.A., A. Polacin, C. Süß: A comparison of conventional and spiral CT with regard to contrast and spatial resolution: An experimental study on the detection of spherical lesions. J. Comput. Assist. Tomogr. 1994 (in press)
27. Costello, P., D.E. Dupuy, C.P. Ecker, R. Tello: Spiral CT of the thorax with reduced volume of contrast material: A comparative study. Radiology 183 (1992) 663–666
28. Naidich, D.: Volumetric scans change perceptions in thoracic CT. Diagnostic Imaging 4 (1993) 70–74
29. Ney, D., E. Fishman, A. Kawashima, D. Robertson, W. Scott: Comparison of helical and serial CT with regard to three-dimensional imaging of musculoskeletal anatomy. Radiology 185 (1992) 865–869

30. Kalender, W.A.: Technical foundations of spiral CT. Seminars in Ultrasound, CT and MRI 15 (1994) 81–89

31. Gmeinwieser, J., A.P. Wunderlich, P. Gerhardt, M. Strotzer: Dreidimensionale Rekonstruktion von atemverschieblichen Organen und Gefäßstrukturen aus Spiral-CT-Datensätzen. Röntgenpraxis 44 (1991) 2–8

32. Napel, S., M. Marks, G. Rubin, M. Dake, C. McDonell, S. Song, D. Enzmann, B. Jeffrey: CT angiography with spiral CT and maximum intensity projection. Radiology 185 (1992) 607–610

33. Rubin, G., M. Dake, S. Napel, C. McDonnell, B. Jeffrey: Three-dimensional spiral CT angiography of the abdomen: Initial clinical experience. Radiology 186 (1993) 147–152

34. Galanski, M., M. Prokop, A. Chavan, C. Schaefer, K. Jandeleit, J. Nischelsky: Renal arterial stenoses: Spiral CT angiography. Radiology 189 (1993) 185–192

35. Prokop, M., C. Schaefer, W.A. Kalender, A. Polacin, M. Galanski: Gefäßdarstellungen mit Spiral CT: Der Weg zur CT-Angiographie. Der Radiologe 33 (1993) 694–704

36. Rüegsegger, P., P. Niederer, M. Anliker: An extension of classical bone mineral measurements. Ann. Biomed. Eng. 2 (1974) 194–205

37. Phelps, M.E., M.H. Gado, E.J. Hoffman: Correlation of effective atomic number and electron density with attenuation coefficients measured with polychromatic X rays. Radiology 117 (1975) 585–588

38. Rutherford, R.A., B.R. Pullan, I. Isherwood: Measurement of effective atomic number and electron density using an EMI scanner. Neuroradiology 11 (1976) 15–21

39. Genant, H.K., D. Boyd: Quantitative bone mineral analysis using dual energy computed tomography. Invest. Radiol. 12 (1977) 545–551

40. Wegener, O.H., P. Koeppe, H. Oeser: Measurement of lung density by computed tomography. J. Comput. Assist. Tomogr. 2 (1978) 263

41. Kalender, W.A., E. Klotz, C. Süß: An integral approach to vertebral bone mineral analysis by X-ray computed tomography. Radiology 164 (1987) 419–423

42. Kalender, W.: Physik und Methodik der Knochenmineraldichtemessung. In: Schild, H., M. Heller: Osteoporose. Thieme Verlag Stuttgart 1991 S. 78–99

43. Kalender, W.A., R. Rienmüller, W. Seißler, J. Behr, M. Welke, H. Fichte: Spirometric gating for measuring pulmonary parenchymal density by quantitative computed tomography. Radiology 175 (1990) 265–268

44. Kalender, W.A., H. Fichte, W. Bautz, M. Skalej: Semiautomatic evaluation procedures for quantitative CT of the lung. J. Comput. Assist. Tomogr. 15 (1991) 248–255

45. Agatston, A., W. Janowitz, F. Hildner, N. Zusmer, M. Viamonte, R. Detrano: Quantification of coronary artery calcium using ultrafast computed tomography. JACC 15 (1990) 827–832

46. Breen, J.F., P.F. Sheedy, R.S. Schwartz, A.W. Stanson, R.B. Kaufmann, P.P. Moll, J.A. Rumberger: Coronary artery calcification detected with ultrafast CT as an indication of coronary artery disease. Radiology 185 (1992) 435–439

Brain and spinal cord – before CT

B.G. Ziedses des Plantes, G. Rosenbusch

Trepanations have been carried out from antiquity. They might not always have been therapeutic but ritual. Despite these ancient attempts, neurosurgery did not see any progress until the nineteenth century. The reasons are that surgery in general had not been developed sufficiently and that neuroanatomy and physiology of the central nervous system only began to flourish after the circulation of the cerebrospinal fluid (CSF) and the localization of function and pathways in the brain and spinal cord became known. Clinicians learned to classify certain dysfunctions topographically. At the end of the nineteenth century, the diagnosis of neurological disorders saw a significant expansion and improvement as a result of elaborate physical examination, the development of CSF analysis and the introduction of ophthalmoscopy (1851) by Helmholtz (1821–1894).

Neurosurgery before the turn of the century

What kind of neurosurgical problems were tackled before the turn of the century? There were decompressions in space-occupying lesions or hemorrhages, and at times drainage of brain abscesses. Intracerebral surgery was very exceptional, but on 25 November 1884 the London surgeon R.J. Godlee operated on a patient suspected, solely on the grounds of symptoms, of having a brain tumor. A walnut-sized tumor was found between the frontal and parietal lobes at the exact location where it had been clinically suspected, and was removed. The patient survived for at least a month.

Challenge for Edison

On 5 February 1896, Thomas Alva Edison (1847–1931) received a cable from the publisher of the 'New York Journal', W.R. Hearst, asking if he could '. . . make cathodograph of human brain'. Edison, the versatile inventor, who contributed extensively to roentgenology, accepted the challenge. At the end of January 1896, Edison had begun experimenting with X-rays. On 14 February 1896, he was *'extremely skeptical'* about any success, attributing his skepticism in part to technical matters and in part to the *'insuperable obstacles'* imposed by the skull itself (according to Shepard 1974).

Would it be feasible to visualize the brain one day? The first radiographic examinations of the skull were performed on brain injuries to localize pieces of metal before surgery. Further progress occurred when skull fractures could be recognized, but this was only possible after skull radiographs had been analyzed in great detail and the confusing lines, shadows and orifices assigned anatomically. To overcome the intricate anatomy of the skull, it was necessary to learn how to take radiographs in standard projections that permit a differentiation of fracture lines from cranial sutures and of other pathological changes from normal structures.

Cushing, the founder of modern neurosurgery

On 6 November 1896 Harvey Cushing (1869–1939), the celebrated American neurosurgeon, took a radiograph of the cervical spine of a patient with Brown-Séquard-syndrome and later (1925) described the circumstances as follows:

'It was in that fall of 1896 that I went to Johns Hopkins and made the first roentgenograms that were taken there, with the aid of a decrepit and perverse static machine as big as a hurdy-gurdy and operated in the same way, by turning a crank. My first paper submitted for publication contained an account of a case of gunshot wound of the spine with plates showing a bullet which a Baltimorean had planted in the body of his wife's sixth cervical vertebra. I once showed these pictures to Dr. Cole and he expressed himself as astonished that such good plates of a spine could have been taken in 1896; but I do not know whether I told him, as I shall now confide to you, that the plates were the result of exposures averaging 35 minutes. And I may add that the pictures which were reproduced were not those of a single experience, for I think the patient was given as many as half a dozen sessions at least, before plates were secured which were sufficiently good for reproduction. Needless to say, she was a most cooperative patient.

Subsequently a Willyoung coil was purchased which I think had a spark gap of 2 or 3 inches. With this coil and the aid of many bottles of rodinol (I do not know whether rodinol is anything more than a memory for the few grey heads in this audience), I spent many weary hours for the next year or two in an improvised dark room off from the old amphitheatre at the Johns Hopkins Hospital developing roentgen-ray plates in which no one at the time took any very great interest. Certainly none of us could have had any possible conception of the increasingly important role the roentgen-ray was to play in clinical diagnosis and treatment!'

Schueller and the bony skull

The skeletal cranium could show secondary signs that allowed conclusions on the underlying pathology. Tumors of the hypophysis could lead to erosion and enlargement of the sella turcica, hydrocephalus through increased intracranial pressure to a thinning of the calvarium, and an acoustic neurinoma to a dilatation of the internal auditory canal.

The Viennese Arthur Schueller (1874–1957) (Fig. IV, 23) was an expert in this type of plain-film diagnosis. He was a close coworker of G. Holzknecht, who performed fundamental investigations in photographic techniques and interpretations, based on a close relationship with clinical studies, anatomy and pathology, and is considered as one of the founders, or at least pioneers, of neuroradiology. An exactly defined projection technique to visualize the mastoid processes – important to recognize its inflammation – was developed by Schueller and bears his name.

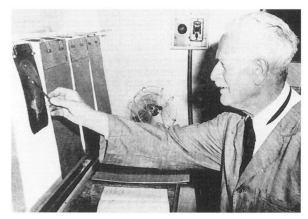

Fig. IV, 23. Arthur Schueller (1874-1957). Viennese radiologist, one of the fathers of neuroradiology. Interpretation of plain films. Emigration to Australia.

Air – a new era

Skull radiographs of patients with brain tumors sometimes showed a presumptive tumor density, although this was more often an accidental finding. In 1916, in a follow-up examination on 100 proven brain tumors, G. Heuer and W. Dandy (Fig. IV, 24) found radiographic skull changes in only six cases; they were related to changes in the skeleton and were therefore of secondary nature due to erosion or displacement. All things considered, this was a dismal result.

Walter Dandy (1886–1946) thought that the ventricles could provide important information when filled with an appropriate contrast medium, because brain tumors would change the ventricles either directly or indirectly, by displa-

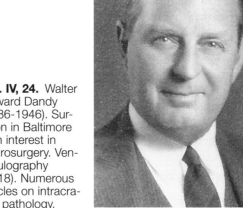

Fig. IV, 24. Walter Edward Dandy (1886-1946). Surgeon in Baltimore with interest in neurosurgery. Ventriculography (1918). Numerous articles on intracranial pathology.

cement, compression or infiltration. In his preliminary studies he filled the brain ventricles of a dog with a contrast medium.

To be used on humans, the substance should possess good radiographic properties, be neither irritant nor toxic, and in addition be easily absorbed and discharged. The early contrast media he used on his dogs, such as thorium, sodium, iodide, kollargol, and bismuth nitrate and subnitrate, always killed the animal.

A solution of the contrast medium problem finally came from a comment made by the celebrated American surgeon William Stewart Halsted (1852–1922) that visceral gas seemed to have the particular property to 'perforate' bones in the Roentgen image. Thus, in 1918, Dandy replaced the contents of a ventricle with air. Before closure of the fontanelles in infants, he punctured the ventricle via the bone defect; after the fontanelle was closed, he had to drill a small opening in the cranial vault to gain access to the ventricular system. His method, in which he introduced 40–300 ml gas, visualized the lateral ventricle in all patients and the fourth ventricle in two-thirds of the cases. Dandy's 'ventriculography' meant trauma to the brain, but was less invasive and at the same time less dangerous than an exploratory craniotomy (Fig. IV, 25).

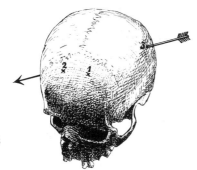

Fig. IV, 25. Puncture sites for ventriculography.
1, 2 = anterior horns
3 = posterior horn
(1926).

In his ventriculograms Dandy had observed that air accumulated on the brain surface, namely in the sulci. From this he concluded that the air must have followed the normal CSF circulation: Monro's foramen, third ventricle, fourth ventricle, aqueduct, Magendie's and Luschka's foramen, cisterna magnum, along the base of the skull, subarachnoid cavity, and sulci. The entire subarachnoid cavity appeared graphically outlined by air. The more completely the ventricles were filled with air, the faster and more detailed the subarachnoid space was visualized.

Based on these observations, Dandy arrived in 1919 at the concept of injecting air into the lumbar dural sac through a lumbar puncture. Indications for such an 'encephalography' were hydrocephalus, brain atrophy and obliteration of the subarachnoid cavity by a tumor. As air ascends, Dandy realized that the position of the body was important during the administration of 20–120 ml of air: the head had to be at least 20° higher than the puncture needle. Because air is absorbed more quickly in the subarachnoid cavity than in the ventricles it could not be traced radiographically after 24 h (Fig. IV, 26–30).

The German Adolf Bingel (1879–1963) developed, according to his statements independently from Dandy, 'encephalography by insufflation of air into the lumbar canal' (1921). Lumbar puncture was, of course, less traumatic than ventricular puncture and understandably prevailed. It is remarkable that Bingel introduced air with the patient in a sitting position, allowing it to enter

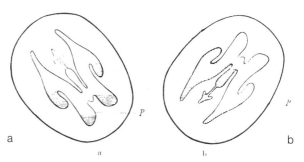

Fig. IV, 26a, b. Possible drainage routes of the ventricles. **a)** Puncture of the anterior horn in an oblique prone position. P = puncture site. **b)** Puncture of the posterior horn in an oblique supine position. P = puncture site (after Dandy, 1926).

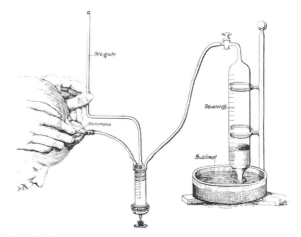

Fig. IV, 27. Device by O. Juengling to perform the ventriculography (1926).

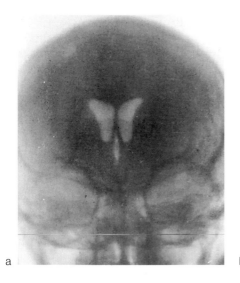

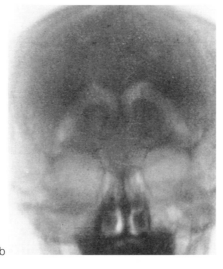

a

b

Fig. IV, 28a-c. Normal ventriculography. **a)** Sagittal projection in supine position. Butterfly shape. **b)** Tomogram in prone position, normal.

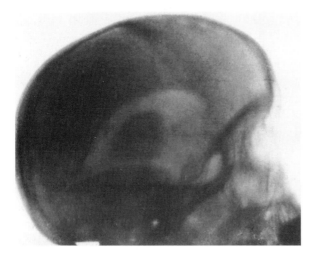

Fig. IV, 28. c) Lateral projection.

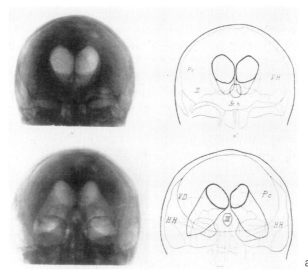

a

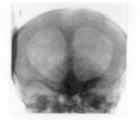

b

Fig. IV, 29a-c. Tomogram in supine position. Anterior horn is symmetrically enlarged. **a)** VH = anterior horn, P.c. = pars centralis, III = third ventricle, St.h. = frontal sinuses. **b)** Tomogram in prone position. Ventricle triangle and posterior horns are also enlarged (1926).

Fig. IV, 30. Lateral view of a considerably enlarged ventricle, somewhat retouched. Third ventricle (a) and foramen of Monro (b).

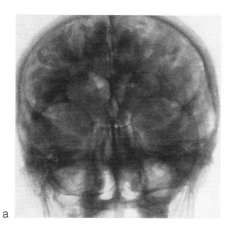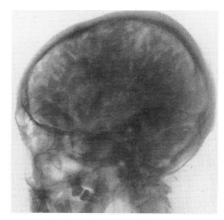

Fig. IV, 31a, b. Pneumo-encephalography and ventriculography. **a)** Sagittal view. **b)** Lateral view.

a

b

mainly the ventricular system. At the same time, he measured the CSF pressure, collected the fluid and introduced air simultaneously in small increments of 5–10 ml up to an amount of 40–60 ml. He also took radiographs during the insufflation of air. The technique was improved further by taking various projections with different distributions of air in the ventricular system, for which the patient sometimes had to assume the most awkward positions (Laruelle 1931, 1933).

In certain cases, such as an occlusion interfering with the filling of the ventricular system, both Bingel's encephalography and Dandy's ventriculography were used (Fig. IV, 31).

Ventriculography and pneumoencephalography marked the beginning of a new era in the surgical treatment of brain tumors and other surgical intracranial diseases. In many cases, it resulted in exclusion or a more precise localization of a lesion; previously more than 50% of brain tumors were impossible to localize, either by clinical examination or by explorative surgery.

Pneumoencephalography was performed differently in various countries, and the technique also differed between clinics as to the amount of air, the projection, and the number of photographs. It was a long time before standardization was realized as to the amount of air to be administered, the direction of projections, and the various positions of the patient. Since the air often had to be maneuvered into the part of the ventricle to be visualized, great efforts were demanded from patients and staff. Supine positions, prone positions, and turning the head of the patient were requested, and often survey views in a sitting position. A variation of the technique was the cisternal puncture or subatlanto-occipital puncture, practised in several clinics.

The examination was extremely unpleasant for the patients, being accompanied by headache,

nausea, hypotension, weakness and perspiration, which only subsided after 3 days. Moreover, the early death rate was high: Dandy had three of 100 patients and Bingel two of 200 patients who died after diagnostic pneumoencephalography. As this was an examination of relatively high risk, the patient had to be hospitalized. Indications and contraindications could only be formulated after considerable experience.

In the fifties and sixties, because air as a contrast medium often proved to be inadequate, Pantopaque, a contrast medium similar to Lipiodol was used by many radiologists for certain diagnostic questions, such as assessment of the third and fourth ventricle or suspicion of acoustic neurinoma. At the end of the examination, the contrast medium had to be maneuvered into the lumbar sack and removed to avoid inflammatory changes of the arachnoid membrane and adhesions in the ventricular system or lumbar sac.

Mechanical precision: Lysholm and Schoenander

In addition to the work of the Viennese Arthur Schueller and Ernst Georg Mayer (1893–1946), the plain film diagnosis of the skull was expanded by the Dutch neurologist Hendrik Willem Stenvers (1889–1973) (Fig. IV, 32). His numerous contributions included the fracture sites of the optic foramen, the inflammation of the frontal sinuses, and the petrous bone with its complex content (Fig. IV, 33) comprising labyrinth and neurovascular canals. A projection with its angulation given in degrees could visualize the petrous bone in such a way that its interior could be assessed and its apex scrutinized for possible erosion caused by a cerebellopontine tumors.

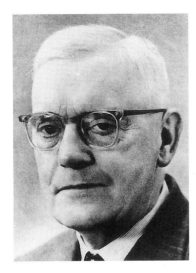

Fig. IV, 32. Henrik Willem Stenvers (1889-1973). Dutch neurologist (Utrecht). Based on experimental studies, he defined the projections of reproducible radiographic views of the petrous pyramid.

obtain the correct standard pictures but also enabling us to supplement these pictures by altering the projection and exposure, thus obtaining a roentgenological analysis of the findings, all according to the judgement of the roentgenologist. This is the art of roentgen examination and must be the outcome of an individual effort.'

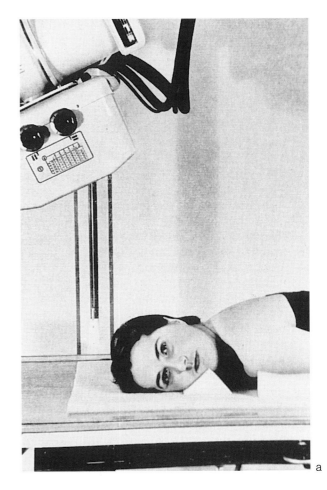

Following the protocol to obtain the exact position for these radiographic views demanded that the technologist, in addition to the physician, had a thorough anatomical and topographical knowledge of the cranial base. Special views of other parts of the skull also required very precise techniques to reproduce the appropriate position of the skull and direction of the central ray consistently.

Based on his experience with complicated and time-consuming projections, the Swedish neuroradiologist E. Lysholm (1892–1947) (Fig. IV, 34) stated in 1931: *'We need certain standard projections according to the clinical problem that can yield maximum information and can form the basis of examination. This is picture making and ought to be a mechanical procedure. We need an apparatus to easily*

a

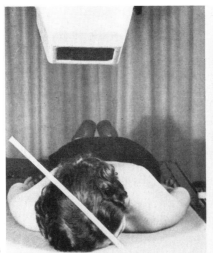

b

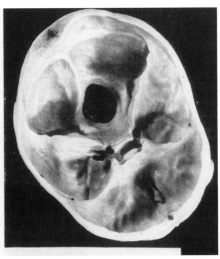

c

Fig. IV, 33a, b, c. Projection and adjustment for a tomogram of the petrous bone after Stenvers (1961).

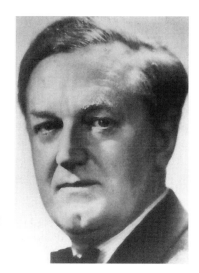

Fig. IV, 34. Eric Lysholm (1891-1947). Swedish neuroradiologist, who designed new devices that achieved exact and reproducible projections of certain parts of the skull.

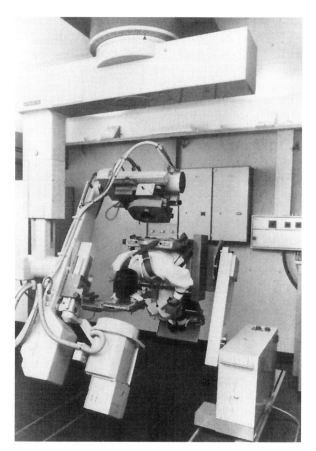

Fig. IV, 36. MIMER with a patient in a chair that can be swivelled 360 degrees.

Lysholm, together with the engineer Georg Schoenander (1894–1958), designed and built an apparatus with the basic feature of an X-ray tube that rotates along an arc around the patient's skull resting on the examination table, with its central ray always directed toward the arc's center. All movements of the X-ray tube could be followed by measuring the different angles of rotation (Figs. IV, 35–37). Lysholm's first apparatus also had built-in mirror so that the examiner could see the patient's chin. This apparatus became famous throughout the world, bore Lysholm's name, and was further refined.

A few projections were later combined with tomography to attain more detailed information. Ziedses des Plantes developed his planigraphy to improve neuroradiological imaging, as already mentioned.

Lysholm was not only interested in technical developments but also in clinical investigations.

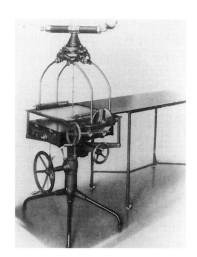

Fig. IV, 35. Early device for radiographic examinations of the skull after Lysholm.

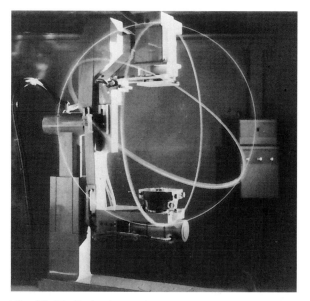

Fig. IV, 37. Projection options with the MIMER.

In monographs, he presented the changes found with various pathologies in ventriculograms (1937–1939). A special somersaulting chair, which was connected to a radiographic stand, was developed to direct small amounts of air into the desired places within the ventricular system. The chair, to which the patient was strapped, allowed a 360° rotation as well as forward and backward somersaulting. Under fluoroscopic guidance, the insufflation of air and its final intraventricular location could be controlled. Lysholm and Schoenander were unswervingly devoted to improve and, at the same time, to simplify this apparatus, which progressed from Mimer I to Mimer III, to be utilized not only for pneumoencephalography, but also for special projections of the skull and tomography. Equipment companies, including Philips and CGR, followed by developing special neurological units.

Lysholm, a coworker of Goesta Forssell, founded the famous and influential Swedish neuroradiological school in Stockholm, which produced men like T. Greitz, E. Lindgren, S. Cronquist, S. Radner, I. Wickbom and K. Lindblom.

New dimensions: visualization of vessels

In the twenties, Antonio Egas Moniz (1874–1955) (Fig. IV, 38) wondered why, despite the great advances in ventriculography, a correct diagnosis was only made in 124 of 392 cases; he also wondered whether it would be feasible to visualize the brain itself radiographically with a positive contrast medium. He considered the possibility of staining the brain by intravenous or parenteral administration of radiopaque substances, or even by injecting such substances intra-arterially. With the latter method or 'arterial encephalography', as called by Moniz in 1927, he was successful, but only after extensive animal experiments to test contrast and toxicity of various substances, such as lithium bromide, strontium bromide, Lipiodol, bromide and iodide salts. Eventually, he used a 25% sodium iodide solution.

For the injection, Moniz exposed the carotid artery and ligated it temporarily. In his first investigations, the vessels showed a very weak contrast. The search for stronger contrast media went on. Around 1931, he turned to the colloidal thorium dioxide, Thorotrast. But already in the early forties, liver cirrhosis and eventual malignant tumors were observed in patients after thorotrast injections because of the RES uptake of the radioactive thorium from the contrast medium. New contrast media such as Diodrast and Umbradil were synthesized, but these could provoke epileptic attacks, pareses and aphasia. Experimental studies showed damage to the blood-brain barrier from these contrast media. It was not until less toxic water-soluble iodide-containing contrast media became available that arteriography of the carotids became a relatively safe examination (Broman et al, 1948, 1950).

Angiography also demanded very exact positioning since pathologic processes had to be diagnosed from the course and calibre of the intracranial vessels, which often showed rather subtle changes secondary to space-occupying lesions. Since the cassettes were changed manually, repeat injections were often necessary to visualize the vessels for a complete image of the circulation and any pathology, particularly pertaining to the evaluation of the smaller vessels. In addition, it was always necessary to take biplane images since many changes could only be seen in one plane. Often a third or even fourth projection was needed to arrive at a definite conclusion. Later, the automatic film changer could take a series of radiographs within a preprogrammed interval of approximately 15–20 s, reducing the amount of injected contrast medium. Cerebral angiography as performed in a neuroradiologic center requires two X-ray tubes and two automatic film changers for simultaneous biplane imaging. By visualizing and assessing large and small vessels, arteriography was capable of detecting tumors, post-traumatic hemorrhages, vessel anomalies and intracerebral hemorrhages.

Since arteriography of the carotid artery often had to be carried out bilaterally, the patient was subjected to the tremendous suffering of two ar-

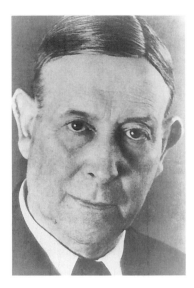

Fig. IV, 38. Antoio Egas Moniz (1874-1955). Neurologist in Lisbon since 1911. Cerebral arteriography for the diagnosis of tumors. Nobel prize awarded in 1949 for leukotomy and cerebral arteriography.

teriotomies. It was not until the introduction of the percutaneous puncture that the examination method was simplified (Figs. IV, 39 and 40). Local trauma to the carotid artery, however, was unavoidable. Through arteriography of the carotid arteries, the vessels of the cerebral hemispheres could now be visualized. From 1953, the vessels of the posterior cranial fossa, i.e. the cerebellum, had been investigated by injecting contrast med-

ium into the vertebral arteries (Takahashi 1940, Berczeller und Kugler 1937, Lindgren 1950). The necessary percutaneous puncture of the vertebral arteries required great experience. Several other methods were formulated later, among them the countercurrent angiography with injection of contrast medium under great pressure into the radial or brachial arteries against the arterial blood flow to achieve retrograde filling of the vessels of the head and neck (Gould et al, 1955).

Since the forties and fifties, carotid angiography had developed slowly but steadily. Eventually, the percutaneous transfemoral arteriography after Seldinger (1952) and the development of preformed catheters for catheterization of the neck vessels reduced the discomfort and complications for the patients (Fig. IV, 41)

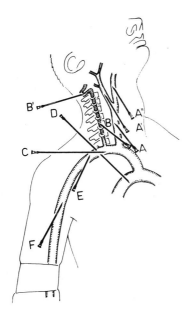

Fig. IV, 39. Percutaneous puncture methods.
A = via a. carotis communis
A' = a. carotis externa
A" = a. carotis interna
B = a. vertebralis
B' = a. vertebralis in the sulcus
C = a. subclavia
D = arcus aortae
E = a. axillaris
F = a. brachialis

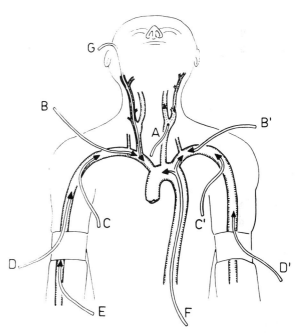

Fig. IV, 41. Methods of catheterization. A = via a. carotis communis (interna and externa), B = a. subclavia, C = a. axillaris, D = a. brachialis, E = a. radialis, F = a. femoralis, G = a. temporalis superficialis

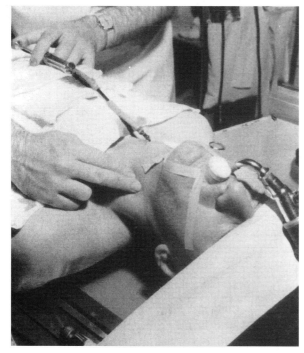

Fig. IV, 40. Carotid angiography. Patient under general anesthesia (1965).

Arteriography of the extra- and intracranial vessels developed into a relatively reliable radiographic method that produced results enabling vascular surgery of the vessels in the neck and in the intracerebral region. On the whole, diagnostic radiology had made much progress, thanks to the countless clinical studies that not only localized the pathology but often determined its nature as well (Figs. IV, 42 and 43).

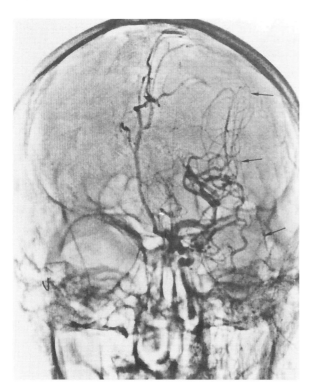

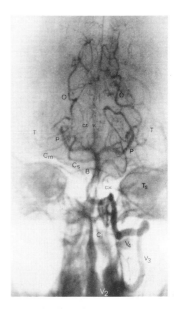

Fig. IV, 43a, b. Normal vertebral angiography. **a)** a.p., **b)** lateral.

Fig. IV, 42. Epidural hematoma in the middle cranial fossa. Biconvex avascular space (arrow). The anterior and middle cerebral arteries are deviated (H.O.M. Thijssen).

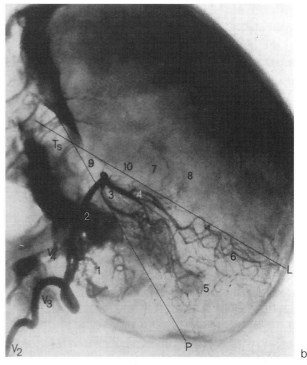

Seeing more by subtraction

In the arteriogram, vessels of the cranial base of the skull were often unidentifiable or difficult to assess in detail because of the encasing bony structure, particularly in the region of the petrous bone. In 1934–1935, the great Dutch neurologist and radiologist B.G. Ziedses des Plantes made this anatomically difficult area accessible with his brilliant concept of subtraction angiography. In this method, first carried out photographically, the difference between two radiographic images is enhanced when one photograph (= mask) is subtracted from another. If the second photograph is an arteriogram, then only the opacified vessels remain, while the bony skull is essentially erased by virtue of 'subtraction'. The success of this technique requires a radiograph, later inverted and used as a mask, taken immediately before the vessel is injected and no patient motion until the angiography is completed. With the introduction of electronic facilities in the eighties (Mistretta, Heintzen), the entire subtraction method can now be performed digitally and is better known as digital subtraction angiography.

Vertebral canal

Vertebral canal and spinal cord became targets of radiologic investigations at the same time as the brain. Myelographies with air were indeed carried out between 1919 and 1921, but the images were hardly if ever interpretable, a difficulty caused by the overlying vertebral column. It was not until two or three decades later with the development of tomography that air myelography was revived and that spinal cord and vertebral canal could be visualized without the interference from osseous structures. The Frenchmen J.A. Sicard (1872–1929) and J. Forrestier (1890–1978) introduced the contrast medium Lipiodol for myelography (Figs IV, 44 and 45). Because Lipiodol was slowly resorbed and could induce arachnoiditis, they initially tried to remove the contrast medium after the examination. Later, synthesized water-soluble iodine containing contrast media (e.g. Abrodil) were used. The patient was examined on a tilting table to achieve visualization of various sections of the spinal canal by gravitational migration. The method is still used for the diagnosis and the assessment of the extent of arteriovenous anomalies of the spinal cord. For selective visualization of the delicate spinal arteries correspondingly fine catheters with preformed tips were necessary.

Isotopes and ultrasound

In 1948, G.E. Moore showed that fluorescein accumulated in brain tumors. Subsequently, he synthesized the radioactive di-iodofluorescein and could localize tumors by gamma radiation. Radioactive isotopes led to a great progress in the diagnostic evaluation of the brain. Used as the first imaging method, brain scans could detect focal cerebral lesions, such as tumors, metastases or inflammations. The introduction of new compounds labeled with radioactive isotopes and the development of specialized imaging devices contributed to this advancement.

In neuroradiology of adults, ultrasound was of importance only in detecting midline displacements, but its results depended greatly on the quality of the examination and it was only used as screening test, particularly in head injuries. In newborns and small infants, however, ultrasound plays a great and still increasing role in neuroradiology.

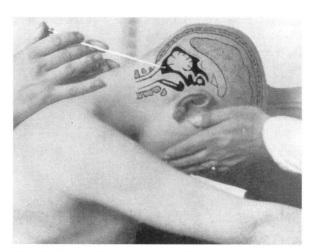

Fig. IV, 44. Position for suboccipital puncture.

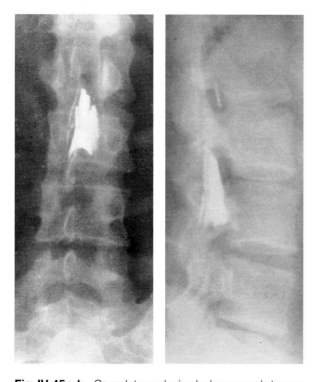

Fig. IV, 45a, b. Complete occlusion by large cauda tumor. Lymphangiocavernoma. **a)** a.p. projection, **b)** lateral projection.

New answer by G.N. Hounsfield to Hearst's request to Edison

In the early seventies, neuroradiology had, from a technical point of view, attained a high degree of perfection in myelography, pneumoencephalography and arteriography, often supplemented by tomography and subtraction. In the fifties and sixties, these methods had expanded the diagnostic range of neuroradiology, particularly in the USA, through contributions by, among others, J.M. Taveras, E.H. Wood, G. Di Chiro, S.K. Hilal, T.H. Newton, D.G. Potts, Mannie Schechter and Merril Sosman (first neuroradiologist in the USA). It had been particularly favorable that in the USA, as in Sweden, neuroradiology had always been part of radiology. Other names to be mentioned are Edward Wing Twining, J. Bull and G. du Bulay in the UK; L. Penning and B.G. Ziedses des Plantes, in The Netherlands; P.E. Chaussé, R. Djindjian, R. Thienpont, H.K.C. Fischgold and Wackenheim in France; H. Richter, H. Krayenbuehl and M.G. Yasargil in

Switzerland; J. Jirout in the Soviet Union; F. Thibaut, in Belgium; and S. Wende, K. Decker, E. Kazner, T. Riechert, W. Toennis and H. Vogelsang in Germany.

Neurosurgery developed considerable after the Second World War, including an increase in vascular surgery of the head and neck, accompanied by a growth of neuroradiology through mutually beneficial interaction between neurosurgery and neuroradiology. At the same time interventional radiology including stereotactic operations have increasingly gained in importance.

Investigations performed by the English engineer Godfrey N. Hounsfield (born 1919) and the English neurologist J. Ambrose in the early seventies led to a new dimension in neuroradiology when computed tomography (CT) made its triumphal entry. Since the discovery of X-rays, CT is the most important development, which has revolutionized diagnostic radiology and, especially, neuroradiology.

Thomas Alva Edison could now have said 'yes' to Hearst's request to take a 'cathodogram' of the brain.

References

Bennet, A.H., R.J. Godlee: Case of cerebral tumour. Lancet 2 (1884) 1090–1091

Berczeller, A., H. Kugler: Freilegung der Arteria vertebralis am Sulcus atlantis. Arch. Klin. Chir. 190 (1937) 810–815

Bingel A.: Zur Technik der intralumbalen Lufteinblasung insbesondere zum Zwecke der "Encephalographie". Med. Wschr. 47 (1921) 1492–1493

Broman, T., B. Forssman, O. Olsson: Further experimental investigations of injuries from contrast media in cerebral angiography. Acta Radiol. 34 (1950) 135–143

Broman, T., O. Olsson: The tolerance of cerebral bloodvessels to a contrast medium of the Diodrast group. Acta Radiol. 30 (1948) 326–342

Bull, J., H. Fischgold: A short history of neuroradiology. VIIIth Symposium Neuroradiologicum, Paris, 1967

Cushing, H.: Discussion. Am. J. Roentgenol. 13 (1925) 10–11

Dandy, W.E.: Ventriculography following the injection of air into the cerebral ventricles. Ann. Surg. 68 (1918) 4–11

Dandy, W.E.: Roentgenography of the brain after the injection of air into the spinal canal. Ann. Surg. 70 (1919) 397–403

Gould, P.L., W.T. Peyton, L.A. French: Vertebral angiography by retrograde injection of the brachial artery. J. Neurosurg. 12 (1955) 369–374

Hauge, T.: Catheter vertebral angiography. Acta Radiol. (1954) Suppl. 109

Laruelle, L.: Le repérage des ventricules cérébraux par un procédé de routine. Presse Méd. 39 (1931) 1888–1891

Laruelle, L.: Le repérage ventriculaire. Rev. Neurol. 40 (1933) 129–149

Lindgren, E.: Percutaneous angiography of the vertebral artery. Acta Radiol. 33 (1950) 389–404

Lysholm, E.: Apparatus and technique for roentgen examination of the skull. Acta Radiol. (1931) Suppl. 12

Lysholm, E., B. Ebenius, H. Sahlstedt: Das Ventrikulogramm, part I. Acta Radiol. (1935) Suppl. 24

Lysholm, E., B. Ebenius, K. Lindblom, H. Sahlstedt: Das Ventrikuologramm, part III. Acta Radiol. (1935) Suppl. 25

Lysholm, E., B. Ebenius, H. Sahlstedt: Das Ventrikulogramm, part II. Acta Radiol. (1937) Suppl. 26

Moniz, E.: L'encéphalographie artérielle, son importance dans la localisation des tumeurs cérébrales. Rev. Neurol. 2 (1927) 72–89

Moore, G.E.: The use of radioactive diiodofluorescein in the diagnosis and localization of brain tumors. Science 107 (1948) 569–571

Pfahler, G.E.: Cerebral skiagraphy. Trans. Amer. Roentgen Ray Soc. 9 (1905) 175–181

Schüller, A.: Die Schädelbasis im Röntgen-Bilde. Fortschr. Roentgenstr. Erg.band 11 (1905)

Schüller, A.: Röntgen-Diagnostik der Erkrankungen des Kopfes. Wien (1912) A. Hölder

Shepard, D.A.E.: Thomas Edison's attempts at radiography of the brain (1896). Mayo Clin. Proc. 49 (1974) 59–61

Sicard, J.A., J.E. Forestier: Méthode générale d'exploration radiologique par l'huile iodée (Lipiodol). Bull. Soc. Med. Hop. Paris 46 (1922) 463–469

Sicard, J.A., J.E. Forestier: L'huile iodée en clinique; applications therapeutiques et diagnostiques. Bull. Soc. Med. Hop. Paris 47 (1923) 309–314

Sjögren, S.E.: Percutaneous vertebral angiography. Acta Radiol. 40 (1953) 113–127

Sjöqvist, O.: Arteriographische Darstellung der Gefäße der hinteren Schädelgrube. Chirurg 10 (1938) 377–380

Stenvers, H.W.: Über die Bedeutung der Radiographie des Felsenbeins für die otologische Diagnostik. Arch. f. Ohren-, Nasen- und Kehlkopfheilkunde 103 (1919) 162–172

Stenvers, H.W.: Röntgenologie des Felsenbeins und des bitemporalen Schädelbildes. Julius Springer, Berlin 1928

Takahashi, K.: Die percutane Arteriographie der Arteria vertebralis und ihrer Versorgungsgebiete. Arch. Psychiat. 3 (1940) 373–379

Walker, A.E.: A history of neurological surgery. Hafner, New York 1967

Ziedses des Plantes, B.G.: Planigraphie en subtractie. Röntgenologische Differentiatiemethoden. Thesis, Utrecht 1934

Brain and spinal cord - with CT

H. Becker

Computed tomography (CT) caused a revolutionary change in neuroradiological investigations. Particularly in diseases of the nervous system, there was a need for even more information but also for less invasiveness. Since brain and spinal cord are surrounded by bone, they are far less accessible than other organs of the body.

CT was first used in neuroradiology. It strongly influenced digital processing and imaging, and led to the development of other digital imaging systems. Consequently neuroradiology was given a key position.

Major advances in the diagnostic evaluation with CT were first attained in the head. For the first time, the cerebral parenchyma could be visualized *in vivo*. Direct visualization of a hemorrhage, a cerebral infarct, or a brain tumor had become possible.

The first prototype of a computerized tomograph to investigate the brain was developed by the English engineer Hounsfield (Fig. IV, 16) [13] and was ready for use in September 1971. Because of the round shape of the head and the lack of any movements of its content, the brain seemed to be a particularly suitable organ. The apparatus was set-up at the Atkinson Morley Hospital, which was in the vicinity of Hounsfield's research laboratory near the EMI company. The hospital had a large neurosurgical and neurological department. Ambrose [1] worked there as neuroradiologist. The first patient examined on 4 October 1971 had a brain tumor in the left frontal lobe. Six months later at the Annual Congress of the British Institute of Radiology in London, the method of CT and the already available results of examinations performed on the prototype were presented for the first time. Ambrose had already used intravenous administration of contrast medium to enhance pathologic changes associated with an impaired blood–brain barrier and/or abnormal vessels on CT [7].

From then on, CT was rapidly accepted throughout the world. For example, the first CT scanner in Germany was installed in late June 1974 in the Department of Neuroradiology at the University of Frankfurt, Frankfurt/Main, where the author of this article was privileged to participate in its clinical use from the very beginning [10].

It soon became apparent that CT had an enormous impact on neuroradiology. It became the leading method in the topographical diagnosis of various cerebral diseases. Because it was the only technique for direct visualization of soft tissues, it gained paramount significance in diagnosing brain tumors. From the location of a space-occupying lesion, the measured CT densities, the contrast enhancement and the clinical findings, it was now possible to make a far more disease-specific diagnosis [15] – with the appropriate CT experience. There are, however, nonspecific findings defying a reliable classification; for instance, assigning ring-enhancing structures to a specific diagnosis can be difficult. Nevertheless, after surgery, radiotherapy or chemotherapy, CT has demonstrated its value in monitoring therapeutic effects and in recognizing any recurrence.

CT was the first imaging method that could narrow the differential diagnosis of a stroke. In CT, an acute cerebral hemorrhage is seen as an area of increased density in comparison with normal brain tissue, and an acute cerebral infarct, also in comparison with normal brain tissue, as decreased density. It must be kept in mind that the cerebral infarct becomes visible in its entirety only after 24 h, while the fresh hemorrhage immediately presents as hyperdensity in CT. In the 2nd and 3rd week after the acute insult, the infarct is temporarily isodense (fogging effect) and cannot be seen in the unenhanced CT, especially after disappearance of the mass effect due to the regression of the cerebral edema (Becker, 1979). At this time, the blood-barrier impairment is at its height, resulting in strong enhancement of contrast medium in the infarcted area.

CT is a simple and quick method of assessing the internal and external cerebrospinal fluid spaces. The various forms of hydrocephalus and the related abnormal circulation of cerebrospinal fluid can be visualized in detail. The acute occlusion hydrocephalus is recognizable by a periventricular hypodensity. The aqueduct stenosis shows a distinct discrepancy in the form of a dilated third ventricle and a normally configured fourth ventricle. The communicating normal pressure hydrocephalus is characterized by dilated ventricles and normal external subarachnoid spaces, but a definite exclusion of cerebral atrophy remains difficult, and the decision whether the cerebrospinal fluid should be drained by means of a shunt should be made only after epidural pressure measurements. Atrophy of the brain with loss of cortical and subcortical brain tissue may have many causes. The CT can be performed on outpatients and is well tolerated. In earlier times, a comparable examination result could only be accomplished by pneumoencephalography, which required hospitalization of the patient for a period of about 14 days, was painful and accompanied by symptoms, lasting several days, related to the vegetative nervous system.

Before the introduction of CT, only conventional radiographs could visualize intracranial calcifications. The presence of physiologic and pathologic calcifications was of great diagnostic relevance as a direct or indirect sign of a pathological process. Today, CT is the method of choice to visualize intracranial calcifications. As a result of its high-density resolution, CT can even demonstrate fine calcifications that are not recognizable in radiographs of the skull.

The simultaneous visualization of the surrounding soft tissue structures and subarachnoid spaces in CT allows an exact classification of the calcification. The calcification itself is seen as hyperdense structures, more striking than in conventional radiographic images and almost impossible to miss, and this feature is an additional diagnostic advantage in the early recognition of pathological calcifications in the course of a disease. This helps, for instance, to establish the diagnosis of tuberous sclerosis, which presents with characteristic subependymal calcifications. On the other hand, CT could find calcifications in pathological structures, such as metastases, where hardly, if ever, calcifications were found in earlier conventional radiographic studies. The physiologic calcifications demonstrated in CT are of little importance, although they are seen more frequently than in conventional radiographs. Since pathologic processes are direct visualized, their indirect signs have become less important. Thus, CT is now the essential imaging method to detect, record and classify intracranial calcifications and to determine their significance. Conventional radiography of the skull, formerly performed first in the routine diagnostic evaluation of every case with clinically suspected organic brain disease, has lost its former role as primary examination.

CT is especially suitable for trauma patients to assess the extent of any head injury. As a fast and reliable method, it has attained a paramount role in this field. CT provides information that could not be obtained with any other diagnostic modality in any comparable way. Within seconds, it is possible to visualize extracerebral or intracerebral blood and to separate it from cerebral contusion or edema. At the same time, displacement and compression of the ventricles and subarachnoid space can be recognized. Fractures including depressed fracture fragments as well as intracranial air and foreign bodies can also be visualized. The information provided by CT is only retrievable when the CT images are reviewed at different window settings.

While at the outset, CT was considered as the ideal method of visualizing soft-tissue structures, it soon became apparent that it was also particularly suitable for visualizing osseous structures in high-resolution edge-enhancing bone programs. Since the CT bone density can exceed 1000 Hounsfield units (HU), osseous structures should be reviewed using a wide window setting of the CT number range to encompass the entire range of bone densities. This technique can clearly visualize the calvarium as well as the cranial base. In the region of the calvarium, fractures with fragment displacements, particularly impression fractures, and bone tumors including calvarial metastases can be demonstrated [2]. The complex structures at the cranial base with its numerous foramina, osseous canals, sutures and air-filled spaces can also be visualized in detail.

CT has the advantage of representing a real tomographic method. Only anatomic structures in a specified layer are imaged, and is in contrast to conventional tomography, which suffers from disturbing densities representing blurred adjacent osseous structures. A further advantage is the reduced radiation exposure compared to conventional tomography [3]. As a result of technical developments in CT equipment, the spatial resolution has also been improved so that the most delicate osseous structures, such as the petrous bone, can be assessed in detail. Thus, it has become possible to visualize the auditory ossicles and the osseous labyrinth with cochlea and semicircular canals. CT made pluridirectional conventional tomography of the petrous bone superfluous [16]. High-resolution CT of the petrous bone can reveal dysplasias or obliterative ossification of the cochlea and has become very helpful in the preoperative evaluation for cochlear implantations that can be inserted to restore hearing for individuals with sensorineural deafness (Fig. IV, 46) [18]. The pneumatized spaces in the cranial base, often the sites of infections, are also well visualized by CT. Concerning the paranasal sinuses in particular, it had been shown that conventional paranasal sinus series cannot satisfactorily display the ethmoid air cells and the surgically important ethmoidal infundibulum. Direct coronal sections are used for CT of the paranasal sinuses and are displayed at a window width of 2000 HU, visualizing air, bones and soft tissue structures at extremely different CT densities. By using lower milliampere second settings, the administered radiation dose can be greatly reduced [19].

Conventional radiology only provides a limited diagnostic evaluation of the orbital region. The surrounding osseous structures can be visualized, but not the contents of the orbits. Only intraorbital radiopaque foreign bodies and calcifications could be visualized radiographically. It was customary for diagnostic evaluation to resort to special neuroradiological procedures, such as carotid angiography and orbitophlebography. CT has achieved detailed visualization of the intraorbital soft tissues. With a section thickness of 3 mm, the globe with its vitreous body and lens, optical nerve, extraocular muscles, retrobulbar fat pad, and major vessels can be imaged. The adjacent bones and the surrounding air-filled spaces are simultaneous visualized. The dose to the lens and the risk of radiation-induced cataract is considerably less than in conventional tomographic or angiographic methods. Tumors, arteriovenous malformations, cavernous hemangiomas, anomalies, hemorrhages, trauma, inflammation and endocrine ophthalmopathy can be diagnosed with CT. But establishing a definite diagnosis can be difficult on the basis of the CT images alone, even after administration of intravenous contrast medium. In addition to axial sections taken parallel to the course of the optic nerve, coronal sections are indicated, particularly for processes of the orbital floor or roof [9].

In addition to intravenous administration of contrast medium for disclosing an impaired blood-brain barrier and vascular malformations, efforts have been made to increase the diagnostic value of CT by outlining the subarachnoid space with contrast medium. Non-ionic water-soluble contrast media as well as air were used, primarily to improve the visualization of the basal cisterns. This technique became feasible with the introduction of high-resolution CT developed for bone imaging. With the intrathecal administration of contrast medium, it was possible to detect intracisternal causes of disorders of the cranial nerves. Furthermore, anomalies and malformations of the subarachnoid spaces could be better recognized, and arachnoid cysts directly visualized. Since the relationship between the intracisternal course of the cranial nerves and basilar vessels can be superbly delineated, the method could also be used for the evaluation of neurovascular compression syndromes [8].

For a detailed image of the cerebellopontine cistern, air cisternography was used because of the effective contrast provided by subarachnoid

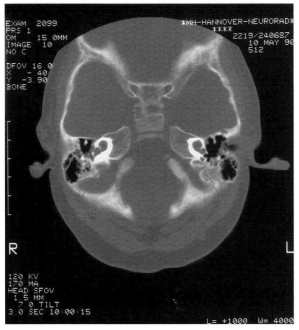

Fig. IV, 46. Bone CT: bilateral Mondini's malformation of the cochlea.

air surrounding cerebral and nervous structures, with a difference of 1000 HU. After lumbar puncture with intrathecal instillation of air, the patient was placed in such a position that the air accumulated in the cerebellopontine cistern. Under normal circumstances, the entire internal auditory canal is filled with air, outlining facial and vestibulocochlear nerves as well as the anterior inferior cerebellar artery, and often also the intracisternal segment of the trigeminal nerve. This method was primarily used to delineate intracanicular acoustic neurinomas. False-positive findings could be caused by arachnoid adhesions [17].

Great efforts were made to improve the scope of CT by developing the appropriate software that can reformat the measured data points into any plane for review. This led to the reconstruction of sagittal, coronal or oblique images from a series of axial tomographic sections [21], with the third dimension to be added mentally. Soon, software was developed for three-dimensional (3-D) reconstruction (Fig. IV, 47). The 3-D images are computed from contiguous or overlapping axial sections, typically of 3mm thickness. The number of tomograms required for 3-D reconstruction depends on the size of the object to be visualized. Often the routine axial CT sections are adequate. If a CT examination is specifically obtained for 3-D visualization, the radiation dose can be reduced (e.g. 60 mA instead of 510 mA). Within 5 min, a standard 3-D surface image is computed from the acquired data. The computation time depends on the number of tomographic sections to be reconstructed. This displayed standard surface image can then be rotated in increments of 1 degree around each spatial axis at the press of a button. A continuous rotation is also possible and enhances the illusion of three dimensionalty, which

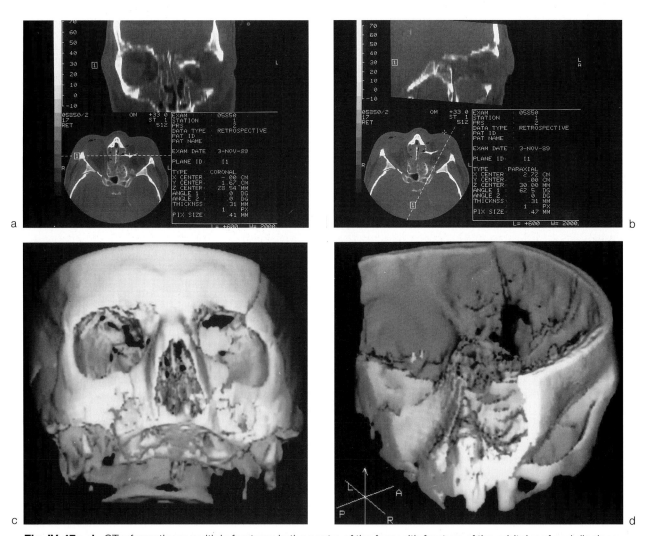

Fig. IV, 47a-d. CT reformations: multiple fractures in the centre of the face with fracture of the orbital roof and displacement of a bone fragment into the left orbit. **a)** Coronal 2D CT, **b)** Sagittal 2D CT, **c)** and **d)** 3D CT.

is further enhanced by displaying structures closer to the viewer brighter than those further away. This shading of the object surface can be manipulated.

The 3-D CT has been found to be very useful in the three-dimensional rendering of the skeleton. A representative axial CT section is selected to serve as reference for the region of interest. Only pixels that exceed a selected threshold value on the Hounsfield scale are used for the subsequent calculations performed on-line using the computer of the CT installation or on a separate workstation.

The three-dimensional rendering of soft tissues is more difficult, with the achievable three-dimensional visualization best for tumor tissues exhibiting strong contrast enhancement or containing calcifications. In the field of neuroradiology, three-dimensional CT has been successfully applied for the spatial representation of the complex osseous structures of the cranial base, facial bones, and spine. Three-dimensional visualization seldom provides new diagnostic insight since the clinically relevant information can usually be extracted from the conventional two-dimensional CT images. However, the topographic anatomy is better appreciated with 3-D CT, making it easier to communicate the diagnosis to the referring and treating physicians. In particular, surgeons have become very interested in using 3-D images when planning operations because of the afforded spatial view of the surgical site. Color coding can be used for better separation of different structures for the simultaneous visualization of bones and soft tissues. In addition to a 3-D image display, it is now possible to fabricate bone models from the CT data (Fig. IV, 48).

The introduction of CT has not only revolutionized diagnostic imaging, but has also influenced therapeutic modalities. In neurosurgery, stereotactic surgery has benefited from the precise image information now available. Surgical techniques have been modified to perform stereotactic operations under CT guidance, which is achieved by locating intracranial target points with excellent spatial accuracy and by transferring the registered target points of the CT coordinating system to the stereotaxic coordinating system. The CT-adapted stereotaxis has not only advanced surgical therapy but also interstitial radiotherapy of brain tumors with radioactive seeds [20]. Moreover, CT has also become essential in radiotherapy planning to calculate the exact isodoses of the radiation fields in relationship of the tumor volume [6].

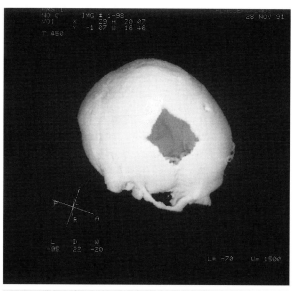

a

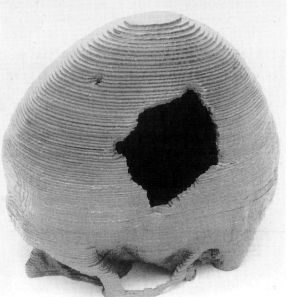

b

Fig. IV, 48a, b. 3D CT **(a)** and bone model **(b)**: status post trepanation of the right parietal calvarium. Tomogram before planned bone grafting.

A new dimension in CT was attained by the continuously increasing the speed of CT scanners, making it possible to obtain dynamic CT examinations. With this technique, serial CT-images can be obtained in the same tomographic plane immediately following bolus injection of contrast medium. By recording the inflow and outflow of the contrast medium, the perfusion of the brain vessels can be visualized and the cerebral blood volume computed [11].

The regional cerebral blood flow measurement with the stable xenon-enhanced CT follows the principle of a dynamic CT [12]. Using a gas-handling system and a supplied software, the cerebral blood flow can be measured and displayed at high spatial resolution. The patient inhales 33% stable xenon in oxygen through a breathing mask and two baseline scans are obtained at three standard levels, which have been selected from the digital topogram. Beginning after approximately 1 min of xenon-oxygen inhalation, an adequate saturation of arterial blood is reached, and four enhanced scans are obtained at each level over an interval of approximately 4 min. The density values are measured in HU at each level using standard regions of interest at each level and, using a dynamic scan program, the time-dependent xenon concentration is calculated. In addition, the end-expiratory xenon concentration, which is proportional to the xenon concentration in the arterial blood, is continuously registered. These values are used to compute a CT-analogue flow image of the cerebral section examined, referred to as flow map.

Film documentation is obtained at a fixed level of +50 HU and a fixed window of 100 HU. The grey tones of the CT image is transformed into a color scale corresponding to the natural color spectrum, from violet (0 ml/100g brain tissue/min) via green (50 ml) and red (75 ml) to white (100 ml and above). Moreover, in each selected region-of-interest, the regional circulation can also be expressed in ml/100g/min.

After determining the resting cerebrovascular blood flow, a second study was performed after intravenous injection of 1 g of acetazolamide to determine the cerebrovascular reserve capacity. This carbonic anhydrase inhibitor leads to acidosis, which causes dilatation of the cerebral vessels and an increase in the flow velocities of approximately 47% above the baseline levels. This acetazolamide-induced vasodilation can determine the hemodynamic relevance of vascular stenoses or occlusions. Assessing the cerebrovascular reserve is of particular importance for planning vascular bypass surgery in patients with cerebrovascular diseases. It is possible to differentiate between thromboembolic or hemodynamic causes of cerebrovascular diseases (Fig. IV, 49).

After establishing the technical foundations that enabled CT of the body, CT has assumed an important role in the evaluation of the spine, virtually making discography and phlebography superfluous and dramatically reducing the number of myelographies, particularly for the diagnosis of degenerative disk disease.

The spine is examined by means of the section-scan technique, i.e. the image reconstruction is

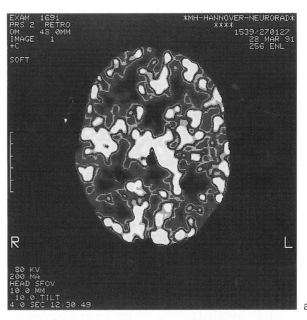

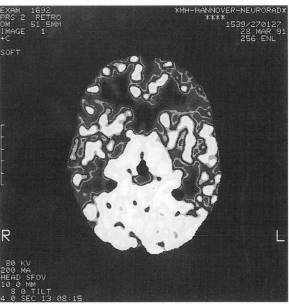

Fig. IV, 49a, b. Xenon CT: reduced cerebral reserve capacity in the supply area of the internal carotid arteries caused by occlusion of the left internal carotid artery and filiform stenosis of the right internal carotid. **a)** Cerebral blood flow at rest, **b)** after stimulation with acetazolamide.

confined to the region of the spine, which improves the image resolution. To improve the spatial resolution further, thin sections, for instance 3 mm in width, should be selected. For optimal presentation of the anatomical relationships and accurate measurements, the axial sections should be parallel to the disk space or vertebral end plates, to be achieved by angulating the gantry as deemed necessary from the lateral topogram. The axial sections are reviewed at different window settings on the monitor and density measurements are performed. Multiplanar reconstruction from the axial sections can be obtained in any orientation desired. By means of a edge-enhancement bone program, the osseous structures can be selectively displayed. A bolus injection of contrast medium is used to enhance tumors (neurinomas, meningiomas, metastases, angioblastomas) and vascular anomalies as well as to differentiation scar tissue from recurring disk herniation.

For a better assessment of the spinal cord, particularly in the thorax region, the intrathecal administration of water-soluble, non-ionic contrast medium is recommended and a CT-myelography is obtained. The increased density of the cerebrospinal fluid (CSF) clearly outlines the cord and the nerve roots in the CT image (Fig. IV, 50). It is particularly suitable to perform a CT-myelography immediately following a conventional myelography, often adding useful information. The CT-myelography should be performed after the lying patient was rotated several times to avoid layering of contrast medium in the subarachnoid space. For the CT-myelography of the lumbosacral region, the prone position is recommended, so that the contrast medium can accumulate along the anterior contour of the epidural space and in the anterior nerve root sleeves.

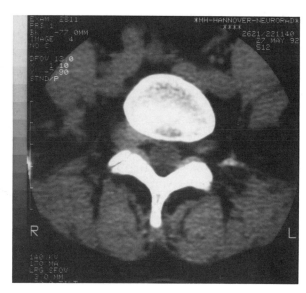

Fig. IV, 51. Spinal CT: herniated disk at L5/S1 with cranial extension and compression of the right L5 nerve root.

Spinal CT is largely used in the diagnosis of disk herniation. With CT, it was possible to visualize the intervertebral disk directly (Fig. IV, 51). Disk protrusion and herniation can be well visualized, and the relationship between herniated disk tissue and the nerve roots can be well delineated. Other degenerative changes, such as spondylotic osteophytes or spondylarthrotic changes and narrowing of the bony spinal canal, can also be assessed. In many cases, this eliminates invasive myelography, which usually requires hospitalization because of its known side effects.

CT is also used in spinal trauma. In general, CT follows after conventional radiographs have been obtained as screening examination. Any fractured region can be targeted for assessment by CT, which can determine the presence of a retropulsed bone fragment, a hemorrhage in the spinal space or a traumatic disk herniation. CT has the advantage of visualizing soft tissue structures as well as osseous structures, which, however, have to be reviewed at different window settings. Frequently, the extent of the injury revealed by CT is often more extensive than suspected from the conventional radiographs.

The simultaneous imaging of injuries to the paravertebral soft tissues and the possibility of imaging other regions of the body (abdomen, thorax, skull) at the same time without changing the position of patients with multiple injuries are additional advantages of CT.

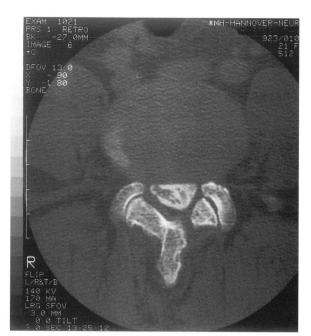

Fig. IV, 50. CT-Myelography: arachnopathy with adhesion of the nerve roots of the cauda equina. Postoperative changes following surgery for left herniated disk L4/L5 18 years ago.

Vertebral fractures, particularly those occurring in the cervical and thoracolumbar regions, frequently are at risk of having retropulsed vertebral fragments that could lead to compression or injury of the spinal cord. CT can very accurately locate fracture fragments in the vertebral canal and is clearly superior to conventional radiography. Spatial relationships can be even better visualized by using the data of the axial sections for the reformation of images in different planes. Moreover, 3-D CT was found particularly valuable in complex vertebral fractures. Three-dimensional CT can visualize the intraspinal fragment only when the 3-D reformation includes the spinal canal. Translation injuries with torsion and dislocation are particularly suitable for 3-D visualization because its intricate visualization of anatomical relationships (Fig. IV, 52). In addition to fractures, dislocations are also clearly visible. There is a direct relationship between the plane of the fracture and the plane selected for reformation. If the fracture is in the sagittal plane, a 3-D CT with rotation around the X axis is appropriate. If the fracture is in the coronary plane, it is sensible to take a 3-D CT around the X axis if only one vertebral body is to be examined. If several vertebral bodies and their interrelationship are to be evaluated, a rotation around the Z axis is indicated. For a fracture in the axial plane, 3-D CT has no advantage and a sagittal or coronary 2-D CT reformation will suffice [5].

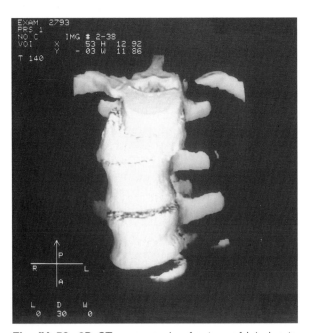

Fig. IV, 52. 3D CT: compression fracture of L1 due to translation and rotation trauma as well as burst fracture of L3.

A new CT technique is the spiral CT. It requires a CT scanner that can continuously rotate over a multitude of the usual 360° rotations. These scanners employ slip rings to transmit the high voltage from the generator to the X-ray tube and to transfer the measured data to the computer. With accurately controlled transportation of the patient table at a predetermined constant speed, the anatomic volume of interest is measured in a spiral scanning geometry. The table feed per 360° rotation typically is one axial section width, this means that in a 1-s scan for a 10-mm section thickness the recording speed is 10mm/s, whereby continuous data acquisition of up to 30 s has been possible so far. Motion artifacts that occur from direct reconstruction of data obtained from a spiral path are eliminated by linear interpolation of data points from the volume data set. With a special image reconstruction algorithm, planar CT tomograms are computed from the available raw data obtained in spiral geometry [14]. The high tube load during volume scanning is a limiting factor, and the method is primarily suitable for clinical tasks requiring a low radiation dose. The indications in the neuroradiological field are not yet established. The possible applications include, for example, trauma patients to shorten the examination time within the CT scanner and improved visualization of vascular malformations by taking advantage of the higher contrast enhancement achieved after bolus injection of contrast-medium bolus. In addition, the spiral volumetric data can be used for 3-D reconstructions.

Within the last few years, magnetic resonance imaging (MRI) has had an enormous impact on the spectrum of CT indications. The pathological findings are easier to recognize in the MR image as a result of the high signal difference between healthy and pathological structures. In many cases, MRI has proved to be more sensitive than CT. The diagnosis of brain tumors should primarily rest on MRI today. The detection of infarcts, particularly in the brainstem and cerebellum, is more successful and precise with MRI. This is also true for sinus thromboses, arteriovenous malformations, inflammation, degenerative brain diseases and congenital anomalies. Diseases in the region of the orbit can also be examined better and with more detail with MRI. Delayed symptoms after head injuries or after intracranial hemorrhage are now indications for MRI. Moreover, MRI has become the examination of choice for the diagnostic evaluation of the spine. With its increasing work capacity and the optimization of its image quality, MRI has more and more taken over the diagnosis of disk herniation.

Despite all these advantages of MRI, there are still diseases that need to be investigated by CT. For instance, the differential diagnosis of a cerebrovascular accident (CVA) is easier and faster with CT, which can determine whether the paralysis is caused by hemorrhage or infarct. The essential feature of an acute hemorrhage is its CT visualization shortly after the acute event. CT is also able to confirm the presence of fresh blood in the subarachnoid space and to suggest its site of origin. Preoperative angiography can be directed to the vessel most likely to be involved. CT remains the method of choice for acute head trauma. Its prompt diagnosis of traumatic intracranial hemorrhages enables rapid live saving interventions. CT is superior to MRI in visualizing osseous structures. With high-resolution edge-enhancing bone program, CT can clearly and accurately delineate traumatic bone changes. Functional examinations, such as required for detecting post-traumatic CSF fistulae, can be performed after intrathecal administration of a non-ionic water-soluble contrast medium, and are also an indication for CT. Postoperative follow-up studies in suspected complications should be carried out by CT because of its short examination time and its easy detectability of hemorrhages and abnormal CSF circulation.

CT remains the method of choice for the visualization of intracranial calcifications. Accurately demonstrated calcific structures can be an important component for a diagnostic classification. Thus, the indications for CT have changed under the influence of MRI during recent years. In neuroradiology, CT has increasingly become the primary modality for the diagnosis of acute conditions as well as for the visualization of osseous and calcific structures.

References

1. Ambrose, J.: Computerized transverse axial scanning (tomography). Part 2. Clinical application. Br. J. Radiol. 46 (1973) 1023–1047
2. Becker, H., D. Norman, P.D. Boyd, R.S. Hattner, T.H. Newton: Computed tomography in detecting calvarial metastases: a comparison with skull radiography and radionuclide scanning. Neuroradiology 16 (1978) 504–505
3. Becker, H., H. Grau, H. Hacker, K.W. Ploder: The base of the skull: a comparison of computed and conventional tomography. J. Comput. Assist. Tomogr. 2 (1978) 113–118
4. Becker, H.: CT fogging effect with ischemic cerebral infarcts. Neuroradiology 18 (1979) 185–192
5. Becker, H.: Neue Aspekte in der Wirbelsäulendiagnostik durch die dreidimensionale Darstellung im CT (3-D CT). Psycho 16 (1990) 219–224
6. Berninger, T. H. Becker, H. Gräfin Vitzthum: Computertomographische Verlaufsuntersuchungen bei Strahlentherapie von Hirntumoren. Strahlentherapie 160 (1984) 549–566
7. Bull, J.W.: The history of computed tomography. In: Contribution à l'hstoire de la neuroradiologie europienne. Ed. by E.A. Cabanis. Pradel Paris 1989
8. Galanski, M., G. Fahrendorf: Hochauflösende Kontrast-CT-Zisternographie. Quo Vadis CT. Hrsg., C. Claussen, R. Felix. Springer Berlin 1988
9. Gonzalez, C.F., M.H. Becker, J.C. Flanagan: Diagnostic imaging in ophthalmology. Springer New York 1986
10. Hacker, H., H. Becker: Die klinische Erprobung des Siretom.
Electromedica 43 (1975) 56–61
11. Hacker, H., H. Becker: Time controlled computed tomographic angiography. J. Comput. Assist. Tomogr. 1 (1977) 405–409
12. Haubitz, B., H. Becker, K. Holl, N.M. Nemati: Regionale Hirndurchblutungsmessung mit der Stable-Xenon-Computertomographie. TW Neurologie Psychiatrie 5 (1991) 299–313
13. Hounsfield, G.N.: Computerized transverse axial scanning (tomography). Part 1. Description of system. Br. J. Radiol. 46 (1973) 1016–1022
14. Kalender, W., W. Seissler, E. Klotz, P. Vock: Spiralvolumetric CT with single-breathhold technique, continuous transport and continuous scanner rotation. Radiology 176 (1990) 181–183
15. Kazerner, E., S. Wende, Th. Grumme, O. Stochdordh, R. Felix, C. Claussen: Computer- und Kernspintomographie intrakranieller Tumoren aus klinischer Sicht. Springer Berlin 1988
16. Köster, U.: Computertomographie des Felsenbeins. Thieme Stuttgart 1988
17. Kricheff, J.J., R.T. Pinto, R.T. Bergeron, N. Cohen: Air CT-cisternography and canalography for small acoustic neuromas. Am. J. Neuroradiol. 1 (1980) 57–63
18. Laszig, R., R.D. Battmer, H. Becker: Hochauflösende Computertomographie als ergänzende Voruntersuchung zum Cochlear Implant. HNO 34 (1986) 429–433
19. Marmolya, A., E.J. Wiesen, R. Yagan, C.D. Haria, A.C. Shah: Paranasal sinuses: low-dose CT. Radiology 181 (1991) 689–691
20. Mundinger, F., W. Birg: CT-stereotaxy in the clinical routine. Neurosurg. Rev. 7 (1984) 219–224
21. Unsöld, R., C.B. Ostertag, J. de Groot, T.H. Newton: Computerreformations of the brain and skull base. Springer Berlin 1982

Torso

P.E. Peters

'Your treating physician suspects that you have a disease of the suprarenal glands, we therefore need a special roentgenologic examination to assess the size and shape of your suprarenal glands. The examination is slightly uncomfortable but not dangerous. I would like to explain its procedure to you.

Today, we will give you a laxative, because the intestines must be absolutely clean. Tomorrow you cannot have breakfast. We will then ask you to take the knee-elbow position as when children crawl, do you understand? Then I will inject a local anesthesia near the os coccygis and subsequently I will introduce a thicker needle between the rectum and sacrum. I will introduce the needle and place the index of my left hand into the rectum in such a way that I am certain that I will not damage the rectum.

As soon as the needle is in the correct position, we will pass 800–1200 ml pure oxygen from an oxygen cylinder through the needle. The gas distributes around the adrenal glands so that they are outlined in the radiograph. You will only notice a somewhat numb pressure, you need not feel more – except for the puncture, of course. This method is called pneumoretroperitoneum.

The method just described was performed by an American roentgenologist for the first time in 1947 and had been adopted throughout the world [1]. We ourselves have performed some 500 of such examinations without serious complications. So you do not have to worry . . .'

Thus, or similarly, were patients prepared for a radiographic examination of the adrenal glands in the early seventies. It did not mean you did not have to worry afterwards, but there was no alternative.

The diagnostic evaluation of the adrenal glands and other regions have dramatically changed after Hounsfield and Cormack developed computed tomography: many distressing, unpleasant, stress causing procedures could completely be replaced by painless imaging [2, 3]. The diagnostic certitude increased and new options arose in diagnosis and therapy. The two developers were awarded the Nobel Prize for Medicine in 1979 for their pioneering innovation in medical imaging.

In the following contribution, the revolutionary progress of computed tomography of the torso will be illustrated by typical examples. Such a demonstration must be fragmentary because of the considerable diagnostic spectrum. Current textbooks on computed tomography comprise a thousand or more pages [4]. To illustrate this progress, I will refer to radiological methods that have partly or completely been replaced by computed tomography, as, for instance, the aforementioned pneumoretroperitoneum.

Thorax

The radiographic examination of the chest is the most frequent and best known examination in medical imaging. Lungs, heart, mediastinum, major vessels and bony thorax including thoracic spine are visualized by plain radiographs. The density of the air-containing lungs is so different form the density of the heart and mediastinum as well as from the density of the ribs that almost optimal imaging conditions are met for plain film radiography.

The fundamentals of the diagnosis of chest diseases are essentially unchanged since the discovery of X-rays, except for improvements of the X-ray tubes (smaller focal spots), better films and intensifying screens (less radiation exposure, better image quality) and the change from the positive (black on white) image of our ancestors for the more favorable negative (white on black) image.

The cardinal problem of projection radiology has remained: the superposition of normal and pathological structures. By obtaining an additional exposure in a second plane and by applying the rules of image analysis, we succeeded in assigning the pathologic finding an approximate location within the chest, but this was by no means accurate. This uncertainty led to the development of tomography [5], now referred to as conventional tomography to be distinguished from computed tomography (see contribution by Stieve).

The spatial assignment of pathological and normal structures in the conventional tomogram of the lungs is remarkably successful due to the high contrast between the aerated lungs and pathologic densities. These favorable conditions apply even more for computed tomographic imaging, which has a far higher intrinsic contrast resolution than conventional tomography. In addition, computed tomography adds the third plane – the transverse section – to the diagnosis of the chest and, by means of the window technique, allows the assessment of the air-containing lungs, mediastinal structures and bony thorax from the same set of data. Furthermore, multiplanar reconstructions of high quality can be obtained with the modern volume-scanning technique.

Already with conventional radiographic techniques, it was tried to disclose the third plane by means of transverse tomography through the body. The comparison between such a transverse tomogram dating from 1959 and the modern computed tomogram clearly reveals the diagnostic quantum leap instated by computed tomography (CT) [6] (Fig. IV, 53a,b).

The diagnostic gain through CT in comparison to conventional radiography, including conventional tomography, can generally be divided into three categories:

In category 1, structures and lesions not visualized with conventional techniques are made visible by CT. The diagnostic advantage is rather impressive.

In category 2, normal and pathological structures are visualized better with CT than with the conventional radiographic methods. Most examples encountered in diagnostic imaging of the chest fall into this category. Here the benefit is not so much in the detection of diseases but in the treatment planning (surgery, radiation) and posttherapy follow-up.

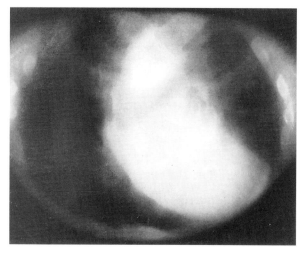

Fig. IV, 53a. Transverse tomogram of 1959 [6]. According to the caption, bronchiectasis on the left.

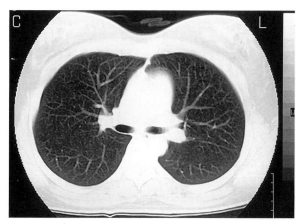

Fig. IV, 53b. Cross-section CT directly below the carina. Displayed at pulmonary window. Normal finding.

In category 3, anatomical and pathological structures are only imaged differently than with conventional radiographic methods. Fortunately, this situation is hardly ever encountered in CT of the chest. Without diagnostic and/or therapeutic benefit, CT should not be used because of its higher radiation dose in comparison with conventional radiographic techniques. Judgement should therefore be exercised when ordering a CT examination. Practicing the ALARA principle ('as low as reasonably achievable'), the choice of imaging method is always determined by the outcome of an analysis of benefit versus risk. CT examinations are not indicated for clinical questions that fall into the third category.

Lungs

Conventional radiology can visualize the air-containing lungs rather well. Pathological changes, such as infiltrations, nodules and atelectasis, are seen as easily identifiable densities. Physicians of all disciplines are comfortable reviewing conventional chest radiographs and are conversant with the interpretation of such images. Even laypersons are familiar with chest films, often from their own experience. Whenever a medical ambience is to be conjured in the movies or on television, chest films are in the hands of the main character or on the view box in the background. While the urinary glass was the characteristic feature of physicians in the Middle Ages, the radiograph (usually of the lungs) is their symbol today. In relation to the conventional radiographs of the chest, CT of the chest is less known and not as popular.

The one projection obtained as part of the conventional radiographic examination of the chest is in contrast to the approximate 30–40 sections comprising the CT examination of the chest, usually displayed at two different window settings and adding up to 60–80 images for review. The cross-section anatomy of CT is extremely accurate but its interpretation needs thorough practice.

Radiologists have learned to reconstruct a complete mental image from many 1-cm slices, a task fraught with difficulties for clinicians not trained in image interpretation. The modern spiral CT scanner offers the possibility of three-dimensional reconstruction relegating processes previously performed inside the observer's head to the computer. Particularly fascinating is the dynamic analysis of a series of tomograms in cine mode, creating the impression of traveling with a movie camera through the thoracic cavity. Spatial assignment of pathological processes to anatomical structures has obviously been facilitated by such a dynamic analysis.

Imaging of the chest should still begin with the conventional radiograph. Despite the mentioned favorable imaging conditions for conventional radiography, including conventional tomography, there are findings demonstrated by CT that are completely absent in radiographs of the conventional technique (category 1). Small pulmonary metastases and early opportunistic infections are two examples to be mentioned.

Small pulmonary metastases

The importance of detecting pulmonary metastases in oncologic patients is obvious. Depending on the initial disease, the demonstration of pulmonary metastases may have various therapeutic consequences:
– initiation of chemotherapy
– referral for surgical resection
– termination or modification of chemotherapy
– cessation of curative therapy of the primary tumor.

In view of this clinical background, the CT examination is indicated when the conventional chest radiographs are normal and when presence or absence of pulmonary metastases determines the course of further treatment. Pulmonary metastases are frequently located subpleurally and can be hidden, in the conventional chest radiograph, by the superimposed structures of the bony thorax (Fig. IV, 54). Metastases adjacent to vessels, another common site for pulmonary metastases, cannot be differentiated from vascular structures on conventional radiographs.

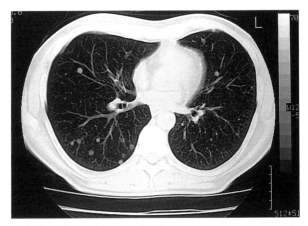

Fig. IV, 54. Multiple small pulmonary metastases, partly subpleural, partly perivascular. Cross-section CT through the hilar region.

As a rule of thumb, it can be stated that in conventional radiology, including tomography, nodular densities can only be reliably recognized if they exceed 15 mm in diameter [7]. In CT, in contrast, pulmonary nodules can be detected with certainty with a diameter of 3 mm onward. Furthermore, CT has proven to discover more nodular lesions in addition to already known pulmonary metastases [8, 9].

With respect to establishing the nature of pulmonary nodules, CT, by means of density measurements and demonstration of calcium, is somewhat more reliable than conventional radiography, but in many instances, a diagnosis cannot be reached and surgical resection of the lesion in question or a CT-guided biopsy are required to obtain a histological diagnosis.

Opportunistic pulmonary infections

Within the scope of an aggressive chemotherapy or after transplantation with immunosuppressive therapy, the patients often develop high fever without a detectable cause on conventional chest radiographs. We could show in a clinical study that unremarkable findings on a technically adequate conventional chest radiograph on the day of the CT examination does not exclude an early pulmonary infection. The initially very small lesions of a pulmonary mycosis found adjacent to vessels are of particular concern [10]. An early diagnosis of these processes is clinically relevant, since it leads to a targeted bronchoalveolar lavage (BAL) for early demonstration of pathogenic organisms and timely initiation of the appropriate therapy (Fig. IV, 55a,b).

Staging and therapy planning

The majority of CT examinations of the chest belong to category 2, performed to improve the definition of a lesion already seen on conventional radiographs. An example would be a large pulmonary nodule detected on a plain chest radiograph. Within certain limits, the CT analysis might determine its nature. The presence of calcium in a certain arrangement probably indicates a benign lesion (e.g. status post tuberculosis), while irregular and spiculated margins are considered to be a sign of malignancy. The literature has extensively contributed to this problem in which the boundaries of such an assessment are discussed [11]. This example should only illustrate how density measurements and form analysis of CT findings can contribute to the choice of therapy (Fig. IV, 56).

Bronchiectases were diagnosed by bronchography prior to the CT era. The instillation of an oily or water-soluble contrast medium via bronchial catheters or via a flexible fiberoptic bronchoscope indeed affords beautiful images, but it is associated with potential hazards and elicits cough attacks, making it a rather unpleasant

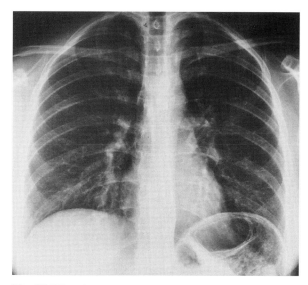

Fig. IV, 55a. Acute myelocytic leukemia. Fever in aplasia. Conventional chest tomogram without pathologic findings.

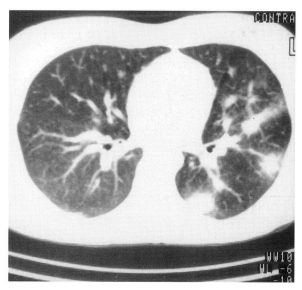

Fig. IV, 55b. Thorax CT taken the same day. Mostly left basal multiple, ill-defined peripheral infiltrates. Aspergillosis diagnosed by bronchoalveolar lavage (BAL).

radiographic examination. The painless and quick CT examination of the affected pulmonary region shows the dilatated bronchi and thickened bronchial walls clearly by using high-resolution technique (HRCT) (Fig. IV, 57).

This category also includes examinations performed for staging bronchogenic carcinomas and other malignant tumors. CT can also demonstrate anomalies of the pulmonary vessels after bolus injection of intravenous contrast-medium, noninvasively without angiography.

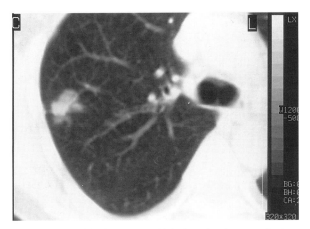

Fig. IV, 56. Well-demarcated lobulated pulmonary lesion, approximately two cm in diameter and of heterogeneous density, with discrete pleural reaction. Not seen in earlier chest radiographs. A 60-year-old female patient without risk factors. CT diagnosis: suspected peripheral bronchial carcinoma. Histologic diagnosis: tuberculoma.

The list of pulmonary conditions that are better visualized by CT than by conventional radiography can be lengthened at will. Diffuse parenchymal diseases, inhalation damage, occupational diseases such as pneumoconioses, emphysema, trauma and postsurgical changes are all included in the list. All conditions mentioned here are generally suspected on the basis of history, clinical examination and plain radiographs and are referred for further investigation by means of the noninvasive CT. Exact morphologic imaging and topographic assignment is essential for any therapy planning, either by surgery or radiotherapy.

Pleura

Pleural fluid is a frequently encountered finding in conventional radiography and usually can be further evaluated by conventional means, possibly supplemented by an ultrasound examination. A CT examination is indicated when the cause of the pleural effusion is unknown. Conventional radiographic techniques cannot differentiate pleural empyema from a subpleural lung abscess. Other diseases of the pleura, such as mesotheliomas and metastatic tumors, often present first through the associated pleural effusion and can only be localized and differentiated from peripheral pulmonary lesions by means of CT.

CT plays a special role in patients with documented or suspected asbestos exposure. The asbestos-induced discrete fibrous lesions along the

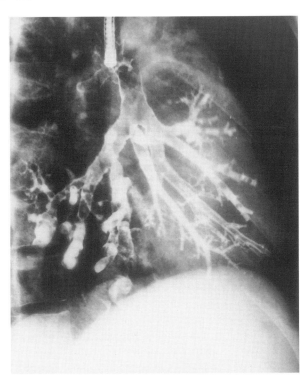

Fig. IV, 57a. Bronchography through a flexible fiberoptic bronchoscope: saccular bronchiectases.

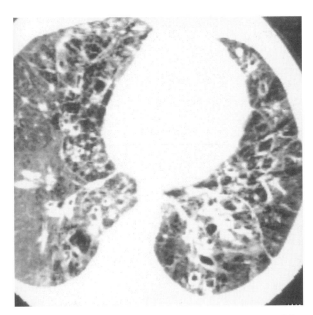

Fig. IV, 57b. Bronchiectases in the CT. Thickening of the bronchial walls. Dilatation of the bronchi. Increased interstitial septation.

parietal pleura (pleural plaques), often partially calcified, are extremely well identified on CT, whereby the transverse sections are clearly superior in detecting plaques along the mediastinum and in the paravertebral region. In the majority of cases, the morphologic findings are confined to the pleura. Asbestos-related pulmonary changes ('asbestosis') can be assessed by reviewing the images at levels suitable for visualizing the lung parenchyma. CT of the chest is of great importance in the classification of this occupational disease and in the early diagnosis of asbestos-induced malignant mesotheliomas [12].

In general, a pneumothorax is reliably diagnosed on conventional plain radiographs. Critically ill patients, who are frequently post-traumatic or postsurgical, can only have their radiographs taken supine in AP projection. In addition, these patients often have indwelling tubes and drains and are covered with surgical dressings. In these situations, localized air accumulations along the anterior pleural space can easily be overlooked, and any CT examination performed on these patients should be scrutinized for an occult pneumothorax. Furthermore, intensive-care patients, who show inadequate improvement while on artificial respiration, should undergo CT early to discover pneumothorax, atelectases and/or early signs of acute respiratory dyspnea syndromes (ARDS) [13, 14] (Fig. IV, 58).

film-screen systems and mediastinal filters can make the cardiac silhouette more transparent, we still have to rely on secondary signs, such as displaced mediastinal lines, to diagnose a pathological process in this region. Conventional tomography is suitable for visualizing the bronchial system without superimposed structures. Opacification of the esophagus and the major mediastinal vessels can reveal indirect signs of a mass in the mediastinum.

Various methods of air insufflation ('pneumomediastinum') have been advocated to differentiate the relevant mediastinal structures radiographically. Using the cervical approach, a pneumothorax needle is introduced laterally into the neck at the level of C4/C5 and directed into the paravertebral space [16]. After aspiration (to exclude a vascular puncture) 400–1000 ml oxygen or carbon dioxide is insufflated, with the neck compressed so that the gas will flow downward into the mediastinum. Other authors recommend a retroxiphoidal instillation [17] as well as transsternal and parasternal techniques [18] or paravertebral punctures [19]. Suprasternal techniques with special needles have also been

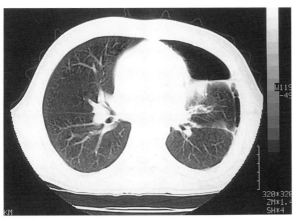

Fig. IV, 58. Compartmentalized left anterior pneumothorax. Status post thoracotomy.

Mediastinum

'With a dorsoventral X-ray beam, the roentgen image shows the normal mediastinum as homogeneous shadow, which is only transparent in the superior region, the so-called vascular band, while the shadow of the heart remains opaque.' [15].

This statement from a textbook published in 1963 also applies to conventional radiology today. Though high-kV technique, appropriate

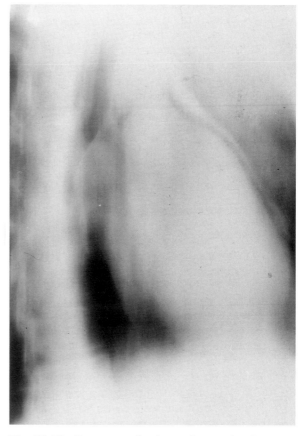

Fig. IV, 59. Pneumomediastinum. Conventional sagittal tomography. Small anterior thymic remnant.

mentioned (Fig. IV, 59). All pneumomediastinal methods have in common that they are invasive, have limited diagnostic value and carry a high risk. It is therefore not surprising that this technique has now been abandoned completely as a result of the current availability of CT. It is now part of medical history as so many other methods that were once useful for both patients and physicians.

The increase in diagnostic information obtained from CT is quite revolutionary, even from the standpoint of a critical analysis from a scientific historian. For the first time, the complex structures of the intrathoracic spaces could be observed directly and not indirectly as signs displayed by neighboring organs. For today's physician, this has become the daily routine of practicing medicine and I will restrict myself to a few examples to illustrate the diagnostic gain.

Mediastinal masses

The first indication of a mediastinal space-occupying process is broadening of the mediastinum seen in plain radiographs. CT can discover the anatomic structure from which the space-occupying process has developed. Though CT will not make a histologic diagnosis, the nature of a pathological space-occupying process can be deduced with some accuracy from its shape and localization. In cases of lipomatosis, CT can establish the diagnosis from morphological and density measurements and spare the patients further examinations.

The diagnosis of lymphadenopathy is as problematic in the mediastinum as it is in other regions of the body. The size of the lymph node is the only criterion used as evidence of a pathologic finding. Currently, it is impossible to distinguish nodal metastasis from lymphadenitis. The metastatic involvement of normal-sized lymph nodes also escapes computed tomographic detection since the internal structure of the lymph node cannot be resolved with presently available techniques. In a randomized prospective study of 155 patients with a non-small cell bronchogenic carcinoma, conventional radiography discovered only 9% of the histologically confirmed nodal metastases in the mediastinum, but CT was found to have a sensitivity of 52%. Though considerably better than conventional radiography, CT is also hampered by the fact that it does not recognize mediastinal nodal metastases in nearly every other patient [20].

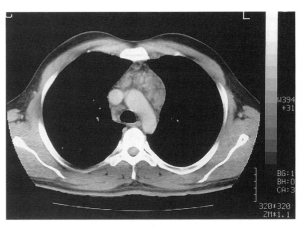

Fig. IV, 60. M. Hodgkin. Multiple enlarged lymph nodes in the anterior mediastinum and right paratracheal region. Contrast enhanced chest CT.

The accuracy is significantly higher in lymphomas because of more extensive nodal enlargements (Fig. IV, 60).

Tumors of the thymus or thymic hyperplasia already appear as a mass in the fatty tissue of the anterior mediastinum if the diameter of the thymus exceeds 1 cm. Statistically, 10–15% of these 'thymomas' are malignant, but there are no reliable CT criteria to characterize this group. The evidence of an infiltrative growth in the surrounding tissues is the only reliable finding of a thymus carcinoma.

The computed tomogram can easily recognize mediastinal cysts due to their configuration and water content.

Vascular processes

The arterial and venous vessels of the mediastinum can be visualized after intravenous administration of contrast medium. The main vessel is the thoracic aorta and its branches. The uncomplicated dilatation on the basis of arteriosclerosis is characterized by an increase of its lumen up to 4 cm, numerous mural calcifications, and a tortuous, elongated course. The true thoracic aortic aneurysm, generally also on the basis of arteriosclerosis, measures 5–10 cm in diameter or even more. The risk of a rupture correlates with the diameter: an aneurysmal diameter between 5 and 10 cm is given a 10% risk, which increases to 50% if the diameter exceeds 10 cm [21].

The dissected aortic aneurysm can be reliably diagnosed with modern fast CT scanners or with spiral CT scanners.

The therapy is determined by the site of the dissection. Type B of the aortic dissection involves the descending aorta, begins distal from the origin of the left subclavian artery, and has a more favorable prognosis. Type A involves the ascending aorta and may affect the origins of the coronaries and brachiocephalic vessels. CT examination aims at identifying the entry point and, if possible, at assessing the dissection up to the re-entry point. In a few cases, thoracic angiography might be necessary for the exact determination of the extent of the dissection, but the primary diagnosis rests on the contrast-enhanced computer tomography (Fig. IV, 61).

Fig. IV, 61a-d. Dissecting aorta aneurysm, type B. Spiral CT with automatic contrast-medium injection.

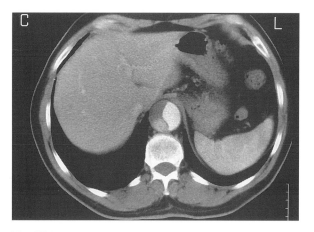

Fig. IV, 61b. Difference in flow in the true and false lumen below the level of the diaphragm. Partial thrombus formation.

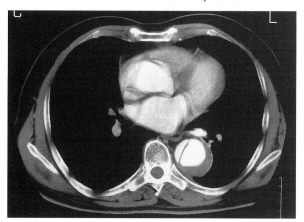

Fig. IV, 61a. Descending aorta. Dissection membrane clearly outlined. Good blood flow in both lumina. Mural thrombus laterally and dorsally.

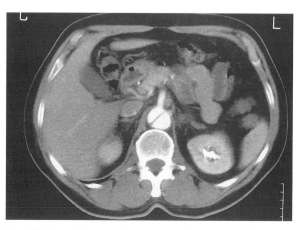

Fig. IV, 61c. The superior mesenteric artery originates at the apparent true lumen.

In young patients, traumatic pseudoaneurysms are the most commonly encountered of thoracic aneurysms. They are almost exclusively caused by blunt chest trauma (deceleration trauma). The tear usually involves the aorta in the region of the isthmus. The changes can be extremely discrete and should be primarily evaluated by angiography. The chronic pseudoaneurysms that might develop from an aortic tear can be an incidental finding in CT.

Heart

CT can assess the heart and its cavities just as detailed as the major mediastinal vessels. Because of cardiac motions, short scan times or ECG-triggered scanning is necessary. Apart from research

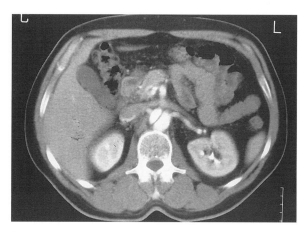

Fig. IV, 61d. The right and left kidney arteries are supplied by different lumina.

projects, there are relatively few indications for CT of the heart. In part, this is the result of the excellent features of echocardiography and, in part, it is related to the rapid progress of magnetic resonance imaging. So far, pathologic CT findings of the heart have usually been incidental, found during other examinations. Typical examples are pericardial effusion, pericardial infiltration as manifestation of malignant disease and post-traumatic hemopericardium. Targeted CT examination of the heart is indicated when a tumor of the cardiac cavities (e.g. atrial myxoma) is suspected, but these questions are increasingly solved by magnetic resonance imaging.

Ultrafast computed tomography

The ultrafast CT scanner has extremely short scan times and has been specifically designed for computed tomographic cardiac examinations. A deflected electron beam rotates around the patient. The absorption values are recorded in a fixed detector ring and are reconstructed with standard cross-sectional reconstruction algorithms. The value of this type of CT would be the detection of calcium in the coronary arteries, considered by some investigators a useful technique for assessing calcified plaque formation in asymptomatic subjects and in patients with coronary artery disease and for studying the natural history of coronary artery disease and the effects of intervention on its course [22]. The American Heart Association, however, has issued the statement that *based on available evidence, clinical use of ultrafast computed tomographic imaging to screen patients for coronary artery disease is not justified at this time'* [23].

Thoracic wall

Flat bones following a curvature (e.g. skull, pelvis and rib cage) are difficult to assess in conventional radiology. Fractures and other pathological processes are easily overlooked, even in oblique views and under rotating fluoroscopy. Transverse CT solves the problem, and it can accurately diagnose complex fractures of the ribs and sternum. In addition, CT can identify pathologic processes of the thoracic wall and separate them from pleural and pulmonary processes (Fig. IV, 62).

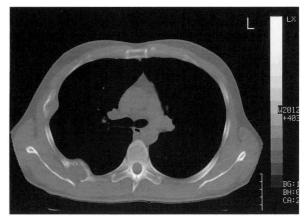

Fig. IV, 62. Non-Hodgkin lymphoma of the ribs in AIDS. Expansion and destruction of the affected ribs on the right seen in the bone window. Medial displacement of the pleura. Definite extrapulmonary process.

Abdomen

A conventional radiograph of the abdomen shows surprisingly little of the abdominal organs. This is due to the fact that muscles, intestinal wall, major vessels and abdominal organs differ little in their water content and therefore do not differ in their X-ray attenuation. Only lucencies caused by intestinal air and a few fatty structures interrupt the monotonous image. Already at an early date, researchers had recognized that abdominal radiography could only be improved by selectively changing the radiation absorption in the individual organs. Through this need radiographic contrast media came into existence, with the first experiments carried out as early as 1896 [24].

The change of the absorption was achieved by medication with a high atomic number (positive contrast media), either systemically administered (kidney and gallbladder) or introduced locally into existing hollow organs (esophagus, stomach, small intestines, colon).

Vascular radiology came later in the form of iodine-containing contrast media, used for arteries, veins and lymphatic system.

In addition, gaseous contrast media were insufflated into real or potential anatomic spaces in manifold ways to achieve, for instance, a pneumoperitoneum or pneumoretroperitoneum. Structures surrounded by the instilled gas (negative contrast medium) became visible.

Finally, in 100 years of diagnostic radiology of the abdomen, we have learned to interpret the few available natural contrast structures in context with the clinical findings. Changes in the intestinal air content and air-fluid levels with the patient upright or in the left lateral decubitus position became established findings for the ileus diagnosis, essentially still valid in the age of CT [25]. Equally valuable is the evidence of free intraperitoneal air as an indication for a possible perforation of a hollow organ.

Despite these few indisputable successes in the radiological diagnosis of abdominal diseases, the abdomen remained a map with many uncharted areas to the early radiologists. Only with the advent of CT and sonography, this region of the body could be unveiled for a more detailed imaging diagnosis. Nowadays, the number of conventional gastrointestinal radiographic studies, including barium studies, is decreasing throughout the world, while all section imaging methods, particularly sonography, are increasing. Endoscopy has also been a decisive factor in the decline of gastroenterologic radiology.

In line with the general theme of this retrospective historical contribution, only those organs and regions will be presented in which CT has considerably increased our knowledge, has become more reliable, and/or has definitely simplified the diagnostic procedures for the patients. It will be necessary to separate CT from sonography and magnetic resonance imaging, and to address the role of these two other tomographic methods in the evaluation of abdominal diseases in relation to CT. These remarks cannot replace complex differential indications, but are meant to show a general pattern that applies to most abdominal organs.

Computer tomography versus sonography in the diagnosis of abdominal diseases

Sonography is customarily the first choice in diseases of the abdominal cavity. The method does not use ionizing radiation, is widely available, and has excellent diagnostic results at the hands of an experienced examiner. Sonography is adversely affected by air (intestinal gas), bones and adiposity. It is for those reasons that not all regions of the abdominal cavity yield sonographic results of adequate diagnostic quality. Sonography depends on the experience and level of training of the examiner. The enormous popularization of the technique, which can be found in every practice and hospital, does not (yet) mean that its operators are all well trained. But this issue has already been addressed. Quality assurance regulation as already established for radiology in the 'Röntgen-Verordnung' (Roentgen Regula-

tions, Federal Republic of Germany) of 1987 are also considered for sonography.

CT, in contrast, employs ionizing radiation, is not as widely available, and definitely more expensive. It should therefore be reserved for problems unresolved by sonography, or for situations requiring reproducible cross-section images of the abdomen (e.g. therapy monitoring, therapy planning).

Computer tomography versus magnetic resonance imaging in the diagnosis of abdominal diseases

At this time, there is no good reason to replace CT with magnetic resonance imaging in the routine diagnostic evaluation of the abdomen, except in situations precluding the administration of iodine-containing contrast media or the use of ionizing radiation associated with computer tomography. There is some research evidence that magnetic resonance imaging is superior to CT in the diagnosis of focal liver lesions, but this approach has not yet been adopted in the clinical setting.

Magnetic resonance tomography operates without ionizing radiation, but it is less available and more expensive than CT. Respiration, intestinal peristalsis and any movement affect the quality of the obtained image, but these problems are being resolved by shorter acquisition sequences. Considering the unusually rapid development of magnetic resonance imaging, it can be predicted that both methods will offer abdominal examinations of comparable quality in the near future. Then, magnetic resonance imaging might be favored by virtue of its lack of absent radiation exposure. Currently, the image quality of abdominal CT is generally better and subject to less interference than the image quality obtained with magnetic resonance imaging; the majority of clinical questions are therefore examined by CT.

Gastrointestinal tract

The entire gastrointestinal tract from esophagus to colon is considered the domain of conventional radiology and endoscopy. The small intestine is a notable exception and is only claimed by radiology since no endoscopic alternative exists to its radiologic evaluation.

The strength of CT is its ability to demonstrate the other side of the intestinal viscera that is not accessible radiologically or endoscopically: the thickness of the intestinal wall, an extrinsic process, or an infiltrative process that arises from the intestinal lumen and extends into the surrounding structures or vice-versa. For instance, the surgeon is interested whether an already confirmed esophageal carcinoma extends into adjacent structures. Are important vessels eroded? Are the crura of the diaphragm infiltrated? Has the tumor invaded the tracheobronchial system? Is lymphadenopathy present? Can distant metastases be demonstrated in the liver or lungs? The decision whether the tumor can be resected or will benefit from curative radiotherapy or whether only palliative treatment is indicated, depends to large extent on the outcome of the computed tomographic staging (Fig. IV, 63).

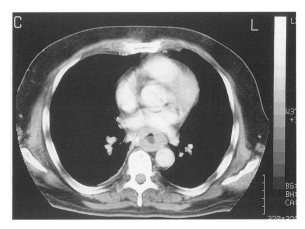

Fig. IV, 63. Esophageal carcinoma. Distinct circular thickening of the wall. Fluid level in the dilated esophageal lumen above the carcinoma. Tumor separated from the left atrium and aorta by delicate fat planes. Contrast-enhanced chest CT.

Similar considerations are true for tumors of the stomach and colon, even though CT only offers an unsatisfactory answer to the important question as to the presence of regional metastatic lymphadenopathy.

The assessment of the thickness of the intestinal wall by CT can be of value in the diagnosis of edema, hematomas, inflammatory wall processes, or radiation-induced enteritis, but CT rarely plays a role as primary diagnostic modality of diseases of the gastrointestinal tract. The notable exceptions to this rule are blunt abdominal trauma and the acute abdomen (see below).

Hepatobiliary tract

Prior to cross-sectional imaging, the liver, the largest abdominal organ, was just a homogenous shadow in the right upper part of the abdomen. Its increase in size could be recognized by the displacement of adjacent organs. Structures within the liver, e.g. tumors, cysts or metastases, could only be detected after they had reached a considerable size. Oral cholecystography and intravenous cholecystocholangiogram could visualize the gallbladder and biliary ducts. Selective angiography of the hepatic arteries as well as direct and indirect splenoportography opened the vascular system of the hepatic artery and portal vein for diagnostic purposes.

This 'uncharted region' on the radiological map of the abdomen was investigated meticulously with the newly arrived CT. Today, CT of the liver and biliary tract belongs to the most important medical measures. It has become essential for therapy planning, therapy monitoring, and prognostic evaluation of many diseases. Its spectrum comprises CT examination of the liver without contrast medium (unenhanced CT), CT after intravenous bolus injection of contrast-medium (enhanced CT) and CT angiography with selective injection of contrast medium into the hepatic artery or into the superior mesenteric artery for indirect visualization of the portal vein.

Either technique of CT angiography is only used in cases considered for resection of metastases. With the new fast spiral CT scanners, selective visualization of the hepatic artery and its branches as well as the portal vein can be achieved after peripheral intravenous injection of contrast medium. The majority of CT examinations of the liver consist of unenhanced sections without intravenous contrast medium followed by enhanced sections after bolus injection of contrast medium.

The first examination in the diagnostic evaluation of focal hepatic lesions is sonography, which has a high accuracy for lesions down to the size of approximately 1.5 cm. The advantage of CT is its precise anatomic assignment of the lesion and its ability of providing characterizing criteria for differential diagnostic consideration, such as measuring its density, and assessing its contour and vascularity. Common dysontogenetic cysts in the liver can be recognized with great accuracy in CT examination. The diagnosis of cavernous hemangiomas of the liver, observed in approximately 10% of adults, can be established in 55% of the cases on the basis of their characteristic enhancement pattern in computer tomography [26]. Both conditions are primarily benign focal hepatic lesions that can simulate metastases in patients with known malignant disease.

The list of focal hepatic lesions includes focal nodular hyperplasia, liver adenoma, hepatocellular carcinoma, cholangioma, focal hepatic lymphoma and hepatic abscesses. A presentation of their differential diagnostic findings would fall outside the scope of this contribution. As a general statement, CT decisively contributes not only to the detection but also to the classification and differential diagnosis of focal hepatic lesions. The exact determination of the lesion's location also allows CT-guided biopsy to obtain a histologic diagnosis (Fig. IV, 64).

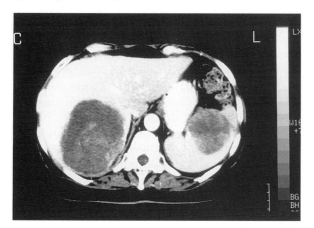

Fig. IV, 64. Advanced ovarial carcinoma with metastases to liver and spleen. Contrast-enhanced CT of the upper abdomen. The stomach is outlined by a diluted barium sulphate solution.

In diffuse hepatic diseases, the role of CT is less defined. Fatty infiltrations of the entire liver (hepatic steatosis) or sections of the liver can be recognized by decreased global or regional density values caused by a difference in photon absorption. In contrast, liver diseases with an excessive iron deposition, such as hemochromatosis or hemosiderosis, can be diagnosed by an increase in density values. In liver cirrhosis, changes in shape and size of the liver can be documented as well as a possibly associated ascites or splenomegaly.

Imaging of the gallbladder and biliary ducts lies in the domain of sonography. Special indications are reserved for CT, usually related to the biliary ducts. Dilatation of the intrahepatic biliary ducts can easily be diagnosed sonographically, but to discover its underlying cause can be difficult. In addition to endoscopic retrograde cholangiopancreatography (ERCP), CT is indi-

cated in this situation. The biliary obstruction must be localized first before any conclusions as to its etiology can be drawn. Ductal obstruction in the vicinity of the papillae often indicates a papillary or pancreatic tumor. The biliary carcinomas generally originate at the confluence of the intrahepatic ducts (Klatskin's tumor), but can be more proximal and infiltrate the liver, making a differentiation from other hepatic neoplasms difficult [27].

Spleen

In addition to the liver, the spleen has become accessible for detailed analysis by sectional imaging. CT has made the clinically difficult assessment of the size of the spleen simple. In addition, CT can visualize focal lesions of the spleen (cysts, metastases, manifestations of lymphomas), accessory spleens and traumatic splenic rupture.

Pancreas

'The pancreas belongs to the organs in which diseases cause considerable problems both clinically and roentgenologically' [28].

This statement is unfortunately still true today. The innovative methods of the sixties, such as pneumotomography of the pancreas, intraoperative pancreatography and direct splenoportography, have now been abandoned. The indirect determination of pancreatic enlargement by means of hypotonic duodenography is still available for cases with specific preoperative questions. Today's armamentarium comprises sonography with direct visualization of the pancreas, ERCP with direct visualization of the pancreatic duct, and CT with direct imaging of the entire pancreas and its surrounding structures. The diagnostic accuracy of CT for pancreatic carcinoma is 95%; however, nothing has changed the dismal prognosis of this tumor [29]. Furthermore, while surgical patients survive on average for only 11–21 months, patients with unresectable tumors live only 3 to 5 months after the diagnosis [30]. An elaborate Japanese study reported that 0.4% of 2194 patients with a surgically treated stage T1a pancreatic carcinoma had a 5-year survival rate of 86% [31]. As mentioned, the improved accuracy achieved with CT has not been equalled by any improvement in the prognosis of pancreatic carcinoma, which now is the fourth leading causes of tumor deaths in the USA. Its diagnosis always comes too late. These

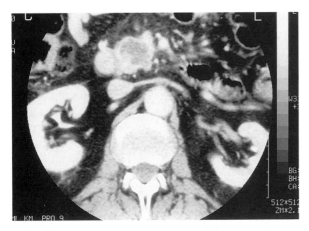

Fig. IV, 65. Carcinoma of the head of the pancreas, 2.5 cm in diameter, unresectable. Contrast-enhanced CT of the pancreas, section thickness 5 mm.

discouraging and dismal facts should not let us forget that computed tomographic evaluation of the pancreas has brought a considerable improvement for patients with benign pancreatic diseases (Fig. IV, 65).

Acute pancreatitis and its complications can be well recognized by CT, which has been found to be of value to guide the therapeutic decisions, together with the clinical and laboratory parameters. Edematous pancreatitis usually has a good prognosis, but the prognosis worsens if pancreatic necroses or phlegmonous extensions are demonstrated by CT (Fig. IV, 66).

In patients with chronic pancreatitis, CT can demonstrate the extent of calcifications and pseudocysts. Furthermore, it can diagnose acute episodes and secondary complications of the disease.

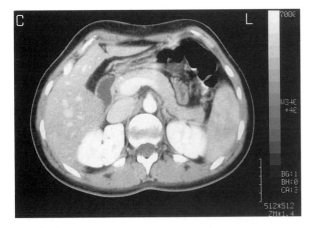

Fig. IV, 66. Acute pancreatitis, edematous type. Harmonic enlargement of the entire pancreas. Slight accentuation of the left anterior renal fascia. No necrotic areas.

Abdominal wall and peritoneal cavity

Computed tomographic cross-section imaging has made pneumoperitoneum dispensable. The normal contents of the abdominal cavity and the most important pathological findings are differentiated from one another by means of their intrinsic contrast. It has been proven to be of great value to opacify the intestines with a diluted liquid solution of contrast medium (barium sulphate or iodine-containing contrast medium). The patient drinks one to two liters of this solution 1–2 h prior to the examination. The subsequent CT cross-sections allow assessment of the major abdominal organs, but can also show intraperitoneal abscesses, foreign bodies or tumors. Knowledge of the normal peritoneal spaces and the typical fluid pathways, mainly origination from the pre-CT era, is imperative for the diagnostic evaluation of the abdominal cavity [32]. But being cognizant of the surgically altered anatomical compartments is also important for the correct interpretation of postoperative accumulation of fluid [33]. Nowadays, after the clinically suspected pathological accumulation of fluid has been confirmed, it is usually followed immediately by CT-guided drainage. Interventional radiology can select a puncture route that avoids damage to neighboring organs (e.g. intestines), thanks to the accurate anatomic display of CT. Hernias, tumors and hemorrhages of the abdominal wall can be identified by CT and their extraperitoneal location can be clearly outlined.

Retroperitoneum

The classic major structure of the retroperitoneum is the psoas muscle, which can be identified in a well-exposed AP supine plain radiograph of the abdomen. A complete unilateral loss of the lateral psoas margin does not bear great diagnostic meaning since it could be caused by a slight scoliosis of the lumbar spine. Segmental loss of the psoas margin, on the contrary, can be considered a secondary sign of a pathological process. We learn from anatomical studies that the retroperitoneum can be divided into three compartments, namely the anterior and posterior pararenal space, and the perirenal space. In CT, these spaces can be recognized clearly so that the image analysis of anatomical spaces can be used to predict the pattern of distribution of pathological fluid concentrations. As a result, the pneumoretroperitoneum, discussed earlier in this contribution, belongs to the history of our profession.

The most important anatomical structures of the retroperitoneum are aorta, inferior vena cava, retroperitoneal lymphatic system, kidneys, adrenal glands, and urinary tracts.

The major vessels of the retroperitoneal spaces can be demonstrated by angiography, which firmly remains in today's diagnostic arsenal. Non-invasive CT allows assessment of the aorta and its branches after intravenous administration of contrast medium. In contrast to angiography, it does not only visualize the patent vascular lumen, but also calcium in the aortic wall and any mural thrombotic deposits that might narrow the lumen. With three-dimensional reconstruction of the data points supplied by spiral CT, the reviewer can compute and observe angiographic images from every angle (CT angiography) [34].

Anomalies of the inferior vena cava, thromboses or venous collateral circulations can be diagnosed after peripheral injection of contrast medium so that the direct visualization of this vein (cavography) is rarely indicated today (Fig. IV, 67).

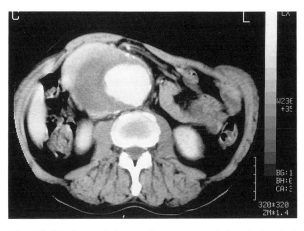

Fig. IV, 67. Large infrarenal aneurysm of the abdominal aorta. Diameter approximately 11 cm, true lumen approximately five cm. Mural calcifications of the aneurysm. Large excentric lamellated mural thrombus.

Assessment of the retroperitoneal lymphatic system can present problems. Large retroperitoneal lymphomas in lymphoproliferative diseases can be diagnosed correctly and monitored easily during therapy. The diagnostic accuracy is considered by some investigators to be somewhere between 68 and 100%. The high accuracy mainly applies to the bulky lymphadenopathy, as typically found in non-Hodgkin lymphomas. Less sa-

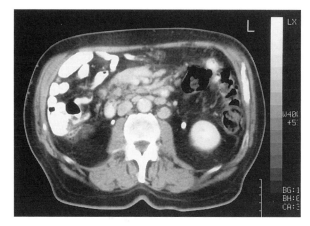

Fig. IV, 68. Non-Hodgkin lymphoma. Multiple enlarged lymph nodes in the retroperitoneum and in the mesenteric root.

tisfactory results have been observed in nodal metastases and in Hodgkin disease. The size of the lymph nodes is the only criterion of malignancy just as in the mediastinum. The internal structure cannot be observed [35] (Fig. IV, 68).

Thus, staging exploratory laparotomy for the evaluation of the lymph nodes is still needed in tumors with a predilection for retroperitoneal nodal metastases. Furthermore, a few patients with normal lymph node status by CT and sonography will still undergo lymphography to reveal diseases in normal-sized lymph nodes.

Kidneys

The outline of the kidneys, which are surrounded by fat in Gerota's capsule, is well seen in an AP supine plain radiograph of the abdomen. Conventional tomography can help to eliminate overlying intestinal gas. The delicate calices and infundibula of the intrarenal collecting system, renal pelves, ureters and bladder can be demonstrated in remarkable detail after intravenous injection of contrast medium. But this excretory urography is less suitable for evaluating processes in the renal parenchyma unless such a process has led to a mass effect on or infiltration of the pelvicaliceal system. These questions are best solved by cross-sectional imaging, such as sonography and CT. Excretory urography remains the modality of choice to detect subtle pathological changes of the pelvicaliceal system. Imaging of the kidneys follows an orderly approach, whereby CT is primarily indicated to demonstrate and, in case of malignancy, to stage space-occupying processes. In addition, it can reveal causes of urinary obstructions due to extrinsic processes (e.g. lymph nodes or tumors in the lower pelvis), and assess extrarenal processes which have invaded the kidneys or arisen from the kidneys.

By means of density measurements, analysis of wall contours, and enhancement after intravenous administration of contrast medium, a disease-specific differentiation of various renal masses can be achieved with high accuracy. A retrospective review of patients who had a nephrectomy for suspected renal cell carcinoma revealed a positive predictive of 96% for renal CT when three or more characteristic findings were present [36]. Renal angiography is no longer indicated for strictly diagnostic reasons, but it remains important to solve complicated questions related to therapy planning, as encountered with carcinoma in a solitary kidney (Fig. IV, 69 and 70).

Staging according to the TNM system is decisive for both therapy and prognosis. CT determines the size of the tumor (T) accurately, but determining the nodal involvement (N) is a little less accurate. Assessment for distant metastases (M) is again very accurate but requires scintigraphy, conventional radiology, and CT. The typical tumor spread into the renal vein and possibly into the inferior vena cava can be diagnosed by CT.

The transitional carcinoma of the collecting system in its early stages is limited to the mucosa and therefore not seen by CT. As soon as it infiltrates the kidneys or the surrounding fatty tissue (stage III), it will be demonstrated by CT. In addition to renal tumors, the spectrum of conditions diagnosed by CT includes lymphomatous infiltration of the kidneys, and the acute and chronic inflammatory processes.

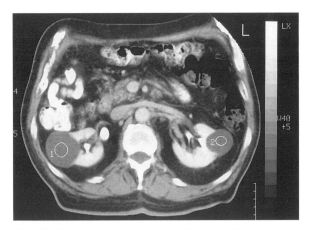

Fig. IV, 69. Cortical renal cysts, bilaterally. Density measurements in areas 1 and 2 yielded 6.1 and 3.5 HU, respectively, consistent with water equivalent cyst contents. No enhancement after administration of intravenous contrast medium.

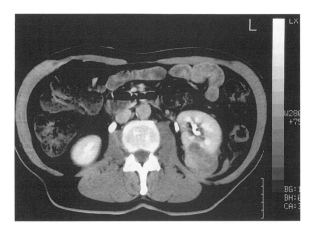

Fig. IV, 70. Renal-cell carcinoma at the posterior periphery of the kidney. Contrast-enhanced renal CT. Indistinct demarcation of the tumor from normal renal parenchyma, with heterogeneous uptake of contrast medium by the tumor.

Adrenal glands

The diagnostic quantum leap brought about by the introduction of CT is quite impressive if today's diagnostic state is compared to the cumbersome, painful and risky measures of the pneumoperitoneum. The adrenal glands are small organs in the retroperitoneal fatty tissue, measuring approximately 2–4 cm in length and 5–7 mm in diameter. Its surrounding fat allows the computed tomographic visualization in nearly 100% of the patients. A diameter increase of 5 mm can be recognized in CT with the appropriate thin-section technique (Fig. IV, 71).

The adrenal glands can serve as an example that solving an old problem with a refined diagnostic technique can create a new problem. Many adrenal masses have been observed as incidental findings in patients who have neither an abnormal adrenal function nor a tumor with a predilection for adrenal metastases. These incidentally found hormone-inactive tumors are called 'incidentalomas'. Pathoanatomically, they represent hormonally inactive adenomas which are found in 2–8% of all autopsies. These benign tumors usually do not need therapy. However, the situation becomes problematic in cases with an extra-adrenal malignant tumor that has the propensity for metastatic spread to the adrenal glands. CT cannot differentiate between a hormonally inactive adenoma and a metastasis, and CT-guided biopsy or surgery with histologic

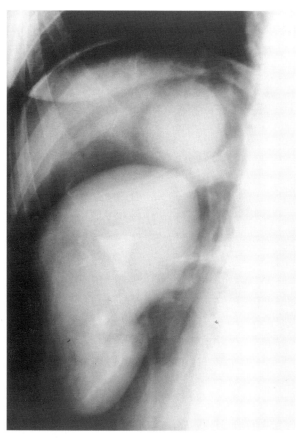

Fig. IV, 71a. Pneumoretroperitoneum. Adrenal tumor, right side.

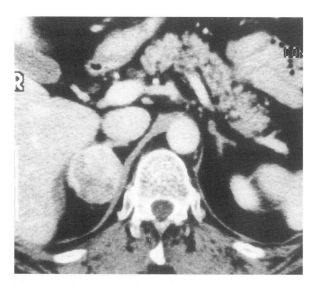

Fig. IV, 71b. Hormonally inactive adrenal adenoma (approximately 4 cm in diameter). Left adrenal gland is seen as an inverted "Y" and morphologically inconspicuous. Contrast-enhanced adrenal CT. Section thickness 3 mm.

examination is necessary in these cases. Despite its lack of specificity, CT is the primary examination for imaging adrenal tumors and for localizing extra-adrenal pheochromocytomas [37].

Blunt abdominal trauma – acute abdomen

For a long time, the radiological armamentarium for patients with blunt abdominal trauma or acute abdomen consisted of AP supine and left lateral decubitus plain radiographs of the abdomen [25]. These simple means, together with clinical examination and auscultatory evaluation of the bowel sounds, could narrow the possible causes of the acute abdomen rather well. Considering its speediness, availability and simplicity, this diagnostic approach has not yet been surpassed and for this reason it still belongs to today's diagnostic arsenal.

The increased availability as well as technical advances of CT scanners led to a new role of CT in traumatology, with emphasis on injuries of the abdomen and pelvis [38].

In previous chapters, we have demonstrated the detail and anatomic accuracy afforded by CT to depict the organs of the abdomen and pelvis, and it is indeed only logical to apply this technique to trauma patients. In collaboration with traumatologists, a triage concept has been developed to decide whether the patient should be examined by CT or immediately sent to the operating room. According to this concept, hemodynamically unstable patients will undergo surgery since the delay incurred by the diagnostic investigations could influence the prognosis unfavorably. Hemodynamically stable patients, in contrast, immediately undergo CT of all regions of interest as quickly as possible. Preferably, contrast medium should be administered and a dynamic technique used. This approach demonstrates intraperitoneal and extraperitoneal accumulation of fluid as well as lacerations of liver, spleen, pancreas and kidneys. By virtue of the accuracy of the CT findings, any necessary surgical intervention can be more targeted than emergency surgery without this diagnostic information. Today, many traumatologists frequently decide to observe hemodynamically stable patients who have intra-abdominal injuries demonstrated by CT and to monitor the injured organ regularly by sonography or CT. In this way, unnecessary splenectomies and partial hepatic resections can be avoided.

This concept has particularly prevailed in renal trauma. Approximately 85% of all renal injuries are inconsequential. CT can recognize contusion, small lacerations, intrarenal hematomas, or small subcapsular hematomas. These injuries can be managed conservatively. Even parenchymal injuries with extravasation of urine, large subcapsular hematomas, and complete lacerations do not require urgent surgery as long as the response to conservative therapy can be monitored by follow-up CT [39]. The progress of trauma surgery has resulted in fewer organ resections, an advancement made possible by computer tomography (Fig. IV, 72).

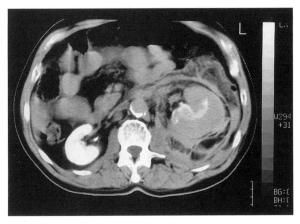

Fig. IV, 72. Rupture of the left kidney. Massive bleeding into the perirenal space. Thickening of Gerota's fascia. Enhancement of perfused remnants of lacerated renal parenchyma after administration of contrast medium. Successful conservative therapy.

Pelvis

Before the CT era, organs of the pelvis did not belong to the radiologist's domain. The gynecologist's palpating finger, the urologist's cystoscope, and the surgeon's and gastroenterologist's rectosigmoidoscope have evaluated this region diagnostically. CT had, until recently, not caused a spectacular change. There are, however, reports that attach considerable importance to magnet resonance imaging.

While CT only showed a limited success in diagnosing abnormalities of the intrapelvic organs, it has made a great contribution to the evaluation of the bony pelvis. The complex anatomy of the bony pelvis and hips cannot be demonstrated well by conventional radiography. Today's treatment of pelvic fractures is hard to imagine without the aid of the transverse tomographic plane made possible by CT.

Musculoskeletal system

In the Royal Library at Windsor Castle, Leonardo da Vinci's collection of anatomical drawings include drawings from 1487 to 1489 that anticipate today's computed tomographic visualization. They were called 'corpo transparente', the quasi CT of early anatomists, as illustrated in the diagram of a leg measured and cut into sections [40] (Fig. IV, 73).

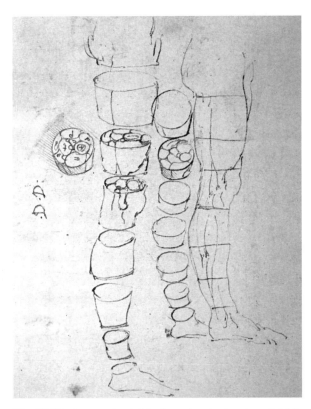

Fig. IV, 73. Leonardo da Vinci, anatomic drawings (1487-1489). "Corpo transparente" - CT technique [40].

Five hundred years after Leonardo da Vinci, the means are in place for the transparent technique to evaluate disorders of the musculoskeletal system. Of interest is that the very first image taken with Roentgen's 'neuer Art von Strahlen' also evaluated the musculoskeletal system.

From the abundance of all conceivable applications, three categories will be presented to illustrate the expanded diagnostic dimensions: tumors of the soft tissues, tumors of the bones, and traumatology.

Primary soft-tissue tumors are statistically rather infrequent and the majority are benign. They must be differentiated from hematomas or muscle ruptures, often occurring with athletic

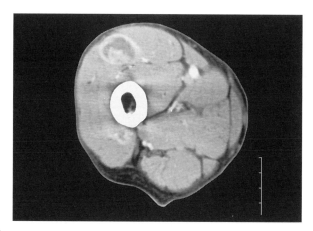

Fig. IV, 74. Liposarcoma of the left thigh. After administration of contrast medium, ring-shaped enhancement of the pseudocapsule but also heterogeneous enhancement in the center of the tumor.

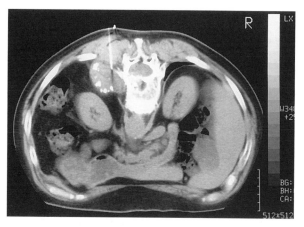

Fig. IV, 75. Left paravertebral spindle-cell sarcoma, amorphous calcifications. Diagnostic confirmation after CT-guided biopsy in prone position. CT with biopsy needle in place.

activities, and from abscesses or cellulitis. This differentiation is therapeutically relevant. CT can define the exact location and site of origin, and can contribute to the specific diagnosis by density measurements and the enhancement pattern following intravenous injection of contrast medium (Figs IV, 74 and 75).

In bone tumors, all relevant conclusions with respect to a specific diagnosis and presumed benign or malignant nature are drawn from the analysis of conventional radiographs. CT (and MRI) can only outline any intramedullary expansion and soft tissue extension. CT has replaced angiography, which used to provide this information.

In traumatology, fractures and dislocation involving complex anatomical regions can clearly be demonstrated on the transverse sections of CT, which has resulted in better treatment and improved outcome. Classical examples are pelvic fractures, separations of the sacroiliac joints, fractures and dislocation of the hip and calcaneal fractures. In these cases, three-dimensional reconstruction has proved to be of great value for orthopedic surgeons, who can get a better perspective of the pathological changes. The increasing number of requested three-dimensional reconstructions suggests that this type of presentation not only has aesthetic appeal but also informative content that simplifies the surgeon's task [41] (Fig. IV, 76).

On the basis of CT data sets, custom-made hip replacements and tumor protheses are commercially manufactured. Computer-assisted surgery and medical CAD/CAM (computer-assisted de-

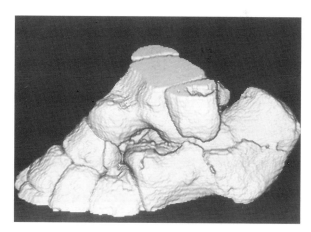

Fig. IV, 76. Comminuted calcaneus fracture. 3D reconstruction from a CT data set.

sign, computer-assisted manufacturing) are developments based on CT.

Spine

The spine consists of closely interrelated bony structures, ligaments, intervertebral discs, and spinal cord with its efferent nerves. The bony structures are visualized clearly in conventional radiology. The vertebral canal and root sleeves of the efferent nerves can be radiographically visualized after intrathecal administration of contrast-medium (myelography). Imaging of the spine by these established imaging methods has been expanded by CT (and MRI). The possibility of cross-sectional visualization of nonosseous structures has reduced the number of invasive myelographies worldwide.

The importance of CT of the vertebral column will be illustrated by two clinical examples: diagnosis of vertebral disc herniation and osteodensitometry. It is now generally accepted that MRI is superior for many imaging applications of the spine and many indications for CT have already been delegated to MRI.

Backache is one of the most frequent clinical complaints. The conventional plain radiographs afford a reliable assessment of form, height and alignment of the vertebral bodies, and frequently show osteophytes, disc space narrowing and degenerative changes of apophyseal joints.

CT adds transverse sections to these findings, revealing whether spinal canal or foramina are narrowed by osseous overgrowths. Moreover, these transverse images can directly visualize and assess the intervertebral disc, and demonstrate whether a protrusion or a herniation is present. Lumbar CT is one of the most frequent examinations performed in radiological practice. In the past, the question of a herniated disc had to be resolved by myelography but today this is no longer necessary. To evaluate persisting pain after diskectomy ('failed back surgery syndrome'), myelography is combined with CT (CT-myelography) to obtain the best imaging contrast possible. If minimally invasive treatment of the vertebral disc (nucleolysis, suction, laser coagulation) is planned, the fibroid annulus is examined by diskography supplemented by subsequent CT (CT-diskography) (Fig. IV, 77).

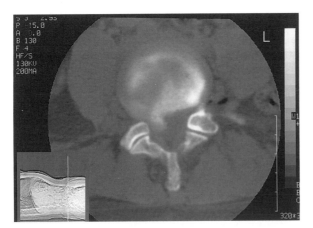

Fig. IV, 77. CT-diskography after injection of contrast medium into the disk. Right lateral disk herniation at L4/L5 with rupture of the annulus fibrosis (in collaboration with Dr. Castro, Orthopedic University Clinic, Muenster, Germany).

Osteodensitometry, also called quantitative computed tomography (QCT), consists of selective density measurements of the trabecular bone of three lumbar vertebrae and calibrated against a reference phantom outside the body. The calculated bone density is compared to values of a collective standard matched for age and gender. This allows an individualized treatment of the many forms of osteoporosis and an objective assessment of its effectiveness [42, 43].

Summary

CT of the torso has revolutionized the clinical history of diagnostic imaging of many diseases in a very short period of time. Above all, patients profit from this revolution since many painful and risky measures can be entirely replaced by CT. The patients benefit further from the painless and better computed tomographic diagnosis, reflected in a better outcome of their disease. The improved diagnostic accuracy means that surgery can be more elective, in addition to being performed at an earlier stage of the disease and to becoming more precise. But there are also situations in which exploratory surgery (exploratory laparotomy) remains the procedure of choice. Finally, minimally invasive operations can be performed, made possible in part by an accurate computed tomographic diagnosis or in part by direct CT guidance. In conservative treatment, the extent of the disease is assessed at the beginning of the therapy and its course monitored under CT.

Physicians from all disciplines benefit from an improved diagnosis made by CT due to accurate visualization of pathological lesions. Only by seeing the local extension into the surrounding tissue and by recognizing the possible complications, it is possible to have a rational therapeutic concept. Multicentric studies of rare diseases can be conducted due to the reproducible image documentation of CT. Despite the justified enthusiasm for this technique, all the more understandable when one thinks back and remembers the pre-CT era, it should not be overlooked that CT uses ionizing radiation. The radiation exposure of all CT examinations is, as a rule, greater than that of a plain radiograph. The higher radiation exposure is justified if the CT examination can diagnose or confirm a disease or eliminate a differential diagnostic possibility. In addition, CT is indispensable in planning surgical, conservative or radiation treatment and in monitoring the therapeutic outcome.

References

1. Ruiz Rivas, M.: Generalized subserous emphysema through a single puncture. Am. J. Roentgenol. 64 (1950) 723

2. Cormack, A.M.: Representation of a function by its line integrals with some radiological applications. J. Appl. Physiol. 34 (1963) 2722–2727

3. Hounsfield, G.N.: Computerized transverse axial scanning (tomography): Part I: Description of system. Br. J. Radiol. 46 (1973) 1016–1022

4. Lee, J.K.T., S.S. Sagel, R.J. Stanley: Computed Body Tomography with MRI Correlation. Raven Press New York 1989

5. Ziedses des Plantes, B.G.: Een bijzondere methode voor het maken van röntgenfoto's van schedel en wervelkolom. Ned. Tijdschr. Geneesk. 75 (1931) 5218–5222

6. Gebauer, A., E. Muntean, E. Stutz, H. Vieten: Das Röntgenschichtbild. Georg Thieme Verlag Stuttgart 1959

7. Crow, J., G. Salvin, L. Kreel: Pulmonary metastasis: a pathologic and radiologic study. Cancer 47 (1981) 2595–2602

8. Mintzer, R.A., S.R. Malave, H.L. Neiman, L.L. Michaelis, R.M. Vanecko, J.H. Sanders: Computed vs. conventional tomography in the evaluation of primary and secondary pulmonary neoplasms. Radiology 132 (1979) 653–659

9. Muhm, J.R., L.R. Brown, J.K. Crowe, P.F. Sheedy, R.R. Hattery, D.H. Stephens: Comparison of whole lung tomography and computed tomography for detecting pulmonary nodules. Am. J. Roentgenol. 131 (1978) 981–984

10. Roos, N.: Persönliche Mitteilung

11. Siegelman, S.S., N. Khouri, F.P. Leo, E.K. Fishman, R.M. Braverman, E.A. Zerhouni: Solitary pulmonary nodules: CT assessment. Radiology 160 (1986) 307–312

12. Staples, C.A.: Computed tomography in the evaluation of benign asbestos-related disorders. Radiol. Clin. North Am. 30 (1992) 1191–1207

13. Mirvis, S.E., K.D. Tobin, I. Kostrubiak, H. Belzberg: Thoracic CT in detecting occult disease in critically ill patients. Am. J. Roentgenol. 148 (1987) 685–689

14. Wall, S.D., M.P. Federle, R.B. Jeffrey, C.M. Brett: CT diagnosis of unsuspected pneumothorax after blunt abdominal trauma. Am. J. Roentgenol. 141 (1983) 919–921

15. Anacker, H.: Erkrankungen des Mediastinum. In: Klinische Röntgendiagnostik innerer Krankheiten. Bd. I Thorax. Haubrich R, Springer Verlag Berlin (1963) 586–624

16. Tricomi, G., G. Capaldo: Pneumomediastino posteriore. Ann. Ist. Forlanini 13 (1951) 133

17. Baccaglini, M.: Rilievi di tecnica sul retropneumoperitoneo, con particulare riguardo alla possibilita di ottenere il pneumomediastino. Radiol. med. (Torino) 28 (1941) 247

18. Sansone, G., A. de Maestri: Visualizzazione simultaneo del mediastino posteriore et anteriore dopo insufflatione peridurale. Minerva pediat. 3 (1951) 332

19. Paolucci id Valmaggiore, G., E. Giacobini: Voies d'acces pour l'application du pneumomediastin. Presse med. 59 (1951) 1222

20. Webb, W.R., C. Gatsonis, E.A. Zerhouni, R.T. Heelan, G.M. Glazer, I.R. Francis, B.J. McNeil: CT and MR imaging in staging non-small cell bronchogenic carcinoma: report of the Radiologic Diagnostic Oncology Group. Radiology 178 (1991) 705–713

21. Posniak, H.V., M.C. Olson, T.C. Demos, R.A. Benjoya, R.E. Marsan: CT of thoracic aortic aneurysms. Radiographics 10 (1990) 839–855

22. Janowitz, W.R., A.S. Agatston, M. Viamonte: Comparison of serial quantative evaluation of calcified coronary artery plaque by ultrafast CT in persons with and without obstructive coronary artery disease. Am. J. Cardiol. 68 (1991) 1–6

23. AHA Medical/scientific statement: Potential value of ultrafast CT in persons with and without obstructive coronary artery disease. Circulation 87 (1993) 2071

24. Haschek, E., T.O. Lindenthal: Ein Beitrag zur praktischen Verwertung der Photographie nach Röntgen. Wien. klin. Wschr. 9 (1896) 63–64

25. Swart, B., G. Meyer: Die Diagnostik des akuten Abdomens beim Erwachsenen – ein neues klinisch-radiologisches Konzept. Radiologe 14 (1974) 1–57

26. Freeny, P.C., W.M. Marks: Hepatic hemangioma: Dynamic bolus CT. Am. J. Roentgenol. 147 (1986) 711–719

27. Baron, R.L.: Computed tomography of the biliary tree. Radiol. Clin. North Am. 29 (1991) 1235–1258

28. Anacker, H.: Krankheiten des Pankreas. In: Klinische Röntgendiagnostik innerer Krankheiten. Bd. II Abdomen. Haubrich, Springer Verlag Berlin (1966) 319–374

29. Clark, L.R., M.H. Jaffe, P.L. Choyke, E.G. Grant, R.K. Zeman: Pancreatic imaging. Radiol. Clin. North Am. 23 (1985) 489–501

30. Livstone, E.M., H.M. Spiro: The pancreatic cancer problem. World J. Surg. 8 (1984) 872

31. Ichikawa, M. zit. bei Grundmann, R. In: Palliative Krebstherapie. Pichlmaier H. Springer Verlag Berlin (1991) 481–502

32. Meyers, M.A.: Dynamic Radiology of the Abdomen. Springer Verlag New York 1976

33. Kumpan, W.: Computertomographische Analyse postoperativer abdomineller Kompartments. Eine Vergleichsstudie an 100 Patienten mit abdominellen Abszessen. Radiologe 27 (1987) 203–215

34. Napel, S., M.P. Marks, G.D. Rubin, M.D. Dake, C.H. McDonell, S.M. Song, D.R. Enzmann, R.B. Jeffrey jr: CT angiography with spiral CT and maximum intensity projection. Radiology 185 (1992) 607–610

35. Peters, P.E., K. Beyer: Querdurchmesser normaler Lymphknoten in verschiedenen anatomischen Regionen und ihre Bedeutung für die computertomographische Diagnostik. Radiologe 25 (1985) 193–198

36. Curry, N.S., J. Reinig, S.I. Schabel, P. Ross, I. Vujic, R.P. Gobien: An evaluation of the effectiveness of CT vs. other imaging modalities in the diagnosis of atypical renal masses. Invest. Radiol. 19 (1984) 447–452

37. Dunnick, N.R.: Adrenal imaging: current status. Am. J. Roentgenol. 154 (1990) 927–936

38. Gay, S.B., C.L. Sistrom: Computed tomography evaluation of blunt abdominal trauma. Radiol. Clin. North Am. 30 (1992) 367–388

39. Federle, M.P., J.A. Kaiser, J.W. McAnich et al: The role of computed tomography in renal trauma. Radiology 141 (1981) 455–460

40. Da Vinci, L.: Anatomische Zeichnungen aus der königlichen Bibliothek auf Schloß Windsor. Prisma Verlag Gütersloh 1979

41. Martinez, C.R., T.G. di Pasquale, D.L. Helfet, A.W. Graham, R.W. Sanders, L.D. Ray: Evaluation of acetabular fractures with two- and three-dimensional CT. Radiographics 12 (1992) 227–242

42. Montag, M., M. Dören, H.M. Meyer-Galander, Th. Montag, P.E. Peters: Computertomographisch bestimmter Mineralgehalt in der LWS-Spongiosa. Normwerte für gesunde perimenopausale Frauen und Vergleich dieser Werte mit der mechanischen Wirbelsäulenbelastung. Radiologe 28 (1988) 161–165

43. Reinbold, W.D., H.K. Genant, E. Dinkel: Vergleichende Knochendichtemessung bei gesunden Frauen und Frauen mit Osteoporose. Radiologe 28 (1988) 152–160

Chapter 5

The invisible light manipulated

Evolution of X-ray technology by interaction of physicians and engineers

Introduction

G. Rosenbusch, E. Ammann, M. Oudkerk

'All we elderly people have to do to realize the enormous difference between former times and the present is to look back on our own youth. We can still remember the time when the steamship and the locomotive took their first feeble steps. Filled with doubt and amazement, we heard the tale of how light itself could 'paint pictures' and make them visible to the human eye; that the mysterious new force called 'electricity' could spread news through entire continents and across the isolating oceans at the speed of lightning, that the same force produced solid metals from their liquid solutions and was able to expel the night with the light of day! Which of us today is still astonished about such natural occurrences? Without them, our young people could hardly imagine leading a civilized life, in a time when, based on Reuleaux's calculation, numerous 'iron workers' labour day and night in the service of each and every civilized human being, when millions of people who only yesterday were separated by vast distances are brought together every day, and immeasurable quantities of goods are transported over land and sea, through the mountains and across their peaks and valleys at a previously unthinkable speed by the harnessed forces of nature, when the world-spanning telegraph alone no longer satisfies all of our communication needs and must give way to transmission of the living word through the telephone and retreat to those wild expanses where transmission of the human voice is limited by the confines of nature, when the latest fruit of the cross-fertilization of natural science and technology, electrical engineering, has in the course of its rapid development opened up more and more new fields to mankind for further research and useful application of natural forces.'

Thus spoke Werner von Siemens (1816–1892) in his address entitled 'The Scientific Age', held at the 59th Convention of German Natural Scientists and Physicians on 18 September 1886.

The Industrial Revolution began in England around the middle of the 18th century. Initialy, machines were invented to enable faster and cheaper weaving and spinning. These early machines were simple devices which could replace specific manual actions. They were usually designed by people who regarded their previous work as overly strenuous, time-consuming or tedious. Without any knowledge of physical laws, they merely sought improvements in a purely empirical manner.

Numerous attempts had already been made to harness steam as a source of energy for some time. However, not until 1769 did James Watt succeed in building the first steam engine which really worked. Following further development and an increase of its efficiency, the steam engine made it possible to replace manual labour with machines. It was then used in mining to transport large quantities of water out of mines in order to be able to penetrate deeper below the Earth's surface. The steam engine attained great importance in the field of public transport; the steamship and the locomotive began their triumphant journey. Both rail and steamship travel initially served to transport passengers.

Figuratively speaking, distances became 'shorter', which was also a necessity, since more and more people began to commute between their homes and place of work. On the other hand, these means of transportation were also increasingly used to transport ore, coal and agricultural products as well as industrial goods. Further development of railway and steamship travel became possible only after corresponding progress had been made in mechanical engineering. Machines had to be constructed for the manufacture of various different parts. Improvements in the quality of the iron and steel used were also necessary. Large steel mills like the Krupp steelworks were founded and experienced an unexpected boom. If you just stop to consider that the railway network had to span thousands of kilometers and that locomotives, rail cars and coaches, ship's hulls and agricultural machines all had to be built, it becomes clear to what extent the steel industry then prospered.

The population of all European countries increased dramatically in the 19th century. Many cities, e.g. Berlin, London and Vienna, grew so fast that they tripled or even quadrupled in size within a single year. The cities were places of refuge for the impoverished rural population.

Faster public transport and industrial manufacture also made it necessary to transmit messages or orders more quickly. In 1837, the American inventor Samuel Morse introduced the first functioning telegraph and in 1844 a test line was set up between Washington DC and Baltimore, Maryland.

Werner von Siemens considered telegraphy to be an exceptionally important branch. Following his studies at the Berlin Artillery and Engineering College, he improved the telegraph. Together with Johann Georg Halske (1814–1890), he attempted to achieve a new design, for which purpose he founded his own electrical engineering company in 1847. Telegraphy was the basis for this firm's further investigations and enterprises. In electrotechnical development, the telegraph represented the first major and extensive application to everyday life. Siemens and Halske continued to introduce important innovations, such as insulation for electrical cables and the double-T armature for inductor telegraphy. As a result, they received orders for the establishment of worldwide telegraphic communications.

Although many people were engaged in the study of electromagnetism, Werner von Siemens is generally regarded as the actual discoverer of the electrodynamic principle. Instead of a permanent steel magnet, he employed an electromagnet or solenoid. The special shape and winding of the armature led to improved utilization of the magnetic field. The electric motor was conceived around the middle of the 1860s and has been available for general use since the 1880s. By transmitting electric power over great distances, people were no longer dependent on remaining close to the site of the electric power plant. Werner von Siemens immediately recognized the significance of the electric motor for exploiting electric power in industry. Electric vehicles such as electric locomotives, trams and electric drills are just a few examples of the many possibilities involved. Electric light also became generally available within a few decades.

While preoccupation with the subject of electricity chiefly represented a form of entertainment and amusement until the beginning of the 19th century, this topic now began to take on an increasingly important dimension in everyday life. On the one hand, this meant that technology began directing questions to science to obtain more fundamental knowledge and explain certain phenomena which in turn lead to improvements and further developments. This necessitated a level of education offered only at the universities or newly established technical colleges. The engineering profession had come into being. The humanities or liberal arts thus had a serious rival. This paved the way for what was later referred to as two cultures, each going its own separate way without any knowledge of the other, as antagonists instead of as partners. On the other hand, the accounting profession was also called on to provide calculations of manufacturing and marketing costs. Finally, politicians laid the framework within which technological developments were to take place.

In Germany, which had hardly participated in world trade since the 16th century, great and successful strides were undertaken to catch up with technological developments, especially those that had taken place in England. A large share of this development can be directly attributed to individuals such as Borsig, Krupp and Werner von Siemens.

During the second half of the 19th century, industrial production rose in several countries at an annual rate of 6%. This flowering of technology and the natural sciences was accompanied by upheavals in daily life. These developments allowed the underprivileged classes to participate in the mainstream of political life. Their participation in cultural affairs was also promoted through newspapers and books.

The year 1895, the year in which Roentgen made his trail-blazing discovery, already possessed a sound economic and technical base, especially in the field of electrical engineering. It is therefore not surprising that numerous small companies were already manufacturing X-ray systems. However, in the course of time, this broad base narrowed to include only those large, electrotechnical enterprises that possessed both the expertise and the laboratories required to produce and further develop new findings. The laboratories, particularly, were of paramount importance in achieving progress in the manufacture of X-ray equipment.

This chapter describes the development of X-ray technology, including the endless amount of work and inventive genius which were necessary to reach our current position. Today's radiological systems result from the co-operation between numerous subdisciplines united under one roof in an 'X-ray company', and at the same time represent the chief means by which such a firm distinguishes itself.

Interaction and ideas from radiologists, medical technical assistants, engineers and managers bring innovation: the demands and wishes voiced by medicine, radiation protection and radiobiology as well as new components and techniques from the most divergent technologies, e.g. mechanical engineering with vibration science, statics and dynamics, materials science, electrical engineering with high-voltage and high-power technologies, motor drives, control and automation engineering, electronics, data processing and communication engineering, optics, air conditioning technology, vacuum technology, manufacturing technologies, software science, testing and quality control procedures, tool making and construction of jigs and fixtures, organization,

project engineering, transport, installation and service procedures, legal frameworks and procedures, standardization, physics, operational research and organizational procedures must all work together hand-in-hand in such a way that a single X-ray system can be handed over to the physician for use as a diagnostic tool. As a result, technical achievements are seldom accomplished by individuals working in the foreground, but rather, result from the efforts of a large team whose members constantly stimulate each other.

In the past, and to an even greater extent, in the future as well, one goal of technology has always been to perform examinations in such a way that the patient is subjected to as little discomfort as possible. Lesions must be discovered as early and reliably as possible and effective therapeutic tools must be created which are as non-invasive as possible. Further aims include a reduction in the medical team's workload and cost-effective use of the 'tool' to keep the costs of examinations as low as possible. In the final analysis, it is the quality of the diagnosis, and therefore, the patient who benefits the most from technological improvements and innovations.

X-ray tubes

E. Ammann, G. Rosenbusch, M. Oudkerk

'*The X-ray tube is by far the most important component for the success of X-ray examinations. The more outstanding its quality, the better the results ... One can say that two-thirds of all X-ray technology is a tube question.*' This statement by Albers-Schoenberg in 1903 still applies. However, it was a long road to today's high-performance tubes.

W.C. Roentgen's tubes: ion X-ray tubes

In his experiments, which finally led to the discovery of X-rays, Roentgen used gas ion tubes (Fig. V, 1) (Prellwitz, 1974 [36]; Rønne and Nielsen, 1986 [38]). These were cathode ray tubes as used by H. Geissler, J.W. Hittorf, W. Crookes and Ph. Lenard in their fundamental experiments. The basic structure of these tubes was identical: a cylindrical, spherical or pear-shaped glass vessel contained two fused-in electrodes roughly at right angles to one another. The tubes were evacuated to approximately a millionth of normal atmospheric pressure. By applying high voltage between both electrodes – the negative electrode is the cathode, the positive the anode – positively charged ions of gas were accelerated through the electric field to strike the cathode, from which electrons were released, which in turn generated X-rays, on striking the glass wall of the tube. The degree of rarefaction of the air or gas in the tube and the voltage applied determined the magnitude of the tube current. If electrons in large numbers strike the glass bulb then the tube life is short. The glass melts when a very low limit for cathode rays is exceeded because the energy expended when electrons collide is largely converted into thermic energy (99%) and only about 1% into X-rays. Roentgen's first publication (28 December 1895) states

that he first experimented with tubes with cathodes made out of a round aluminium plate emitting electrons that struck the glass surface facing it.

Platinum anticathodes

The X-ray exposures taken under such conditions suffered from blurring, because the X-rays did not come from a concentrated focal spot but from the relatively large curved glass surface. In addition the exposure times were very long, as the intensity of the rays emitted from the glass wall was low. As early as his second publication of 9 March 1896, Roentgen reported that he had introduced a small inclined platinum plate into his discharge tubes in the path of the emitted electrons. This third electrode, or anticathode – fitted opposite the cathode – increased the yield and intensity of the X-rays. Platinum has a high atomic number and a higher melting point than aluminium. Roentgen's finding led to improved metallic anticathodes being fitted in the tubes, thereby increasing their thermal load capacity and the yield of X-rays. In his second communication, Roentgen also reported that a platinum anticathode emits considerably more X-rays than an aluminium plate. For some weeks he had also been successfully using a discharge apparatus, in which a concave mirror made of aluminium acted as a cathode and a platinum plate fitted in the centre of the curvature inclined at 45° to the axis of the mirror acted as an anode. Such tubes with a concave cathode had also been used for some time to study gas discharges (Figs. V, 2–V, 4). Roentgen, therefore, used known principles in his investigations.

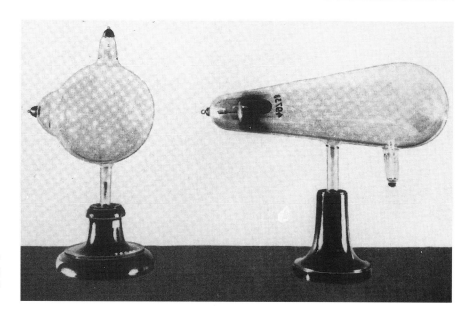

Fig. V, 1. 1895: Hittorf X-ray tube (collection of X-ray tubes belonging to Roentgen in the German museum).

The observations described by Roentgen were also put to practical use in X-ray examinations: the electrons were emitted from the cathode mirror [P 2] and focussed onto a platinum plate inclined at 45°, causing the X-rays to originate from a focal spot. They were relatively intense because of the high atomic number of platinum.

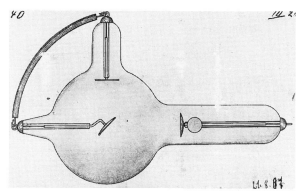

Fig. V, 3. Drawing of an ion X-ray tube, 1897: anode on the top, anticathode with 45° angle made of platinum in the centre and concave cathode on the right-hand side. Such a design had already been proposed by W.C. Roentgen.

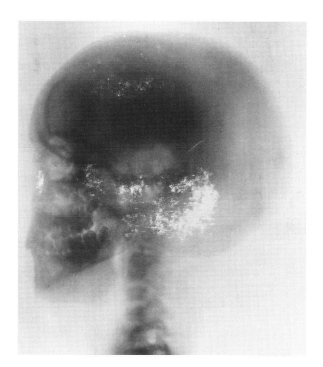

Fig. V, 2. 1896: Radiograph by Reiniger, Gebbert and Schall of a skull of a living person, taken with a Reiniger, Gebbert and Schall inductor of 15 cm spark length; exposure time 11 min [40] (damaged by water in the archive).

The anode and anticathode were electrically connected to prevent the anticathode becoming negatively charged because of the electron flow. The glass wall was also subjected to less stress, so that the lifespan of the tubes was prolonged.

Distribution of radiation intensity

In Roentgen's third communication, dated 10 March 1897, he reported that the intensity of the radiation was nearly the same in all directions in an imaginary hemisphere on the anode plate and that Lambert's law did not apply as it

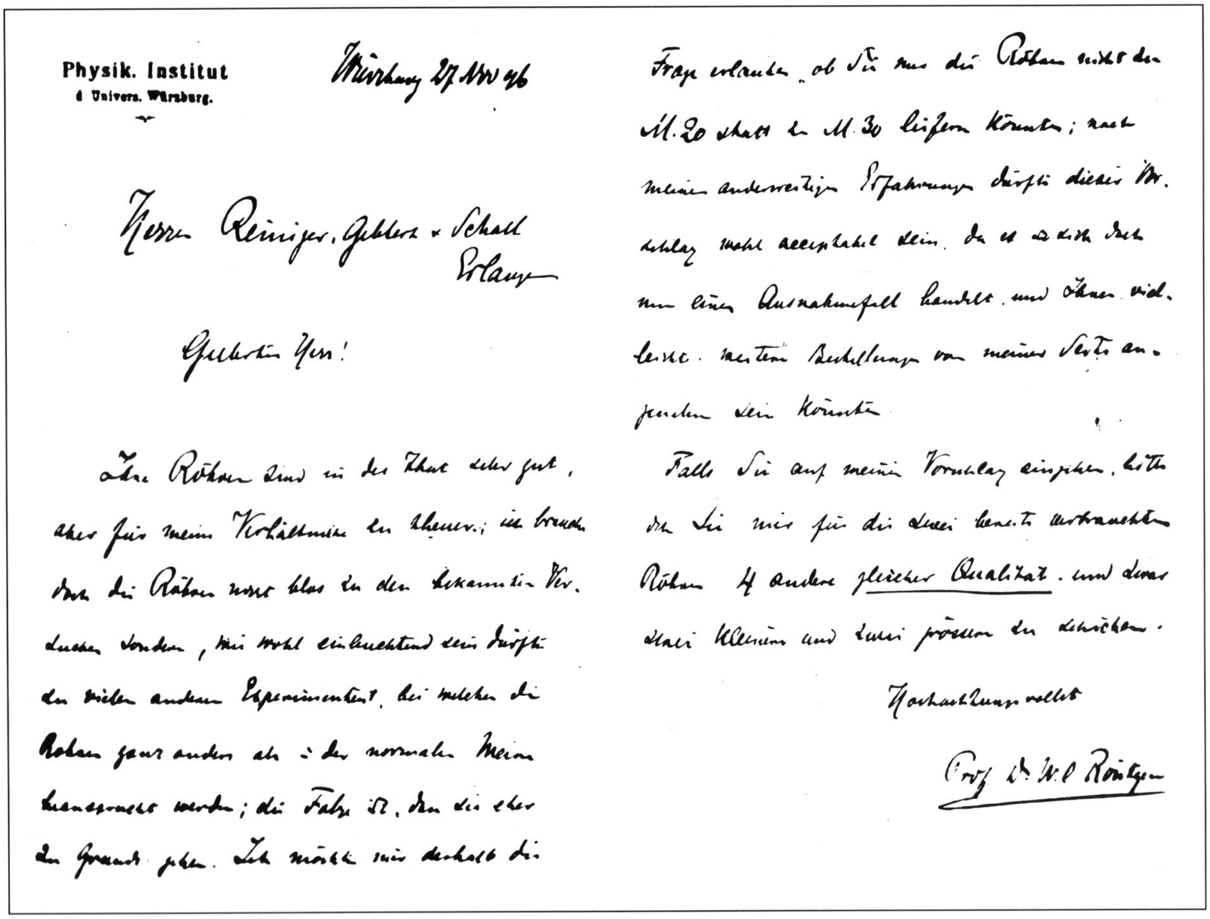

Fig. V, 4. Letter by Professor Roentgen to Reiniger, Gebbert and Schall in Erlangen, dated Wuerzburg, 27 November 1896. Translation: *Physics Institute, University of Wuerzburg. Dear Sir, Your X-ray tubes are indeed very good, but too expensive for my situation; after all, I need the X-ray tubes not only for known experiments but also, as should be obvious, for many other experiments which put much more wear on the X-ray tubes than is normal; consequently they are ruined earlier. For this reason, I am taking the liberty of asking whether you could sell me the X-ray tubes for 20 Marks instead of 30 Marks. From experiences I have had elsewhere, this proposal should be quite acceptable, since it is an exceptional case and you might perhaps be interested in further orders from me. In the event that you accept my proposal I would like to ask you to replace the two X-ray tubes already used with four others of the same quality – namely two smaller and two larger ones.Sincerely yours, (signature) Prof. Dr W.C. Roentgen.*

did in light emitters. He proved this by pinhole camera exposures of the focal spot: the more the angle of the beam examined approached the tangent to the anode surface, the smaller the focal spot became; however, the density did not decrease. He also clearly observed a dose reduction in the marginal zones of small anode angles of less than $10°$, now called the Heel effect. He expressly recommended the use of small anode angles to improve definition, but to avoid the range of a few degrees.

The tubes were manufactured in all kinds of shapes and sizes (Fig. V, 5). Auxiliary spheres were intended to ensure a larger volume for better constancy of gas ions. The glass should not be too thick on the exit side of the X-rays, as the absorption of rays would be too high, with corresponding attenuation. Lindemann therefore produced a glass of relatively low atomic weight materials that was more transparent to X-rays.

Gas ions determine radiation hardness

The quality of the radiation depended upon its hardness, which was affected by residual gases in the tube and the efficiency of the spark inductor. Low pressures of 0.005 mbar (0.5 Pa) required a high operating voltage and produced 'hard' radiation. Higher pressures of 0.015 mbars (1.5 Pa) required a low operating voltage and produced 'soft' radiation. The gas ions de-

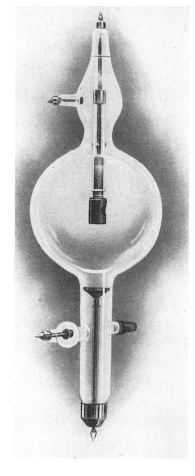

Fig. V, 5. 1913: Reiniger, Gebbert and Schall ion tube for the REKORD apparatus, with very small focal spot, also to be used with induction apparatus and electrolytical interrupter. Platinum anticathode (price 76 Marks): for higher output in rapid sequence exposure technique, an anticathode of iridium is recommended (price 96 Marks); the diameter of the glass sphere is approximately 190 mm [40].

The French physicist P. Villard introduced osmotic regeneration using palladium in 1897. The palladium tube had to be heated with a flame. Hydrogen was conducted by osmosis into the X-ray tube, making the radiation softer.

Another regeneration device – introduced by C.H.F. Mueller in 1898 – was made of activated carbon or mica ('mica regeneration'). Traces of gas and water were bonded between the individual layers and were only released on heating. Activated carbon releases gas into the vacuum much more easily than mica, so that only slight heat was needed to regenerate the tubes.

H. Bauer succeeded (1908) in regenerating tubes using a capillary tube filled with mercury. A second tube was connected to the side and sealed at both ends with plates made of a permeable clay-like material, which admitted air but not mercury. The mercury column could be raised and lowered by remote operation of a rubber ball. The entry of gas into the tube could thus be precisely controlled. This so-called Bauer valve was a major contribution to the lengthening of tube life.

Tubes with automatic release of gases were developed to simplify the work of radiologists. As the resistance in the tube increased and therefore the voltage rose, sparks passed through a small tube initiating the release of gas. The width of the spark gap could be adjusted according to the required degree of hardness.

The consumption of gas ions had already been slowed by the introduction of the anticathode, because the glass was subject to less stress and therefore less gas ions were absorbed. Larger tubes with a corresponding increase in the volume of gas residues have not prevailed in practice.

creased in number during operation because of absorption by released metal atoms. The gas deficit could be compensated for at first but only by increasing the voltage, which meant that the X-rays increasingly hardened, were of shorter wavelengths, with more energy, and thus more penetrating. 'Regeneration' was therefore applied to soften 'hard' tubes. It was based on one of two principles: the release of gas from gas-combining substances inside the tube by treatment from the outside, or the supply of gas from the outside [P1]. A device to regulate the degree of hardness was a very important component of ion X-ray tubes.

Even before Roentgen's discovery, William Crookes in England used potash, a hygroscopic powder, to regenerate his tubes in discharge experiments. Potash, which releases gas when heated, was placed in a thin tube connected to the X-ray tube. Roentgen, at an early stage, also used lime tree charcoal to regenerate his tubes. Carbon required only slight heating to release gas into the vacuum.

Tantalum or tungsten instead of platinum?

Platinum was a considerably better anode material than aluminium. The melting point of platinum is 1755°C whereas that of aluminium is 660°C. But platinum was also far from being the best material. Platinum was replaced by tantalum [P 6] in 1906. Tantalum indeed has a slightly lower atomic number than platinum, yet it has a considerably higher thermal load capacity due to its melting point of almost 3000°C.

It was known for a long time that tungsten has a very high melting point of almost 3380°C and an atomic number of 74. Unfortunately it could not be shaped in a suitable manner into an electrode until 1904 when a Siemens patent [P7] was granted. However, it took a further 5 years (1909) until the tungsten anode became a practical proposition. F. Dessauer's 'BLITZ' with a tungsten anticathode tube could achieve exposure times of 0.01 s. Up to the present time, tungsten has remained the basic material for anodes.

Focal spot size and extrafocal radiation

Using a pinhole camera, Roentgen had already established in his third communication that, in a *'correctly designed'* tube which was not too *'soft'*, the radiation came from a spot, 1–2 mm in size, where the cathode rays strikes the platinum plate. The existence of extrafocal radiation, as it is called today, was also recognized. This is emitted at low intensity from the platinum plate outside the focal spot and also from the glass wall.

How is the heat dissipated?

High thermal loads on the anodes require long breaks in operation, for which reason, early attempts were made to dissipate and compensate for the *'accumulating thermal masses'* on the anticathode (Gocht, 1914; s. Fig. I, 23) and to prevent it becoming too intensively hot and incandescent.

In the high-metal-content tubes, the anticathode was enlarged by solid or tubular metal masses, by which more heat was absorbed and dissipated into the surroundings [P 3, P 5]. The larger amount of metal also ensured a comparatively constant vacuum by releasing gas. The MAMMUT tube from Mueller had a particularly voluminous copper anticathode to increase the heat capacity.

In the low-metal-content tubes, the anode was cooled by air or carbon dioxide, by water or a combination of different coolants. The rib-shaped configuration of the anticathode head ensured better heat distribution, whereas a hole drilled in the anticathode shaft close to the focal spot improved heat exchange by permitting a flow of air, carbon dioxide or water (Fig. V, 7).

The anticathode of a water-cooled tube [P 4] formed the bottom of a vessel filled with water. The circulation of the hot water next to the anticathode over a relatively wide connecting tube to the water reservoir had to be guaranteed. Water was preferred as coolant since it is a better conductor of heat than air. A further development was the boiler tube which used the latent heat of evaporation for cooling. It is known that each gram of water evaporating requires 536 calories (2251 J) of heat. This tube delivered relatively constant radiation.

There was a large variety of different types of tubes in the first two decades after the discovery of X-rays, because numerous companies developed their own models. Despite its many weaknesses, the ion tube was a governing factor in X-ray technology for almost 20 years. The book Development of the Ion X-ray Tube by Paul Rønne and Arnold B.W. Nielsen (1986) [38] provides a good picture of which paths were followed to improve it and what developmental work was undertaken.

High-vacuum tubes

Although much was achieved with the tungsten anode, the deficiencies and limitations of the existing ion tube remained, as summarized by W. Coolidge (Fig. V, 6), an employee of General Electric in 1913 (Coolidge, 1914, 1914/15; Coolidge and Charlton, 1945 [8, 9, 10]).

– *With low discharge currents the vacuum gradually improves, with a consequent increase in the penetrating power of the rays produced.*
– *With high discharge currents there are very rapid vacuum changes, sometimes in one direction and sometimes in the other.*
– *If a heavy discharge current is continued for more than a few seconds the target is heated to redness and then gives off so much gas that the tube may have to be reëxhausted.*
– *If the temperature of the standard copper-backed target is allowed to get up to bright redness, a rapid deposition of metallic copper begins to take place on the bulb.*

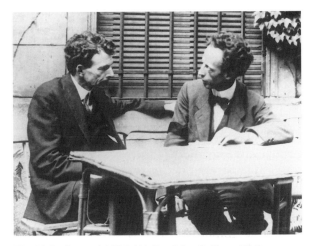

Fig. V, 6. Around 1921: W. Coolidge (left) and F. Dessauer (right) in discussion.

– Of the tubes tested, very many have failed from cracking of the glass in the zone around the cathode.

– The focal spot on the target in many tubes wanders about very rapidly.

– While it is relatively easy to lower the tube resistance by means of the various gas regulators, it is a relatively slow matter to raise it much.

– No two tubes are exactly alike in their electrical characteristics.

– When operated on a periodically intermittent current, even though it be of constant potential, the tube, of necessity, gives a very heterogeneous bundle of primary Röntgen rays.

Cooling there – heat here

A few years before Roentgen's discovery, experiments showed that incandescent metals emit electrons in a vacuum. This finding was soon applied to X-ray tubes. Experiments had already been performed in 1905 by A. Wehnelt and Trenkle to generate cathode rays independent of gas ions. This tube was not suitable for medical applications because the tube voltage was too low. Residual gas ions affected emission and operation. The vacuum had to be very high, four to five orders of magnitude better than in the ion tubes, so that the tubes were also called 'gas-free tubes' or 'electron tubes'.

In 1911/1912 J. E. Lilienfeld (Lilienfeld and Rosenthal, 1911/12 [34]) described and patented an 'X-ray tube of arbitrarily and instantaneously adjustable hardness independent of vacuum' (Fig. V, 7). It had a filament (G) which was fed by a filament transformer (Tr). The cathode (K) consisted of an aluminium cylinder which was lined on the inside with quartz and contained a perforated cathode facing the anode (A) located above. A potential of a few kilovolts existed between the cathode and the filament–adjusted with the resistor (W). The electrons emitted from the filament struck the perforated cathode, exciting secondary electrons that were accelerated towards the copper anode which had a platinum coating. A rectified tube voltage was applied between the filament and anode. This tube was equipped with water cooling. Advantages were initially seen in the two-stage discharge, as a focused electron beam generated a small focal spot, and in the homogenizing effect of the perforated cathode.

Only one year after Lilienfeld in 1912, R. Fuerstenau combined the filament with the cathode in the tube named after him, which, however, operated with the vacuum still customary for ion

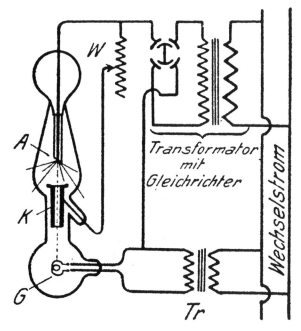

Fig. V, 7. 1911: Principal sketch of the Lilienfeld X-ray tube [24]. It had a filament (G) which was fed by a filament transformer (Tr). The cathode (K) consisted of an aluminium cylinder which was lined on the inside with quartz and contained a perforated cathode facing the water-cooled anode (A) located above. A potential of a few kilovolts existed between the cathode and the filament – adjusted by the resistor (W).

tubes. Fuerstenau believed that gas ionization was important, so his tube lacked the high vacuum as the decisive criterion and therefore received no practical acclaim. The Lilienfeld tube, on the other hand, was a popular and much-valued tube for several years, despite its complicated mode of operation.

The American engineer W.D. Coolidge (1914, 1914/15) [9, 10] reported in 1913 on 'A powerful roentgen ray tube with a pure electron discharge', a paper which was also immediately published in German in 'Fortschritte der Roentgenstrahlen'.

Coolidge had already replaced the aluminium cathode with an incandescent tungsten wire filament. This provided him with the interesting possibility of obtaining electrons directly from a hot controllable cathode. Coolidge stated that he had been prompted by I. Langmuir's work. The electron emission of hot tungsten wires was also stable and reproducible at a very high vacuum and it would indeed be advantageous to free the cathode wires from their residual gas. The New York radiologist L.G. Cole (1914) [6, 7] presented the new type of tube during an official dinner. The incandescent cathode tube enabled the anode voltage, and thus the hardness of the radiation, to be independently adjusted from the anode current. The power was more than ten times increased compared with the ion tube. Exposures became reproducible and radiation exposure was reduced at the same time, primarily because the need for repeated exposures as a result of poor image quality lessened. The principle of Coolidge's incandescent cathode in a high vacuum is used exclusively in X-ray tube design to the present day. The development of the Coolidge tube would not be conceivable without the preliminary work of O.W. Richardson, J. Elster, H. Beitel, A. Wehnelt and I. Langmuir.

The surgeon and line focus

One day G. Katsch, a physician for internal medicine, had lunch with his cousin Otto Goetze (1886–1955) (Fig. V, 8), also a young surgeon, at the University in Halle in 1917. Katsch complained about unsharp radiographs. Goetze, who had occupied himself with radiological studies of operated stomachs, knew of E. Regener's (1917) [39] ideas, and wondered about a solution. In Goetze's opinion, a surgeon had to have a good understanding of engineering, and he found the solution for an increased output of the focal spot without increasing its optical size: the line focus (Fig. V, 9) [26, P9]. A roughly square optical focal spot (Fig. V, 10) was generated by the projection of a rectangle with a length ratio of 3:1 on a 20° slope.

The old established Mueller company started to design experimental high-vacuum tubes with

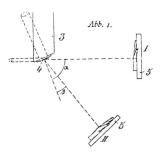
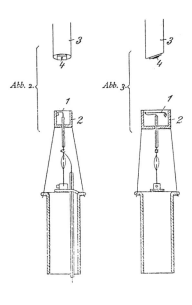

Fig. V, 9. 1918: Sketch of a patent [P9] of Dr Otto Goetze for the line focus which has been in use in practically all diagnostic X-ray tubes up to the present day. Dr Katsch, a physician for internal medicine, lamented about blurred radiographs to the young surgeon Goetze in Halle on their way to lunch. Goetze knew of a paper by Regener (1917) [39] and thought about a solution to Katsch's complaint. The company CHF Mueller in Hamburg started to design a tube in 1917 and Dr Chaoul in Munich performed the first clinical tests in the summer of 1919. He testified that the new tube with line focus showed impressive results in the recognition of detail.

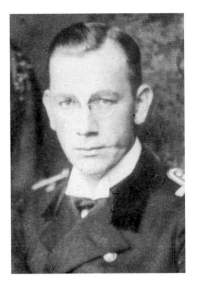

Fig. V, 8. Otto Goetze (1886–1955) Professor of Surgery who worked in Halle, Frankfurt/M, and Erlangen. He cared very much about engineering sciences. Radiographs were a very important part of his daily surgical activity. Inventor [P9] of the line focus. This portrait from 1919 was donated by his daughter Dr Ortrud Goetze in Fuerth.

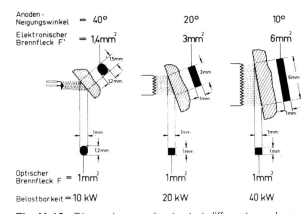

Fig. V, 10. Dimensions and output at different anode angles of an optical focal spot of 1.0; output increases from 10 kW to 20 kW and 40 kW. The round focal spot (40°/10 kW) was replaced by the line focus (20°/20 kW) in 1923. A spot-film focus (10°/40 kW) was introduced in 1963 [44].

a line focus. H. Chaoul was able to take the first clinical radiographs in Munich in 1919 and found that this tube provided very-high-definition images. However, it took another 3 years until this tube became commercially available as the MEDIA tube with line focus or 'Goetze focus'. Goetze's ideas were significant for the realization of smaller foci with increased loadability.

The fact that two different aspects – motion blurring and spatial resolution – were important in imaging caused G.C. Kucher [P 10] and his team to build a tube with two focal spots, a large high-power focal spot for full format exposures and a small one for fine detail reproduction (Fig. V, 11). This double-focus principle was available in 1923 as the DOFOK tube. Initially this tube was designed with a round filament, although the patent included both filament designs for round and line focus.

Radiation protection in and on the tube

There were attempts to provide radiation protection at the turn of the century. The first protective devices originate from F. Dessauer (Fig. V, 6), who surrounded the anticathode with a tube shield which had a lateral window for the exit of the X-rays. The beryllium window from Siemens [P11] prevented the creation of secondary radiation by absorption of electrons.

A. Bouwers (Fig. V, 14) [3, 29] developed the METALIX metal glass tube in 1927. Only the tube ends and the exit port for the X-rays were made of glass, the rest of the tube being of a chromium iron alloy. This tube was additionally surrounded by a lead cylinder. A cross-section of the Siemens TUTO tube housing is shown in Figs. V, 12 and V, 61.

The 'Roentgen KUGEL' (s. Fig. V, 55) came on the market in 1933. It was a single tank unit housing the tube and the high-voltage transformer in a metal sphere only 22 cm in diameter. This tube could be operated at 60 kV and 10 mA. This was only possible because oil was used for both insulation and heat dissipation. This Siemens KUGEL served in many medical practices and hospitals for half a century.

Rotating anode tube

Motion blurring, particularly of chest and internal organs, caused by respiratory movements, pulsation of vessels and peristalsis, was not only disturbing to the eye when assessing exposures

Fig. V, 11. 1923: Double focus X-ray tube made by Kucher of Phoenix, the X-ray tube factory in Rudolstadt, Thuringia.

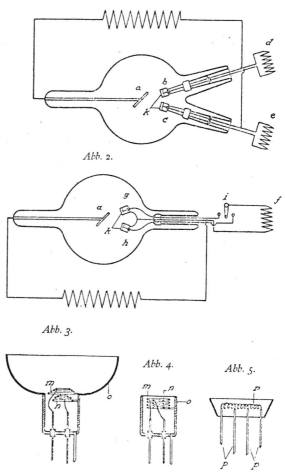

Abb. 2.

Abb. 3.

Abb. 4.   *Abb. 5.*

Fig. V, 11a. Sketch from the patent [P10]. X-ray tube with high-vacuum and two or more independently controlled filaments which generate X-rays in the anticathode of different focal spot sizes. The idea was to provide a small focal spot with high-detail resolution in fluoroscopy besides a powerful focal spot for radiographs. Most diagnostic X-ray tubes still use this principal, especially in angiography.

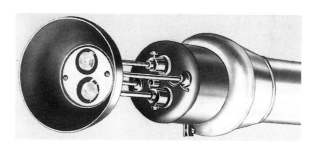

Fig. V, 11b. Cathode design with two spiral filaments.

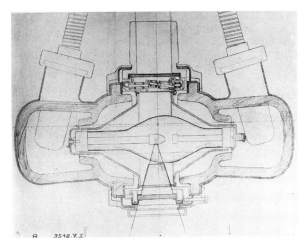

Fig. V, 12. 1931: Drawing of the TUTO tube housing assembly with radiation protection, designed by Siemens.

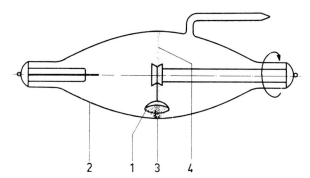

Fig. V, 13. 1897: R.W. Wood proposed a rotating X-ray tube [13]. The cathode (1) remains in place by force of gravity while the glass sphere (2) rotates around the cathode. The electrons hit the glass wall to create the focal spot (3). The heat generated is now distributed in a focal spot track during rotation (4).

but also affected the diagnosis, so that certain lesions were detected with less accuracy, or not at all. If the tube was to contribute to the reduction of motion blurring, its capacity had to be increased to achieve shorter exposure times. Of course, factors such as focal spot size and radiation hardness, which essentially influenced image quality, had also to be considered. The electrons emitted by the filament in high-vacuum tubes heated the anode after a few exposures to such a degree that even the high melting point of tungsten of more than 3400 °C and the line focus design were not sufficient to withstand high emissions. For optic–geometric reasons, electrons had to be deflected only onto a very small area of the anode.

Cooling the focal spot by rotating the anode

A technical milestone had been reached in X-ray tubes with the tungsten anode, line focus and double focus. Only one solution brought further progress, in which the anode material was moved beneath the focal spot, and therefore mechanically provided heat transfer. Only in this fashion could the heat capacity be increased without exceeding material-dependent temperature limits.

As early as 1897, when it was still customary to decelerate the cathode rays in the glass bulb, the American R.W. Wood proposed a mechanical solution, in which the cathode rays struck glass that was cold or cooled-down by rotation of the glass bulb (Fig. V, 13). Platinum came into use as anode material at the same time, so this idea was not pursued. In 1910, W.C. Kaye (1910) [31] re-

ported on an ion X-ray tube he had built with a rotating anticathode made of platinum and in 1914, E. Pohl attempted to increase the heat capacity of the anticathode of radiation therapy tubes by relative movements of cathode or anticathode [P 8].

A year later, following a proposal by E. Thomson (Coolidge, 1915) [11], General Electric attempted the construction of a rotating anode tube. It was already very similar to our present-day rotating anode tube principle, which has generally been adopted for standard tubes. It consisted of an eccentrically arranged cathode and a flat anode disk, rotating at 750 revolutions per minute, with a focal spot track diameter of approximately 2 cm. At that time it was still not possible to manufacture larger and thicker tungsten disks. This prototype was not robust enough for diagnostic purposes.

The first laboratory prototype of a rotating anode tube from Siemens in 1927 should also be mentioned among these attempts. Experiments were also undertaken with high-temperature radiation cooling in the development of these tubes (Ungelenk, 1934) [45]. Physical measurements showed that the heat dissipation from a surface increases to the fourth power of the absolute temperature. This means that, if the anode temperature is doubled, it would be possible to increase the heat dissipation capacity 16-fold. This trail-blazing finding by Siemens using high-temperature radiation cooling is applied in all rotating anode tubes nowadays.

A. Bouwers (1929, 1963) [4, 5] (Fig. V, 14), the great Dutch radiophysicist, who at first worked at Philips and later at De Oude Delft, is acknowledged to have designed and built the first com-

Fig. V, 14.
Albert Bouwers, Professor Dr., Dr. h. c. (1893–1972), worked at Philips in the Roentgen and high-voltage laboratory from 1920 on. He was the father of the initial load theory (continuous falling load during an X-ray exposure) and designed the first usable rotating anode tube [4]. In 1941, he joined N.V. Optical Industries 'De Oude Delft' as chief engineer, developing and producing mass fluorography cameras such as the ODELKA and the CINELIX for the recording of cine runs. [5]

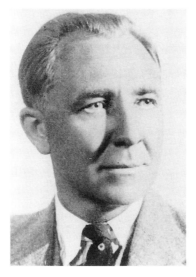

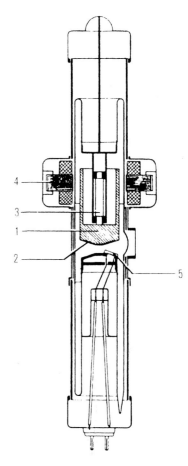

Fig. V, 15. 1929: ROTALIX X-ray tube designed by A. Bouwers (Philips) for clinical use, shown in a sectional view [4]. The anode (1) was made of a copper cylinder with an angled area for the anode consisting of a tungsten ring (2). The copper cylinder served as a rotor (3) and was built into the X-ray tube. Outside the X-ray tube was the stator (4) to drive the anode. The filament of the cathode (5) was opposite the rotating anode, eccentrically mounted so that electrons hit the tungsten ring of the anode to generate X-rays.

mercially available rotating anode tube in 1929. It was a tube with tungsten–copper anode and a radiation protection tube housing called the RO-TALIX tube (Figs. V, 15 and V, 16). The anode – a tungsten ring embedded in a solid copper cylinder – was rotated by an induction motor. The rotor was connected directly to the anode inside the vacuum of the tube, the stator was housed outside the tube. Rotating anode tubes have been continuously developed since 1929. The ROTALIX tube could only be operated to temperatures of a few hundred degrees centigrade, and was therefore not suitable for high continuous output.

The PANTIX tube

A. Ungelenk (1934) [45, 46] took a major step forward in 1933 with the PANTIX tube (Figs. V, 17 and V, 18). An anode disk made of solid tungsten, mounted on a thin molybdenum shaft running on ball bearings was used in series production for the first time. The drive was with 50 Hz line frequency and brought the tungsten disk to just on 2800 revolutions per minute. The 80 mm anode disk permitted the effective use of high-temperature radiation cooling. In addition, the high voltage was fed into the tube housing for the first time through insulated high-voltage cables. The PANTIX tube had built-in airflow cooling using a fan and was characterized by its high level of safety for both patient and medical staff. A focal spot of 1.2 allowed an output of

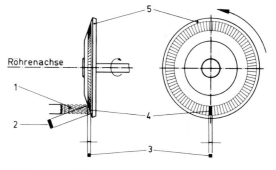

Röhrenachse

1 Elektronenstrahl	4 Brennfleck
2 Wahre Brennfleckfläche	5 Wolframteller
3 Wirksame Brennfleckgröße	

Fig. V, 16. Principal of a rotating anode tube [44]. (1) electron beam, (2) actual area of the focal spot (electronically), (3) optical focal spot, and (4) focus location on (5) the tungsten anode disk.

20 kW at an exposure time of 0.1 s; 40 kW was reached with a focal spot of 2.0. The heat radiating surface of the 80 mm anode disk and the useable heat capacity matched the lower radiological demands in those days, taking into consideration the necessary cooling periods. Thus almost unlimited flouroscopy and radiography was possible.

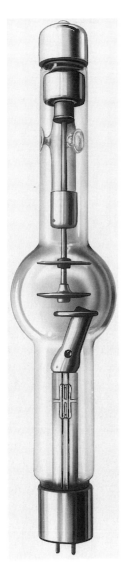

Fig. V, 17. 1934:
Siemens introduced the rotating
anode X-ray tube with a tungsten
anode disk, using high-temperature radiation cooling [45];
focus 1.2 (air-cooling outside the
glass envelope).

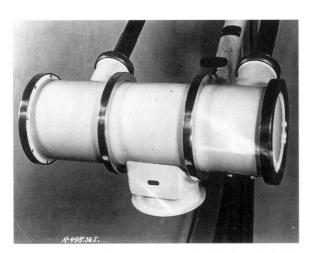

Fig. V, 18. 1949: An oil-filled X-ray tube housing assembly
(HAUBE) for the PANTIX P20/40ö rotating anode tube with
two focal spots of 1.2/20 kW and 2.0/40 kW (the tube window is at the bottom of the picture).

In later years, further increases in output resulted from the use of tungsten anode disks
with larger diameters and, in addition, higher rotational speeds. Increasing the track radius of the
focal spot produced a further increase of heat
capacity and detail resolution.

X-ray cinematography

Since the beginnings of radiography, physicians
have attempted the display of moving objects
with cinematography. Relatively high radiation
exposure occurred in this case, because the radiation could not be switched off during film transport from one image to the next.

A PANTIX tube with a 100 mm anode was developed in 1937 for X-ray cinematography. For
dose reasons, but also to thermally relieve the anode, this was switched synchronously with the
shutter-open phase of the cine camera. The mechanical switches customary at that time allowed,
at the most, one to two exposures per second. A
grid-controlled cathode, switching without delay,
was therefore developed. The 'pull' of the continuously applied high voltage was neutralized
by a negative voltage of 1–2 kV between the filament and the cathode head. The electrons were
held back in the cathode. The tube emitted radiation only when the grid voltage was turned off. It
was now possible to prolong the cine run by 25%
at the same output and dose level.

Hard radiation technique – why?

By the forties, the tube voltage had been increased to 125 kV, to 150 kV by 1952 and, finally, in 1959, to 200 kV. The high kV technique
(Wachsmann et al, 1952; Gajewski, 1953) [25,
48] gained in importance primarily for chest
X-rays. Hard radiation penetrated the ribs, so
that pathological lesions of the lungs behind
them could be visualized on the X-ray film. However, the anode disk diameter was also increased
to 100 mm at this time, which made special demands on the rupture strength of tungsten at
such high rotational speeds. In addition, the
cooling of the tube and tube housing was
changed from air to oil (Fenner, 1953) [19]. A
focal spot output of 30 kW could thus be
achieved. These tubes with oil cooling at increased output had become smaller, since the
oil served simultaneously as an insulator. The entire unit comprised the tube, stator for the drive
of the anode disk, tube protective shield and

connection of the high-voltage cables, was called the 'tube housing assembly'.

The dual-angle anode

The double focus has been available in rotating anode tubes since 1945. In the early fifties, the need for different focal spot sizes arose, to assess fine details better where necessary. The solution was the Silbermann patent [P14] which was granted in 1954 and implemented in the first commercial product, the BIANGULIX tube, in 1957. K. Silbermann's idea was to make the anode disk with two different angles, e.g. 10° and 19°, and to install two filaments into the cathode for each individual focal spot track. The large angle of 19° is required to expose the large cassette format of 14×17 inches in full. Naturally the small angle is used for spot films, to radiograph very fine details (Pressler, 1959) [37]. A positive side effect was an increased lifespan of the tube, since two filaments and two focal spot tracks were operated one at a time in one tube. The lifespan of the focal spot track was determined by its roughening due to heat. It led to a drastic drop in dose, so that the radiation intensity of the tube decreased and longer exposure times therefore became necessary. W. Frik (1959) [22] ascertained, through extensive investigations, that the 40 kW focal spot is suitable for fluoroscopy.

Increasing the anode disk speed to 8500 revolutions per minute – three times the line frequency – provided further improvements in detail resolution and penetration capacity. This new tube – Super ROTALIX – was available in 1959 with focal spots of 0.6 at 14 kW and 1.2 at 50 kW (Fenner, 1956; Fenner and Joachim, 1957; Kuntke, 1957; Roeck and Milne, 1978; DIN/IEC, 1981) [15, 20, 21, 32, 41].

The focal spot size of X-ray tubes was standardized at a much later date. The electronic focal spot on the anode was elliptical, because the anticathode was inclined and the filament circular. The electronic focal spot on the anode became rectangular only on introduction of the line focus – the edge length could therefore be measured in millimetres, corresponding to the power density in the anode material: watts per square millimetre (W/mm^2). However, the optical focal spot, which can be documented on an X-ray film with a pinhole camera, was important for image quality. It should be roughly square. The tolerances in the manufacturing process of glass tubes were of course very large, so that edge lengths with a 100% increase were not infrequent. IEC, the International Electrotechnical Commission, in conjunction with the Deutsche Industrie Norm, DIN, defined a new focal spot nominal value without dimensions. Each number, according to DIN/IEC 336/1981 [15], has been defined with maximum dimensions in width and length as well as the associated measuring procedure: for example, a focal spot with a nominal value of 1.0 may be a maximum of 1.4 mm wide and 2.0 mm long.

Several metals compounded

It was metallurgy that made possible the next innovation in the design of X-ray tubes: the element rhenium. This was discovered in 1925 by I. and W. Noddack and O.C. Berg in Hamburg and has an atomic number of 75. It is therefore better than tungsten, and has a melting point of 3180°C [P15]. Tungsten anodes with an addition of 5–10% rhenium (Elsaß, 1962) [18] suffered less roughening and crater formation in the focal spot track (Fig. V, 19). Rhenium was a very expensive material and could therefore not be used in all tungsten anode disks, although the radiation yield was increased and thus the value of the tube. The anode disk was also redesigned by applying an alloy layer of tungsten-rhenium of about 2 mm thickness to a thick layer of molybdenum. The X-radiation is produced in the tungsten-rhenium layer. The advantage of this composite anode was the good heat-storage capacity of molybdenum, which, however, is only half as heavy as tungsten. Thus a larger volume of material could be achieved without a weight increase.

Why is the weight of the tube or anode so important? Different dose rates are required for fluoroscopy and radiography. Fluoroscopy is used for orientation and functional examination and radiography for filming. Both are combined in spot filming. Since this is performed with a high kilowatt output and with the shortest possible exposure time, the anode must rotate with the highest possible revolutions per minute. This, however, reduces the lifespan of the ball bearings. No rotation is necessary in fluoroscopy because of the low output of a few hundred watts. So the rotating anode is stopped by the high speed starter directly after each exposure [P 12]. However, since the transition time from fluoroscopy to radiography must be short, the filament must be heated to high emission within about 1 s and the rotating anode disk must be accelerated to full speed simultaneously. The high-

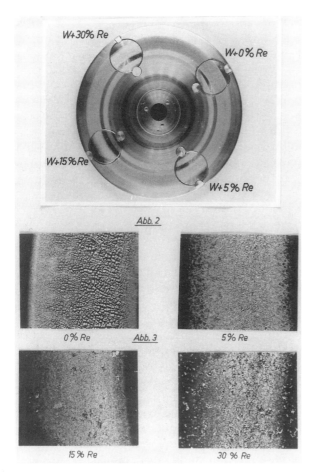

Fig. V, 19. 1960: A rotating anode of rhenium tungsten alloy (SRW laboratory memo V-Lab E/NE from 5 July 1960). The top figure (Abb. 2) shows the test arrangement and the four bottom figures (Abb. 3) the surface of the pieces magnified. The pure tungsten piece without any rhenium (0% Re) shows a significant decrease in dose output and a very rough surface.

speed starter has to overcome the inertia of the anode disk. Accordingly, the lighter the anode disk, the faster is its acceleration. This innovative anode disk design is called the RTM anode (rhenium, tungsten, molybdenum). With a speed of 8500 revolutions per minute, and the proven dual angle or BIANGULIX principle according to Silbermann [P14], this tube had a small focal spot of 0.6 at 30 kW and a large focal spot of 1.0 at 50 kW. Two BIANGULIX Rapid versions were combined with the small 0.6 focal spot: focal spot 1.3 at 100 kW or 1.8 at 150 kW.

Angiography and overtable tubes: a new challenge

The need to further increase the available energy never diminishes, even 100 years after Roentgen's discovery of X-rays. Thus, in 1969, the back of the RTM disk was blackened [P 18] thereby increasing the dissipation of heat. Overtable tubes needed higher tube output to compensate for the unfavourable geometry of source-film distances between 1.20 and 1.50 m. These systems are used particularly in gastrointestinal diagnostics. Not only economic pressure forced physicians to examine more patients in less time but also angiography, the imaging of vessels with contrast medium, became increasingly frequent, requiring higher tube outputs. Thus the black layer on the back of the RTM anode with a disk diameter of 100 mm was replaced by solid graphite (Figs. V, 20 and V, 21) [P 16]. This so-called CALOREX anode was introduced in 1973 primarily for angiographic examinations, but also on overtable units for radiography, spot films and tomography (Friedel and Haberrecker, 1973) [23]. Graphite is only a tenth as heavy as tungsten and has an excellent heat-storage capacity.

The anode of such a highly efficient overtable work station had to be warmed slowly to prevent radial cracking of the disk (Fig. V, 22) and bursting of the anode (Dietz, 1974) [14]. One of the ways to achieve this was by switching fluoroscopy on before an examination. This was not advisable, however, because of radiation safety considerations. Another solution was to choose exposures that required minimal energy to be carried out first but this was not often feasible. During daily radiological practice, all kinds of exposures are needed at different times of the day. It was quite possible that the first exposure of the day might be a lumbar spine, carried out with a cold anode. The lifespan of tubes was therefore limited, because the disk became cracked. To avoid these cracks, K. Dietz [P 17] had slots machined into the anode disk during manufacture (Fig. V, 23). Anode stress was thereby relieved and high-energy exposures on a cold anode were possible. This anode became available in 1972 and made a significant contribution to radiation hygiene as well as to the lifespan of the tube.

There was a particular need in neuroradiology to visualize very fine intracranial vessels. This challenge led to the design of the OPTILIX tube (Crolla et al, 1979) [12], which became available in 1976. Apart from reducing the size of the focal spot, there was only one alterna-

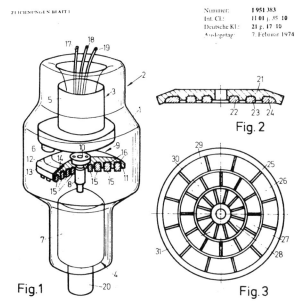

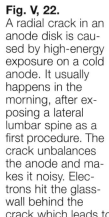

Fig. 2

Fig.1   Fig. 3

Fig. V, 20. 1969: Drawing from a patent [P16] of an X-ray tube with increased heat storage capacity using graphite on the back of the anode disk.

Fig. V, 22.
A radial crack in an anode disk is caused by high-energy exposure on a cold anode. It usually happens in the morning, after exposing a lateral lumbar spine as a first procedure. The crack unbalances the anode and makes it noisy. Electrons hit the glass-wall behind the crack which leads to the destruction of the tube [14].

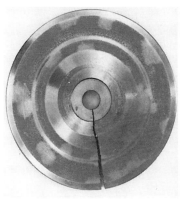

Fig. V, 23. 1971: Stress-relieved anode [P17]. The disk has many slots. This prevents radial cracks under heavy exposure (high kWs), such as an exposure of a lumbar spine on a cold anode.

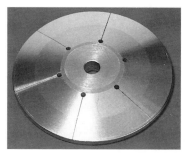

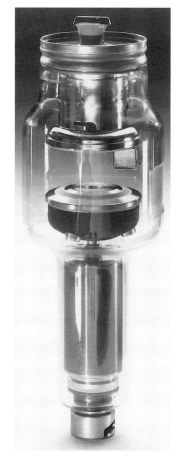

Fig. V, 21.
1982: CALOREX anode disk [P16] for a POLYPHOS single-tank generator with a focal spot 1.3/30 kW at 50 Hz or 1.0/30 kW at 60 Hz or two focal spots 0.5/20 kW and 1.0/50 kW at 200 Hz.

tive, namely to increase the speed of the anode disk. Since the output of the focal spot depended among other things upon the square root of the speed, doubling the speed resulted in an output increase of approximately 40%. However, this effect can also be utilized in reverse, namely reducing the focal spot size while maintaining the output. Thus it was possible by state-of-the-art power electronics to build a high speed starter for 300 Hz, equal to 17 000 revolutions per minute.

This very high anode disk speed allows the operation of focal spots of 0.2 at 12 kW and of 0.6 at 50 kW. The smallest vessels can now be imaged, even magnified, with high contrast (Crolla et al, 1979; Gould and Genant, 1981) [12, 27].

Fluoroscopy with three-dimensional impression: stereoradioscopy

Stereo images were known from photography even before the discovery of X-rays. It was therefore not surprising that experiments with stereo

X-ray images were immediately undertaken. However, a successful breakthrough was never achieved, although those who could see the stereo images three-dimensionally were enthusiastic about them. Engineers created a new design in the eighties: the OPTILIX tube was built into a tube housing assembly that allowed a mechanical angular shift of the focal spot position [P 22] at a frequency of up to three images per second: the STEREOLIX tube. The focal spot offset was 25 mm and produced outstanding stereo exposures with a magnification factor of two, primarily in neuroradiology but also in gastrointestinal diagnostics with double contrast. The stereo technique found no general use in fluoroscopy.

A further difficulty in angiocardiography was that the coronary arteries were not only thin but also moved in the same rhythm of the systole and diastole with velocities of up to 200 mm/s (Berger, 1961) [2]. Image intensifiers with 7-inch diameters are sufficient for cine radiography to display the heart. Therefore, the anode disk angle could be reduced to around 8°, corresponding to the system geometry. Short exposure times of only a few milliseconds and a small focal spot at high tube output are required to display these fast-moving coronaries with the smallest possible motion blurring. Reducing the angle to 8° enlarges the area of the electronic focal spot in which the power is converted while at the same time the size of the optically effective focal spot is decreased. A focal spot of 0.6 at 40 kW and 0.8 at 100 kW was achieved.

Ceramics instead of glass

The thermal loading of the X-ray tube was extreme, and so new materials were tested. The Super-ROTALIX ceramic tube came on the market in 1979 (Hartl, 1990) [30]. Here glass could be replaced by a metal–ceramic combination. These two materials could be produced with higher precision than glass. Manufacturing glass tubes is indeed a skilful art.

Fine focus for angiography

The first three-focus tube for angiography was built in 1981. This tube had two line focal spots, the smaller one of which could even be made smaller by applying a negative voltage to the cathode head. This was made possible by a cathode design like the one used for the grid-controlled PANTIX tube as used in 1937. In the cine mode, the selected voltage is so high (2.8 kV) that no electrons escape from the cathode, even though the tube voltage is switched on.

If a grid voltage with a value of a few hundred volts only is applied, the emerging electron beam is compressed somewhat more in the breadth than in the length. In this way the optically effective focal spot is reduced in size and can also be used for fine focus or as a microfocal spot for super-selective angiography and magnification techniques.

Expansion of angiography and angioplasty

The eighties once again brought innovations through a variety of requirements for angiography and computed tomography. There were also therapeutic advantages for the patient, namely, interventional procedures for treating stenotic blood vessels. Cardiac and vascular diseases have increased sharply in industrialized countries and are responsible for almost 50% of deaths. Angiography and catheterization techniques to dilate vascular stenoses, whether of the coronary or peripheral vessels, offer the patient a more comfortable and less invasive therapy than surgery, and at even lower costs.

Multidirectional views with isocentric patient positioning was necessary to visualize a stenosis clearly and perform quantitative evaluations. On the other hand, the length of time that a catheter remained in the blood vessel represented a medical risk for the patient. All technical efforts were aimed at simplification and to accelerate the course of the examination, so that the heat storage capacity of the tube once again reached technical limits. From 1985 onwards, angiographic systems were equipped with a tube with an anode disk diameter increased to 120 mm. Its anode angle was adapted to 12° for large image formats of the PUCK film changer of 35 × 35 cm as well as the 40 cm input field diameter of the X-ray image intensifier, and the heat storage capacity was increased to 10^6 Ws (1 MJ). Thus there were practically no forced waiting times caused by thermal limits during angiography or angioplasty of a patient. This was an essential contribution, among many other measures, to reducing the risk for the patient. In this tube, the focal spots of 0.6 at 40 kW and 1.0 at 70 kW were available for general angiography and focal spots of 0.4 at 40 kW and 0.8 at 80 kW for angiocardiography.

Helical fluid bearings instead of ball bearings

In 1964, Muijderman (1964) [35] proposed a completely new principle in his dissertation on helical fluid bearings (Fig. V, 24) [P 21]. The first tube using a helical fluid bearing – the MAXIMUS ROTALIX Ceramic – for angiocardiography special procedure rooms was introduced in 1989 (focal spot 0.5 at 45 kW and 0.8 at 85 kW) (Behling, 1990) [1].

Bearing noise is now no longer perceptible. Rotation is switched on only once a day and is continuous. Previously, braking after each exposure or exposure series prolonged the life of the ball bearings.

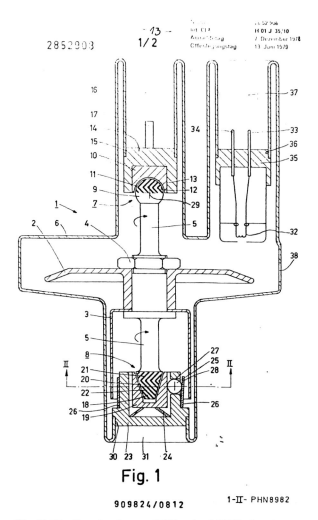

909824/0812   1-Ⅱ- PHN8982

Fig. V, 24. Drawing from a 1978 patent [P21] showing an X-ray tube with a liquid spiral bearing. Philips introduced such a tube for angiocardiography in 1989.

A special case: computed tomography – a return to the fixed anode?

Computed tomography examinations were always a high-energy technique with regard to the tube. The first computed tomograms were taken in the early seventies with a 4-kW fixed anode tube which had to cope with an energy of 1.2 MWs for one scan. It was soon replaced by rotating anode tubes. The year 1987 brought the DURALIX tube supplied over high tension slip rings, a dual innovative thrust in computed tomography. On the one hand, the tube could now rotate around the patient without interruption and, on the other hand, it had a flying focal spot, which was significantly simpler than the proposal by B.J. Mayo in 1975 [P 19]. Both the scan time and the examination time could be shortened by a factor of 5 with the software innovation of the spiral CT modality which followed later.

An electron gun (Fig. V, 25) [P 20] is used by Imatron. The anode is indeed stationary and forms a ring around the patient but, at the same time, is operated in accordance with the rotating anode principle. The difference is that the electron beam is moved over the stationary anode. Pulsed power up to 200 kW and continuous power up to 20 kW is now available with a single scan time of less than 50 ms. This X-ray tube technology opens up new possibilities for computed tomographic examinations of the thorax and abdomen as well as in paediatrics, where motion blurring is usually a problem.

Overload warnings

X-ray tubes are technical 'works of art'. They are expensive and must be protected against damage. Many generator circuits, even in the late thirties (KODIAPHOS), served exclusively to protect against overload. Simple devices to indicate energy levels, which usually displayed a percentage value, were available in the seventies. LOADIX [50] was introduced in 1973: a photo cell senses the anode disk temperature. An optical signal is displayed according to the traffic light principle of green–amber–red if a pause is required. Green means unobstructed work. Amber lets an exposure or scene that has begun run to the end, in order to wait for green before starting a new exposure. Red means that the temperature has exceeded the permitted value, which as a rule leads to damage or even destruction of the X-ray tube.

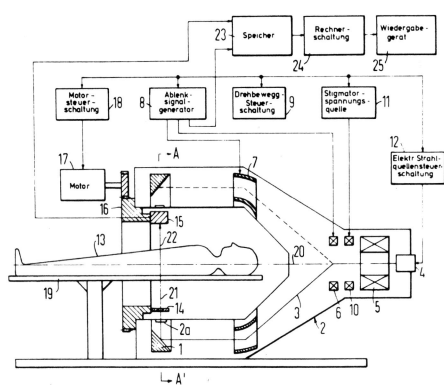

Fig. V, 25. 1977: Drawing from a patent [P20] for an X-ray tube system for ultrafast computed tomography examinations or the so-called electron beam tomography (EBT).

POLYPHOS generators directly indicated the waiting time. For the first time, medical staff could read the waiting time between two exposures if the tube had reached its thermal limit.

Breast cancer and X-ray tubes

Besides angiography which began its rapid spread in the seventies, another medical milestone should be mentioned: the soft radiation technique known as 'mammography' (Salomon, 1913; Goynes et al, 1931; Seabold, 1931; Vogel, 1932; Lame and Pendergrass, 1947; Warren, 1950; Egan, 1960, 1988) [16, 17, 28, 33, 42, 43, 47, 49]. Breast cancer had been a challenge to radiology for decades. The diagnosis requires not only extensive medical knowledge, but also radiographs with good soft-tissue contrast, low motion blurring and enormously high perceptible detail to characterize microcalcifications, beyond ten line pairs per millimetre. The beam spectrum, existing focal spot sizes and film-screen systems were unable to meet these requirements, without mentioning the high radiation exposure to the breast.

The contribution of the tube designers will be the only facet discussed here. In 1966, Gros (s. Fig. II, 50) referred to the advantageous, characteristic, inherent radiation of molybdenum,

but it was not until 1970 that a completely innovative tube was used for mammography. This tube was of a single-pole design, operating from 25 kV to a maximum of 50 kV. It had a metal sheath, a beryllium window [P 11, P 13] and a molybdenum rotating anode. The radiation spectrum was filtered additionally by molybdenum. In this way, contrast-reducing, high-energy radiation was reduced, but the characteristic inherent radiation could be used fully for imaging.

Radiation exposure could be reduced to an acceptable value, and a first compromise was reached between focal spot size, system geometry and tube output. The mammography tube was also being constantly developed further. While retaining, or even increasing, the output, the optically effective focal spot could be decreased in size. So, today, focal spots of 0.3 and smaller are used for routine and screening examinations.

Outlook

Only the major milestones in the development of the X-ray tube have been sketched here. The many small improvements that led to these milestones, and made them possible, should not be forgotten. There was not room here to consider X-ray tubes for radiotherapy, material testing or crystallography.

Single-pole tubes will come into use in conventional radiological procedures. This means that only one single high-voltage cable will run to the anode or cathode.

Rapid changes in tube current, precise switching of a dose value and eliminating the waiting time between fluoroscopy and exposure and vice versa are unfortunately not yet implemented in routine applications. The combination of an electronically controlled electron gun with a continuously rotating anode is taking its time.

Patents

P 1   DRP 91 028 vom 24. März 1896, Siemens & Halske: Hittorfsche Röhre mit Vorrichtung zur Entlüftung nach dem Malignanischen Verfahren.

P 2   DRP 97 491 vom 24. Juli 1897, Rzewuski: Einstellung der Elektroden an fertigen Fokusröhren zur Optimierung der Strahlenintensität.

P 3   DRP 100 298 vom 7. Okt. 1897, Hirschmann (Berlin): Röntgenröhre.

P 4   DRP 113 430 vom 21. Mai 1899, Walter Föhre: Röhre mit justierbarem Vakuum (C.H.F. Müller): Röntgenröhre mit durch Wasser gekühlter Antikathode.

P 5   DRP 114 455 vom 9. Nov. 1899, M. Levy, Fabrik Elektr. App. Berlin: Röntgenröhre mit aus verschiedenen Stoffen zusammengesetzter Antikathode.

P 6   DRP 156 746 vom 25. Nov. 1903, Siemens & Halske: Röntgenröhre mit Tantal-Elektrode.

P 7   DRP 165 138 vom 8. Nov. 1904, Siemens & Halske: Röntgenröhre mit Wolfram-Elektroden.

P 8   DRP 376 359 vom 11. Feb. 1914, E. Pohl: Über Relativbewegungen von Kathode und Antikathode.

P 9   DP 370 022 vom 2. Feb. 1918, Dr. Otto Goetze in Frankfurt a.M.: Verfahren und Glühkathodenröntgenröhre zur Erzeugung scharfer Röntgenbilder (Strichfokus).

P 10   DP 406 067 vom 17. Feb. 1923, Georg Conrad Kucher, Phönix Röntgenfabriken Rudolstadt: Glühkathoden-Röntgenröhre mit hohem Vakuum (2 oder mehrere unabhängig voneinander geheizte Kathoden).

P 11   DP 473 930 vom 27. Okt. 1925, Siemens Reiniger-Veifa Ges. für med. Technik: Röntgenröhre mit einem nahe um den Brennfleck herum angeordneten Blendenkörper (mit großem und geringem Absorptionsvermögen, P-Anspruch 4: aus metallischem Beryllium).

P 12   USP 2 242 182 vom 24. Nov. 1939, J.C. Brown (GE): DC Braking for Rotating Anode x-ray tube.

P 13   USP 23 120 567 vom 8. Jan. 1941, Z.J.   Atlee & H.W. Brackney (GE): Vakuum tight brazed beryllium window x-ray-tube.

P 14   DP 956 708 vom 1. Okt. 1954, Karl Silbermann, SRW: Drehanodenteller für eine Drehanoden-Röntgenröhre (2 Winkel auf Anodenteller).

P 15   DP 1 270 192 vom 30. Juli 1960, Karl Silbermann, Siemens AG: Drehanoden-Verbundteller für Röntgenröhren (Rhenium).

P 16   DP 1 951 383 vom 11. Okt. 1969, R. Friedel und W. Wiche (Siemens): Röntgenröhren-Drehanode mit einem Verbundkörper aus einem Schwermetallteil und wenigstens einem Graphitteil und Verfahren zu ihrer Herstellung.

P 17   DP 2 112 672 vom 16. März 1971, K. Dietz, A. Lehnert, K. Silbermann, A. Elsas, G. Appelt: Röntgenröhren-Drehanodenteller (radiale Einschnitte im Anodenteller).

P 18   DP 2 201 979 vom 17. Jan. 1972, R. Friedel, R. Lauterbach (Siemens): Verfahren zur Herstellung einer geschwärzten Schicht auf Drehanoden von Röntgenröhren.

P 19   DP 2 538 517 vom 27. Aug. 1975, B.J. Mayo, EMI: Radiologisches Gerät.

P 20   DP 2 708 612 vom 28. Feb. 1977, E. Watanabe, Japan: Vorrichtung zur Gewinnung eines Röntgenstrahlenbildes in einer Querschnittsebene eines Objektes.

P 21   DE 2 852 908 vom 7. Dez. 1978, J. Gerkema und E.A. Muijderman (Philips): Drehanodenröhre (Gleitlager mit Spiralrillen und GA-Lagerschmierung).

P 22   (PGM) G 8 304 046 vom 14. Feb. 1983, M. Grübl (Siemens): Röntgenstereoaufnahmeeinrichtung.

References

1. Behling, R.: The MRC 200: a new high output X-ray tube. Medica Mundi 35 (1990), 57
2. Berger, A.: Zum Problem der Bewegungsunschärfe im Röntgenbild der Lunge und des Herzens. Röntgen-Bl. 14 (1961), 369
3. Bergmüller, H.: Pre- and early history of the x-ray tube. Medica Mundi 35 (1990), 7
4. Bouwers, A.: Der Brennfleck einer Röntgenröhre und seine Belastbarkeit – Eine Metallröntgenröhre mit drehbarer Anode. Fortschr. Röntgenstr. 40 (1929), 284
5. Bouwers, A.: Verleihung der Röntgenplakette. Röntgen-Bl. 16 (1963), 234
6. Cole, L.G.: Note of the diagnostic and therapeutic value of the Coolidge tube. Arch. Roentgen-Ray 164 (1914), 368
7. Cole, L.G.: Vorläufige Mitteilung über die diagnostische und therapeutische Verwendung des Coolidge-Rohres. Fortschr. Röngenstr. 22 (1914), 29
8. Coolidge, W.D.; E.E. Charlton: Roentgen-ray tubes. Radiology 45 (1945), 446
9. Coolidge, W.D.: Röntgenröhre mit reiner Elektronenentladung. Fortschr. Röntgenstr. 22 (1914) 18
10. Coolidge, W.D.: A Powerful Roentgen Ray Tube with a Pure Electron Discharge. Phys. Rev. 2 (1913) 409–430 Übersetzte Zusammenfassung Ref. 9

11. Coolidge, W.D.: A Summary of Physical Investigation Work in Progress on Tube and Accessories. Am. J. Roentgenol. 2, Nr. 11 u. 12 (1915) 881–892

12. Crolla, D., A.L. Baert, K. Römhildt, J.L. Termote: Routinemäßige Hochqualitätsvergößerungsangiographie mit Puck 24- oder AOT 35-Blattfilmwechsler und Mikrofokus-Hochleistungs-Röntgenstrahler OPTILIX. Electromedica 47 (1979), 89–97

13. Dietz, K.: Altes und Neues über Röntgen-Röhren. Sonderdruck für Siemens-Reiniger-Werke AG Erlangen aus: Röntgenpraxis, S. Hirzel Verlag, Stuttgart 1964

14. Dietz, K.: Die Röntgenröhre im diagnostischen Einsatz. Sonderdruck Heft 1 und 2 aus Röntgenberichte 3 (1974), 1 und 3

15. DIN/IEC 336/1981: Standard für Brennfleckbezeichnung und Toleranzen der Brennfleckgrößen.

16. Egan R.L.: Experience with mammography in a tumor institution. Evaluation of 1000 studies. Radiology 74 (1960), 894

17. Egan, R.L.: Breast imaging. W.B. Saunders Comp., Philadelphia, 1988

18. Elsaß, A., Th. Zimmer: Höhere Belastung von Drehanodenröhren durch Verwendung von legierten Anoden. Fortschr. Röntgenstr. 97 (1962), 511

19. Fenner, E.: Die thermischen Belastungsgrenzen von Ölhauben für Diagnostik-Röhren. Röntgen-Bl. 6 (1953), 308

20. Fenner, E.; H. Joachim: Bestimmung der Brennfleckgröße aus der geometrischen Unschärfe. Fortschr. Röntgenstr. 87 (1957), 109

21. Fenner: Lochkamera-Aufnahmen der Brennflecke von Röntgenröhren. Elektronik 5 (1956). München, Franzis Verlag

22. Frik, W.: Detailerkennbarkeit und Dosis bei der Röntgendurchleuchtung. Hüthig, Heidelberg 1959

23. Friedel, R., K. Haberrecker: Leistungssteigerung bei Drehanoden-Röntgenröhren, Electromedica 41 (1973) 198

24. Fuchs, F.: Elektrische Strahlen und ihre Anwendung (Röntgentechnik). H. 3 von Dannenmann, F. (Hrsg.): Der Werdegang der Entdeckungen und Erfindungen. Verlag R. Oldenburg, München und Berlin 1922

25. Gajewski, H.: Die Grundlagen und Anwendungsmöglichkeiten der Hartstrahlentechnik. Röntgen-Bl. (1953) 53

26. Goetze, O.: 37. Herr Otto Goetze – Frankfurt a.M.: Eine scharf zeichnende Coolidgeröhre mit bandförmigem Brennfleck. Zitat aus Separatdruck der Verh. Dtsch. Röntgenges. 11 (1919)

27. Gould, R.G., H.K. Genant: Quantitative and Qualitative Comparison of Two Microfocus-Tube Imaging Systems. Radiology 138 (1981) 195

28. Goynes, J., D.F. Gentil, B. Guedes: Sobre la Radiografia de la Glandula Mamaria y Valor Diagnostico. Arch. Espan Oncol. 2 (1931), 111

29. Hartl, W.: X-ray tubes: an introduction. Medica Mundi 35 (1990) 4

30. Hartl, W: Thirty years of the Super Rotalix. Medica Mundi 35 (1990) 21

31. Kaye, G.W.C.: Über die Verteilung der Röntgenstrahlen einer Fokusröhre. Fortschr. Röntgenstr. 15 (1910) 50

32. Kuntke, A.H.G.: Untersuchungen über die Änderung der Röntgenstrahlen-Ausbeute an Drehanoden-Röntgenröhren, Fortsch. Röntgenstr. 87, (1957) 397

33. Lame E.L., E.P. Pendergrass: An addition to the technic of simple breast roentgenography. Radiology 48 (1947) 266

34. Lilienfeld, J.E., W.J. Rosenthal: Eine Röntgenröhre von beliebig und momentan einstellbarem, vom Vakuum unabhängigen Härtegrad. Fortschr. Röntgenstr. 18 (1911/12) 256

35. Muijderman, E.A.: Spiral grove bearings. Dissertation, Techn. Univ. Delft 1964

36. Prellwitz, F.: Zur Geschichte der medizinischen Röntgenröhren. Röntgenpraxis 27 (1974), 17, 38 und 92

37. Pressler, K.: Erfahrungen mit der Doppelwinkelröhre. Fortschr. Röntgenstr. 90 (1959) 25

38. Rønne, P., A.B.W. Nielsen: Development of the Ion X-ray Tube. Acta Historica Scientiarum Naturalium et Medicinalium, Bibliotheca Universitatis 1986

39. Regener, E.: Über die Schärfe der Röntgenbilder und ihre Verbesserung. Münch. med. Wschr. 64 (1917) 1518

40. Reiniger, Gebbert und Schall: Elektro-Medizinische Apparate und ihre Handhabung. 6. Auflage, Erlangen, 1897

41. Roeck, W.W.; Milne, E.N.C.: A highly accurate focal spot camera Laboratory and Field Model. Radiology 127 (1978), 779

42. Salomon A.: Beiträge zur Pathologie und Klinik des Mammakarzinoms. Arch. Klin. Chir. 101 (1913), 573

43. Seabold, P.S.: Roentgenographic diagnosis of diseases of the breast. Surg. Gynecol. Obstet. 53 (1931), 461

44. Silbermann, K.: Hochleistungsröhren, Röntgen-Bl. 17, (1964), 284

45. Ungelenk, A.: Eine Drehanodenröhre mit Hochtemperatur-Strahlungskühlung. Fortschr. Röntgenstr. 49 (1934) 162

46. Ungelenk, A.: Eine Röntgenröhre mit Drehanode und Hochtemperatur-Strahlungskühlung. Intern. Radiolog. Kongreß in Zürich, (1934) Berichtsband 2

47. Vogel, W.: Die Röntgendarstellung der Mammatumoren. Arch. Klin. Chir. 171 (1932), 618

48. Wachsmann, F., K. Breuer, E. Buchheim.: Grundlagen und Ergebnisse der Hartstrahltechnik. Fortschr. Röntgenstr 76 (1952), 728

49. Warren S.L.: A roentgenologic study of the breast. Am. J. Roentgenol. 24 (1930), 113

50. Wolter, I.: LOADIX – ein System zur thermischen Überwachung von Röntgenstrahlern. Electromedica 45 (1977), 73

Generators

E. Ammann, G. Rosenbusch, M. Oudkerk

Prior to Roentgen's experiments, three types of devices to generate high voltage were familiar in physics institutes: electrostatic generators, Tesla (high-frequency) transformers and Ruhmkorff inductors.

Electrostatic induction machines were used for electrotherapy and later to generate X-rays; however, they were not really powerful enough for the latter purpose and were abandoned (Fig. V, 26). On the other hand electromedical equipment had already been used for the purpose of electrostimulation by Watson in Great Britain as early as 1837, and was produced by Werner von Siemens starting in 1847.

In 1891 the Croatian-born physicist and electrical engineer Nikola Tesla (1856–1943) developed a high-frequency AC transformer. Called the 'Tesla transformer' in honour of its inventor, this achievement was followed by a mercury interrupter in 1898. The Tesla transformer functioned according to the oscillating circuit principle with two air-core coils (Fig. V, 27).

The Scotsman Campbell Swinton (1863–1930) used a Tesla transformer to run a self-contrived X-ray tube with which he took his radiographic exposures on 7 January 1896. In the same year Thomson and the General Electric Company manufactured X-ray generators using Tesla transformers. Due to its lack of iron, this generator was lighter in weight than an inductor and had a more compact design, making it easier to transport. Siemens and Halske also utilized this feature [P 9].

Roentgen stated in his second report paragraph 19 that:

'It is often advantageous to connect a Tesla apparatus (capacitor and transformer) between the discharge device supplying the X-rays (i.e. the tube) and the Ruehmkorff (inductor).... The tube is sub-

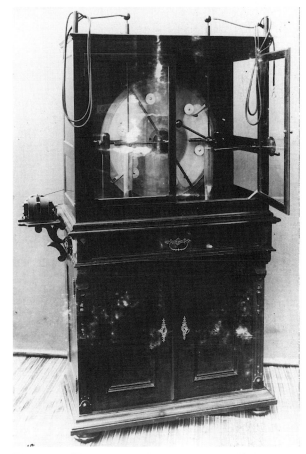

Fig. V, 26. Electrostatic induction machine with lead storage batteries and motor drive designed by Toplar in 1901. This principle for generating X-rays was abandoned.

jected to less wear and tear because it doesn't heat up so much and sparking seldom occurs. Furthermore, tubes which have an insufficient or excessive vacuum, and therefore fail to function properly with

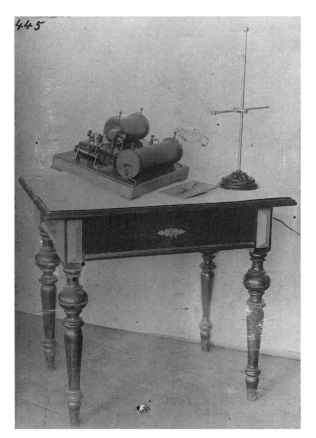

Fig. V, 27. 1896: A Tesla instrumentarium for generating X-rays.

the Ruhmkorff inductor alone, still supply useful X-rays with the Tesla transformer.'

Based on his first report, Roentgen used a Hittorf vacuum tube which was exposed to the discharge of a large Ruhmkorff inductor. Heinrich D. Ruhmkorff (1803–1877) was born in Hannover and became a mechanic. He then established a workshop in Paris in which he manufactured, among other things, electromagnetic instruments. It was here that he designed and built the first induction coil in 1848 (Grossmann, 1912; Fuchs, 1922; Walter, 1926; Hackl, 1929) [23, 29, 30, 60].

Inductors

It might be said that the history of induction (see table I, 1) [49] began with Stephen Gray (1666–1736) who first distinguished between conductors and insulators in 1729. In 1733, Charles F. Dufay discovered the electric charge, later classified as positive and negative

charges by Georg Ch. Lichtenberg (1742–1799) in 1778. In 1755, the American Benjamin Franklin (1706–1790) proved that no charge is present inside a virtually closed and charged vessel and the Swede Johann Carl Wilcke (1732–1796) explained electrostatic induction in 1757.

In 1775, Alessandro Volta (1745–1827) demonstrated the first electrostatic generator capable of producing current of approx. 10 millionths of an ampere at voltages of 30–100 kV.

A chemical cell as an electric power source was introduced by A. Volta in 1800. The link between the magnetic field and electric current was proven in 1820 by H. Ch. Oersted, and in 1832 the Englishman Michael Faraday (1791–1867) discovered electromagnetic induction. Ruhmkorff used this law of induction in the design of his inductors, which were later utilized by Roentgen for his experiments.

In 1844 Werner von Siemens (Siemens, 1966) [56] experimented with a self-made voltaic inductor by attempting to alleviate his brother Friedrich's toothache through the application of electric shock therapy to the root of his tooth.

'The pain (caused by the shock through its root) was at first enormous, but then it suddenly stopped. By summoning the immense willpower my brother Friedrich had always been endowed with, he then went on to treat the rest of his teeth.... Unfortunately, the toothaches gradually began to return on the second day. Although further electrotherapy alleviated the pain when repeated, the effects of this technique abated more quickly with each treatment until they had been altogether eliminated.'

Between 1848 and 1850 Siemens and Halske delivered seven voltaic inductors as medical sliding induction devices for a price of twelve thalers each. A total of 450 such devices were sold between 1855 and 1865.

For the second London World Fair held in 1862 Siemens and Halske constructed a large voltaic inductor featuring a 95-cm-long, 6-cm-diameter iron core and a secondary coil with 299 188 turns of a 0.14-mm-thick, silk-wound copper wire with a length of approx. 10 755 metres.

'The capacitor consists of a 15 000 cm² tinfoil separated by layers of varnished paper. With our design (differing from Ruhmkorff's), it has only minimal influence on the spark gap, but it considerably reduces the intensity of the primary spark.'

Two Daniell cells with fresh and potent nitric acid were used as a power source. With good cells, a spark gap of 39 cm could be attained and with six cells, a spark gap of 58 cm.

Inductor design

Several hundred turns of insulated copper wire measuring 2–3 mm in diameter were wrapped around an iron core. This coil was then connected to a DC current source, e.g. a lead storage battery, via an interrupter. Another well-insulated coil, the secondary coil, comprising thousands of turns of 0.1–0.2-mm-thick copper wire was located over the primary coil. The two wire ends of the secondary coil were routed to an X-ray tube and connected in parallel to a spark gap (Fig. V, 28).

The first X-ray exposure in history occurred at the University of Pennsylvania in February 1890. The X-ray Museum Guide in Lennep reports that A. W. Goodspeed wanted to photograph the spark of a Ruhmkorff inductor. Before the photographer, a certain Mr Jennings, left the laboratory, he placed his fare, namely two coins, aside and watched several more trials with the discharge tube. Both men were dismayed to see that nothing came of the exposures except for a picture of two round shadows. When Roent-

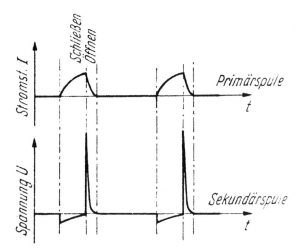

Fig. V, 28b. If the contact closes, the current I in the primary coil (P) increases and decreases rapidly when the contact opens. A voltage is induced in the secondary coil (S) when the contact closes and therefore soft radiation is produced in the cathode of the ion X-ray tube by the reverse current. During opening of the contact, the voltage induced has a higher value and produces X-rays in the anticathode if the polarity is correctly applied [26].

gen's discovery of X-rays later became known, they repeated this experiment to verify their earlier X-ray of the coins, which they had, of course, originally failed to recognize for what it was.

The inductor per se was already a familiar device in physics departments around 1895. One question remained unanswered for Roentgen: can a constant discharge potential produce X-rays or do they result only from fluctuations in potential?

Lead storage batteries (accumulators)

Accumulators were used as a power source for these inductors. Lead storage batteries [31] were studied by G. Planté (1834–1889) in 1859, who discovered the 'forming' process. In 1881 Faure increased the capacity of storage batteries by applying 'active material' to their plates. The capacity of storage batteries is specified in ampere hours (Ah) and indicates the length of time for which a given current can be discharged from a storage battery until it is empty. The positive plate was coated with minium (Pb_2O_3) and the negative plate with lead oxide (PbO). This prepared the battery for artificial forming. Volkmar improved the effectiveness of lead storage batteries operated with dilute sulphuric acid by the use of a lead plate grid design.

Fig. V, 28a, b. Inductor

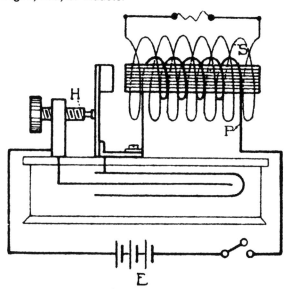

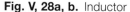

Fig. V, 28a. 1922: Principal schematic [23] of an inductor. H.D. Ruhmkorff built the first one in 1848. The core of thin iron rods carried the primary coil with 100–400 turns. It was connected via an interrupter to a lead storage battery (E). The interrupter was a so-called Wagner hammer with platin contacts (H) or a Foucault mercury interrupter for less powerful inductors. Rotary mercury or electrolytic interrupters were used for powerful inductors. The secondary coil had 40 000–200 000 turns. The induced voltage was high when the contact opened and a little lower when the contact closed, causing a reverse current ('closing light').

Why interrupters?

The current path leading from the lead storage battery to the primary coil of the inductor is routed via an interrupter, thus generating the high voltage in the secondary coil.

Platinum interrupters

Roentgen used a Depréz interrupter (Fig. V, 29). The contact was opened by the magnetic field of the induction coil and closed again by spring force. Since high currents had to be switched – in the case of Roentgen's inductor 20 A – platinum was chosen as the contact material. It oxidized minimally and had a high enough melting temperature to withstand the spark on break. However, a capacitor still had to be inserted par-

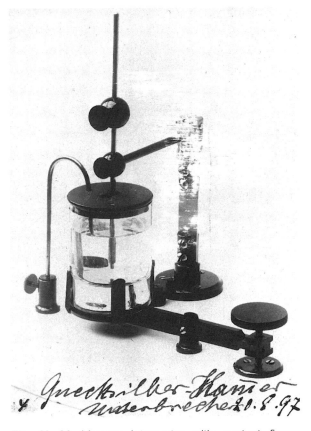

Fig. V, 30. Mercury interrupter with contact finger, 20 August 1897.

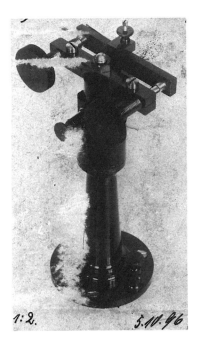

Fig. V, 29. Depréz interrupter, 5 October 1896. Original photograph – damaged by water.

allel to the two contact points to ensure reasonably good functioning. Its efficiency and performance life were quite limited. For this reason the search for better interrupter designs continued.

Mercury interrupters

Mercury was used as a contact material. Béclère and von Drault in Paris as well as Tesla in New York and Siemens and Halske in Berlin manufactured these interrupters (Figs. V, 30–32), which

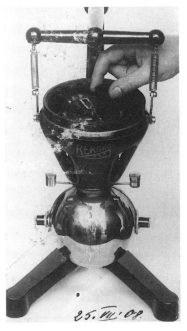

Fig. V, 31. 1908: The REKORD interrupter was based on the principle illustrated in Fig. V, 32 (measuring the oil level).

Fig. V, 32. Cross-section of a mercury petroleum interrupter [30]. A cast iron pot was mounted on the axle of a 1/3 horsepower motor. A layer of mercury was put in the pot, and the rest filled with petroleum. A hard rubber roll with metal sections was mounted within the pot. The interrupter began working when the motor rotated the pot and the mercury crept up the wall under centrifugal force, until it touched the metal sections in the rubber roll. When the contact opened, the spark was extinguished by the petroleum in the pot (Sanitas, RGS).

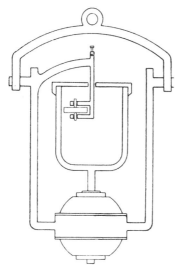

Wehnelt electrolytic interrupters

The improved, electrolytic interrupters developed by A. Wehnelt [P 2] had the advantage that the cleaning of mercury and contacts was no longer required. Wehnelt described the function of his idea in his patent specification as follows (Figs. V, 33 and V, 34):

'If an electric current is transmitted through an electrolyte with two electrodes of unequal surface area while applying a voltage considerably higher than the opposing polarization voltage, the well-known light and heat phenomena first studied by Davy and then by Planté and many others appear. . . . A lead plate (b) and a platinum wire (c) sealed in a glass tube (d) are immersed in a beaker (a) filled with diluted sulphuric acid. The glass tube is then filled with mercury to conduct the current to the platinum wire (c).'

again required a capacitor to attenuate the switching spark. Their chief advantage was the uniformity of interruption. Furthermore, with a synchronous drive, an AC voltage could be utilized as a power source. However, the motor required a power of 1/3 HP (250 W).

Interrupters using petroleum as an insulating material required frequent cleaning. A. Hackl (1929) [30] reported how this was done:

'After the petroleum has been poured off, the remaining mercury is placed on a cloth. The mercury is then pressed through the cloth by hand so that any contamination, especially particles of soot, remains trapped in the cloth. In order to prevent mercury poisoning, the person performing this procedure always had to carefully wash his hands afterward.'

Another development used gas as an insulating material instead of petroleum. Contact segments were made of a resistant nickel alloy and the interrupter was connected to the gas line in order to replace the air inside with gas.

These contacts could be adjusted from the outside so that longer or shorter current intervals could be switched. The mercury was cleaned in the same manner as with the petroleum interrupters; the contacts were filed off to free them of residue caused by the gas combustion. The interrupter designed by Reiniger, Gebbert and Schall was the most commonly used version.

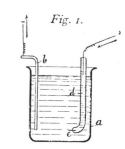

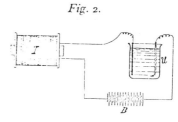

Fig. V, 33. A. Wehnelt applied for a patent for an electrolytic interrupter on 3 January 1899 [P2]. The interrupter was widely used in inductor systems.

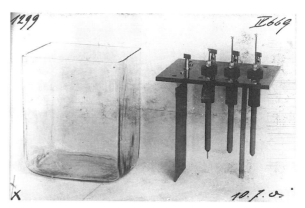

Fig. V, 34. July 1901: Triple Wehnelt interrupter. The cover plate (right) held three electrodes and was inserted in the glass beaker (left) filled with dilute sulphuric acid.

The advantages lay in simplicity, no wear and tear on parts, exact and uniform interruption at high frequencies of up to 1700 Hz, frequency adjustable via voltage level, direct connection to 100 V or higher municipal lighting mains, and finally simple AC/DC conversion.

The function of the Wehnelt interrupter was based on heating the platinum tip, producing an insulating steam jacket around the tip, which interrupted the current. The primary winding of the inductor then induced a high voltage, resulting in a sparkover between the platinum tip and the electrolyte. This separated the steam jacket into its oxygen and hydrogen components and caused the gas mixture to explode, again bringing the electrolyte in contact with the platinum tip. The platinum tip then heated up again and the cycle was repeated. This interrupter required no servicing and could be adapted to the required radiation hardness using the Walter circuit (Grossmann, 1912; Walter, 1926) [29, 60]. The optimum switching frequency in X-ray operation was 30–40 interruptions per second.

The stability of the current was, however, greatly dependent on the temperature of the electrolyte. Noise level was also quite high and sound absorbing (i.e. muffler) casings were already being offered at that time (Grossmann, 1912) [29].

Power supply, interrupter, and inductor were interconnected to an X-ray generator, as one would put it in modern standardized terms. The exposure times were set with switches in the primary circuit (Figs. V, 35 and V, 36).

O. Glasser (1959) [27] quotes the Journal of Electrochemistry **2**(24), 523, of 20 March 1896 as follows:

'Equipment for generating X-rays according to Roentgen's principle.

In response to numerous inquiries on the arrangement, power consumption and costs of reliable equipment for the performance of Roentgen's experiments, we turned to Siemens and Halske, Berlin, for information and, thanks to the obligingness of this firm, are now able to report the following:

The simpler technique, associated with many drawbacks (unsteady light, bursting of vacuum tubes, etc.), involves the use of an inductor with a sparking distance of at least 15 cm (with slow current alternation) and a mercury interrupter or some other type of self interruption.

According to the price list published by Siemens and Halske, the total price for this system was 716 Marks.

This device was powered by only five Bunsen cells or five small storage batteries. However, in places where a

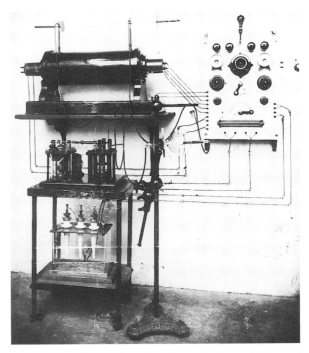

Fig. V, 35. A complete Roentgen instrumentarium of 1903: a 60-cm inductor for stereo fluoroscopy, triple Wehnelt interrupter, and controls and switches mounted on a marble panel.

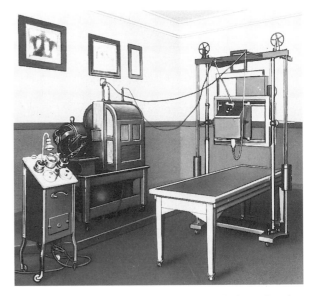

Fig. V, 36. An X-ray examination room of 1910, showing on the left hand side the IDEAL apparatus with a rotary, high-voltage rectification system (Fig. V, 51) and the inductor. High-voltage cables lead to the ion X-ray tube with protective housing mounted in a tube stand over the examination table. The stand was mobile and the tube holder could be brought into any position for vertical or horizontal beam direction.

lighting power plant, block station, DC generator or lead battery with a 65–120 V EMF is available as a source of electricity, it is advisable to select a method which, in contrast to the one above, will ensure that the fluorescence remains steady and calm and the vacuum tubes burst much less often. This can be accomplished by replacing the mercury interrupter with a rotating interrupter driven by an electric motor. For this purpose the primary current must have a voltage of at least 50 V; however, the inductor sparking distance with slow current alternation needs only to be approximately 7 cm and, when the rotating interrupter is applied, roughly 2–3 cm.'

The total price for such a system is 616 Marks. 300 Marks for the inductor, 180 Marks for the motor and interrupter, 16 Marks for two evacuated glass spheres (X-ray tubes) and 120 Marks for regulating resistors, switches and installation.

'Siemens and Halske recommend fresh eosin silver plates as photographic plates (procured from Reichardt and Stoll, Berlin, Hollmannstrasse 17).'

Glasser (1959) [27] continued:

'Looking back to 1896, serial production of X-ray equipment kept pace with the progress made throughout radiology and it must be said that industry at the time responded to the enthusiasm of X-ray researchers with an unbelievably resounding echo. The production of radiological equipment during the early years of radiology was no less romantic than the actual discovery of X-rays and its acceptance throughout the world.'

Chief components were thus a spark inductor and an interrupter for operating an ion X-ray tube.

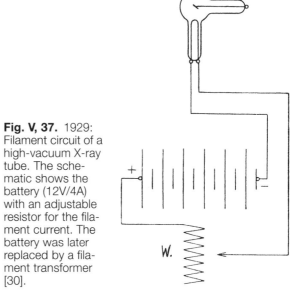

Fig. V, 37. 1929: Filament circuit of a high-vacuum X-ray tube. The schematic shows the battery (12V/4A) with an adjustable resistor for the filament current. The battery was later replaced by a filament transformer [30].

In 1913 Coolidge introduced the high-vacuum X-ray tube (Fig. V, 37). This increased the stability and reproducibility of the radiation while at the same time boosting the tube power. The following years brought a number of technical improvements of individual components, which primarily served to reduce the exposure time. With his 'single-spark machine' ('BLITZ'), F. Dessauer managed to reduce the exposure time to only 10 ms (Fig. V, 38).

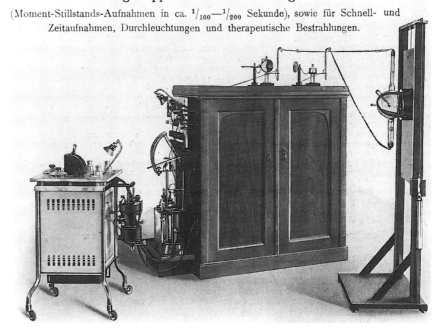

Röntgenapparat für Einzelschlag-Aufnahmen.

(Moment-Stillstands-Aufnahmen in ca. $1/100$—$1/200$ Sekunde), sowie für Schnell- und Zeitaufnahmen, Durchleuchtungen und therapeutische Bestrahlungen.

Fig. V, 38. 1906: Roentgen apparatus for single-pulse operations. The control console is on the left hand side with the REKORD interrupter; the inductor cabinet is in the middle with a spark gap on top; on the right hand side, the X-ray tube is mounted on a wall stand. Built especially for chest radiographs, exposure times of 10 ms could be achieved.

Transformers

In 1866 Werner von Siemens discovered the dynamoelectric principle governing the conversion of working power to electric current without the use of permanent magnets; 1878 witnessed the commissioning of the first AC generator, followed in 1892 by the first large-scale three-phase generator, which at 750 revolutions per minute delivered an output of 39 400 volt amperes (VA) and supplied a current of 14.5 A with a voltage of 1575 V. Thus DC, AC, and three-phase lines replaced lead storage batteries as power sources.

A transformer is used to change or convert AC voltages and currents. It functions according to the law of induction and has a closed iron core and at least one primary coil and one secondary coil. By selecting the number of turns in the secondary coil, a voltage of over 100 000 V or, as we call it in radiology, 100 kV, can be obtained from a line voltage of approximately 100 V.

In 1897 Hermann M. Lemp of General Electric became the first engineer to replace the inefficient inductor with a transformer (Grossmann, 1912) [29]. Since the polarity was constantly reversed with AC voltage, he designed a device that generated only single pulses with uniform polarity. General Electric applied for a patent on this innovation in 1897, and this was finally granted in 1904.

In the same year, Siemens built the first X-ray generator featuring a high-voltage transformer which, following considerable improvements, was introduced to the market in 1908 as the 'IDEAL' apparatus (s. Fig. V, 36).

In 1904, Franz J. Koch had the idea of reversing the negative half-wave so that it could also be used to generate radiation. This will be explained in more detail in the section on high-voltage rectification.

For country doctors and hospitals not hooked up to electric power plants, transportable transformers capable of being connected to an in-house generator for the purpose of taking X-ray exposures were already being manufactured as early as 1907. Driven by a gasoline engine, these 'dynamos' supplied electricity both for the X-ray generator and for the lighting of the operating room. At the ICR held in Amsterdam in 1905 the American Homer C. Snook was quoted as saying '. . . *the day of the induction coil is passing*' (Grigg, 1965) [28]. Snook had previously designed a high-voltage rectifier with which the ion tube could be operated more efficiently by employing an autotransformer

and a single-phase high-voltage transformer. One of these units was installed at Jefferson Hospital in Philadelphia in 1907 and a second one at Johns Hopkins in Baltimore, where it was used for routine clinical work until 1946. In 1910 Snook was granted a patent for his high-voltage rectifier. Snook was probably also the first to use an autotransformer to adapt the tube voltage or 'hardness' as it was commonly referred to at the time. In 1916 he expanded the primary coil of the transformer to include 30 taps after the high-vacuum tube had made its way into the X-ray room.

In 1912 the generation of high voltage with high-frequency AC current was explained by Siemens employee Gustav Grossmann in his book Introduction to X-ray Technology (Grossmann, 1912) [29]. We will be dealing with this technique devised by Tesla in more detail in connection with the years 1935, 1958 onward, as well as in the section on rectification and single-tank generators.

According to this publication, Siemens and Halske's high-voltage transformers had a threefold subdivided primary winding to attain different tube voltages ranging from 20 to 120 kV. These transformers operated at an efficiency of at least 98%.

A patent (Fig. V, 39) [P 14] of great importance to X-ray generators, the first three-phase circuit, was drawn up at the Siemens and Halske laboratory by its engineer Karl Lasser (Fig. V, 40) and applied for on 29 July 1915.

The single-phase application for radiology and the use of high-vacuum valve tubes with hot-cathodes as rectifiers were also patented.

On 26 January 1916, Karl Lasser (1916) [39] held a memorable presentation at the Berlin Medical Association, in Berlin, on the subject of 'The generation of X-radiation in the new tube and special generators for its diagnostic and therapeutic use.'

The Coolidge high-vacuum tube required a filament transformer (s. Fig. V, 37), i.e. a transformer that transformed the line voltage in such a manner that the tungsten filament of the cathode could actually be 'heated' in the truest sense of the word. This meant that a specific current must flow through the filament to heat it in a manner similar to the familiar light bulb.

Lasser explained:

'In order to obtain equipment which meets practical demands, we must take precautions to ensure that we will be able to adjust the operating voltage within wide limits, comfortably operate the control equipment, and observe the measuring instruments. These addi-

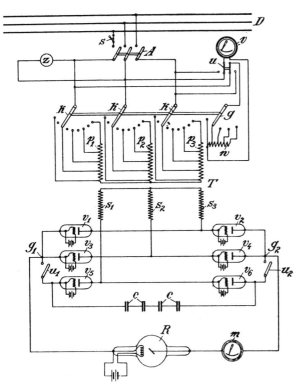

Fig. V, 39. 1915: Schematic of a three-phase, six-pulse X-ray generator for high-vacuum X-ray tubes from the Lasser patent [P14]. High-vacuum valves (v1–v6) were proposed to rectify the high voltage of the transformer (T). The kV selection was performed by the selector (K) via taps from the primary transformer coils (p).

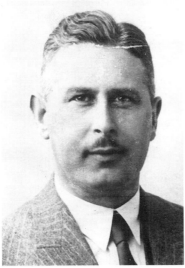

Fig. V, 40.
Karl Lasser (1884–1954) worked as engineer at Siemens and Halske in the Roentgen Laboratory. He invented the three-phase X-ray generator in 1915 [P14]. Later, he was in charge of the technical sales organisation of SRW in Erlangen.

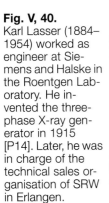

tions led to the development of a very simple new instrumentarium...', a 4-kW, single-phase generator. Lasser demonstrated that using this new tube for fluoroscopy at 4 mA, he could now also vary the 'hardness' or voltage without altering the current. The voltage first equalled 40 kV

or 6 Wehnelt and then 70 kV or 10 Wehnelt. The voltmeter thus could be calibrated according to either the Wehnelt or the Christen scale.

'Practical experience will tell whether we will later be able to do without the old hardness scale . . . or whether the electrical unit of voltage measurement, the volt, will take its place.'

How right he was. Today we still speak of 'kV' as the unit of measurement for tube voltage in diagnostic radiology.

Then came the next experiment:

'The next step was obviously to investigate the question of whether a radiogram could be produced with constant hardness at identical quality if an exposure of the ankle is taken at 5 mA and 10 s and then repeated at 10 mA and 5 s. The result you see in the exhibited foot X-rays shows complete agreement. Thus, within certain limits we can take an exposure of equal quality under varying conditions by altering the factors of the milliampere–seconds product, which in this case equals 50.'

It was thus realized that the time and the milliampere settings have an inverse, mutual influence with regard to image quality. As a result the expression 'mAs product' – i.e. the amount of the charge – was coined. In the case of moving objects, time is of course the most important factor.

Lasser continued:

'The question may rightly be asked, why we didn't develop this technique at an earlier date using ion tubes? We could not venture to do so, since due to its inconstant character, any "softening" of the X-ray tube was tantamount to a short-circuit.'

The key to the new circuit was that the rheostatic control used in older types of generators was replaced by the 'windings ratio control' on the transformer. Regarding the question of rectification, Lasser further explained that rectification was no longer required for a hot cathode X-ray tube.

'This is due to the fact that, by increasing the heat capacity and surface of the anode, we ensured that the tungsten block could not reach a temperature capable of causing an emission of electrons. . . . It might also be mentioned here that due to its simplicity and many applications the new generator also offers many benefits to field X-ray stations since all radiological tasks usually must be performed with relatively limited means at such locations. This generator does not require a large number of tubes featuring different degrees of hardness, which together with their transport packaging require an excessive amount of space when taken along. Instead, only two hot-cathode high vacuum tubes, one of which serves as a spare, are required.'

Lasser used two single-phase transformers in a V circuit instead of a 3-phase transformer to produce a 6-pulse wave shape at the X-ray tube with the help of six high-voltage rectifier tubes.

'Multiple-tube operation can also be performed using this generator; all you have to do is connect the tubes parallel to each other like incandescent lamps in a lighting system. Of course, special precautions must be taken to provide for system shutdown using a high-voltage switch. The tube current of each individual tube can then be regulated separately by simply altering the filament current.'

'It might have struck you during the last experiment that the tungsten block came to glow very quickly despite the fact that the heat capacity of its long stem and fairly solid block is quite considerable. Due to the continuous electron bombardment caused by the high-DC voltage, the above condition occurs faster and more intensely than we can perceive in the diagnostic tube. However, this is irrelevant here, since we now operate our X-ray tube with a DC voltage produced by high-vacuum rectifiers instead of with the AC voltage used in the experiments that we demonstrated earlier.'

Lasser demonstrated the Universal generator: 'As you can also see on the control console, a timer with an automatic switch is implemented so that we can also perform extremely accurate, short exposures.' He then concluded his experimental presentation with the following words:

'I have just introduced you to a new frontier of physics and technology which the physicist discovered and researched and the engineer entered to pave the way so that it can be exploited for the common good. I am confident that the time is near when the physician will be in full possession of this new technical territory and able to take up the fight against illness and death with improved weapons.'

Apparently a lively discussion then followed, which has been handed down to us in written form. G. Bucky (s. Fig. V, 85):

'I don't think it's arrogant of me or that I'm underestimating the intellect of the audience if I assume that not everyone here understood all of this presentation. It is, however, perhaps interesting for you to hear some of the benefits which we physicians and radiologists are able to obtain from this new gasless Siemens and Halske X-ray tube. Those radiologists who see the main emphasis of their work in the manual skills associated with taking X-ray exposures now stand in front of an open grave into which they must cast all their skills. They must bury everything they were once proud of, since it is really not difficult to prophesy that in the future they will be able to obtain the most outstanding X-ray images without previous knowl-

edge or experience. In my opinion, these 'radiologists' must now despair of the future.

But – and here comes the BUT – for those radiologists who have sighted on higher goals and regard the technical capabilities involved only as necessary equipment and not as the final cause of their special science, this presentation was a revelation. Because now we finally come to a method of generating X-rays which, I would like to say, is supported by a mathematical basis. Everything we did in radiology until now using the old tubes was just patchwork.... A similar situation existed with X-rays. The radiation which we generated comprised a mixture of different rays, varying in wavelength, character, and the type of effect which they produced. Now all of a sudden a generator will be placed in our hands which can generate X-rays of outstanding purity... produce images with a specific type of radiation... not more beautiful... (but) with a definite penetrating capacity.... These are the benefits and great progress offered by the new technique... One disadvantage... the simplified technique... of producing the most superb X-ray images without previous knowledge or experience will persuade an ever increasing number of physicians to purchase X-ray equipment. This may lead to discrediting radiology, since this science demands more than technology alone.'

Bucky closed his contribution to the discussion by saying: 'These possibilities may develop to the point where this simple generator would tempt untrained persons to practice radiotherapy and apply excessive doses of radiation. Such a situation must be avoided under any circumstances.'

H. Gocht (s. Fig. I, 23) then claimed the floor: 'Concerning this very interesting presentation, I would just like to say a few brief words as an old practitioner. As you know, I have been working in the field of radiology since 1896.... The biggest surprise that we experienced in our time was the rectifiers, which freed us from the use of inductors. Today, the demonstration which we witnessed represents... a milestone in radiology.... Believe me when I say that, as an X-ray man I was thrilled to hear that such performance and adjustment capabilities are possible.'

He continued:
'To be able to exactly set the current intensity with a particular hardness without any dependence on that hardness ... and vice versa ... is a truly great achievement. I am especially happy about the fact that I am now so-to-say sitting at the source here in Berlin, and will therefore be able to witness and participate in the further development.'

Two witnesses of history in the making, Bucky and Gocht, provided us with a very vivid impression of this event.

Setting the tube voltage and the tube current

For the purpose of diagnostics, an epoch-making patent (Fig. V, 41) [P 16] was registered in 1916. Since the hardness of a hot-cathode tube depends on the tube voltage and the intensity of radiation depends on the tube current, it is possible to control the hardness regardless of the intensity. A severe drop in the voltage of the high-voltage system could, however, cause a tube overload which, in accordance with the patent claim, must be prevented: following a change in the tube current the excitation or winding ratio of the high-voltage transformer had to be adapted so that the tube voltage remained constant. This discovery and its implementation have remained important until this very day, and were refined by Siemens with ever increasing precision through the use of closed loop control circuits during the 1970s.

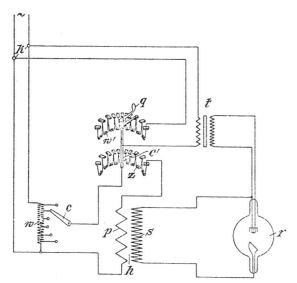

Fig. V, 41. Schematic of a 1916 Siemens patent [P16] to select kV and mA values for a high-vacuum X-ray tube (r). The selector (q) works synchronously and adjusts the filament current via the transformer (t) and the primary voltage for the transformer (h). This was an important protection measure against tube overload.

High-voltage insulation

Friedrich Dessauer (s. Fig. I, 29) worked on the problem of high-voltage insulation in transformers which were equipped with an iron core and still insulated in air. His discovery in 1918 made it possible to reduce the maximum voltage between the winding and the iron core by at least 50% [P 18].

In the mid-twenties, hard rubber cylinders were used in addition to air insulation between the primary and secondary windings. However, around the end of the twenties oil began to move in as the major insulating and cooling medium used in radiology [30]. As mentioned earlier it had already been used to extinguish sparks in mercury interrupters.

The patent registered by Harry F. Waite (Grigg, 1965) [28; P19] in 1920 shows how oil can be used both for insulation and for cooling purposes. At Siemens, B. Doering and G. Grossmann (1923) [18] also experimented with inductors and transformers filled with thick oil in 1919. However, not before 1926 was the HELIODOR high-voltage transformer available for delivery, and then with thin-oil insulation.

In 1924, the POLYPHOS featuring four hot-cathode valves in a Graetz circuit was introduced to the market: this was a genuine 'two-pulse' generator. The firm of Koch and Sterzel in Dresden developed a high-performance diagnostic generator with an output of 40 kW which was initially installed at the University Medical Clinic in Breslau in 1927. As Kurt Leistner (1928) [40] from the Koch and Sterzel Laboratory then reported:

'Recently, radiology has increasingly turned away from the high-kV technique originally made possible by the introduction of the double film. Because of the enhanced image detail they offer preference is given to X-ray images taken with a relatively low tube voltage.'

H. Chantraine (1927) [16] was quoted on soft-radiation exposures of the lung using high mA values. Since, however, the amount of radiation decreases in proportion to the square and cube of the tube voltage, the power requirement increases considerably. For this reason a three-phase transformer in a delta/star-configuration connected to six valves in a Graetz rectification circuit was selected. Leistner explained that it was advisable to follow the proposal made by H. Franke (1927) [21] and characterized the tube voltage with the term 'peak voltage'. This article also described the lead spinning top used to measure the switching time. This was a widely used method up to the sixties, since the voltage pulses were thus imaged on film. The number of pulses for a given line frequency and rectifier circuit could thus be counted to check the exposure time. High output levels obtained with three-phase generators yielded acceptable loads for power plants which did not allow single-phase operation at high output levels due to the resulting voltage drop. The special SIMPLEX valves used were supplied by the firm C. H. F. Mueller AG in Hamburg who also provided the MAMMUT–MEDIA X-ray tube. The timer applied could not switch reproducibly short exposure times; therefore the shortest possible exposure time was limited to 20–30 ms.

Thus began the 'performance race' for X-ray tube focal spots. Rotating anode tubes, particularly those designed according to the high-temperature radiation cooling technique used by Siemens after 1927, replaced fixed-anode tubes. Only these tubes combined with three-phase generators kept the focal spot sufficiently small to optimize the geometric unsharpness with that of motion blur caused by the exposure time and motion of the object.

In 1928, Siemens introduced the GIGANTOS diagnostic X-ray generator to the market. This unit featured a maximum tube current of 2000 mA at 80 kV in a six-pulse, three-phase circuit and a high-radiation output (Fig. V, 42).

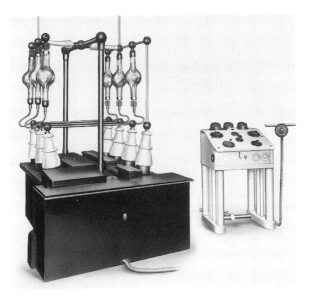

Fig. V, 42. 1928: SRW three-phase X-ray generator. The transformer in an oil container is on the left and mounted on top are the six high-vacuum valves for the six-pulse rectification. The control console for the generator is on the right.

'Quality' at all times

Vacuum technology and generators are very closely linked. Thus for example a Siemens protocol dated from 4 August 1930 documents how product quality was controlled in the test laboratory:

'The Test Lab determined that the Pertinax strips of the limit switches in the Gigantos switching frame are too long and therefore collide with the chain. The Engineering Dept. checked to see whether the deficiency was caused by engineering or manufacturing.'

And further:

'During the inspection of the Gigantos, problems cropped up with the high vacuum valves at voltages above 100 kV. The rectifying valves must always be run up to this voltage over a long time with slowly increasing voltage. Three valves have been returned to the factory as unusable, although only one of them could be designated defective by the factory.'

Quality demands control, and so this report continued:

'It was decided from now on to test the motor relay in the test room for correct timing. This requires additional work . . . since an mAs meter must be installed each time in order to make comparisons.'

A protocol dated 7 May 1931 also reveals concern for the customer and the company's image:

'The Test Lab has been complaining that no wiring diagrams can be obtained for non-standard systems, meaning special customized systems. Since the delivery of these systems is normally urgently required, hand-drawn sketches must be used. As these rather primitive documents do not make a very good impression on the customer, the Dept. is using its influence to have the Design Dept. provide schematics according to engineering specifications. Applications to that effect should be duly made with specific deadlines by the Dept.'

And that is still the daily bottom line in industry today. Each piece of equipment must be checked thoroughly. The complexity of products and systems has increased in the meantime and many more people are involved now than was the case in 1931 or before. This approach constantly inspired everyone to design and manufacture better products for the good of the patient and thus for everyone's good sooner or later.

Quality of radiation and dose

As far as three-phase transformers were concerned the scientific discussion reached full swing during the following years. C. Niemann and W. Zeyss (1932) [48] from the Medical Technical Laboratory of the Siemens and Halske factory in Berlin wrote about the advantages of the three-phase generator. Names like Chantraine, Leistner and H. Franke were mentioned here once again. The chief aspect was the question of whether or not an increased dose could be obtained through additional smoothing by high-voltage capacitors.

The main emphasis was placed on the methods of measurement and the laboratory findings obtained during the years 1927 and 1928, which were obtained using a single-pulse generator, a two-pulse generator, and a DC voltage generator [P 21]. The dose rate of the three-phase generator must therefore lie between that of the two-pulse and that of the DC voltage generator. A previously known interdependence between dose rate and tube voltage was rediscovered:

'The emitted radiation changes at high voltages in proportion to the square of the tube voltage, while a decrease in the tube voltage increases the exponent, which can then assume ever higher values.'

Leistner (1928) [40] postulated an increase in efficiency of 22% if six valves were used for rectification instead of only four and one of 27.4% if DC voltage were to be used. While these values were indeed confirmed, a comparable radiation quality would make it necessary to reduce the voltage with a three-phase generator, leaving an increase in efficiency of only 10–15%. On the other hand, and here is the benefit for the focal spot using a three-phase generator, focal spot output is uniformly distributed, thus yielding a further gain, so that the three-phase generator yielded an output which was 30–40% higher. The additional circuitry and hence costs involved were weighed against the gain in image quality and the reduction of the patient's exposure to radiation.

Small generators as well as large generators

In the tug-of-war between costs and patient benefits, the market remained big enough for both types of generators during the course of the next 50 years (Bischoff and Gellinek, 1965) [9]. Was this the end of the road for the development of the transformer? Of course not. In 1933 Siemens designed a line-voltage equalizer, the PUGNO-VANONI regulator (Pugno-Vanoni and Reimann, 1933) [50], which among other things increased the reproducibility of the tube voltage.

In the same year, a small generator was offered which eventually became an X-ray legend: The 'Roentgen-Kugel' or 'Siemens Kugel' (Kugel meaning sphere or globe).

Despite this fact, much discussion and intense work continued to be devoted to the subject of powerful generators for very short exposure times since screen technology had also made great progress, thus requiring shorter exposure times. K. Bischoff (1935) [12] therefore posed the question: 'To what extent can three-phase technology decrease the exposure time?' The

answer was that it requires 50% less exposure time than radiography with a two-pulse generator. Yet another argument in favour of image quality was found for the three-phase transformer.

After Philips had introduced the MEDIO D with a high-voltage switch for two workstations integrated in the high-voltage transformer tank, the Siemens HELIPHOS came out with three further improvements in 1941: Four rectifier tubes were installed immersed in oil in the transformer tank for rectification purposes, and as had already been the case with Philips, the workstation switch was included as well. The generator was additionally equipped with a new type of voltage-regulating transformer featuring a collector-type slide-way equipped with carbon brush wipers so that the fluoroscopic and radiographic voltage could be continuously adjusted. These carbon brush wipers were simultaneously used to compensate for fluctuations in the line voltage. And finally this generator featured the TUTOMAT circuit: Exposure data were set to match the anatomical regions being X-rayed, thus simplifying the operation considerably. In addition, pre-exposure display of the mAs value was offered to account automatically for the voltage drop resulting during an exposure. This was just one more example of how important competition was in achieving progress.

In 1944 K. Bischoff [P 25] patented a display and control device (Fig. V, 43) to set and pre-indicate technique factors of the generator. K. Franke (Fig. V, 44) and his team implemented this idea step by step for all examinations beginning in the late sixties: A programmed technique with 'organ selection'. Figure V, 45a shows the control console of all OPTIMATIC generators with which technique factors could be selected freely to override preprogrammed organ parameters if necessary (Schmitmann et al, 1971; Steiner et al, 1973) [53, 57]. The control and power electronics cabinets of the constant potential generator PANDOROS OPTIMATIC (Ammann, 1974; Schmitmann and Ammann, 1973) [6, 54] is shown in Fig. V, 45b.

A further reduction in size of these bulky cabinets and control consoles was achieved in the eighties by applying microprocessor technology, high-frequency power electronics, and touch screen controls (Fig. V, 46).

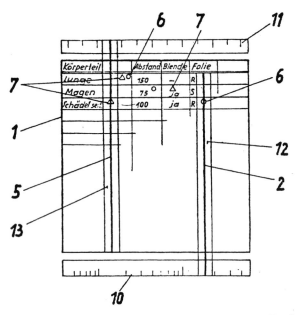

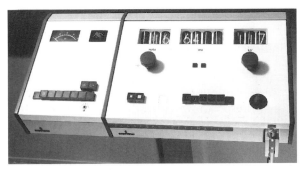

Fig. V, 45a. 1972: Control console for an OPTIMATIC generator with power circuits of 50, 100, and 150 kW, free selection and electronic analogue computer for technical factors (kV and mAs) scaled to exposure points, automatic overload protection for all focal spots, and satellite consoles in time-sharing operations. Since 1972, all Siemens generators have been equipped with a closed-loop control system for the tube voltage (kV) and with service support function [22, 53, 57].

Fig. V, 43. K. Bischoff and E. Leuteritz filed a patent [P25] in 1944 to simplify the selection of kV and mAs. Names of body regions and organs were displayed along with the associated technical factors and markers (6, 7). A bar (5) could be moved across to position it over a marker (7). The kV value was indicated on the scale (11) and set automatically. A second bar (2) was used likewise for the mAs marker (6) and the mAs value on the scale (10). This was an important patent leading to the organ-specific programmed techniques.

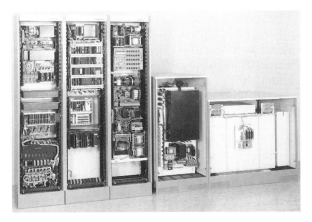

Fig. V, 45b. 1972: PANDOROS OPTIMATIC. From left to right, the first generator cabinet contained a high-speed starter and the system distribution centre; the middle cabinet contained the electronic analogue computer, the kV and mA control circuitry and the automatic exposure control system. The third cabinet contained the power distribution, filament circuitry, and stabilisers for the internal voltage supply. The high-voltage transformer cabinet and the tank for the high-voltage control triodes are on the right. It was a 150-kW constant potential generator with closed-loop circuitry for tube voltage and current. Any of four X-ray tubes of up to 150 kW could be used in pulsed operation with up to 500 frames per second. Shortest exposure time was 0.3 ms and 1 ms with IONTO-MAT 7 [6, 54].

High-kilovoltage techniques

In 1949 J. Meiler (1949) [43] reported from the Radiological Laboratory of Siemens–Reiniger in Erlangen on the effect which different high-voltage transformers and their rectifier circuits had on image quality and tube load. His research had been completed in 1944, but the end of the war

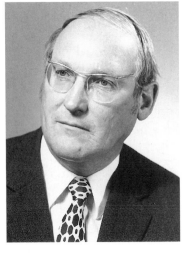

Fig. V, 44. Kurt Franke (born 1920), Doctor of engineering sciences, Chief Engineer and Director of Generator Engineering at Siemens in Erlangen (retired 1982). He simplified control functions via automation of fluoroscopy, tomography, cine application, spot-filming with image intensifiers and digital subtraction angiography. He brought high-frequency generators based on inverter technology and microelectronics into production in 1978. Since 1987, all Siemens diagnostic generators have been based on this technology.

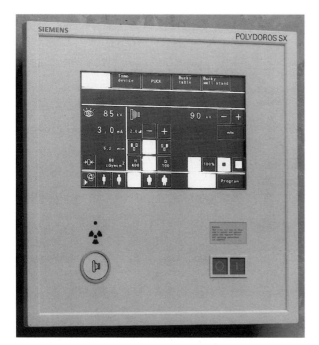

Fig. V, 46. Control console in 'touch screen' technology for the POLYDOROS SX (1993), a microprocessor-controlled high-frequency generator (80 kW) for fluoroscopy, radiography and digital imaging. Figure V, 47 shows its high-voltage transformer unit.

apparently postponed its publication. Meiler's findings again demonstrated that three-phase and capacitor buffered generators such as the KODIAPHOS require only about 5% more energy than a DC generator.

Hence, a distinction was now made between small-, medium-, and high-output generators. Meiler again wrote in 1950 [44] that transformers and tubes must to an ever-increasing extent have high-kV capability, since a trend towards tube voltages exceeding 100 kV or even 120 kV was becoming more and more apparent. New grids for the reduction of scattered radiation as well as suitable films and intensifying screens had become available.

Meiler devised the following comparison table for equivalent exposures:

Table V,1a. Meiler's comparison table [44]

Wave shape of tube voltage	6-pulse	4-pulse
Output requirement	0.75	1
Rated output of rotating anode tube (kW)	1.5	1
Exposure time	0.5	1
Patient exposure to radiation	0.8	1
Line-voltage drop	0.6	1

The answer to Meiler's question must therefore be that the six-pulse mode of operation has distinct advantages. Readers interested in historical details may wish to refer to the literature (Biermanns, 1949; Müller, 1950; Küchler, 1956) [8, 37, 45, 46, 47] for further particulars.

In 1956 the 40th anniversary of the three-phase generator was fittingly celebrated at Siemens–Reiniger by the introduction of a new 12-pulse generator, the TRIDOROS 4. In his presentation on that occasion, K. Bischoff (1956) [10] recalled how in 1927, Chantraine and Gutzeit had pleaded for the use of an extremely 'soft-radiation' i.e. low-kV technique for chest radiography. Low-ripple, DC voltage, three-phase current and a six-pulse circuit represented the only solution to the question of how the required amount of radiation could be obtained in connection with tolerable exposure times and focal spot dimensions at 2000 mA. On the high-voltage side the TRIDOROS 4 used a star and a delta circuit in order to obtain a tube voltage with a theoretical pulsation of only 3.5%. An alternative circuit patented by K. Franke [P 30] was also available for this purpose. Bischoff explained:

'Considering these substantial advantages, one can only be amazed that the three-phase generator took such a long time to gain ground on the single-phase generator and, that even today, two-pulse generators belonging to the same performance and price class as the three-phase generators are still being manufactured (the American and British medical industries do not offer a three-phase generator even today!). Especially with regard to the high-voltage part, the volume has been reduced to the point where these units can be installed directly in the examination room . . . (still) the maximum operating voltage has increased by almost 50% during the preceding 30 years . . . 150 kV must constitute a reasonable limit for the purpose of practical diagnosis.'

Thus the TRIDOROS 4 was a 100-kW generator featuring 3-ms exposure time and rapid serialography for angiographic sequences of up to six images per second. It therefore provided enough extra output for improved rotating anode tubes, which first became available in 1962 with 100-kW output at a 1.3 focus and using a 150-Hz high-speed starter.

Transformers (Braun and Seidel, 1969) [14] designed for radiological equipment represented a speciality because X-ray tubes require a very high output for only a fraction of a second, defined as the kW level measured at 0.1 s. Thus the high-voltage transformer had to be rated for a brief output of up to 100 kW in the radiographic mode and a continuous output of 300 W in the fluoroscopic mode.

Since 1970 voltage-regulating transformers have been used in a new application: due to the carbon rollers that tapped the current directly from the auto-transformer coil, specific adjustment of the voltage was possible during the exposure. This meant that the initial load proposed by A. Bouwers (1933) [13] could now be realized practically for the first time. Siemens' OPTIMATIC generators were all operated with a continuously falling load to enable the shortest possible exposure time at a constant tube voltage (Schmitmann et al, 1971; Schmitmann and Ammann, 1973) [53, 54].

Chopper or inverter technology

In 1958 SRW conducted laboratory experiments on chopper technology, which during the seventies successfully established itself in modified form for use in high-frequency X-ray generators. At that time three-phase line voltage was fed through silicon rectifiers to an IGNITRON chopper and the resulting AC voltage was then fed to a two-pulse high-voltage transformer unit. The IGNITRON was an electronic switch for high currents which was switched on, or as the technicians put it 'ignited', by a small control current.

Siemens Elema exhibited the first high-frequency generator, the MOBIL XR with 20 kW output, at the ICR in Rio de Janeiro in 1977. This innovation remained unrivalled for some time. The fundamentals of transformer engineering and power electronics have been completely revised since that time [P 36, P 37, P 38]. The operating frequency increased from the line frequency (50 Hz) to a range of 3000 to 5000 Hz. This demanded new core materials with lower eddy current losses, resulting in considerably reduced core cross-sections. As a result it became possible to reduce the structural size of the high-voltage transformer (Fig. V, 47) as far as the new plastic and oil insulation allowed.

The year 1977 represented a genuine turning point in generator engineering which would later be outdone by only two subsequent improvements: W. Kuehnel (1986) [38] and P. Tichy at Siemens in Erlangen developed in 1988 a generator for computer tomography which operated at a frequency inaudible to the human ear and yielded a constant output of 4 kW. This was a genuine contribution to increased efficiency since it enabled examinations at a much higher patient throughput. Of course a completely new type of X-ray tube had to be designed and manufactured

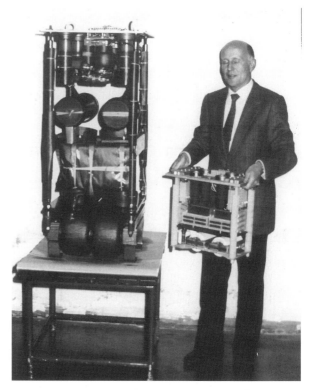

Fig. V, 47. The size of high-voltage transformer units changed in 1984: Conventional 100 kW (left); G. Wiede (right) carries a high-frequency 100 kW unit for the POLYDOROS.

for this purpose. Both of these innovations were first used in the SOMATOM PLUS computer tomography unit.

In 1990 the American firm Bennet introduced another innovation by increasing the operating frequency to 100 kHz although this initially worked only with 30 kW in the radiography mode without fluoroscopy.

The trend is clear: transformer and generator engineering are closely linked both to the innovations achieved in connection with the X-ray tube and to medical requirements for reproducibility and stability of examination conditions, especially of those conditions that influence contrast and perceptibility of details in spatial and time structures. Image quality, but also exposure of patients and medical teams to radiation, space and power requirements, noise level, durability, reliability, and costs have played an important role in the development of an X-ray generator.

High-voltage rectification

Spark gap or rotating rectifier for an ion X-ray tube (with reverse current or 'closing light')

The operation of ion tubes (s. Fig. V, 4) depended on the polarity, and was therefore also dependent on the connection of the lead storage battery. The current flowing through the primary coil of the inductor (s. Fig. V, 28) from the battery is rhythmically interrupted and produces the 'opening' voltage in the secundary windings. When the current path is closed again a smaller voltage is generated by the reverse current. This reversal of voltage means that the anticathode becomes the cathode and radiation is emitted from the actual cathode – the so-called 'closing light' (Grossmann, 1912) [29].

This could be prevented by using a plate-to-point spark gap like the one patented in 1901 [P 3] (Fig. V, 48). It could also be replaced by a valve tube, particularly when using high-power inductors through which current of more than 5 mA flow (Betriebserfahrungen, 1913) [7]. An inductor could, thus, also be operated in an AC network with an electrolytic interrupter.

As early as 1904 Siemens delivered an X-ray generator featuring a high-voltage transformer

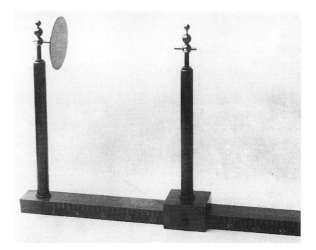

Fig. V, 48. 1901: Spark gap to prevent a reverse current by operating an ion X-ray tube on an inductor.

and rotating high-voltage rectifier that utilized the negative half-wave of the AC voltage to generate radiation in the ion tube. The requirement of ensuring that the rectifier movement was synchronous to the AC voltage placed very high demands on the mechanical precision. Figures V, 49 and V, 50 show an X-ray system of 1920 and the operating principle of the rectifier circuit.

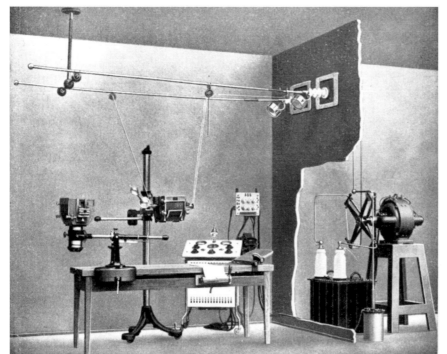

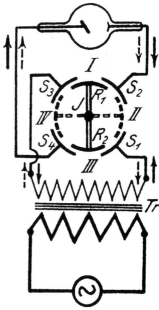

Fig. V, 49. HELIOPAN R generator, tube stand with water-cooled ion tube in protective housing. Open high-voltage leads descend from the ceiling. The generator control console and panel are at the back; the high-voltage transformer and the motor with mechanical cross-arm high-voltage rectifier are on the right (produced between 1920 and 1927).

Fig. V, 50. High-voltage cross-arm rectifier [23]. The tube was better preserved and provided sharp images with good contrast.

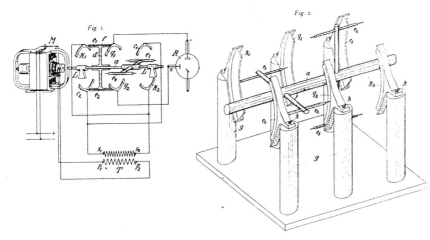

Fig. V, 51. Schematic from a 1909 patent for a high-voltage rectification system for use on transformer-operated X-ray tubes [P4]. According to this, the rotating rectifier was smaller in design because the connecting rod was arranged parallel to the axle of the motor-driven contacts. A generator using this patent is shown in Figure V, 36: IDEAL apparatus

The American H.C. Snook also developed rotating rectifiers. He operated an ion tube hooked up to an AC transformer using a mechanically rotating rectifier powered by a synchronous motor. Snook manufactured this device in quantity and introduced it to routine clinical practice in 1907.

In Europe improvements were incorporated in the production starting with the IDEAL generator in 1908, followed by a patent [P 4] in 1909 which represented a considerable improvement of high-voltage technology (Grossmann, 1912) [29] (Fig. V, 51):

Instead of a two-pole motor, a four-pole version which ran at only half the rotational speed was used. Thus it proved sufficient to double the number of contacts. Axis-parallel high-voltage contact rods were used to simplify the insulation of the shaft considerably. Operation in oil was proposed to utilize the higher dielectric strength, which in turn led to smaller dimensions, and hence smaller structural design. Furthermore contacts did not produce any harmful ozone when immersed in oil. And finally, in order to make the vessel oil-tight as well, the patent also suggested that even the motor should be operated immersed in oil.

A number of additional patents [P 5, P 7, P 8, P 11, P 13] followed in the years leading up to 1911.

Reports (Betriebserfahrungen, 1913) [7] on practical experience dated from 1913 stated:

'Operational experience with X-ray systems: Dr Pasche, an experienced X-ray specialist from the Insel-Spital in Bern, has been working with our X-ray generator (with rotating high-voltage rectifier) for some time and considers it to be an ideal instrument for every X-ray physician. He confirmed that our instrumentarium prolongs the life span of X-ray tubes which . . . is important. Thus, for example, approx.

1500 exposures were taken with a single Mueller water-cooled tube. At the same time, Dr Pasche worked only with medium-hard and hard tubes; he did not use soft tubes at all. Likewise Dr Oetiker in Wengen (Switzerland), who takes some 250 exposures per year with our rectifier, has been using the same three X-ray tubes for approx. two years.'

At the tenth Radiological Convention held in Berlin in 1914, Siemens presented their Universal X-ray system featuring a tube voltage of 150 kV and rotating rectifiers.

High-vacuum valve

The Coolidge high-vacuum tube no longer required a rectifier. This was initially considered to be an advantage by K. Lasser (1916) [39]. Even today, small units such as used in dentistry, operate in this manner. In 1914 Dushman of General Electric designed the KENOTRON, a glass valve with a heated cathode, which first became available as a serially manufactured product in 1926 (Grigg, 1965) [28]. To better utilize the X-ray tube, Lasser also used vacuum valves with hot cathodes in his generator (s. Fig. V, 39). In 1917 Siemens patented a new circuit [P 17] in order to double the voltage by combining a high-vacuum valve and a capacitor. This configuration could also be expanded to a high-voltage cascade. In 1928 GIGANTOS was launched as a three-phase generator with six valves (s. Fig. V, 42) to generate a tube current of up to 2000 mA at 80 kV.

High-vacuum valves were initially operated in air and, starting in 1940 (Philips MEDIO D), were integrated in the transformer tank immersed in oil. Not until the mid-fifties did Siemens, gradually followed by other manufacturers, begin to replace valves with semiconductor rectifiers (made from selenium or silicon).

Switching and control valves

The tube output could be continuously increased especially due to the rotating anode tube. In 1933 this triggered the development of a switchable high-voltage valve at Siemens. The idea was to install such a switching valve on the secondary side in a high voltage capacitor generator so that very short exposure times could be switched repeatedly. Already by mid-1934 a 55-kW output could be switched for an exposure time of 100 ms with a 100-Hz high-speed starter for the X-ray tube. The development of the switching valve was often revised because the grid control circuit was unfavourable and the voltage drop was much too large. The target was to reach a value of 2000 mA. Finally in 1938 the KODIAPHOS generator was introduced with a minimum exposure time of 3 ms.

In 1962 Siemens developed a high-voltage control triode (140 kV/2000 mA), which in 1973 served in the PANDOROS OPTIMATIC generator for angiography (s. Fig. V, 45). At this point the tube output had risen to 150 kW. Furthermore a tube current of 2000 mA and an exposure time of 0.3 ms had also been attained (Schmitmann and Ammann, 1973; Ammann, 1974) [6, 54]. The control valve also provided good service in computer tomography by keeping the tube voltage constant during the scan time.

Selenium rectifier

Vacuum components were subject to an ageing process which resulted in a limited life span. Furthermore vacuum tubes were so expensive that laboratory trials in search of new materials were started as early as 1950: Selenium (Brunke, 1949) [15] turned out to be the most suitable material when properly designed as a semiconductor rectifier. Already in mid-1951 a semiconductor rectifier could be operated under laboratory conditions, immersed in oil at 220 kV and 30 mA. It took another year before higher currents could be managed (Fig. V, 52). In 1953 the STABILIPAN became the first therapy generator with selenium rectifiers. Between 1953 and 1956 Siemens invested a great deal of development work and resources before diagnostic X-ray generators with selenium rectifiers could be manufactured in series.

Fig. V, 52.
A major breakthrough in minimizing the size of the high-voltage rectification system brought the selenium semiconductor rectifier. Wear and tear in rectifiers was a thing of the past. The filament transformer for the high-voltage rectifier disappeared.

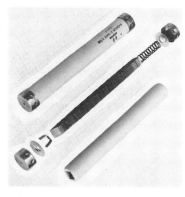

Siemens introduced and designed this rectifier in 1952. The first rectifier was 170 mm long and could withstand a voltage of 5 kV at a continuous current of 11 mA which led to a pulse current of 340 mA.

These rectifiers were much smaller than high-vacuum valves and bore the name 'solid state semiconductor rectifiers'. Although this is a sturdy component, the semiconductor was occasionally destroyed by excessively high voltages. In 1955, Bischoff reported on the introduction of the solid state semiconductor rectifier to radiology (Bischoff, 1955) [11]:

'The now generally accepted method of rectifying high voltage, i.e. using vacuum tubes, has only been in use for some 30 years. Prior to this development, rectification was performed almost exclusively with the aid of rotating rectifiers. The chief advantages which led to this transition to the high-vacuum valve were its noiseless operation and, above all, the lack of arcing. The latter was an especially serious drawback to the use of the mechanical rectifier and represented a considerable source of danger to the connected X-ray tubes. However, it was more or less taken in stride that the virtually indestructible mechanical rectifier had been replaced by a much more sensitive component offering only a finite life span. . . . The high-vacuum valve . . . possesses a number of undesirable attributes. First of all, the necessity of providing a filament circuit for the hot cathode involves no small expenditure for insulating transformers and balancing components . . . [and] space requirement . . . [and] source of danger for the X-ray tube . . . following the failure of a valve. The solid state semiconductor rectifier developed during the last 25 years represents a type of rectifier which would appear to be perfectly ideal for today's interests.'

The selenium rectifier wafer was described in full detail. Due to its extremely small structural form [P 26], the volume of the high-voltage transformer tank was further decreased. However, as it later turned out, extremely high tube currents of more than 1000 mA could not be operated in a reliable way (constant current of 175 mA/cm^2).

Siemens decided in 1955 to develop selenium rectifiers which could be installed following failure of a high vacuum rectifier. Of course, changes in the circuitry also had to be implemented so that the modified internal resistance conditions could be adapted accordingly.

Silicon rectifiers

At the end of the sixties 'soft radiation' techniques with high tube currents was again in demand for angiography. It then became necessary to turn to silicon (Shields, 1955) [55] although, this move involved two disadvantages:

The silicon rectifier wafer could not be operated immersed in transformer oil nor could it withstand overloads even in the case of extremely short voltage peaks such as those unavoidable when X-ray tubes arc. Resistors or capacitors were therefore required to balance the voltage across each rectifier. This made rectification more expensive, but represented the only solution to the problem of being able to control high tube currents.

Around the end of the seventies much smaller high-frequency transformers were equipped with correspondingly smaller silicon rectifiers. However, the latter were pressed in plastic so that they could be inserted in printed circuit boards via a two wire connection. These 'Si diodes' are still used in all high-frequency generators today, and have more than proved their value. Their structural volume amounts to only a fraction of that of the selenium rectifier, with a considerably lower voltage drop.

A wide array of rectifier circuits was used in X-ray generators (Müller, 1950) [45, 46]. For single-tank generators selenium [P 29] (Fig. V, 53), and later on silicon rectifiers, yielded decisive improvements in performance.

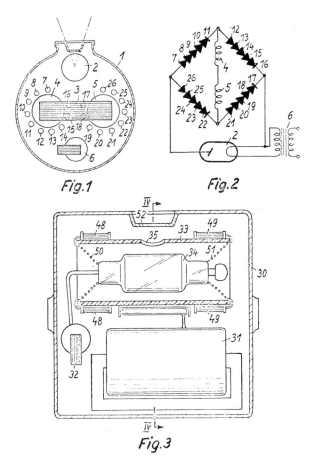

Fig. V, 53. J. Seidel filed a patent [P29] in 1957. He arranged the semiconductor rectifiers within a single-tank unit with two-pulse rectification. This patent led to a new direction in building single-tank units and even today this principle is used for high-frequency single-tank units from 700 W (for dental X-ray machines), up to 50 kW. Fig. 1 shows the single-tank unit (1) with the X-ray tube (2) and the filament transformer (6). The high-voltage transformer with two secondary coils (4, 5) and the high-voltage two-pulse rectification system (7–26). In Fig. 3 a different view shows the rectification system arranged around the X-ray tube (34) and filament transformer (32). The high-voltage transformer (31) is below the X-ray tube and the rectification system (48, 49) surrounds the X-ray tube on the cathode and anode side.

Transformation of the high-voltage rectifier

In 1897 C. Liebenow [P 1] patented a circuit featuring unipolar cells functioning as an AC/DC converter, but this was never put to practice in radiology.

The transformation of the rectifier used for ion tubes ranged from the plate-to-point spark gap to the mechanical cross-arm rectifier with motor drive used to prevent the closing light caused by the reverse current. Coolidge brought out the high-vacuum tube in 1913, thus providing the basis for the high-vacuum valve and the triode or tetrode as a high-voltage switching valve in the twenties. In 1956 the high-vacuum valve was replaced by the selenium semiconductor rectifier, and at the end of the sixties by the silicon rectifier. Noise, wear-and-tear, and large structural volume were all problems which now belong to the past: The rectifier has undergone a technical metamorphosis despite its virtually unchanging function.

Single-tank generator

As early as 1919 the American Harry F. Waite (Grigg, 1965) [28; P19] had the idea of installing the transformer and the X-ray tube in a single radiation-protection housing, thus making high-voltage lines in air between them unnecessary.

An American patent [P 20] to that effect was registered in Germany in 1920 (Fig. V, 54). Waite's idea was implemented by several manufacturers. Thus for example, starting in 1933, Siemens manufactured the 'Roentgen KUGEL'. The oil-filled sphere had a diameter of only 22 cm and contained the X-ray tube and the transformer for the filament and tube voltage; a good compromise was 60 kV and 10 mA. It found many admirers over a period of almost 40 years (Fig. V, 55) and enjoyed worldwide popularity because it proved mechanically robust and reliable in unfavourable climates.

In 1935 single-tank generators were built featuring high outputs of 80 kV at 50 mA, which could also be used for fluoroscopy. They were dubbed 'Roentgen cameras'. This designation

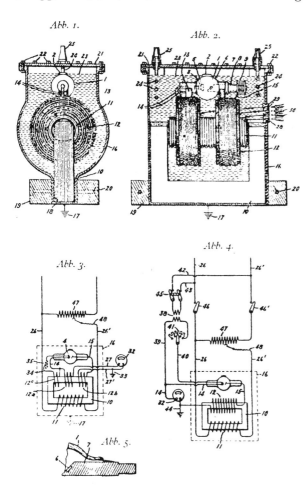

Fig. V, 54. Based on H.F. Waite's 1919 patent for a single-tank generator which contains the X-ray tube and the high-voltage transformer in an oil-filled tank, the International General Electric Company Inc. in New York filed a patent in 1920 [P20] for a single-tank unit. Fig. 1 shows a cross-sectional picture of their proposal and Fig. 2 a longitudinal cross-section. Figs 3 and 4 are principal schematics and Fig. 5 shows a cross-section of the anode of the X-ray tube. A proposal to operate X-ray tubes in oil to avoid the corona effect on the cables between tube and inductor had already been proposed in 1896. The oil itself would also serve as a cooler for the tube. The tube was built with radiation-absorbing lead glass, but the window (2) was radiation-translucent. The core of the transformer (10) in Fig. 3 carried the primary coil (11) and the secondary coil (12) which could be separated into two separate windings (12a and 12b). The tube is mounted on the transformer with isolating materials and the leads from the transformer to the tubes (14 and 15) are directly connected. The material of the tank (16) is metal and grounded (17). The oil (23) is cooled via a pipe (24) which carries a cooled liquid. The primary connection to the transformer (26') is impervious to oil. Figs 3 and 4 show the schematic with all the parts outside the single-tank unit, for example, the mA meter (32) and an adjustable resistor (47).

Fig. V, 55. 1933 Siemens 'Roentgenkugel' ('roentgen sphere') was first built in 1933 and became the universal single-tank generator, manufactured for some 40 years.

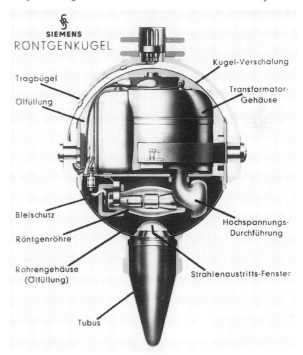

Fig. V, 55a. The cross-section shows on top the connection to the transformer (the German terms are translated in a clockwise direction) sphere housing, transformer housing, high-voltage connection from the transformer to the X-ray tube, radiation window, cone to point at and keep a specific focus–skin distance, oil-filled sphere, X-ray tube, lead protection within the sphere, oil-filled space, support arm. The tube output was 60 kV at 10 mA and the diameter of the sphere was 220 mm.

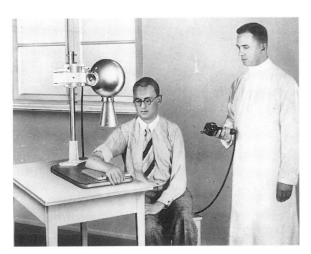

Fig. V, 55b. Forearm exposure with a portable Siemens 'Roentgenkugel' in 1935.

again points to the age-old question of whether the production of X-ray exposures represents a special discipline of photography or is the responsibility of physicists and physicians.

The year 1956 represented yet another milestone for single-tank generators. X-ray image intensifiers for surgery made it possible to view X-ray images without dark adaptation. During that same year Philips brought the BV 20 surgical stand onto the market (s. Fig. V, 175). This stand comprised a C-arm with a single-tank generator mounted on one end and an X-ray image intensifier mounted on the other end. This made it possible to perform fluoroscopy quickly and easily either in the operating room or in the emergency ward. The unit was mounted on a trolley and could be moved around the patient, eliminating any turning of the patient to obtain the medically required perspective.

Single-tank generators had been in use for some time in dentistry, either for exposures of individual teeth (Fig. V, 56) or for the panoramic view. On one hand, the STATUS X [P 22], a versatile X-ray system for 55 kV, was used to record tooth status (Fig. V, 57); on the other hand, the RENODOR was used to take intraoperative radio-

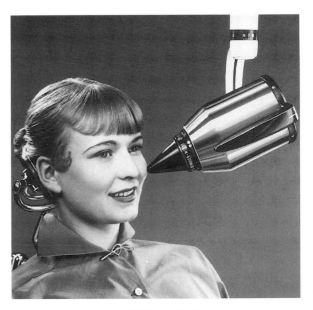

Fig. V, 56. The HELIODENT (50 kV–7 mA) is a classic dental X-ray unit manufactured from 1955 until 1966 and still used today in high-frequency technology.

Fig. V, 57. The STATUS X panorama dental unit was manufactured from 1966 until 1974.

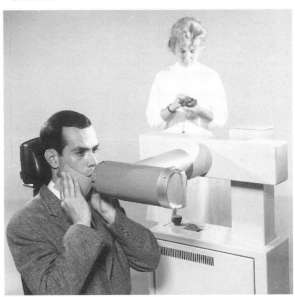

Fig. V, 57a. Patient positioning for a panoramic radiograph of the mandible.

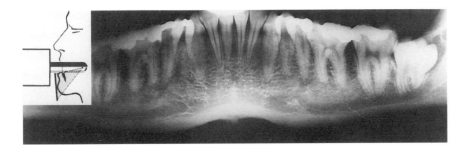

Fig. V, 57b. Principle of the specially designed X-ray tube and a radiograph of the teeth in the mandible.

graphs of kidney stones (Leusch, 1970; Albrecht, 1972) [4, 41]. Even exposures of the shoulder joint (Tölle, 1972) [58] were produced on an experimental basis.

Due to their practicality and to the fact that they no longer required high-voltage cables for the X-ray tube, single-tank generators were soon put to use by the World Health Organisation (WHO) (s. Fig. V, 106) and by the military, who had been interested in the concept of field X-ray units since 1896.

In 1960 Siemens' engineering staff achieved yet another breakthrough: the single-tank NANOPHOS weighed only 27 kg, was compact in size, contained a high-voltage transformer with selenium rectifiers in a two-pulse circuit, and a special rotating anode tube with a focus of 0.8 which attained a remarkable power output (60 kV at 100 mA or 125 kV at 50 mA). This generator was utilized widely as a stationary unit mounted on a floor stand with a Bucky table and Bucky wall stand or as the NANOMOBIL mobile unit. It found widespread use in hospital wards and ICUs, since the high tube voltage was optimally suitable even for high-kV chest radiographs. This was especially important considering the fact that chest radiography of immobile or bed-ridden patients in hospitals had increased dramatically over the past 2 to 3 decades.

But many ambitious engineering attempts had failed. For example in 1967 a NANOPHOS was powered by a set of car batteries via a mercury turbochopper for the purpose of radiography. This functioned without a hitch except for the fact that suitably fast battery chargers were not then available and the batteries' storage capacity was sufficient for only a few radiographs. Part of the problem involved the high power consumption of the IONTOMAT. Due to its extremely high insulation requirement, it had to be designed with amplifier tubes in old-fashioned radio technology. As a result the cathode filaments absorbed a considerable amount of energy from the batteries. With the idea of being able to take radiographs without a power connection, a technical solution was devised but proved inadequate for the wide variety of radiographs required in routine clinical practice. The dream of having a mobile X-ray system independent of the hospital power supply remained unrealized for the time being.

Another decade elapsed before the MOBIL XR was introduced at the 1977 ICR in Rio de Janeiro. Microprocessor technology (Ammann and Schwarzmann, 1990) [5], semiconductor electronics, and high-frequency, high-voltage technology made it possible to again take old ideas and finally put them into practice. This mobile unit was battery-powered and featured motor-driven wheels and a 20-kW single-tank generator.

The principle of high-frequency generators (Kühnel, 1986; Krestel, 1988, 1990; Hoxter and Schenz, 1991) [32, 34, 35, 38] was intensively studied and expanded to increasingly higher power levels. Thus in 1978 the 30-kW POLYPHOS, and only a year later the 50-kW POLYPHOS with two foci (Fig. V, 58) followed in rapid succession. These single-tank generators were designed for fluoroscopy and radiography on tilting tables and Bucky units.

In 1990/91 the single-tank generator was also introduced by Picker and Siemens for use in computer tomography. The inverter principle made it possible to connect the system to either a single-phase or a three-phase power supply since the line voltage was rectified and energy was stored in a capacitor. This DC voltage was inverted to obtain a high-frequency AC voltage. It was then fed to a single-phase, high-voltage transformer which, due to the high frequency, only required a tiny core. It was then rectified and smoothed on the high-voltage side to ensure that a tube voltage

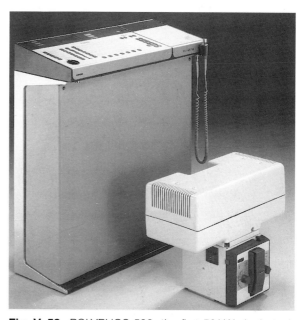

Fig. V, 58. POLYPHOS 500: the first 50 kW single-tank generator (1980) with collimator (in the front). The tank contains the high-voltage and filament transformer, high-speed starter for 200 Hz, and a 50 kW X-ray tube. The control console (at the back) contains the electronics and controls for fluoroscopy, automatic exposure control system and organ programs as well as free selection of kV and mAs.

with a very low high-frequency pulsation was generated.

The inverter principle for single-tank generators originally operated at frequencies of 3–7 kHz, and in 1982 was also introduced for generators with outputs of 80 and even 100 kW, although not with the single-tank design.

High-voltage lines and cables

For many years inductors were connected to X-ray tubes by means of wires suspended in air as can be seen in many older photographs (Figs. V, 59 and V, 60, also s. Figs. V, 27, V, 36, V, 38, V, 49, V, 91 and V, 110). The patient therefore had to be positioned in such a way that these un-insulated high-voltage lines did not come too close to the patient or physician. The technology of manufacturing cables with high-voltage insulation had not then been perfected, although the need was certainly strong enough. Another factor was the frequent need to change tubes (s. Fig. V, 75) in order to adapt the radiation hardness to the job at hand.

This leads us back to Waite, who in 1919 had had the idea of completely eliminating high-voltage lines by combining the high-voltage transformer and the X-ray tube in a single housing. The Coolidge tube (1913) was of course a prerequisite. However, the physicians' unabating desire for yet more power in the focal spot soon placed limits on the single-tank generator as well.

In Germany, 1926 brought a turning point. Siemens introduced the first superficial X-ray therapy unit for 12 kV. This unit had a high-voltage cable between the transformer and the tube (Ebersberger and Morkel, 1968) [19]. Based on this high-voltage cable, Siemens developed the cables for the TUTO tube housing in 1931 (Fig. V, 61). In 1936 high-voltage connectors were introduced to make it easier to separate the transformer from the tube (Figs. V, 62 and V, 63). A long-held desire of production and service departments had thus finally been fulfilled.

Cables had textile sleeves, natural rubber insulation, and tin-coated copper wires as leads. Air pockets posed the greatest problem. Due to

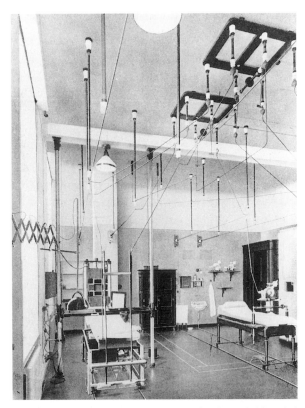

Fig. V, 59. Diagnostic X-ray room in St. Georg's Hospital in Hamburg in 1915: The open high-voltage lines can be clearly seen supporting the different ion X-ray tubes, from the ceiling.

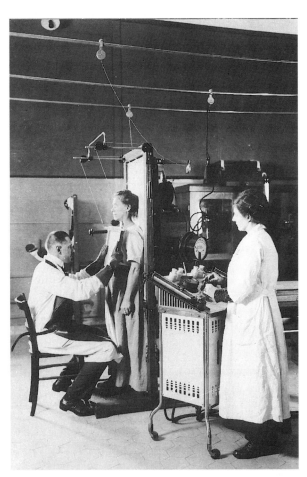

Fig. V, 60. Fluoroscopy room in the University Women's Clinic in Erlangen, 1918.

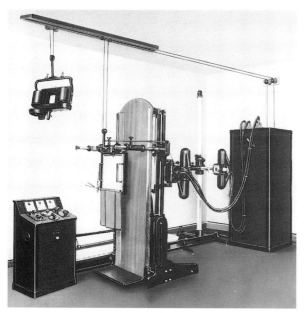

Fig. V, 61. The first diagnostic X-ray system in 1933 with high-voltage cables between the high-voltage transformer on the right hand side and the tube housing assembly. Two X-ray tubes are supported by the generator TUTO HELIO-PHOS, one by the floor stand and the second by the TELE-PANTOSKOP, a tilting table with screen and lead rubber protection. A serial exposure device according to Berg was mounted on the ceiling with a counterbalanced system. This was necessary to examine patients in any angled position between horizontal and vertical. The X-ray tube in the housing was air cooled and the high-voltage cables were not detachable from the tubes. Radiation protection was provided by cones and lead-shielded tube housing as well as the lead rubber leaves.

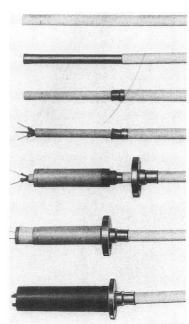

Fig. V, 63. Production steps in a COCIR standardized 75 kV high-voltage connector in 1967. This process took about 30 min. This connector is still used today for both ends of the transformer and the tube [19].

Fig. V, 62. High-voltage cable connector: oil insulation was not used before 1936, so the connection to the transformer and cable was made of porcelain to be used in air. The cable and the tube were undetachably connected [19].

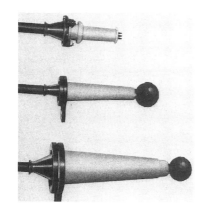

the high field strengths on the surface of the copper wires, air pockets resulted in a corona discharge which produced ozone. This ozone was aggressive, and therefore caused small cracks in the rubber, which in turn intensified the corona to the point where the insulation ruptured and damaged the cable beyond repair. Therefore special attention had to be devoted to the combination of materials, and to the extruder used to encase the conductor in its insulating material.

The solution was finally discovered in 1932 by the Siemens employee Mrs E. Bormann, who patented her discovery as the 'OZONEX principle' [P 24]. The cable contained several individually insulated copper conductors that fed the current from the filament transformers to both filaments of the cathode in the X-ray tube.

In 1949 a high-voltage cable rated at 150 kV was designed for the high-kV technique and was exhibited at the ICR in London in 1950. At the same time the cable diameter could be reduced to 27 mm. This was an important contribution to improved flexibility and a great help to system designers. The textile sleeve was finally abandoned and replaced by a rubber sleeve.

At the end of the fifties natural rubber, which had been imported from the Sunda islands (in the then Dutch colonies), was replaced by artificial rubber such as BUNA or EPR. This had two important advantages: The new material was less sensitive to ozone and, above all, compatible with copper so that the copper leads now no longer had to be tin coated. The diameter of the new cable was further reduced to 23.5 mm, resulting in improved durability under bending stress. Furthermore it was now 'twistable', i.e. could withstand rotational movement or twisting in its longitudinal axis. This point was also welcomed by both system designers and technologists.

Cable terminals and connectors were internationally standardized by the Comité de Coordination des Industries Radiologiques (COCIR). This standardization has been of lasting benefit to all X-ray system users.

Finally, in 1961, a four-pole, high-voltage cable with a standard plug was developed to connect the grid-controlled double-focus tubes for the cine mode in angiocardiography. After having been replaced by the advent of secondary-controlled generators like PANDOROS in 1973, and abandoned altogether after the introduction of the POLYDOROS high-frequency generator in 1984, the grid-controlled X-ray tube experienced a renaissance in 1987 with the introduction of digital pulsed fluoroscopy. Digital pulsed fluoroscopy represented a significant contribution on the part of industry toward decreasing patient exposure to radiation by 50%, especially during interventional procedures. At the same time the quality of the fluoroscopic image was actually improved with respect to motion blurring.

The reduction of cable diameters always was, and is still, an important concern. Thus in 1968 the Siemens cable for a 75-kV single-pole tube voltage had a diameter of only 15 mm. A semiconductive rubber layer located above the inside conductors and below the metal wire mesh at ground potential were two more ideas that helped increase the insulating strength. Today manufacturers of high-voltage cables can be found in almost every country. Although expensive, this component is important for the operational and electrical safety and reliability of each and every X-ray system. Excess filament current can damage or destroy an X-ray system, and movement of the unit can result in inadmissible bending of cables. For this reason, each individual manufacturer of tubes, X-ray systems, and generators must work closely with the cable manufacturer in developing his own high-voltage cable and approving it for operation.

One challenge remains: To replace this specially developed and (due to low production quantities) extremely expensive product with a standard power or communications engineering product, or even with single-tank designs.

This is an example of how just one of the components of an X-ray system was developed. Such systems contain hundreds of other components for each of which a comparable history could be narrated. Each individual component must be tested in its specific X-ray environment. This is because sooner or later in the vacuum of every X-ray tube, arcing will occur, causing more or less high-energy transient waves. They may in turn impair the function of components to the point where the cost advantage and potential damage must be carefully evaluated when procuring spare parts.

Measurement of hardness

The term 'hardness' has many meanings. Here it is not meant to be the physical hardness of a material or of the human will in a physical or psychic sense, but rather a new characteristic. Fuchs [23] wrote in 1922: *'Roentgen determined that the penetrating power of X-rays increases in proportion to an increase of the vacuum in the tube and in proportion to the resulting application of higher voltages across the tube.'*

In 1912 Grossmann [29] wrote:
'In order to solve a wide variety of tasks, the radiologist must have radiation exhibiting every degree of hardness at his disposal . . . to take a radiograph of the hand which clearly displays the bone structure, very soft radiation is required, while an exposure of the pelvis can only succeed with extremely hard radiation.'

Three different types of tubes were then assigned to various indications. Following Roentgen's discovery it had become customary to refer to the hardness of the radiation according to the corresponding tube type with its degree of evacuation.

Again G. Grossmann (1912) [29] wrote:
'The tubes normally referred to as soft are those which are suitable for taking photographic exposures of a child's thorax, the hands and the teeth. Medium-hard tubes permit photographic exposures of extremities, an adult thorax, the skull and the pelvis of non-corpulent persons. Hard tubes must be used for exposures of the pelvis of corpulent persons, the hip joint, the spinal column, kidney stones etc.'

The spark gap as a means of measurement

Since the applied voltage on an ion tube must increase in proportion to its hardness, the tube voltage also constitutes a measure of the radiation hardness. It was also common knowledge that the distance between two electrodes in air – e.g. metal point and metal plate or two points – was a measure of the voltage level. In other words the length of the spark gap which the inductor voltage feeding the ion tube can bridge over is a measure of the tube hardness. A 'spark meter' already existed in 1896: Inductors were equipped with a plate on the negative side and an adjustable point on the positive side where the distance between the two electrodes was read off (s. Fig. V, 35). This distance was thus a measure of the hardness in centimetres.

This was a coarse measure, since the sparking distance for a fixed voltage is very strongly influenced by the quality of the air and the shape of the electrodes. Thus B. Walter (1926) [60] wrote: *'The Association of X-ray Tube Factories has decided to use as electrodes for the spark gap two spheres measuring 25 cm in diameter. According to the specifications made by the Association, with a sparking distance of 6 cm, the voltage across the tube should equal 162 kV and at 7 cm 185 kV.'* It is incredible that this sphere gap remained the most accurate means of measurement available in the X-ray laboratory until well into the 1970s [21]. Taking the air pressure and temperature into account, a high-voltage accuracy equal to 2% of the peak voltage could be attained.

Comparing the brightness of fluorescent images

As early as 1898, scales with numbers and products such as the AKINOMETER or SKIAMETER developed from the KRYPTOSKOP, existed. According to Grossmann (1912) [29] the most widespread scale at that time was the hardness scale devised by Walter [60] and later published in 1926.

A lead disk had 8 holes, each of which was covered with a platinum plate of a different thickness, ranging between 0.005 and 0.64 mm. A fluorescent screen was then laid on top of this and covered with a lead-glass plate. Note that a consciousness of the need for X-ray eye protection already existed in 1902! The number of holes that could be perceived as illuminated under the X-radiation were referred to as the Walter unit (W unit), which was then used as a measure of the radiation's hardness.

Thus, the measurement of hardness had already become practicable in the radiological practice by the turn of the century. This was also an important tool for assessing the correct exposure time. In Basel, Klingelfuss coined the term *'characteristic of a tube'* to designate the degree of hardness at a defined current of 1 or 0.5 milliamperes as the specific hardness.

Benoist used the relative comparison of the luminous intensity of a fluorescent screen. This device comprised a silver disk and an aluminium sector ring made with 6 steps varying from 2 mm to 8 mm thick. These sector fields were numbered. The degree of hardness was specified in Benoist–Walter (BW) units.

The KRYPTORADIOMETER, after Wehnelt, was based on Benoist's device and used a 5 x 20-mm cutout in a lead plate. This plate was covered with a 0.09-mm-thick silver plate. A 16-cm long adjustable aluminium wedge (1–11 mm) was located above the upper part of the cutout. This device had made it possible to define continuously the degree of radiation hardness as early as 1903. Table V,1 indicates associated degrees of hardness, published by G. Grossmann (1912) [29].

These methods utilized the fluorescent screen and a relative comparison of two different irradiated materials. The actual tube voltage was not measured, although a relationship did, of course, exist.

In Bern, Th. Christen (1914) [17] used the half-value layer to describe the hardness. In Erlangen, Reiniger, Gebbert and Schall produced

Table V,1. Measurement of radiation hardness in 1912 [29]

		Soft radiation				Medium-hard radiation		Hard radiation	
Benoist	B	2	2.5	3	4	5	6	7	8
Benoist-Walter	BW	1	2	3	4	4.5	5	5.5	6
Walter	W	2-3	3-4	4-5	5-6	6	6-7	7	7-8
Wehnelt	We	1.8	3.3	4.9	6.5	7.3	8	8.8	9.6
Bauer	Bauer	1	2	3	4	5	6	7	8

Table V,2. Measurement of radiation hardness and indicators in 1926 [60]

		Radiation hardness							
Benoist	B	2	2.5	3	4	5	6	7	8
Benoist-Walter	BW	1	2	3	4	4.5	5	5.5	6
Wehnelt	We	1.8	3.3	4.9	6.5	7.3	8.0	8.8	9.6
Walter	W	2-3	3-4	4-5	5-6	6	6-7	7	7-8
Half-value layer (Christen)	C	–	–	0.63	0.75	0.88	1.00	1.18	1.35
Limiting wavelength in angstrom	–	0.9	0.6	0.45	0.35	0.30	0.26	0.23	0.20
Sparking distance in cm	–	1-4	3-6	5-10	6-12	7-15	8-18	10-25	12-30
Indication			A	A	B	B	C	C	

Indication:

A: Teeth, hands, congenital dislocations in infants, child thorax.

B: Adult thorax, extremities, cranium, neck, shoulders in normal persons, hip joint, spinal column and kidney stones.

C: Pelvis, hip joint, spinal column and kidney stones in obese subjects.

this quality meter which was primarily used in radiotherapy. However, in the eighties this principle regained its earlier significance for diagnosis, since it then enabled the non-invasive measurement of voltage in the radiological practice. H. Aichinger (Aichinger et al, 1990) [1] and K. Franke patented [P 41] this kV meter based on the varying transparency of two filters.

Its measurement principle is also used for automatic exposure control and timing purposes.

Radiation spectrum

B. Walter (1926) [60] also cited the X-ray spectrograph, a hardness meter designed by March, Staunig and Fritz in Innsbruck. The radiation spectrum has a limiting wavelength which is related to the maximum tube voltage level. Thus the radiation was transmitted through an approximately 1-mm-thick sodium chloride plate so that a reflection occurred at the inner lattice planes of the plate. Based on the Bragg law (sine of the reflection angle), the tube voltage can thus be determined with an accuracy of 0.4–5.0 kV.

Today spectroscopy is still used in laboratories as the most exact method available for measuring peak high voltage. However, it has no bearing on the shape of the high-voltage waveform. Another drawback is that the voltage can only be measured with very small tube currents, i.e. only in the fluoroscopic mode, since long measurement periods are required. The tube voltage cannot be determined in this manner for radiographic exposures in the kilowatt range.

Comparison of results from various methods

Walter (1926) [60] stated the corresponding degrees of the different meters (Table V,2), whereby Albers-Schoenberg's indications were also utilized.

Lasser [39] stated in 1916: 6 Wehnelt corresponds to 40 kV and 10 Wehnelt to 70 kV.

Bleeder or high-voltage divider

Engineers then began to measure the tube voltage directly by designing a high-voltage divider with resistors, a so-called bleeder. This is an array of ohmic resistors or capacitors connected between the high-voltage line and ground. Part of the voltage is tapped and measured near ground. Siemens and Halske had all types of hardness and dose measuring equipment in their production programme. Therefore, it was not surprising that Siemens Reiniger designed a bleeder that could be inserted between the transformer and the X-ray tube. A voltmeter or a cathode ray oscilloscope was used to measure the voltage. In the second half of the sixties it was recognized that the reproducibility of the tube voltage was very important for consistently high-quality exposures. Beginning with the TRI-DOROS OPTIMATIC generator (Schmitmann et al, 1971) [53], all Siemens generators feature a high-voltage measuring and feedback system which constantly regulates the tube voltage and keeps it at a predetermined value even during radiation emission.

This helped in connection with the mAs setting or the automatic exposure control system and organ programmed settings to prevent the necessity of repeating exposures. Other companies did not follow suit until many years later, and then still did not consistently offer such systems for all generators (Siemens remained the exception!).

The bleeder finally became superfluous as a service tool and, since the eighties, non-invasive kV meters convenient to use have been offered by many companies.

Intensity – not to be confused with hardness

Finally a word about intensity: It should not be confused with the hardness of the radiation. Intensity of a tube depends on its material composition and design, and changes proportional to the tube current at a particular tube-voltage wave shape. The value in milliamperes (mA) is therefore measured and displayed.

In Paris, Gaiffe introduced the d'Arsonval galvanometer to radiology in order to measure the product of milliamperes and seconds (mAs product, s. Fig. V, 68) – i.e. the amount of electricity, which is an important technique factor for good X-ray exposures (Walter, 1926) [60]. Walter put it this way:

'Intensity can now be theoretically explained quite easily if the obvious assumption is made that the amount of X-radiation generated in an X-ray tube within a given period of time is directly proportional to the amount of electricity cast in the form of cathode rays from the tube cathode to its anticathode within the same period of time.'

Exposure time

Due to the low power of the X-ray tube, exposure times were initially very long, actually several minutes (s. Fig. V, 2). In order to estimate the correct exposure time, the radiologist first screened his own hand. This practice resulted in radiation burn (Fig. V, 64). In 1905, a test hand (Fig. V, 65) was introduced for such exposure time estimates. Figures V, 89 and V, 91 show how the exposure was manually switched. Reinforcement of the anode material's thermal strength and an increased radiation emission – the solution was tungsten – made it possible to attain higher outputs and hence shorter exposure times. Standard clockwork time switches were used and, following elapse of the estimated exposure time, the X-radiation was switched off.

Single-pulse roentgen instrumentarium

In 1909 'BLITZ' (translated 'flash X-ray apparatus') was introduced by F. Dessauer [P 6]. This inductor was capable of switching an exposure time of only 0.01 s, enabling sharp exposures of the lung and of the cardiac shadow for the first time. There were two products: the Veifa BLITZ inductor and the Reiniger unipulse inductor, available since 1906.

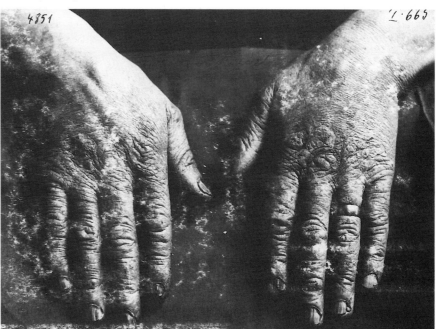

Fig. V, 64. Radiation-burned hands, photographed in 1910. The exposure time was estimated by using the hand as a test object in the fluoroscopy mode.

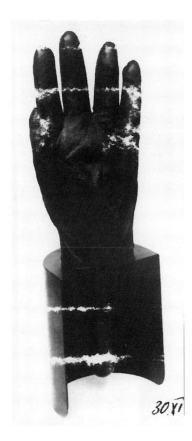

Fig. V, 65.
A standard hand manufactured in 1905 to measure the radiation.

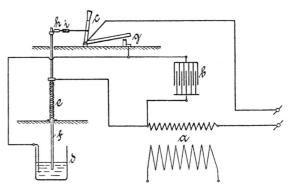

Fig. V, 66. Schematic of F. Dessauer's 1909 patent [P6] to terminate an exposure in an ion tube by a spring-loaded contact.

were suddenly destroyed by the heat, thus interrupting the circuit.

Peak high-voltage and wave shape

'As you no doubt already know, the hardness of the X-radiation emitted by an X-ray tube increases with the tube voltage applied. This voltage increases from zero to maximum value during the first half-wave of the AC voltage and then drops back down to zero. As a result, during the first half-period, the tube first emits softer radiation then increasingly harder radiation until a certain maximum hardness has been attained, after which the emitted radiation becomes softer again. Dessauer correctly realized the fact that radiation of almost constant hardness can be obtained if only the uppermost peak of the AC voltage waveform, i.e. that portion where the voltage least changes, is utilized. Therefore, he planned his 'reform apparatus' with contact segments of small dimensions. As a result, only a very small part of the half-wave was utilized, namely the uppermost peak of the voltage waveform' (Konkurrenz-Apparate, 1913) [33].

This point illustrated the significance of the voltage waveform and its influence on the image character. This was also a trailblazing discovery for the development of generator technology since it demanded better circuitry both for increased dose yield and for short exposure times.

Siemens interviewed radiologists concerning their radiographic technique and received two different answers. The first group described the radiographic technique used by Albers-Schoenberg in Hamburg. On the whole, exposures were taken with a tube current of 10 mA and exposure times of 30–60 s without intensifying screens. The second group worked primarily with the exposure tables compiled by Reiniger,

It was realized in 1913 that the amount of energy thus made available was sufficient for chest radiography but not for stomach radiography or fluoroscopy [P 12]. However, this single-pulse technique was also used with transformers and high-voltage rectifiers. Thus, as described in the literature (Konkurrenz-Apparate, 1913) [33]: *'It was first indicated in 1901 by Klingelfuss and then experimentally tested by Albers-Schoenberg and Walter in 1902...'* Dessauer then picked up on this idea again and developed the single-pulse technique with his inductor, using a mercury switch (Fig. V, 66) which he himself had patented to reach the short exposure time of 10 ms. This switch differed from the method used by Walter and Albers-Schoenberg in 1902 only in that the moving part of the switch was not operated manually but was pulled out of the mercury by a spring. In 1907, Koch used a pistol shot which severed a copper wire. After Dessauer had, as he himself put it, *'created a fiasco'*, he came across the idea of using fuse links as cutouts.

A second patent granted to the Veifa factory (Dessauer) protected the application of fuse links which, after the current was turned on,

Gebbert and Schall which, however, as experience had shown, specified overly short exposure times. At the same time it became apparent that most of the experiments had already been performed with transformer and rectifier systems. Another result was that with a good inductor, 10 mA exposures lasting for 30–60 s, attained a quality comparable to that of the considerably more expensive transformer and rectifier system. Thus in 1913 the exposure tables were mentioned in confidential reports (Vertrauliche, 1913) [59] as follows:

'In conclusion, we would like to announce to you the following information which was kindly placed at our disposal by the Danzig Hospital (Dr Schulz, Table V,3) *comprising the average values taken from 1178 exposures and by the Insel-Spital in Bern* (Dr Paasche, Table V,4); *both of these institutions put our rectifier to good use.'*

An excerpt is shown in Tables V,3. and V,4.

Finally, modified values according to Reiniger, Gebbert and Schall (Vertrauliche Mitteilungen, 1913) [59] are quoted in milliampere seconds in Table V,5 for a tube hardness of 6.5 Walter units.

Timers and the soft-radiation technique

In 1926 Westinghouse manufactured a high-speed circuit breaker and fuses for the generator. The principle used was based on the idea of a releasing magnet with a compound winding.

Table V,3. Technical parameters for a medium-hard tube with an intensifier screen provided by Schulz in Danzig 1913 [59]

Head, anterior view	8 MA	6 s	50 cm distance
Lungs	32 MA	0.75 s	70 cm distance
Gastrointestinal tract	25 MA	1.5 s	70 cm distance
Kidneys/bladder	8 MA	6 s	25 cm distance with diaphragm
Lumbar spine	7 MA	6 s	25 cm distance with diaphragm
Pelvis	8.5 MA	6 s	55 cm distance
Forearm	6.5 MA	3 s	25 cm distance with diaphragm
Metacarpus	8.5 MA	1.5 s	25 cm distance with diaphragm
Knee joint	7 MA	6 s	25 cm distance with diaphragm
Metatarsus	8.5 MA	1.5 s	25 cm distance with diaphragm

Table V,4. Technical parameters for a medium-hard tube without intensifying screen provided by Paasche in Bern in 1913 [59]

Head, anterior view	6 MA	50-70 s	60 cm
Thorax, lungs, rips	30-40 MA	1/10 - 1/20 s*)	120-150 cm
Gastrointestinal tract	20-30 MA	1/10 s*)	70 cm
Kidneys/gallstones	6 MA	1.5 - 2 min.	70 cm
Lumbar region/small of the back	6 MA	1.5 - 2 min.	70 cm
Pelvis and hip joint	6 MA	2-3 min.	70 cm
Arm	6 MA	5-30 s	60 cm
Hand	6 MA	5-10 s	60 cm
Knee	6 MA	1 - 1 1/12 min.	60 cm
Foot, anterior view	6 MA	40 s	60 cm

*) With intensifying screen

Table V,5. Technical parameters for a radiation hardness of 6.5 Walter provided by Reiniger, Gebbert and Schall in Erlangen in 1913 [59]

Head, anterior view	355 Ma/s
Heart and lung	55 Ma/s
Gastrointestinal tract	145 Ma/s
Kidneys and gallstones	555 Ma/s
Lumbar spine	405 Ma/s
Pelvis and hip joint	135 Ma/s
Arm	55 Ma/s
Hand	20 Ma/s
Knee, anterior view	185 Ma/s
Foot	75 Ma/s

(Ma/s corresponds to today's mAs)

From this time on, a timer was installed along with an additional isolating switch, so that the exposure time could be switched for a single snapshot or a rapid series technique. The timer [P 15] (Fig. V, 67) operated independently of the line voltage and the inductor current. Since it operated on the magnetic effect and was triggered by spring tension, this timing relay could be used to set precise switching times ranging from 0.1 to 6 s.

K. Leistner (1928) [40] from the Roentgen factory of Koch und Sterzel AG, Dresden, wrote:

During its recent development, radiology has increasingly turned away from the hard-radiation technique first enabled by the introduction of the double

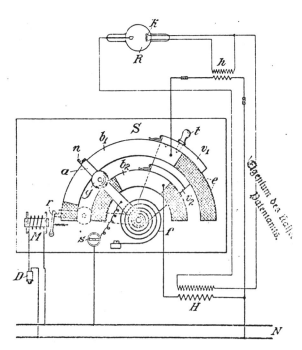

Fig. V, 67. Sketch of a Siemens and Halske patent of 1915. It provides a timer for short exposure times in a generator with high-vacuum X-ray tubes. A pre-contact heats up the filament of the cathode to the appropriate temperature for the selected tube current. The main contact is then turned on to provide the high voltage to the X-ray tube. At the end of the selected exposure time, both circuits are disconnected. This principle has been used in all diagnostic X-ray generators for medical radiographs with short exposure times [P15].

film ... Chantraine emphatically pointed out that soft radiation offers a higher resolution than hard radiation. However, work with low tube voltages has the disadvantage that the dose rate drastically decreases, thus requiring considerably longer exposure times. In addition, the penetration power of radiation decreases. ... In order to attain short exposure times even when soft radiation is used, only one approach can be used: increase the intensity of the tube current to a level which is much higher than the usual amount.'

Thus in 1927, H. Chantraine [16] called for a 2000-mA tube current with approx. 36 kV so that pulmonary diseases could be detected in their early stages with a source-to-image distance of 150 cm. He assumed a value of 200 mAs and, therefore, an exposure time of 0.1 s.

These reports were based on the findings of a three-phase generator built by Koch and Sterzel which was equipped with six high-vacuum rectifier valves yielding an output of 40 kW. It had

been installed in the Radiology Department of the University Medical Clinic in Breslau at the end of 1926. The X-ray tube used was a newly released MAMMUT-MEDIA tube manufactured by C. H. F. Mueller in Hamburg. A new timer for the TITANOS, as the three-phase generator was later named, was capable of switching 20–30 ms accurately. The exposure time was checked by a 'gyroscopic exposure'. A lead disk with a radial slit was rotated as a spinning top on a film cassette. The film was then exposed with preset technique factors. The developed film then showed a number of slits which corresponded to the peak values of the tube voltage. A three-phase six-pulse generator at 50 Hz showed three slits every 10 ms. A spinning top remained in use as a simple method of checking the exposure time well into the seventies.

Since technique factors were already known as the mAs product and the kV value, an mAs meter was developed in the laboratory as early as 1930 (Fig. V, 68). The trend towards the extremely soft radiation technique was demonstrated in 1933 by a three-phase six-pulse generator with 3500 mA at 40 kV, 2000 mA at 60 kV, and 1000 mA at 80 kV. The shortest exposure time was 30 ± 10 ms switching accuracy. A special magnetic time-lag relay had been developed for this purpose. This TRIDOROS also had a line-voltage equalizer, the PUGNO-VANONI regulator (Pugno-Vanoni and Reimann, 1933) [50], with which the tube voltage could be exactly set prior to the exposure. One of Siemens' engineering reports dated 12 December 1933 notes: A rotating anode

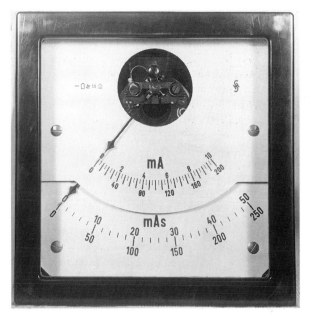

Fig. V, 68. 1950: mA and mAs meter.

tube with a larger anode disk, small focal spot, and a 100 Hertz high speed starter has to be developed for Dr Chantraine. This unit is to be used for long focus-film distance chest radiography with soft radiation and a small focal spot. The anode disk diameter was limited by the speed of rotation and the tensile strength of tungsten. The idea was also mentioned of reducing the speed of rotation to save on wear of the bearings, i.e. decelerate the speed of rotation to increase the life span of the tube. In mid-1934 the tube was available with an 8-cm diameter tungsten anode disk and a 100-Hz high-speed starter for an output of 55 kW at an exposure time of 0.1 s. The 100 Hz were generated by thyratrons, but this solution was very expensive and therefore failed to find general acceptance in radiology.

Trend toward the hard radiation technique

At the end of the forties the trend changed toward the use of higher tube voltages in chest radiography. Suitable scattered radiation grids were built which were moved during the exposure in such a way that the (already very fine) grid lines were 'blurred out' on film. The hard radiation technique especially applied for chest radiography entered the scene. This technique reduced radiation exposure to the patient and the tube load while at the same time improving image quality. Of course this had consequences for tables, stands, high-voltage cables, and the tube housing assembly. Thus for example, grounding the tube housing and dividing the tube voltage into a positive and a negative high voltage value became especially important.

Exposure time of generators, even for rapid serialography at 8 frames per second, could not be forced below 3 ms with electromechanical switching components.

The tube voltage again reached 125 kV and 150 kV. The 180 kV or even higher tube voltage levels often demanded for chest radiography by Swedish radiologists did not meet with worldwide acceptance.

Electronic timer

During the sixties electronically controlled timers were developed which, in conjunction with electronic power switches such as IGNI-TRONS or THYRATRONS, improved the reproducibility of the exposure time while reducing it to only 1 ms. The reduced dose requirement of

film screen combinations also caused permanent problems with the shortest possible exposure time, and hence with reproducible optical film density of chest radiographs. In the USA Picker used a grid-controlled tube for chest stands to enable short and reproducible exposure times.

The mAs relay

The mAs relay patented by C. Niemann, SRW (Fig. V, 69) [P 23] was of course a good solution for improving the reproducibility of exposures. It was introduced by Koch and Sterzel in 1935. It also served as an aid in achieving the organ programmed control of the 1944 Siemens patent [P 25]. The decisive aspect here was that once the tube voltage had been selected to match the required image contrast, it also remained constant even during the exposure. This was made possible by closed-loop control circuits and the use of a tube voltage measuring system which was integrated in all newly developed generators manufactured by Siemens during or after 1971.

Only the use of secondary closed-loop controlled high-voltage circuits could bring exposure times down below 1 ms. The PANDOROS

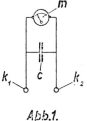

Fig. V, 69.
C. Niemann of SRW in Erlangen filed a patent [P23] in 1928 on a mAs-relay circuit. The tube current is integrated in a calibrated capacitor (c). The spark gap (f) ignites if a specific mAs value has driven up the voltage on the capacitor to a limit. The current through the transformer (i) provides a magnetic force to a lever (r) which had held a spring-loaded contact closed. The exposure is terminated by opening the contact via the lever.

Abb.1.

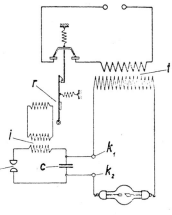

Abb.2.

OPTIMATIC (s. Fig. V, 45) exhibited at the 1973 ICR in Madrid and in clinical test since 1972 switched 0.3 ms fully electronically for tube outputs of up to 150 kW (Schmitmann and Ammann, 1973; Ammann, 1974) [6, 54]. Problems in connection with the shortest possible exposure time for fast film-screen combinations had thus been solved although not without considerable costs and bulkiness. Still, this generator set the standard for the coming decade with regard to the absolute reproducibility of technique factors.

The demand that the exposure time be automated to the point where only the tube voltage and dose required by the image receiving system – i.e. the film-screen combination – need be selected had been expressed by radiologists for some time. Such a measure could help prevent imperfect exposures, and therefore repeated exposures as well, thus making a major contribution to radiation hygiene. Chest radiography with the optical image intensifier (s. Fig. V, 113) was selected as a suitable object.

Automatic exposure control (AEC)

The history of the automatic exposure control (Fig. V, 70) is reflected in the SRW development reports (Entwicklungsberichte, 1938) [20] issued between 1938 and 1948 from which the following texts are quoted:

January 1938:

'(Heinrich) Franke's automatic exposure control system fails (to function properly) due to the fact that the average optical film density which can be measured by a dose chamber cannot be brought into agreement with the required density.'

A development report on the fiscal year March 1940 to February 1941 dated 7 May 1941 reads:

'The problem of the automatic exposure control was again tackled. Proposals made on this subject from various sides were thoroughly discussed in a technical colloquium. A patent was also applied for this year.'

A report written in December 1941 states:

'The status of the trials is being demonstrated in the R Lab. A large-area, radiolucent ionization chamber is being presented on the chest equipment together with the switch gear developed earlier by Dr Franke at C.H.F. Mueller; a new, inertia-free relay circuit is being shown in an experimental version; it is initially planned only for use in mass fluorography equipment for chest examinations; its general application is possible due to the fact that the ionization chamber not only switches off after the total dose has been reached, but also automatically adjusts to the most fa-

vourable voltage without inertia depending on the actual dose rate; the inertia-free voltage control is being demonstrated on the oscilloscope connected in series with the X-ray tube using a power-driven control valve tube' [Editor's note: KODIAPHOS circuit, later PANDOROS].

A development report issued by K. Bischoff in April 1942 then read:

'At the same time, large-scale preliminary trials are being conducted to create a device with a perfect automatic exposure control. This device will not only automatically switch off the radiation once the film has been exposed to a predefined radiation dose, but also automatically set the tube voltage which is correct for the given object. This requires an inertia-free control of the X-ray tube voltage via a high-voltage control valve. Tests have shown that the new type of control valve with cup anode used in the KODIAPHOS is suitable for this purpose. The ionization chamber located between the object and the film influences the grid voltage of the control valve and, therefore, the X-ray tube voltage, to the point where the instantaneous dose striking the film retains a value which is characteristic for the object, regardless of the object thickness, etc. The exposure is interrupted as soon as a given integral dose has been reached. Once the basic possibility of such a control has been determined, the remaining tests and considerations will be devoted to the practical technical design (grid circuit of control valve connected to high voltage or to a single-pole grounded generator etc.).'

An entry from October 1943 read:

'Development has now progressed to the point where a prototype can be built and the construction work can be started. The delay of the electromagnetic switch which causes a variable time error with varying divisions of the mAs product into mA and seconds, is compensated by a new type of circuit (similarly to KODIAPHOS). The large-area ionization chamber, whose metal coating was recently applied using vacuum sputtering at Siemensstadt, exhibits such a tube voltage response that the sensitivity inevitably must be altered via the tube voltage setting. However, at the given tube voltage, no error would be caused by the variable object thickness. The system is in any case useful for mass fluorography of the chest with a fixed tube voltage and should initially be designed for this purpose.'

The impact of the tube voltage response for dose measurements was thus known in 1943. The IONTOMAT was born as a product in 1946. A SRW development report dating from March 1947 read:

'As an attachment for our standard diagnostic systems, a simple automatic exposure control has been developed which automatically terminates the expo-

sure as soon as the film has been exposed to a specific, selectable amount of X-radiation. In contrast to the automatic exposure controls mentioned earlier, the tube voltage is freely selected in the usual manner at the generator. The AEC automatically alters the exposure time so that the average optical film density is correct for an object regardless of the given mA value or any specific object characteristics. The generator switch for the exposure time is turned off by this control via a relay. This AEC thus represents an indispensible tool both for conventional exposures and for mass fluorography. Practical testing of AEC on various different X-ray generators for mass fluorography not only proved its feasibility and convenience. It also showed

benefits which can thus be obtained with regard to an increase in the operating speed (omission of the thickness meter), the prevention of incorrect exposures, and reliable determination of the optimal film density. While the simple automatic exposure control described here is suitable only for time control involving exposure times of as little as 0.1 seconds . . . this simple automatic exposure control can be retrofitted to any X-ray generator.'

In February 1948 the development had basically been completed at SRW, and by 1950 the IONTOMAT had fully established itself on the market (Fig. V, 70b). Similar developments occurred on the American market. Westinghouse had a phototimer based on multiplier technology in 1945. Studying under Paul C. Hodges at

Fig. V, 70a–c. Automatic exposure control system: IONTOMAT.

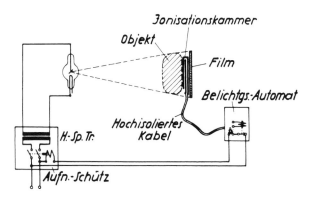

Fig. V, 70a. The principal function of this system is still the same today as it was in 1944. An ionization chamber between object and film measures the dose rate. Highly insulated cables lead a current of a few picoamps to the automatic exposure control unit where the current is compared with a set reference value. When the dose has been reached, the exposure switch in the primary circuitry of the high-voltage transformer opens and terminates the exposure (SRW principle).

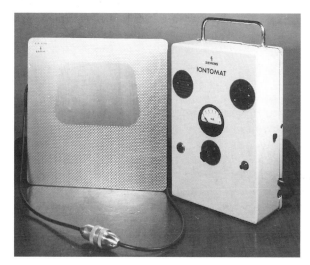

Fig. V, 70b. Ionization chamber (left) and IONTOMAT control electronics (right) for chest radiographs in 1955.

Fig. V, 70c. Proposal for a radiology department with the automatic exposure control system IONTOMAT in 1959. Spot-film device on tilting table (a), Bucky table (b) with an ionization chamber having three measuring fields, Bucky wall stand (c), mass fluorography unit (d) for chest radiographs, workstation selector (e), IONTOMAT control unit (f), and three-phase generator (g) which could serve three or four X-ray tubes.

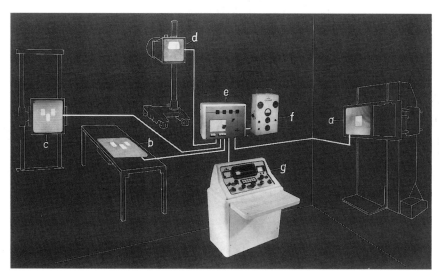

the University of Chicago, Russel H. Morgan designed an automatic exposure control for spot film devices (Krohmer, 1989) [36] in 1948. This achievement was based on an idea conceived by H. Franke in 1923, according to which a 'dominant' exists in every object where the average optical film density is representative for the optical density of the entire film. Figure V, 70c shows an X-ray department with an automatic exposure control system in 1956.

Spot film radiography was predestined for automated exposure control (Gebauer, 1958) [25]. The automatic timing of angiographic exposures on AOT and PUCK film changers followed somewhat later. Further development of the automatic exposure control was characterized by the changes that took place in electronics: The amplifier tube was replaced by transistors and operational amplifiers in semiconductor technology (1970), and finally in 1986 by microprocessor technology.

Ionization chamber and drift compensation

H. Aichinger (1968) [3] introduced a new, shadow-free ionization chamber with three measuring fields in 1968. The technical development status was described by Gajewski (1968) [24] just when technology changed from radio amplification tubes to semiconductors. One serious problem with the automatic exposure control was the DC voltage amplifier, since the ionization chamber supplied currents of only a few picoamperes ($1 \, pA = 10^{-12} \, A$). These DC amplifiers were designed with radio tube circuits and were very susceptible to drift. As a result, in 1971 the amplifier was replaced by semiconductor components and a new control principle was introduced. Closed-loop control systems allowed adjustment of the amplifier to the offset as long as no radiation was present. As a result, no drift was present at the start of an exposure and the drift during the exposure time could be ignored. This considerably increased the quality of OPTIMATIC generators featuring the IONTOMAT 7. The next step for iontomatization was the acquisition and correction of the tube voltage response. Finally, the first microprocessor-controlled automatic exposure control systems, the IONTOMAT P, was commissioned in 1986. Processor technology now made it possible to incorporate any film-screen system which the customer might have so that the tube voltage response of each individual system could be individually calibrated.

Another improvement was the bipolar multifield ionization chamber with preamplifier and a 6-mm chamber. It had thus been made thinner to improve the geometric imaging conditions in tables and stands.

Automatic exposure control (AEC) for tomography

The AEC of tomographic exposures [P 27, P 28, P 32] was of course a special challenge since the exposure time is always strictly specified by the tomography program. Thus only the dose rate can be varied during a tomographic exposure since the required total dose must have reached the film-screen system by the end of the tomographic program. This was first put into effect in 1969 by K. Franke and H. Aichinger (Aichinger and Braun, 1970; Meiler and Aichinger, 1977) [2, 42; P 33, P 39]. The solution was based on a phase-control technique and presented a number of pitfalls to technicians. The pitfalls were not eliminated until 1986 with the IONTO-MAT P. The ionization chamber supplied a current which was proportional to the dose rate. This was attained at a selected tube voltage via a pulse pause modulation technique which could be used with high-frequency X-ray generators like the POLYDOROS S. The required dose can thus be precisely attained in the preset tomographic time.

Automatic exposure control for mammography

The radiation detector for AEC of mammograms had to be located behind the film cassette in order to minimize radiation exposure of the mammae (Säbel et al, 1977, 1979) [51, 52]. The tube voltage response for the extreme soft radiation technique (25–35 kV) had to be corrected by the technician by estimating the given transparency of the mamma. In 1976, H. Aichinger, H.E. Kranberg, and K. Koehler applied for a patent [P 35] on a circuit which enabled measurement of an object's range of contrast. Thus, placing a double detector (Aichinger et al, 1990) [1] behind the film cassette as proposed by Aichinger and Kranberg [P 40] proved quite successful in mammography. Localization exposures for a biopsy could also be taken in two projections with automatic exposure timing for the first time (s. Figs. V, 108 and V, 109). This also contributed to the reduction of radiation exposure and alleviated the work-load placed on the medical staff.

Digital luminescence radiography with automatic exposure control?

Automatic exposure control in connection with storage phosphor technology or computer radiography is controversial yet sensible. Such exposures are normally useful even if the dose fluctuates over a wide range (s. Fig. V, 100). If the dose is too low the image will contain a higher noise level. The physician must decide whether an exposure should be repeated if the diagnostic content is inadequate. However, an excessively high dose cannot be recognized in the image, since an overexposure in the conventional sense, e.g. with film, does not exist here. Hence, an automatic exposure control is very helpful in avoiding the use of unnecessarily high doses.

Automatic exposure control – a contribution to radiation hygiene

Semiconductor electronics and modern generator design have also made two substantial contributions to radiation protection. First of all the necessity of repeating exposures due to technical deficiencies is practically a thing of the past. Even in the case of an arcing X-ray tube the change in dose rate is detected in the ION-TOMAT, and following a brief pause the interrupted exposure is completed. Even such interrupted exposures are normally useful since the film density is properly switched despite the malfunction. On the other hand a combination of two or more X-ray tubes connected to one generator is often encountered. If an X-ray tube inadvertently emits radiation, this is detected by the IONTOMAT P, leading to immediate shutdown of the radiation [P 34]. This feature reduces radiation exposure of patients and medical personnel. And last but not least, the automatic exposure control simplifies operation and data selection considerably. In 1933 A. Bouwers [13] published his theory of temperature distribution in the focal spot from which the idea of initial load control was later derived. In 1958, K. Bischoff [P 31] patented an initial load control which led to the shortest possible exposure time for automatically controlled exposures. Technically speaking it was initially realized in steps and, starting in 1970, for the first time as a continuously falling load (Schmitmann et al, 1971; Franke, 1978; Schmitmann and Ammann, 1973) [22, 53, 54].

Since the seventies, automatic exposure control has been the principal item around which fluoroscopy, spot-film radiography, contrast-medium studies, and the entire field of digital imaging technology were developed by K. Franke's team. It is the principal item in so far as it reliably measures the dose rate and enables uncomplicated operation ensuring consistently reproducible and excellent image quality.

Patents

P 1   DP 103 388 vom 30. Juli 1897, Carl Liebenow, Berlin: Schaltung von Unipolarzellen zur Umwandlung von Wechselstrom in Gleichstrom.

P 2   DP 120 340 vom 3. Jan. 1899, Dr. Arthur Wehnelt, Charlottenburg: Elektrolytischer Stromunterbrecher.

P 3   DP 135 737 vom 21. Sept. 1901, Siemens & Halske Berlin: Verfahren und Vorrichtung zum Betriebe von Röntgenröhren mit Wechselstrom. (Regelbare Funkenstrecke mit Platte-Spitze vor der Ionenröhre).

P 4   DP 225 500 vom 2. März 1909, Siemens & Halske, Berlin: Hochspannungsgleichrichter für Wechselstrom.

P 5   DP 241 614 vom 18. April 1909, Reiniger, Gebbert und Schall, Erlangen: Vorrichtung zum Betrieb von Röntgenröhren mit gleichgerichtetem Wechselstrom mittels eines synchron umlaufenden Stromwenders für den Sekundärstrom. (Ballastwiderstand für den Strom, der nicht durch die Ionenröhre fließt, um Überspannung an der Röhre bei Durchleuchtung zu verhindern).

P 6   DP 250 334 vom 8. Mai 1909, VEIFA-Werke und Friedrich Dessauer, Frankfurt a.M.: Verfahren für Momentaufnahmen mit Röntgenstrahlen. (10 ms Einzelschlagverfahren).

P 7   DP 223 893 vom 29. Mai 1909, Siemens & Halske, Berlin: Hochspannungsgleichrichter für Wechselstrom.

P 8   DP 241 969 vom 2. März 1910, Reiniger, Gebbert und Schall, Erlangen: Vorrichtung zum Betrieb von Röntgenröhren mit gleichgerichtetem Wechselstrom mittels eines synchron umlaufenden Stromwenders für den Sekundärstrom.

P 9   DP 263 053 vom 4. März 1910, Siemens & Halske, Berlin: Verfahren zur Erzeugung von Röntgenstrahlen mittels hochgespannter, der Röhre nur kathodisch zugeführter Teslaströme.

P 10   DP 234 517 vom 2. April 1910, Reiniger, Gebbert und Schall, Erlangen: Vorrichtung zur Messung der Energie der Röntgenstrahlen mittels einer Ionisationszelle.

P 11 DP 236 405 vom 15. Nov. 1910, VEIFA-Werke und F. Dessauer, Aschaffenburg: Verfahren zum Betrieb von Röntgenröhren und ähnlichen Hochspannungsapparaten mit hochgespanntem Wechselstrom.

P 12 DP 262 079 vom 22. April 1911, Siemens & Halske, Berlin: Verfahren zur Erzeugung von Momentaufnahmen.

P 13 DP 259 369 vom 31. Mai 1911, Siemens & Halske, Berlin: Einrichtung zur Regelung der Belastung von Röntgenröhren, welche von einer Wechselstromquelle unter Einschaltung eines Hochspannungsgleichrichters gespeist werden (Variable Kontaktdauer).

P 14 DP 292 596 vom 29. Juli 1915, Siemens & Halske, Berlin: Einrichtung zum Betrieb von Röntgenröhren mit von Mehrphasenstrom gespeisten Hochspannungstransformator.

P 15 DP 293 503 vom 17. Sept. 1915, Siemens & Halske, Berlin: Verfahren und Einrichtung zur Herstellung von kurzzeitigen photographischen Aufnahmen durch Röntgenröhren mit Glühkathode.

P 16 DP 296 464 vom 11. Juni 1916: Siemens & Halske, Berlin: Einrichtung zum Betrieb von Röntgenröhren.

P 17 DP 310 356 vom 8. Feb. 1917, Siemens-Schuckertwerke, Berlin: Verfahren zur Erzeugung hoher Gleichspannung aus einer Wechselspannung.

P 18 DP 339 223 vom 17. Mai 1918, Dr. Fr. Dessauer, Frankfurt a.M.: Reihenschaltung eines Haupttransformators mit einem oder mehreren Hilfstransformatoren.

P 19 USP 1, 334, 936 vom 31. Jan. 1919, H.F. Waite: Oil immersed single tank unit with X-ray tube, filament and high voltage transformer built into one metal box filled with oil.

P 20 DP 416 486 vom 11. Juni 1920 (USA vom 24. Jan. 1919), Intern. General Electric Comp. New York: Röntgenstrahlenapparat mit einer in ein Ölbad eingetauchten Röntgenröhre (Trafo und Röhre im Eintank).

P 21 DP 598 603 vom 3. April 1925, Carl Niemann, Erlangen und Siemens & Halske, Berlin: Verfahren und Einrichtung zur Erzeugung kurzzeitiger Röntgenaufnahmen.

P 22 DP 567 473 vom 25. Feb. 1928, Dr. Walter Hofmann, Erlangen, Siemens-Reiniger-Veifa, Berlin: Glühkathodenröntgenröhre. (Dieses Prinzip wurde bei der STATUS X-Röhre angewendet: geerdete Anode mit Schutzhülle).

P 23 DP 581 160 vom 20. Sept. 1928, Dipl.-Ing. Carl Niemann, Erlangen: Einrichtung für kurzzeitige Röntgenaufnahmen. (SRW: mAs-Relais).

P 24 DP 634 101 vom 2. Juni 1929, Dr. Elisabeth Bormann, Siemens-Schuckertwerke, Berlin: Hochspannungsgummikabel mit im Innern angeordneten halbleitenden Schichten.

P 25 DP 968 848 vom 28. Nov. 1944, Dipl.-Ing. Kurt Bischoff und Ehrhardt Leuteritz, SRW Erlangen: Vorrichtung zur Voreinstellung von Betriebswerten eines Röntgenapparates.

P 26 DP 103 7017 vom 23. Jan. 1956, Johannes Seidel, SRW Erlangen: Trockengleichrichter-Hochspannungseinheit.

P 27 DP 102 4165 vom 9. Juni 1956, Dr. Kurt Franke, SRW Erlangen: Anordnung zur Abschaltung eines Hochspannungstransformators für Röntgenapparate.

P 28 DP 103 1436 vom 18. Juli 1956, Dr. Kurt Franke, SRW Erlangen: Röntgenapparat zur wahlweisen Verwendung mit einem Hilfsgerät, das eine vorgesehene Aufnahmezeit erfordert.

P 29 DP 102 9948 vom 7. Feb. 1957, Johannes Seidel, SRW Erlangen: Röntgen-Eintankapparat.

P 30 DP 104 0138 vom 19. Juli 1957, Dr. Kurt Franke, Siemens-Reiniger-Werke Erlangen: Schaltungsanordnung für Drehstrom-Röntgenapparate: (12-Puls-Schaltung).

P 31 DP 124 5502 vom 18. April 1958, Dipl.-Ing. Kurt Bischoff, Siemens Erlangen: Röntgendiagnostikapparat mit Initiallaststeuerung.

P 32 DP 206 0471 vom 9. Dez. 1970, Jürgen Reimer, Erlangen: Röntgenbelichtungsautomat für die wahlweise Abschaltung beim Erreichen einer vorgegebenen Dosis oder für die Regelung der Dosisleistung.

P 33 DP 240 1774 vom 15. Jan. 1974, Dr. Horst Aichinger, Fürth: Regeleinrichtung für die einem Drehstromverbraucher zugeführte Leistung. (Für Dosisleistungsregelung von Schichtaufnahmen).

P 34 DE 255 0437 vom 10. Nov. 1975, Ing. Herbert Schmitmann, Weiher: Belichtungsautomat für ein Röntgenaufnahmegerät. (Schutz vor zu hoher Strahlendosis).

P 35 DE 261 0845 vom 15. März 1976, Dr. Horst Aichinger, Fürth, Dipl.-Ing. Heinz-Erik Kranberg und Ing. Karlheinz Köhler, Erlangen: Schaltungsanordnung für einen Detektor für ionisierende Strahlung. (Detektor mit mehreren Meßfeldern und Rechenschaltung zur Ermittlung des Kontrastumfanges und Dosisumschaltung).

P 36 DP 280 2450 vom 20. Jan. 1978, Dr.-Ing. Kurt Franke, Siemens Erlangen: Röntgendiagnostikgenerator mit einem seinen Hochspannungstransformator speisenden Wechselrichter und einem die Primärwicklung des Hochspannungsgenerators enthaltenden LC-Schwingkreis (Reihenschwingkreis im kHz-Bereich für Röntgengeneratoren).

P 37 DP 280 2513 vom 20. Januar 1978, Dr.-Ing. Kurt Franke und Dr.-Ing. Gerd Seifert, Siemens Erlangen: Röntgendiagnostikgenerator mit einem seinem Hochspannungstransformator speisenden Wechselrichter, dem ein LC-Schwingkreis zugeordnet ist (LC-Schwingkreis im kHz-Bereich anpaßbar an die Belastung durch die Röntgenröhre).

P 38 DP 281 4320 vom 3. April 1978, Dr. Kurt Franke, Siemens Erlangen: Röntgendiagnostikgenerator mit einer seinen Hochspannungstransformator aus einem Netzgleichrichter speisenden, zwei Wechselrichter aufweisenden Wechselrichterschaltung (Einsatz von zwei Wechselrichtern zur Reduzierung der Welligkeit der Röhrenspannung).

P 39 DE 284 6458 vom 25. Okt. 1978, Dr. Horst Aichinger, Fürth: Röntgendiagnostikgenerator mit einem seinen Hochspannungstransformator speisenden Wechselrichter und einem Regelkreis für die Dosierung. (Für belichtungsautomatisiertes Schichten).

P 40 DE 300 8261 vom 4. März 1980, Dr. Horst Aichinger, Fürth. Dipl.-Ing. Heinz-Erik Kranberg, Erlangen: Röntgendiagnostikeinrichtung mit Mitteln zur Bildung eines Transparenzsignals (Doppeldetektor für Mammographie).

P 41 DE 301 4879 vom 17. April 1980, Dr. Horst Aichinger, Fürth, Dr. Kurt Franke, Erlangen: Vorrichtung zur Messung der Röntgenröhrenhochspannung bei einer Röntgendiagnostikanlage (2 Strahlendetektoren mit unterschiedlicher Filterung und deren Signalverarbeitung).

References

1. Aichinger, H. et al.: Die Belichtungsautomatik in der Mammographie. Electromedica 58 (1990) 61–66
2. Aichinger, H., E. Braun: Belichtungsautomatik für Schichtaufnahmen. Röntgen-Bl. 23 (1970) 400–404
3. Aichinger, H.: Fortschritte in der Technik der Belichtungsautomatik in der Röntgendiagnostik. Radiologe 8 (1968) 233–238
4. Albrecht, K.F.: Urologische Röntgenuntersuchungen. Der Urologe, Springer Verlag, 11. Jg., H. 3 (1972) 140–148
5. Ammann, E., K. Schwarzmann: Microprocess in „smart" Control Consoles. In: Benedetto, A.R. et al. (Ed.): Computers in Medical Physics, AAPM Monograph No. 17, American Institute of Physics (1990)
6. Ammann, E.: Ein neuer Röntgengenerator für hohe Leistung bei sehr kurzer Belichtungszeit. Dissertation, Techn. Universität Stuttgart, 1974
7. Betriebserfahrungen an Röntgeneinrichtungen. Vertrauliche Mitteilungen über Elektromedizin der Siemens & Halske A.G. Wernerwerke Berlin – Nonnendamm, Nr.2 (1913) 28
8. Biermanns, J.: Hochspannung und Hochleistung. Carl Hanser Verlag, München, 1949.
9. Bischoff, K., W. Gellinek: Geräte für die Anwendung ionisierender Strahlen (mit 345 Abbildungen) 121–323. In: Vieten, H. (Herausgeber): Physikalische Grundlagen und Technik Teil 2, Springer Verlag 1965. Gesamtwerk Diethelm, L., O. Olsson, F. Strand, H. Vieten, A. Zuppinger (Herausgeber): Handbuch der Medizinischen Radiologie. Band I, Teil 2, Springer-Verlag 1965.
10. Bischoff, K.: 40 Jahre Drehstromapparate – eine Entwicklung vom Weichstrahlenapparat zum Tridoros 4, dem modernen Großapparat für die Diagnostik mit Spannungen bis 150 kV. Röntgen-Bl. 9 (1956) H. 1, 401
11. Bischoff, K.: Die Einführung des Sperrschichtgleichrichters in die Röntgen-Technik. Fortschr. Röntgenstr. 82 (1955) 117
12. Bischoff, K.: Welche Belichtungszeitverkürzung bringt der Drehstrombetrieb? Röntgenpraxis 7 (1935) H. 1, 40
13. Bouwers, A.: Verkürzung der Aufnahmezeit durch eine neue Belastungsmethode. Fortschr. Röntgenstr. 47 (1933) 703
14. Braun, E., J. Seidel: Hochspannungserzeuger für Röntgenanlagen. Siemens-Zeitschrift 43 (1969) H. 1, 24–29
15. Brunke: Moderne Selengleichrichter. ETZ, VDE-Verlag, Frankfurt/M (1949) 161
16. Chantraine, H.: Über die Weichstrahlaufnahmen der Lunge mit ganz hohen Milliamperezahlen, Fortschr. Röntgenstr. 36 (1927), 700
17. Christen, Th.: Zur Theorie und Technik der Härtemessung. Fortschr. Röntgenstr. Band XXII, Heft 2 (1914) 247–253
18. Döring, B., G. Großmann: Induktoren und Transformatoren mit Dickölfüllung. Strahlentherapie (1923) 213
19. Ebersberger, H., K. Morkel: Entwicklung von beweglichen Hochspannungsleitungen und Endverschlüssen für Röntgenanlagen. Siemens Zeitschrift 42. Jg., H.11 (1968) 920–925
20. Entwicklungsberichte. Siemens Reiniger Werke, 1938 bis 1948, Siemens Med. Arch. Erlangen.
21. Franke, H.: Grundlagen und Technik der Schwer- und Fernaufnahmen. Fortschr. Röntgenstr. 36 (1927), 681
22. Franke, K.: Die neue Generation der Röntgengeneratoren und ihr Einfluß auf die optimale Bildqualität. Radiol. Praxis I (1978) 24–36
23. Fuchs, F.: Elektrische Strahlen und ihre Anwendung (Röntgentechnik). Verlag R. Oldenburg, München und Berlin (1922) H.3 von Dannenmann, F. (Herausgeber): Der Werdegang der Entdeckungen und Erfindungen.
24. Gajewski, W.H.: Der technische Entwicklungsstand der Röntgenbelichtungsautomatik. Radiologica diagnostica 9, H.2 (1968) 239–249
25. Gebauer, A.: Vergleichende Untersuchungen über Vor- und Nachteile der Aufnahmetechnik mit Spannungen von 85 kV bis 150 kV in der Magen- Darm-Diagnostik mit Hilfe der Belichtungsautomatik. Fortschr. Röntgenstr. Band 89, H.5 (1958) 1–8
26. Gerthsen, Ch.: Physik. Springer Verlag, Berlin: 6. Auflage (1960) (1. Auflage 1948).
27. Glasser, O.: Wilhelm Conrad Röntgen und die Geschichte der Röntgenstrahlen. Springer Verlag, Berlin, 2. Auflage 1959 (1. Auflage 1931).
28. Grigg, E.R.N.: The Trail of the Invisible Light. Charles C. Thomas Publisher Springfield, USA, 1965.
29. Großmann, G.: Einführung in die Röntgentechnik. Verfaßt für die Teilnehmer der Siemens & Halske A.G. Charlottenburg 1912.
30. Hackl, A.: Röntgenapparate und ihre Schaltungen. Verlag von Hachmeister und Thal, Leipzig, 1929, Band VIII von Hachmeister und Thals Schaltungsbüchern.
31. Heinke, C.: Einführung in die Elektrotechnik. Verlag von S. Hirzel, Leipzig, 1909
32. Hoxter, E.A., A. Schenz: Röntgenaufnahmetechnik – Grundlagen und Anwendungen. Verlag Siemens Aktiengesellschaft Berlin und München (1991) 14. Auflage
33. Konkurrenz-Apparate. Vertrauliche Mitteilungen über Elektromedizin. Siemens & Halske AG Wernerwerk, Berlin Nonnendamm 2 (1913) 1–6

34. Krestel, E. (Hrsg.): Bildgebende Systeme für die medizinische Diagnostik. Verlag Siemens Aktiengesellschaft Berlin und München, 1988, 2. Auflage

35. Krestel, E. (Ed.): Imaging Systems for Medical Diagnostics. Published by Siemens Aktiengesellschaft, Berlin and Munich, 1990

36. Krohmer, J.S.: Radiography and Fluoroscopy, 1920 to the Present, Radio Graphics 9, No. 6, Monograph (1989) 1129–1153

37. Küchler, R.: Die Transformatoren. Springer Verlag, 1956

38. Kühnel, W.: Der Schwingkreiswechselrichter mit Gegenspannungslast zur Versorgung von Verbrauchern mit gepulstem Gleichstrom. Dissertation, Technische Fakultät der Universität Erlangen-Nürnberg, 1986

39. Lasser, K.: Die Röntgenstrahlenerzeugung in der neuen Röhre und Spezialapparate zu ihrem Betrieb für Diagnostik und Therapie. Berliner klinische Wochenschrift No. 12 und 13 (1916). Sonderdruck des Experimentalvortrags am 26. Januar 1916 in der Berliner medizinischen Gesellschaft zu Berlin, hrsg. von der Siemens & Halske A.G. Berlin.

40. Leistner, K.: Wege zur Steigerung der Leistung von Diagnostik-Apparaten. Fortschritte auf dem Gebiet der Röntgen-Strahlung 37 (1928) 321–328

41. Leusch, G.: Ein neues Röntgenverfahren in der Nierensteinchirurgie. Sonderdruck aus: Der Urologe, Springer Verlag, Ausgabe A, 9. Jg. H.4 (1970) 182–188

42. Meiler, J., H. Aichinger: Automatisierte Dosisregelung während des Schichtablaufes bei linearen Schichten. Röntgen Bl. 30 (1977) 626–635

43. Meiler, J.: Die in der Röntgendiagnostik verwendeten Spannungskurven und ihr Einfluß auf Bildqualität und Röhrenbelastung. Fortschr. Röntgenstr. 72 (1949) 222–241

44. Meiler, J.: Hat der Drehstromapparat wirklich so bedeutende Vorteile gegenüber dem Vierventilapparat? Röntgen-Bl. 3 (1950) 27–39

45. Müller, E.A.: Röhren-Gleichrichterschaltungen und ihre Wirkungsweise. Arch. Techn. Messen. R. Oldenburg, Lieferung 171, April 1950, Blatt T 44 bis 46

46. Müller, E.A.: Schaltung und Wirkunghsweise von Grobstruktur-Röntgenapparaten I: Halbwellenschaltung, 4-Ventil-Graetz-Schaltung, Villard-Schaltung, Liebenow-Greinacher-Schaltung, Zimmermann-Wittka-Schaltung. München: Arch. Techn. Messen, R. Oldenburg München: Lieferung 171, April 1950, Blatt T 74 bis 48

47. Müller, E.A.: Schaltungen und Wirkungsweise von Grobstruktur – Röntgenapparaten II, Erzeugung von Röntgenblitzen und sehr harten Röntgenstrahlen. Arch. Techn. Messen, R. Oldenburg, München, Lieferung 178, Juni 1950, Blatt T 71 bis 72

48. Niemann, C., W. Zeyss: Die Vorzüge des Röntgen-Drehstromapparats. Fortschr. Röntgenstr. 45 (1932) 596–606

49. Pohl, R.W.: Elektrizitätslehre. Springer Verlag, 16. Auflage, 1957

50. Pugno-Vanoni, E., C. Reimann: Ein automatischer Spannungsregler zum Konstanthalten der elektrischen Betriebsbedingungen von Röntgenapparaten. Fortschr. Röntgenstr. 47, H.6 (1933) 707–715

51. Säbel, M., J. Weisshaar, H. Aichinger: Die Belichtungsmessung bei der Xeromammographie. Electromedica 5 (1977) 150–157

52. Säbel, M. et al.: Belichtungsmessung bei der Mammographie mit Film-Folien-Systemen. Electromedica 3 (1979) 127–136

53. Schmitmann, H., E. Noske, W. Sladek: TRIDOROS OPTIMATIC – ein neues Generatorensystem. Electromedica 39 (1971) 83–86

54. Schmitmann, H., E. Ammann: PANDOROS OPTIMATIC – ein Röntgengenerator mit neuen Möglichkeiten. Electromedica 41 (1973) 177–181

55. Shields: Silicon Alloy Junction Diodes for Power Supply Applications. B.T.H. Activities, Rugby, England, The British Thomson Houston Co. Ltd. (1955) 102

56. Siemens, W. von: Lebenserinnerungen. Prestel-Verlag, München, 17. Auflage 1966.

57. Steiner, K., B. Brundin, W. Sladek: Das OPTIMATIC-System. Electromedica 41 (1973) 182–187

58. Tölle, K.-H.: Aufnahmetechnik des Schultergelenkes mit dem Status X. Röntgen-Bl., 25 Jg., H.5 (1972) 192–197

59. Vertrauliche Mitteilungen über Elektromedizin: Über die Expositionszeit bei unseren Röntgeneinrichtungen. Siemens & Halske AG Wernerwerk: Berlin Nonnendamm, August 1913, 6–8

60. Walter, B.: Die physikalischen Grundlagen der medizinischen Röntgentechnik. Verlag von F. Vieweg und Sohn, Braunschweig, 1926

Tables and stands, patient positioning and systems

E. Ammann, G. Rosenbusch, M. Oudkerk

Looking back 100 years, W.C. Roentgen studied the effects of radiation simply by using only a fluorescent screen, a piece of cardboard treated with barium platinocyanide and photographic plates. This allowed the viewing and documentation of X-ray images. Over a period of time, viewing of images from a fluorescent screen was supplanted by the X-ray image intensifier, which resulted in an immensely improved image at lower dose values.

The many different X-ray system designs now in use must be understood from the historical background of the image receptor system and also of X-ray tube design. These two components – the tube and image receptor – are the most relevant with regard to the medical requirements of effective patient positioning, the projection called for, measures to improve image quality – such as compression, collimators, filters, grids and geometry – as well as electrical, mechanical, and radiation protection measures. In addition, the system must also provide an ergonomic ambience for the medical team, and efficient working conditions which must also foster patient comfort. Other issues to consider are size and weight in the interest of simplifying transport and installation, energy consumption, and costs.

Principles for the design of tables and stands

Originally, unit design (Bischoff and Gellinek, 1965) [5] was based on an exchange of ideas with the physician. Over the course of time, however, considerations of engineering, as well as vibration theory and material science, radiation physics, principles of mechanical engineering and manufacturing technology, increasingly influenced the design. Only the physician and medical personnel may perform radiological examinations on a patient, and not the engineer. However, technology provides the impetus for new developments in X-ray tubes, generators, automatic exposure controls, and image receptors. Of course, these are also influenced by the medical and ergonomic situation and economic constraints.

Many system movements must be considered in the design of the tables and stands: the ideal position for the patient would be that of greatest comfort and requiring as little repositioning as possible. The beam should then be adapted to this patient position. However, the examination of certain organs of the body or the control of fluid levels makes it necessary to put the patient into different positions, so that the X-ray beam must be defined and set accordingly. Figure V, 71 illustrates the settings required for an X-ray system. Originally, the patient was examined standing or recumbent; since 1907, examinations in inclined and finally the Trendelenburg positions have also been possible.

Nevertheless, there is an entire series of medical procedures for which a tilting unit is either inadequate or incapable of furnishing the information required. Convenience for the required settings and patient safety have led to a large number of movements which the engineer has had to implement. Figure V, 72 gives examples still found even today in every X-ray system. Movements are performed manually and/or by motor. Lock-in positions, brakes and couplings all help in setting system projections spatially and in relation to the patient. Counterweights hold a mechanical system in position against the force of gravity. Movements must overcome gravity and frictional forces. A number of design elements

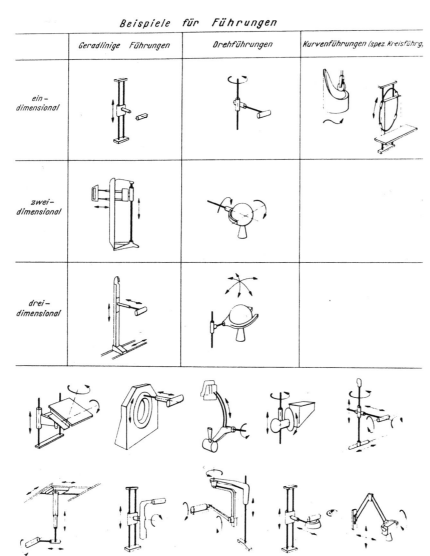

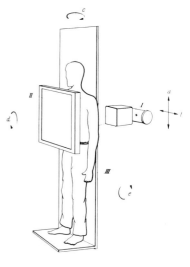

Fig. V, 71. System movements of the X-ray tube (I), the image receptor (II) and the tabletop (III) for patient positioning; direction (a) and (b) refer to longitudinal and transverse movements in relation to the patient, the focus–film distance can vary or can be fixed in a system; (c) rotation around the patient's longitudinal axis; (d) and (e) refer to rotational movements [5].

Fig. V, 72. Basic elements of system movements. Top row: One-dimensional linear movement (left), one-dimensional rotational movement (middle), and one-dimensional curved movement (right). The middle row shows a two-dimensional movement and row three a three-dimensional movement. The lower part of the picture shows 10 examples of a combination of movement elements in X-ray tables and stands. Movements are carried out manually or are motor driven, or both. Clutches, brakes and locking devices are used to keep all the mechanical parts fixed in a specific position [5].

help to implement this: sliding and roller guides, cable, chain and spindle drives, toothed racks, lever devices, transmissions and joints.

Manual versus motor-driven settings have been the subject of many discussions. Manual settings give better control over the speed and position – the operator is 'kept busy' and thus not aware of how much time is needed for the setting. With motor-driven settings, the lack of active participation often gives rise to the impression that 'everything moves too slowly'. It is of course true that motors running at constant speed proved to be too slow for long distances and too fast for fine positioning. A satisfactory solution to this dilemma was found only with the use of speed-regulated motors. This solution has its price, however.

Stands for X-ray tubes and improvements in image quality

Originally, stands with wooden clamps (Fig. V, 73) were used to secure the ion tube. A wooden stand with collimator was built to Immelmann's specifications in 1903 (Fig. V, 74) – one of the first measures to improve image quality. As a result of the collimator, the irradiated volume was reduced, so that less scattered radiation reached the film. The first metal stand was designed in 1905 and the holder for the tube and collimator was suspended with counterbalancing. The collimator could also be used for compression. The first tube with a radiation protective housing appeared in 1906. The exchange of an ion tube

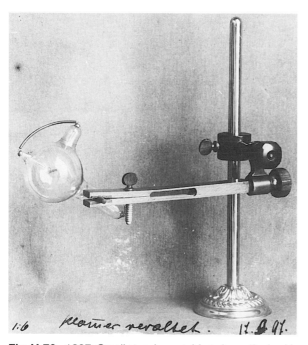

Fig. V, 73. 1897: Small stand on a table to keep the ion X-ray tube in place. The bracket is made of wood.

Fig. V, 75a, b. Centring the focus of an ion X-ray tube in an examination table.

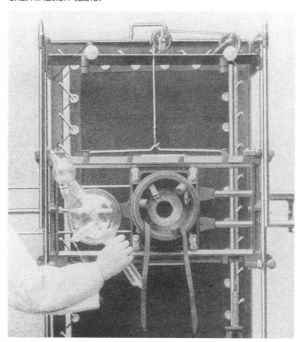

Fig. V, 75a. Exchanging a tube on the KLINOGRAPH tilting table. The tube was held in place with two leather straps. The focus was centred approximately.

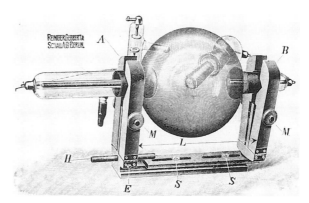

Fig. V, 75b. 1908: Self-centring X-ray tube holder. Each X-ray tube has its own holder and has been centred only once, so the focal spot is always in the same position.

(Fig. V, 75a) was always a challenge because the focus had to be at a specific position but the tube was held in place only with leather belts. In 1908, Reiniger, Gebbert and Schall (RGS) improved the tube holder so significantly that the focus was always centred within the supporting fixture (Fig. V, 75b). This was the first contribution to improved efficiency as it allowed a fast ex-

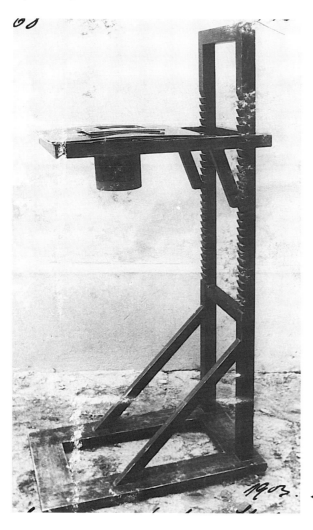

◀ **Fig. V, 74.** 1903: Dr Immelmann's tube stand with collimation system.

change of ion tubes with different beam hardnesses.

Compression

As early as 1902, Siemens and Halske patented a method and an apparatus for compression of soft tissue to improve recognition of detail (Fig. V, 76) [P 1]. Soft parts of the body were compressed with an appropriately large force to reduce the thickness of the irradiated body part in the beam direction and to ensure that the patient did not move. The idea was prompted by poorly visible stones in the bile duct or renal

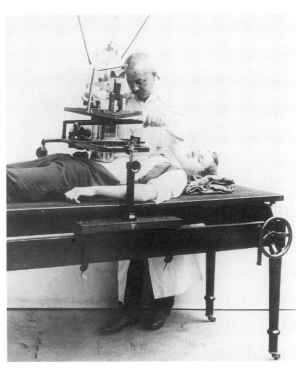

Fig. V, 77. 1905: Collimation and compression device designed by Albers-Schoenberg.

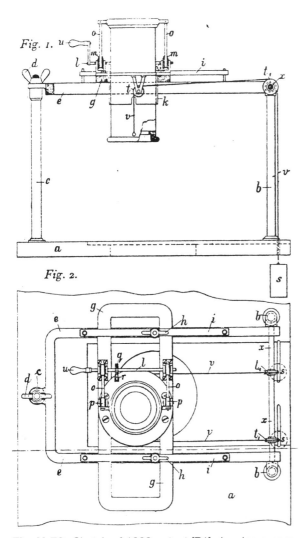

Fig. V, 76. Sketch of 1902 patent [P1] showing a compression device. Compression of the soft organs reduced the mass in the irradiated field and kept the object fixed in position during exposure. This improved image quality, especially when searching for foreign bodies in soft tissue or looking for kidney and gallstones.

stones and by tiny foreign bodies in large soft-tissue masses. The application of this patented method led to a clear improvement in detail recognition. A version used in practice in 1905 by Albers-Schoenberg is shown in Fig. V, 77.

Collimation of the X-ray beam

Controlled collimation improved image quality and made radiation protection possible. Reducing the irradiated object volume results in less scattered radiation on the film, or more generally on the image receptor. As early as 1899, the Boston dentist W.H. Rollins (1852–1929) (Grigg, 1965) [18] proposed an 'internal diaphragm' in the ion tube (Fig. V, 78). The X-ray beam was collimated at a position near the focus, with the possibility of collimating to a still narrower beam using externally mounted leaves. The firm of Reiniger, Gebbert and Schall designed a collimation tube for radiographs of the apex of the lung – the so-called 'LUNGEN-SPITZENBLENDE' according to Groedel (Fig. V, 79; also s. Fig. II, 37). The Berlin company Sanitas introduced the ROTAX universal collimator in 1908, based on the iris principle (Fig. V, 80), for use in radiography, fluoroscopy and radio-

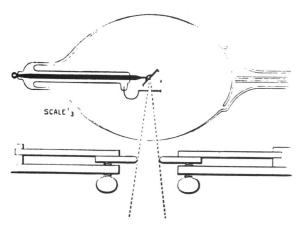

Fig. V, 78. 1899: Internal diaphragm proposed by William Herbert Rollins (1852–1929), a dentist in Boston [18].

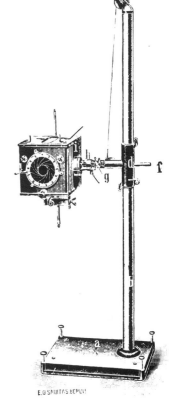

Fig. V, 80. 1908: ROTAX universal box collimator mounted on a stand for radiographs, fluoroscopy and radiotherapy. This system was produced by Sanitas, Berlin [47].

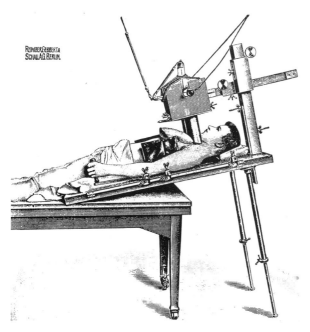

Fig. V, 79. 1908: A collimation system (RGS) according to Groedel III for exposures of the pulmonary apex. This collimation system provided clear and sharp radiographs of the apex, ribs, the calcification of cartilage and the glands. An X-ray tube with two anticathodes and two collimation systems was used to produce one radiograph [47].

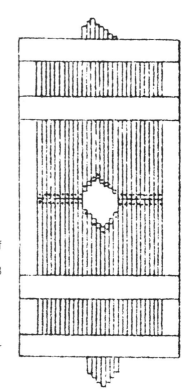

Fig. V, 81. Multileaf collimator for irregular fields designed at the Roentgen Institute of the Rothschild Hospital in Vienna in 1908 [47]. This was especially important for radiotherapy; in diagnostics it was sufficient to apply an iris collimation system or a four-rectangular plate collimation system.

therapy. In the same year, a bar-shaped collimator was introduced by the Radiology Department of the Rothschild Hospital in Vienna; it was used to collimate irregular exposure fields (Fig. V, 81). A collimator with remote control using Bowden cables appeared in 1937 (similar to one shown in Fig. V, 83). This was, in fact, a further development of the multileaf collimator of 1931. It had two pairs of leaves, one close to the focus and one further removed from the focus, producing a well-defined edge in the collimated radiograph. The company SRW introduced automatic collimation in the year 1958, which limited the X-ray beam to the size of the cassette. This eliminated unnecessary radiation exposure to the patient.

A further Siemens contribution in 1994 to dose reduction in angiography is the electronic collimation on a "last image hold" monitor image. The radiologist collimates down to the smallest possible examination field without using radiation.

Light localizer – a tool to define the radiation field without radiation

In 1908, the Vienna company Otto Sommer patented the first light-beam localizer under the name 'Roentgen-Episkop' (Fig. V, 82). In 1938, this was combined with a multileaf collimator, comprising several built-in, coupled, double-slot

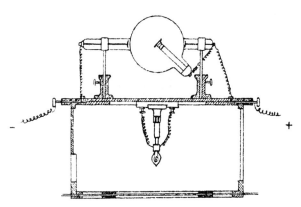

Fig. V, 82. 1908: Light localizer from the Otto Sommer Company in Vienna (DP-Nr. 192 300 and OEP-Nr. 27 146): The focus of the tube and a light source was mounted at the same distance, so that it was called 'isofocal'. The size of the collimation is adjusted with the optical light. By turning the X-ray tube into place, radiographs could be taken with the same field size. (Roentgen-Episkop) [47].

collimators with a depth of 25 cm. Figure V, 83 shows a version of this collimation system dating from the year 1941 and a schematic diagram of the basic principle applied.

Scattered radiation reduction using grids

The Berlin radiologist Gustav Bucky (Fig. V, 85) was responsible for the first honeycomb collimator (Fig. V, 84), introduced in 1912, used to reduce the contrast-impairing scattered radiation in the film. He received a patent on this device in 1913 [P 7]. In 1921, H.F. Waite (Fig. V, 86) [P 8] applied for a patent on a method of grid movement during the exposure, the purpose of which was to blur the grid shadows on the

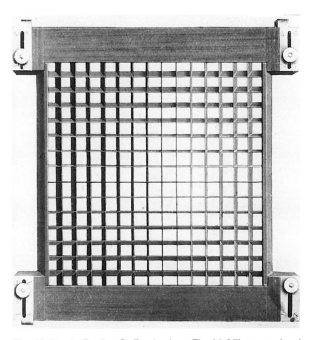

Fig. V, 84. In Berlin, G. Bucky (see Fig. V, 85) recognized the necessity of reducing scattered radiation and applied a honeycomb grid or 'diaphragm' in 1912.

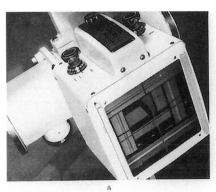

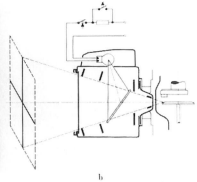

Fig. V, 83. 1938/1957:
(a) Multileaf collimation system from Siemens with a light localizer.
(b) The principal function of this collimation system [5].

Fig. V, 85.
Gustav Bucky (1880–1963), radiologist in Berlin (1910–23 and 1930–33) and New York City (1923–30 and 1933–60), recognized the negative effects of scattered radiation. To improve image quality, he designed a grid (Fig. V, 84 [P7]) which is still essential today.

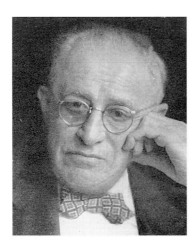

of the twenties, SRW surrounded the open high-voltage supply to the X-ray tube with a grounded metal mesh as a form of protection against unintentional contact (Fig. V, 87). Already in 1931 Siemens showed its high-tension cable solution. Step by step new X-ray systems using cables were introduced (Fig. V, 87). These cables were heavy and were freely suspended between the tube housing and the high-voltage generator (s. Fig. V, 61). Equipment designs had now to cope with the extra pull and the additional

radiograph sufficiently to render them invisible in the image. This made use of a linear grid. A moving grid with initial drive was introduced in 1955, providing the means of controlling the speed of grid movement sufficiently to switch on the X-ray beam at the highest grid speed and continually reduce the grid speed with increasing exposure time. This process eliminated grid shadows on the film with both short and long exposure times.

Protection against high-voltage electric shocks

The problem of working in a fully darkened room for fluoroscopy was discussed in the high-voltage cable section. In the second half

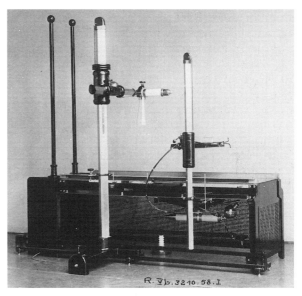

Fig. V, 87. 1932: To reduce the likelihood of electric shock a grounded metal mesh was mounted around the X-ray tube underneath the table.

Fig. V, 86. Sketch of Henry F. Waite's 1921 patent [P8] for a vibrating Bucky diaphragm to reduce scatter radiation. He claimed to turn off the radiation during the endpoint where the grid changed its direction. The moving grid came into clinical routine about 20 years later [18]. Waite (1874–1946) lived in New York and was a physician, inventor and entrepreneur.

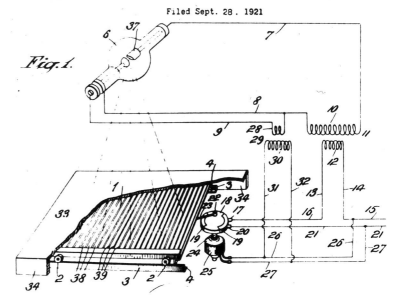

Oct. 16 , 1923.   1,471,081

H. F. WAITE

VIBRATING BUCKEY DIAPHRAGM FOR SCATTERED X-RAY RADIATION

Filed Sept. 28 . 1921

Fig.1.

weight of the tube housings. To this day, problem-free cable runs still represent a serious challenge to every table and stand manufacturer. This development represented a milestone in terms of the protection offered for both the patient and medical staff.

Radiation protection for the examining personnel

As early as 1906, the ion tube was surrounded by shielding. In 1911, however, G. Holzknecht (1872–1931) (s. Fig. I, 15) introduced the 'Distinktor' (palpation spoon). With it, the physician no longer had to use his own hand for palpation in the X-ray beam. This practice resulted in severe radiation burns, leading to finger amputation or even premature death.

The physician was also protected against scattered radiation from the patient by lead cladding. A fluoroscopy system dating from 1940

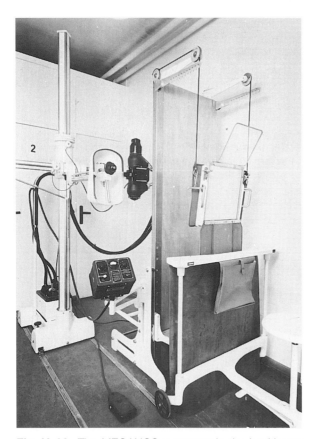

Fig. V, 88. The MEGANOS generator in the healthcare facility of the Wernerwerks F/T of the Siemens factories in Berlin Spandau in 1940. The physician sat in a radiation-shielded mobile cockpit (right) during the fluoroscopy procedure. The control handle to position the tube was also shielded. A cough guard was mounted on top of the fluorescent screen.

(Fig. V, 88) shows that the handle to position the X-ray tube is surrounded by a radiation protection mantle. The physician could work from a sitting position, had a lead-based radiation protection shield in front of him and lead rubber lamella attached to the fluorescent screen. Lead rubber gloves and, above all, the lead rubber apron, are standard protective wear for radiological personnel even today.

Systems for skeletal diagnostics

Diagnosis requires the recognition of fine details. This in turn requires small focal spots with adequate output. High-resolution film-screen combinations are most commonly used. Multileaf collimators reduce the level of radiation exposure to the patient. Operational simplification and the transition to digital imaging, in the interest of avoiding repeated exposures, are now past the experimental stage. Digital images are available whenever and wherever required, even simultaneously at different locations. Quantitative evaluation procedures in orthopaedics and computer-supported surgical planning are at present just beginning. Nevertheless, there is no doubt whatever that their use will increase.

Fluoroscopy and radiography of the hand

The human hand was the first object with which W.C. Roentgen was able to demonstrate the medical relevance of X-rays. By 1896 (Fig. V, 89), radiography of the hand in the X-ray room of the physician had already become routine: the patient placed her hand on the film cassette, which was lying on an auxiliary table. The ion tube, clamped to a stand, was supplied with high voltage via freely running wires from an inductor on the wall. The inductor system was switched on manually and, after the estimated exposure time had elapsed – usually after a matter of minutes – switched off again. Furniture and curtains looked more like normal room furnishings.

Levy-Dorn (s. Fig. I, 16) introduced the ORTHODIAGRAPH (Fig. V, 90) in 1902, which helped to position the focal spot of the tube orthogonally to the fluorescent screen. By 1904, this had developed to a sturdy stand with a collimator which could be inserted between the tube and the fluorescent screen. The use of automatic exposure controls with the skeletal periphery was attempted repeatedly, but this

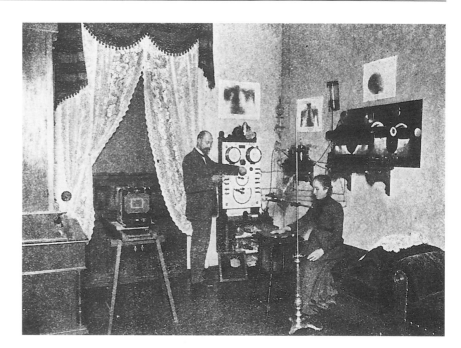

Fig. V, 89. An X-ray room in 1896: The patient is positioned for a hand exposure. The physician (left) looks at his watch for the appropriate exposure time.

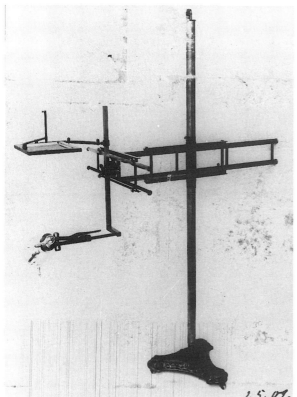

Fig. V, 90. 1902: Mobile ORTHODIAGRAPH devised by Levy-Dorn (s. Fig. I, 16).

method never gained real acceptance. Only with the advent of storage phosphor technology did it become possible to eliminate repeated exposures.

Fluoroscopy and radiography of the lower extremities

Figure V, 91 shows the positioning for an image of the tibia taken in the year 1905. The physician used a mobile X-ray unit in his practice. The exposure time was still under manual control, with the help of a clock.

Figure V, 92 will be familiar to some of us. When buying a new pair of shoes, such an X-ray unit could be seen in shoe stores, to show whether there was sufficient toe room in the shoes. This picture dates from the year 1924, but the store where I once bought my shoes still had such a unit even in the fifties. For reasons of radiation safety, these units have been banned since the sixties.

The development of examination tables and stands

In 1897, simple tables with a wooden table top – but still with stylistic table legs – were used (Fig. V, 93). Images taken around the years 1904/05 reveal an increasing adaptation of the table design to the examination requirements: while wood was still used as the basic material, the supporting fixture for the tube – for reasons of mechanical stability and convenience – was now made of metal. For overtable radiography (Fig. V, 94), a compression cone with variously sized diaphragms was now present as well. Thirty years later, the transition to all metal construction was complete. The wooden table top was, however,

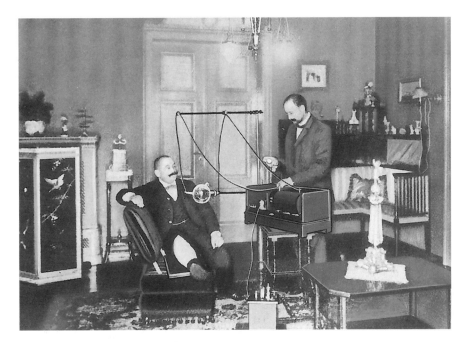

Fig. V, 91. An examination room in 1905 with a mobile inductor X-ray system positioned to take a radiograph of the patient's leg.

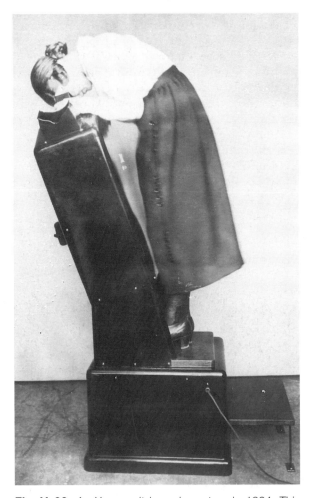

Fig. V, 92. An X-ray unit in a shoe store in 1924. This fluoroscopy unit showed if enough room for the toes was available in new shoes. Such units were in use until the seventies (in Germany, they were made illegal in 1976).

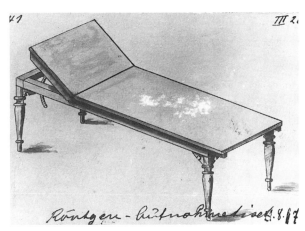

Fig. V, 93. 1897: Table for radiographs.

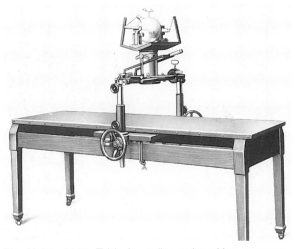

Fig. V, 94. 1905: Table for radiographs with a compression and collimation device according to Albers-Schoenberg (DP 156 389) and made by Siemens and Halske.

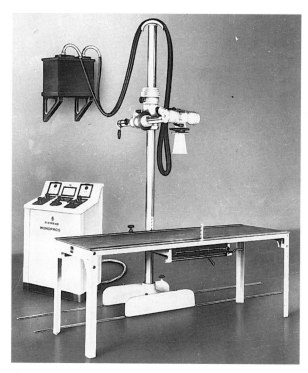

Fig. V, 95. 1943: MONOPHOS generator and Bucky table.

beneath the table top. The stand requires floor rails and functions as the coupling element between the tube and the cassette tray. Profile rails are attached to the long edges of the table top for the attachment of positioning aids and compression devices.

In the late sixties, Bucky tables were equipped with film magazines and directly connected film processors. Magazine technology originated in Japan and the USA (Picker) to overcome personnel shortages. The number of skeletal and Bucky radiographs has increased so dramatically that this technically rather complicated – but very convenient – procedure is now well established. It was no longer necessary to carry heavy cassettes to and from the darkroom. The film from the supply magazine is transported between the screens, which are pressed against the film and, following automatically controlled exposure, transported to the film processor. Figure V, 96 shows the BUCKYMAT, in 1977. Nevertheless, there was still a requirement for simple, compact units with the possibility of linear tomography.

Digital luminescence radiography was further developed in Japan (Fuji) in the eighties to the point that the expensive and relatively complex storage phosphor technology was able to take its place in daily radiographic routine. This technique requires no new table, and it can be used with any cassette tray. Consequently, even Bucky tables with magazine technology are no longer in the production lines of X-ray equipment manufacturers.

still there but now part of a system. The versatility of the tube, by now fully equipped with high voltage and radiation protection was extended. The tube stand travels over the length of the table, and oblique projections are now possible in addition to fluoroscopy and radiography in the horizontal beam direction. Figure V, 95, from 1943, shows the cassette tray with grid installed

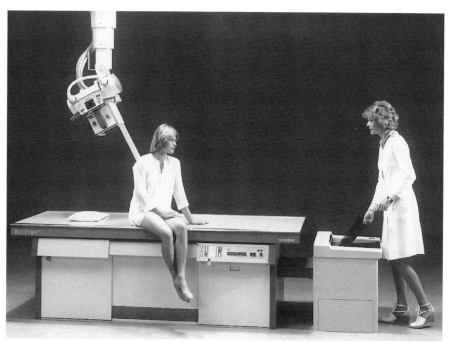

Fig. V, 96. 1973: BUCKYMAT. A radiographic table with magazine technique and connected film processor.

The table top is now made of plastic. It is more homogeneous and has a relatively low attenuation of X-radiation. Carbon-fibre table tops, due to their excessive cost (about ten times that of wooden tables), were unable to prevail over alternative designs except in special procedure rooms, in spite of their low attenuation of radiation and excellent mechanical stability.

The floating table top has travel capability in both the longitudinal and the transverse direction. The underlying principle is not new; as far back as 1896/97, patients were positioned 'floating' on a stretcher between a fixed tube and cassette. In the sixties this principle was taken up again with many Bucky tables, because it represented a considerable simplification for fine positioning. Table top lock-in for the exposure was controlled by electromagnetic brakes. Allowing for the longitudinal and transverse table movements, the distance to the film plane had to remain as short as possible. Curved table tops appeared, which also proved to be more comfortable for the patient than a flat table top. But, to reposition patients confined to bed, flat table tops were again preferred. Purpose, image quality and costs required a compromise.

Stationary stands were, in most cases, floor stands (s. Figs. V, 87, V, 88, V, 95 and V, 117) or floor-to-ceiling stands (Fig. V, 98), requiring guide rails on or in the floor. These had disadvantages: on the floor, they presented an obstacle over which one could stumble if not careful; in the floor, there was the problem of how to clean them. The wish to have the floor free of such obstacles was fulfilled in the sixties. With this step, the freedom of movement of the system also improved. Figure V, 97 represents an early design and a sketch indicating the versatility of a height-adjustable telescope which can travel along and across the ceiling of the room. The 3D stand allows positioning of the X-ray tube (s. Figs. V, 111 and V, 138) or the image intensifier (Fig. V, 138) freely.

Skeletal radiography

Requirement for radiographs of the hand, foot and skull are different from those of the other skeletal parts. In 1909, skeletal radiography was performed predominantly on recumbent patients, using a floating table top. Spinal radiography requires that the settings be made with great care. Cassettes were also developed in long format to be able to display the entire spine on a single film. This in turn made new grids necessary. Uniform optical film density was achieved by the use of filters developed especially for this purpose on the multileaf collimator (Bischoff and Gellinek, 1965) [5]. To minimize

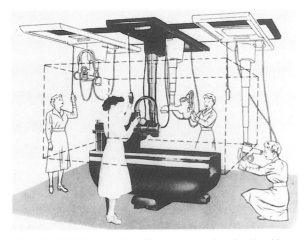

Fig. V, 97. Telescopic ceiling suspension for the X-ray tube shown in a sketch from the sixties [5]. This improved tube positioning and eliminated the rails on the floor as shown in Figure V, 98, which people were inclined to trip over.

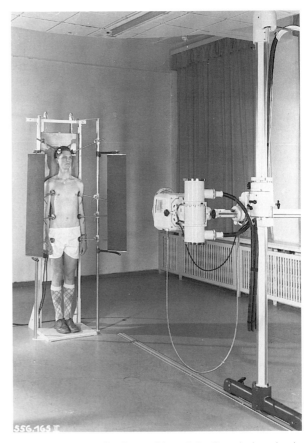

Fig. V, 98. 1955: Radiographic unit for the whole spine in the vertical position. The X-ray tube was mounted on a floor to ceiling stand and the collimation system contained a special set of equalisation filters.

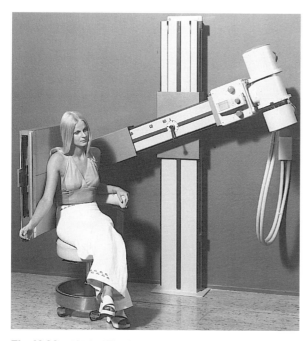

Fig. V, 99. 1973: ATLAS system positioned for a shoulder radiograph. Tube and catapult-Bucky are centred with a variable focus–film distance. The U-arm is height adjustable, counterbalanced, and can be turned into any angled position.

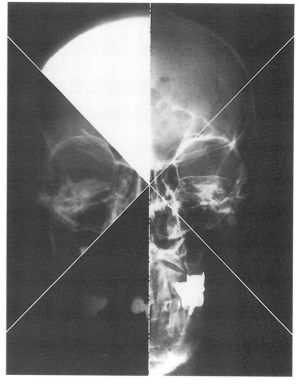

Fig. V, 100. Composite radiographs of a skull phantom. Three film screen radiographs (left) and three digital luminescence radiographs made with the DIGISCAN (right). The top portion is underexposed, the middle portion is correctly exposed, and the lower portion is overexposed. The advantage of digital luminescence radiography is obvious and can avoid retakes, especially in intensive care units.

image distortion, the film-focus distance was extended to 3 m. Figure V, 98 shows a system from the year 1955.

During the seventies, an applications-oriented system configuration (Fig. V, 99) replaced earlier designs. The focus and mid-point of the cassette were centred in a swivel-mounted, height-adjustable and counter-weighted U-arm. Such a system is distinguished by the simplicity of its installation and operation.

Skeletal radiography often requires special projections. For this reason, special units were built in the sixties and seventies, e.g. the ORBIX from Elema (see Fig. V, 103). Its image quality was outstanding and patient comfort was optimal. The settings necessary for good diagnostic quality required considerable knowledge and experience. Consequently, the investment costs for such units were significantly higher than for simple skeletal units where the patient was positioned to the system and not vice versa.

Skull radiography

Figure V, 2 shows a radiograph of 1896. Over 90 years later, Fig. V, 100 demonstrates the superiority of digital luminescence radiography of the skull, on the right, over film-screen radiographs, on the left. The upper two segments are underexposed and the two lower ones are overexposed. Only the two segments in the middle are correctly exposed. This technology is an important contribution to the reduction of radiation exposure and also for speedy diagnosis of chest radiographs in intensive care units.

Going back to the year 1906, the Polyphos company in Munich advertised the PERIDIAGRAPH, after Grashey (s. Fig. II, 3), for fluoroscopy and radiography in different projections without the need to reposition the patient's head (Fig. V, 101). Skull radiography was, of course, also performed on the table, for example, with the Gilmer table of 1910 (Fig. V, 102). Lysholm (s. Fig. IV, 34) – whether consciously or not knowing about Grashey's original idea, developed the well-known Lysholm skull stand in 1925 (s. Fig. IV, 35). In addition to Elema-Schoenander, other companies also manufactured special skull radiography stands, such as Franklin in the sixties.

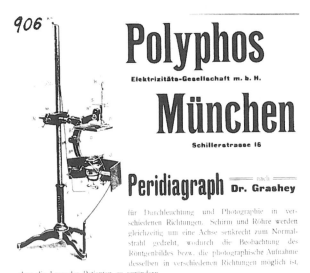

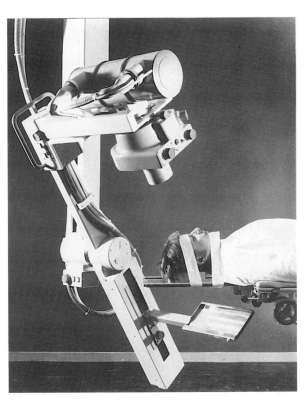

Fig. V, 101. 1906: First C-arm solution for a skull unit, called the PERIDIAGRAPH, devised by Dr Grashey (1876–1950) (s. Fig. II, 3) and manufactured by the Polyphos Company in Munich.

Elema's Lysholm stand was completely redesigned in 1959. The result – MIMER – was a universal skull radiography unit (s. Figs. IV, 36 and IV, 37). It allowed tomograms and also serialography for cerebral angiographies and pneumencephalographies to display the ventricles. The patient was immobilized in a chair, which in turn could be positioned to almost any desired orientation. Computed tomography has, in the meantime, fully replaced this very painful examination procedure, much to the benefit of the patient.

Fig. V, 103. 1971: ORBIX. A special tube cassette stand for radiographs of the skull and extremities manufactured by Elema.

Along with the Lysholm stand, the ORBIX (Fig. V, 103) is still in use as a special unit for skull and skeletal radiography.

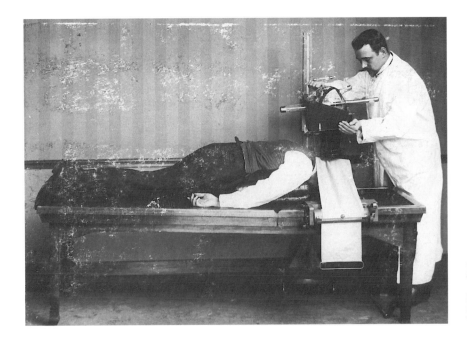

Fig. V, 102. 1910: The 'Gilmer table' for radiographs using compression bands to keep the object in a fixed position.

X-ray examinations in a military environment and for traumatology

Physicians working for the military expressed interest in Roentgen's discovery as early as 1896. Numerous field X-ray units were designed specifically for them (s. Fig. V, 161b). Reliable diagnosis is essential for trauma patients [42] (Rackwitz, 1972) in the operating room, in case there is a need for medical expertise from another location. The methods of positioning, making expo-

sures and communication must all function optimally. This poses constant challenges, because life-saving measures are of the highest priority. Fluoroscopy is needed in the operating room particularly to reposition broken bones. A KRYP-TOSKOP in the operating theatre (s. Fig. V, 174) may have been one solution before the advent of the image intensifier on a mobile C-arm (Fig. V, 104; also s. Fig. V, 175) which provided only an optical viewing system in 1956. A shield served as radiation protection for the physician's head.

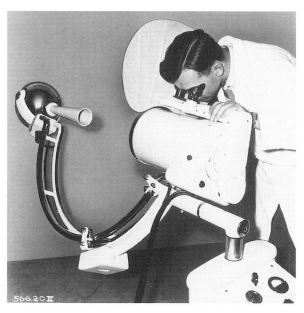

Fig. V, 104. 1956: Surgical C-arm stand containing a 'Roentgen Kugel' and a CHF-Mueller image intensifier and optical output. The physician's head was protected by a lead shield.

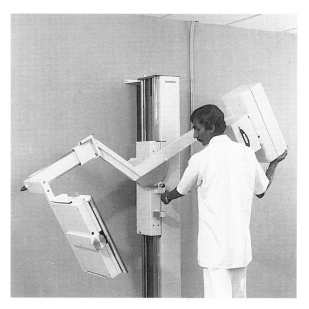

Fig. V, 106. A basic radiographic system BRS according to the World Health Organisation's 1981 specifications. The focal spot in the high-frequency single-tank generator POLYPHOS B (right) is always centred on the Bucky tray on the VERTIX B stand.

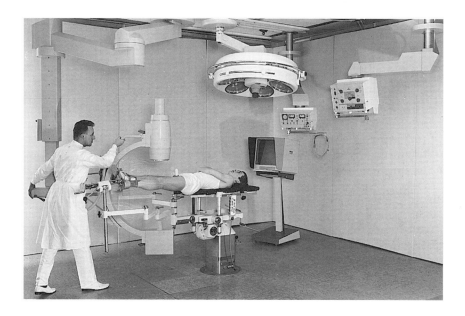

Fig. V, 105. 1968: ARCOSCOP 100 OP. A fixed ceiling-mounted C-arm in the operating room with a 7-inch image intensifier TV system and a single-tank SIREPHOS generator.

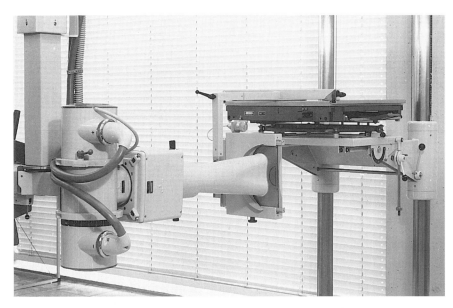

Fig. V, 107. 1966: Mammography stand by the Kreutzer Company. The tube is mounted on a three-dimensional ceiling stand and the multileaf collimator carries a cone as an additional beam-shaping device. The cassette holder contains an ionisation chamber for the automatic exposure control system IONTOMAT.

Television systems finally brought more convenience in the sixties. The C-arm could also be mounted on the ceiling (Fig. V, 105).

For developing countries, the World Health Organisation (WHO) recommends reliable, high-performance radiographic systems to help with the diagnosis of a great variety of disorders (Fig. V, 106). These systems now provide an imaging standard for industrialized nations. They are also appreciated by the military.

Soft-tissue radiography and mammography

The benefit of compression in soft-tissue radiography was recognized even before 1902 (s. Figs. V, 76 and V, 77) [P 1]. Abdominal survey radiograms were also largely made on tilting tables with Bucky tray (s. Figs. V, 77 and V, 94).

Mammography, in fact, presents its own technological challenges, as R.L. Egan was forced to recognize during his lifetime (see the references in the sections on X-ray tubes and generators). Material film and a small focus on a molybdenum anode paved the way for the examination of recumbent patients in the late sixties. Xeroradiography was short lived due to its high radiation exposure level and the geometrical resolution capability required for the diagnosis of microcalcifications.

Special systems were required for positioning and different projections (Figs. V, 107 and V, 109). This led to the introduction of low-dose systems with single-coated films and intensifying screens (Barth et al, 1972) [1] – a truly dramatic contribution to the reduction of radiation dose.

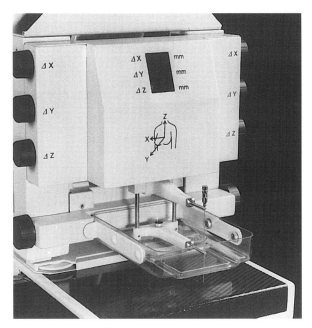

Fig. V, 108. Stereotactic biopsy attachment for the MAMMOMAT 2 in 1988.

Special film processing, compression techniques like OPCOMP, which automatically stops the compression process when optimal exposure conditions are achieved, carbon-fibre material, and the measurement of radiation doses behind the cassette, as well as a constant reduction of the focal spot size with simultaneous increases in output and increasingly sensitive film-screen systems, further contributed to this development. Contrast was enhanced by the use of special grids and refinements in the X-ray tube design. Automatic exposure control systems were capable of switching reproducible optical film density, even in the range of 25–40 kV. This virtually eliminated repeated exposures for diagnosis and biopsy (Figs. V, 108 and V, 109), provided that the most modern tools are applied.

Here too, the future will belong to the digital image (Mosser et al, 1993) [39], and expert systems will be available to the radiologist as additional tools without having to subject the patient to any additional radiation exposure. Early diagnosis and therapy with the best available tools reduce the costs of healthcare and spare family and friends much suffering.

Chest radiography

Chest radiography has been referred to several times in the sections devoted to Tubes and Generators – especially with regard to high and low kV exposure techniques. It (s. Fig. II, 20 and Figs. V, 110, V, 133 and V, 134) comprises 30–50% of all radiographs at many hospitals and therefore deserves special attention. In the seventies, automation led to more cost-effective systems, the so-called chest changer (Fig. V, 111). At high tube voltages, the exposure time had always been a problem. Fine and very slight differences

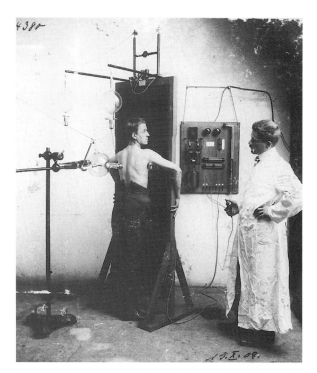

Fig. V, 110. 1908: Apparatus for steroscopic radiographs of the chest and heart.

in density should be clearly recognizable and motion blurring in the entire thorax, caused by the beating of the heart (Berger, 1961) [3], pulsating arteries, respiration, and diaphragm movement, had to be minimized by using exposure times in the millisecond range. This became increasingly

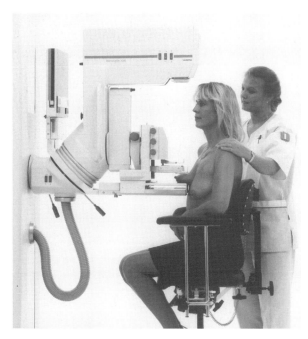

Fig. V, 109. 1994: A state-of-the-art mammography system – the MAMMOMAT 3000. Radiation exposure is reduced, due to the automatic exposure control with a double detector behind the cassette and the Mo/Rh filter combination introduced by Siemens in 1987.

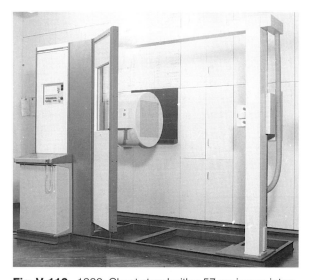

Fig. V, 112. 1982: Chest stand with a 57 cm image intensifier and 100 mm cut-film camera. The high-frequency single-tank generator POLYPHOS provides 30 or 50 kW. The dose applied with the system was a third of a comparable 14 x 17 inch chest radiograph, in a film screen combination at the time [23].

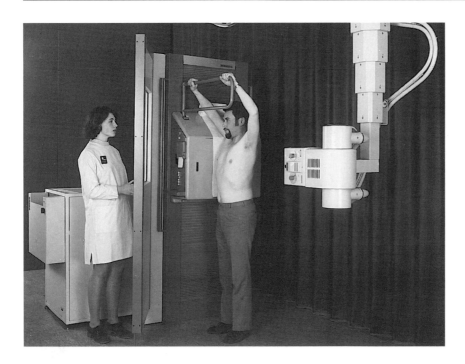

Fig. V, 111. 1973: Chest changer THORAMAT with coupled film processor.

more expensive and was beyond the reach of many mobile units used in the intensive care ward or at the bedside, until high-frequency generator technology solved the problem in 1977. Radiation protection is a high priority for chest radiography. Unfortunately, owing to financial constraints, obsolete X-ray systems are often not removed or properly disposed of. Technical operability alone is no longer a criteria for using a X-ray unit.

Close on the heels of film plates, there followed film-screen systems, optical image intensifiers (ODELKA) with 35 mm cameras (Figs. V, 113 and V, 114), then 57 cm large-format image intensifiers (Fig. V, 112) (Hoxter and Schenz, 1991) [23], rare-earth screens, and finally, in the eighties, digital luminescence radiography, which even permits image post-processing without any additional radiation (Hruby et al, 1992, 1993; Krampla et al, 1993) [24, 25, 33].

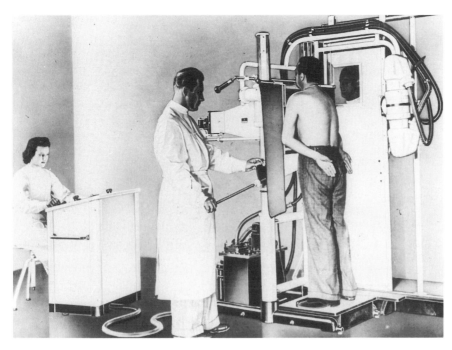

Fig. V, 113. 1938: One of the first units for mass fluorography of the chest (to fight tuberculosis) with an optical image intensifier.

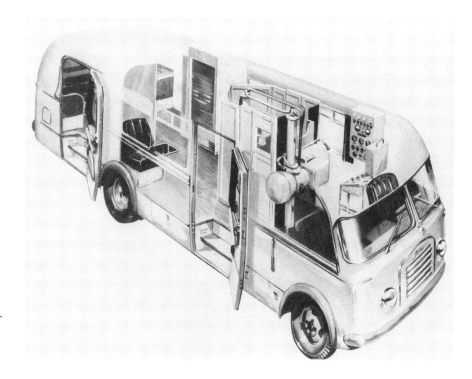

Fig. V, 114. 1960: Mass fluorography unit built into a bus (SRW) [5] to bring the X-ray examination room to the people in rural areas or big factories.

To be able to combat the danger of tuberculosis, from 1937 on, special 'mass fluorography systems' were developed for screening the lungs (Fig. V, 113). Particular emphasis was given to radiation exposure and protection, as well as to the easiest and fastest working procedure for the assistants. The optical image intensifier was a natural choice, because it required a smaller dose than a film-screen combination and also – because it made use of a small format on rollfilm – lower film costs. Mass fluorography systems could also be installed in a bus (Fig. V, 114), suitable for public health offices and for the military. The bus was used in communities without a hospital, in schools, and at large companies for chest screening to detect tuberculosis at an early stage.

Development of the tilting table with spot-film device

Fluoroscopy served for localization and partly also for positioning before an exposure or a series of exposures was taken. Originally, the tube emitted continuous radiation at a low dose rate. A fluorescent screen served as the image receptor. The room had to be completely darkened to view the images on the fluorescent screen. The high-voltage supply was fed via exposed wires from the inductor to the tube. This repre-

sented a significant hazard. The need for greater protection against electrical shock and radiation was apparent.

Tilting table with the tube under the table top

Additional possibilities for examining the recumbent or standing patient were offered with the introduction of the tilting table in 1907 (Figs. V, 115 and V, 116). The KLINOSKOP (Fig. V, 117) featured motor-driven tilting from 1925 on. The fluorescent screen was counterbalanced in every position. The control lever for the collimator was located on the left hand side of the fluorescent screen.

The radiologist Hans Heinrich Berg (Fig. V, 118) (Goerke, 1980) [17] developed the first spot-film device in 1922 (Fig. V, 119). During fluoroscopy, a film cassette was in a parking position, protected from radiation (s. Fig. V, 163). Design engineers have given much attention to this phase of being able to change quickly from fluoroscopy to radiography. Every movement, even that of bringing a cassette from the parked position to the exposure position, results in vibrations which can appear on the film as undesired motion blurring. Counterbalancing was therefore the determining factor for the quality and operating ease of every unit.

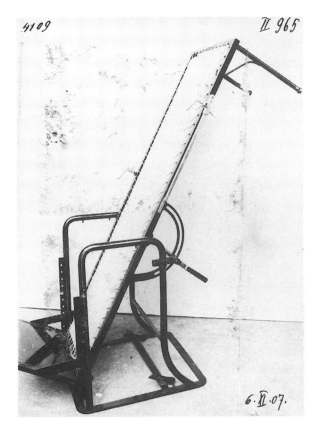

Fig. V, 115. 1907: Tilting table designed to be tilted manually, devised by the engineer Hubert Kress (1886–1936) of Veifa-Werke. (With the merger of Veifa and RGS in 1927 and later with SRW, Kress remained chief engineer in all three companies).

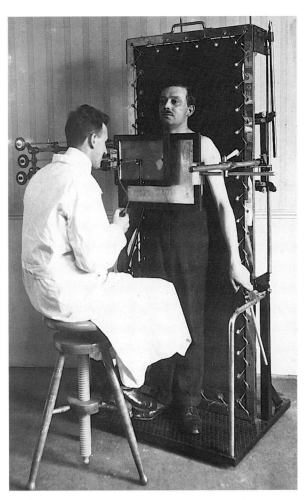

Fig. V, 116. 1907: The KLINOSKOP table with fluorescent screen designed by Kress.

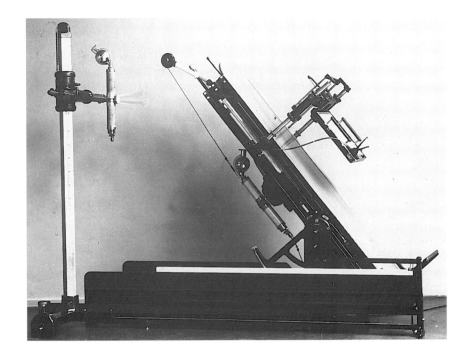

Fig. V, 117. 1920: KLINO-SKOP tilting table. Motor-driven tilting was introduced in 1925.

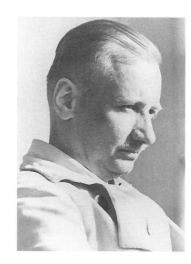

Fig. V, 118.
Hans Heinrich Berg
(1889–1968), Ger-
man radiologist and
professor, contri-
buted design ideas
to a spot-film de-
vice [17].

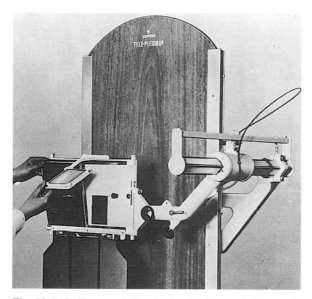

Fig. V, 119. The spot-film device for internal diagnostic
procedures devised by Berg (Fig. V, 118). The device
was manufactured from 1922 until 1934.

But it was also necessary to switch tube parameters between fluoroscopy and radiography
modes, as the tube voltages differed and the
tube current had to be increased substantially
to obtain the required dose within a reasonable
exposure time. Application of the Coolidge principle to tube design allowed the variation of tube
voltage and current over wide ranges, and the
rotating anode gave an increased output. For
fluoroscopy, no rotation was required – this
was to the benefit of the ball bearings and contributed to an increased tube life-span. In summary, then, before taking an exposure, it was
necessary to initiate a number of functions:
bringing the rotating anode up to full speed,
bringing the cathode to a substantially higher

temperature using increased filament current,
setting the tube voltage, corrected according to
the momentary line voltage, moving the cassette
from the park position to the exposure position,
setting the multileaf collimator to the correct exposure format, possibly moving a compression
device in or out, and, finally, setting the scattered
radiation grid in motion to eliminate grid lines
on the film. Originally, the radiologist and technician had to perform all of these tasks manually.
Later, technology contributed to the simplification of the operation by automating these
steps. With the introduction of the automatic exposure control system, over- and underexposed
films were eliminated, because it was now no
longer necessary to estimate the exposure time
by guessing the transparency of the patient.
The goal of simplifying the operation of an
X-ray system was always worth the effort.

Switching the X-ray system from exposure
mode back to fluoroscopy mode also required
time. Above all, the cathode temperature fell
only very slowly to the low value required for
fluoroscopy.

In 1930, a serialography device designed by
Teschendorf was installed in the spot-film device. A four-fold subdivision of the film thus became possible (Fig. V, 120). The spot-film device
in the fluoroscopy system and its ergonomics
were of utmost importance for the radiologist.
The subsequent evolution of spot-film devices
with fluorescent screens is shown in Figs. V, 120,
V, 121 and V, 163. The image intensifier and
optical viewing system could be detached from
the spot-film device (s. Figs. V, 169 and V, 171) to
use the screen for fluoroscopy as an alternative.

The development of spot-film devices followed
more or less the same course with practically all
X-ray equipment manufacturers (Stieve, 1970)
[48]. Significant advantages for spot-film opera-

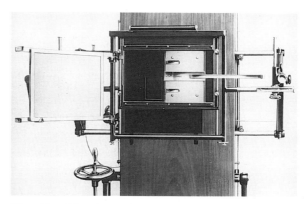

Fig. V, .120. 1930: Spot-film device, designed by
Teschendorf, with subdivisions for a series of exposures.

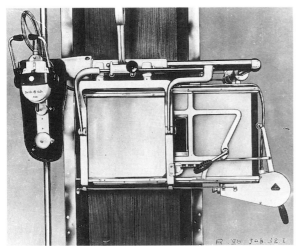

Fig. V, 121. 1934: Spot-film device designed by Albrecht.

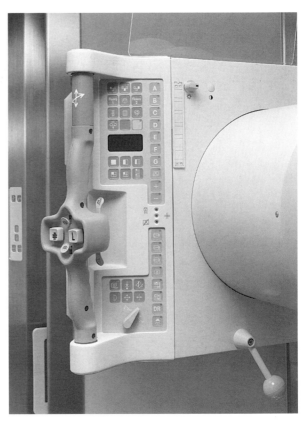

Fig. V, 123. 1991: Controls for the spot-film device used on the SIRESKOP 5 tilting table.

tion came only with the introduction of the image intensifier, as dark adaptation was then no longer required. Spot-film devices now had to be modified (Figs. V, 122, V, 123, V, 173 and V, 177). Documentation took place either on a film cassette or using the cine camera, which had already been introduced for the study of dynamic processes. In 1963, a 70 mm rollfilm camera was adapted.

A tilting table principle proposed by E. Pohl in 1926 is shown in Fig. V, 124. Pohl – a man with many ideas and numerous patents (Bischoff and Gellinek, 1965) [5] – named his unit the OM-NISKOP (Fig. V, 125). A similar table was offered in principle by other X-ray equipment manufacturers (Fehr, 1953; Verse and Weigel, 1954; Strnad, 1955; Morel, 1968; Gajewski, 1970) [10, 14, 38, 49, 52]. The spot-film device with image intensifier could now be operated separately (Fig. V, 126) (Finkenzeller and Schwesig, 1970; Schorr, 1970) [11, 45].

Tilting tables with overtable tubes

Remote-controlled operation became possible in the early sixties with the advent of the television camera and monitor. This system replaced the fluorescent screen and it became possible to work in an examination room with normal daylight. This led to new possibilities for positioning and examining. The classic tilting table, with the tube below or behind the table top and the spot-film device in front of or above the patient, was supplemented by the 'overtable unit'. With this

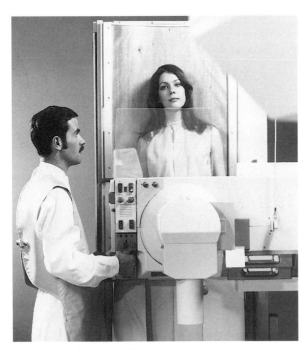

Fig. V, 122. The spot-film device EXPLORAMAT with image intensifier, TV system, and magazine technique for films was introduced in 1973. The magazines for different film sizes are shown on the right hand side of the spot-film device.

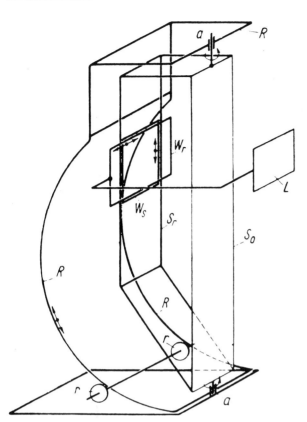

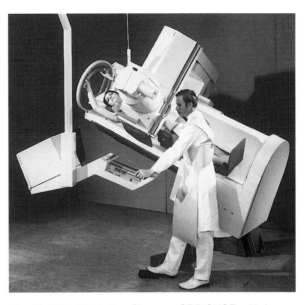

Fig. V, 126. 1968: The Siemens ORBISKOP with image intensifier TV system and remote controls based on Pohl's principle. It is not just a tilting table – the patient could be rotated, and the spot-film device could also be rotated around the patient in any tilting position. Built especially for gastrointestinal diagnostics.

Fig. V, 124. 1926: The principle of Pohl's OMNISKOP (from Albers-Schoenbergs's Roentgentechnik, Rudolf Grashey, ed., Thieme-Verlag, 1941). The table is shown in an upright position with the table top (So) built as a cradle with bearings (a). The whole system can be tilted via a drive (r–R) and carries the spot-film device (L) and the carriage for the X-ray tube (W$_r$).

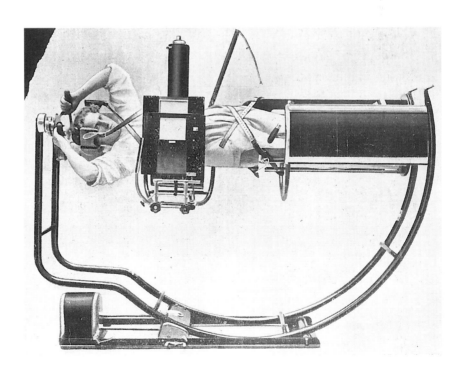

Fig. V, 125. 1935: The OMNISKOP manufactured by the Pohl company.

unit, the tube was located above the patient and the table top and the spot-film device, with the image intensifier, light distributor, television camera, and 70/100-mm camera under the table top. This arrangement brought significant advantages: the patient was now accessible and was no longer 'crushed' by the spot-film device. Only one tube was now required for both spot filming and Bucky radiography. Moreover, it was now possible to set oblique projections and to use the unit as a linear tomography unit. In short, a single examination room could now be used in the morning for scheduled contrast medium examinations and in the afternoon for all Bucky and tomography examinations.

Only the geometry of the imaging system was somewhat inferior to the overtable unit and a higher fluoroscopy output was needed because of the greater film-focus distance. During spot filming, the patient was also subjected to an increase in radiation exposure level due to the absorption of the table top. Since, however, 70/100 mm exposures from the image intensifier required only about a third of the dose, this effect was adequately compensated. More sensitive screens, automated film processing, and automatic exposure controls reduced the radiation exposure level still further (Koehler, 1970) [30]. To this day, both undertable and overtable units have their supporters. But it was in fact the overtable units that initiated a boom in improved

performance of high energy X-ray tubes and generators.

For the first time, outputs of 100 kW and more were in demand. High patient throughput on the overtable unit required tube fans – only for additional cooling. One tube performed the entire day's work, whereas an undertable unit had two or even three tubes (spot-film device, overtable tube for survey radiography on the built-in Bucky tray, Bucky wall stand, and tomography table).

Figures V, 127–V, 130 document the historical evolution. The earliest two special remote-controlled systems (Bischoff and Gellinek, 1965) [5] were those of Jutras in Montreal (Philips) and Chérigié in Paris (Massiot). Jutras's system (Jutras and Ducket, 1958) [28] was a ring stand with overtable tube and a remote-control console separated from the patient by radiation shielding, whereas Chérigié's (1960) [7] was a conventional tilting table with remote controls (Fig. V, 127).

Sensitive palpation was not possible with these tables. Only a remote-controlled compression device was built in. Routine operation since 1958 has demonstrated beyond a doubt that excellent examination results can be obtained by remote-controlled operation, while inclined positions have made new viewing perspectives possible (Fassbender, 1970; Feddema, 1970; Kraemer, 1970; Lohmann, 1970; Van Der Plaats, 1970) [8, 9, 32, 35, 51].

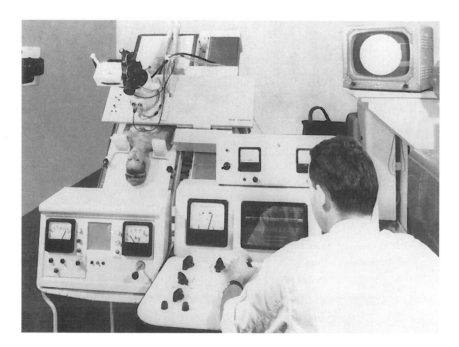

Fig. V, 127. 1958: Remote-controlled tilting table used by Chérigié. Control console for tilting the table and remote compression with an indication of the pressure (left). The spot-film device carries an image intensifier with VIDICON camera and cine camera. This unit was designed by Massiot [5]. Jutras used a Philips-designed, overtable remote-controlled ring stand. The palpation process was replaced with a remote compression device.

At the beginning of the seventies, angiography was in full swing. As a result, the PUCK film changer (Roth et al, 1972) [43], at that time still with two frames per second as a 35 × 35 cm cut film changer, was integrated into the SIREGRAPH (s. Fig. V, 128). With this addition, even abdominal and peripheral angiography could be performed on the remote-controlled tilting table.

The pressure for improved efficiency at the end of the sixties led to the introduction of the magazine technique at the beginning of the seventies: the days of carrying cassettes between the darkroom and the examination room were over. Figure V, 129 shows the SIREMAT [P 16], a fully automatic remote-controlled tilting table with automatic transport of films to the processor

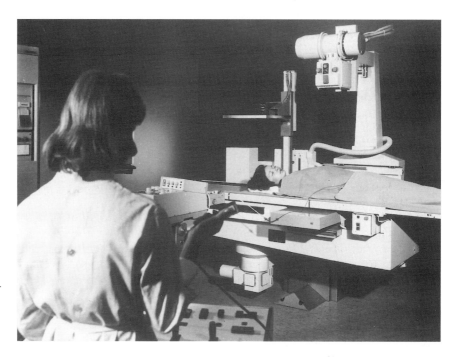

Fig. V, 128. 1971: Remote-controlled tilting table with an additional PUCK film changer under the table for serial angiography up to two frames per second and stepping device (SIREGRAPH A), especially for peripheral angiography.

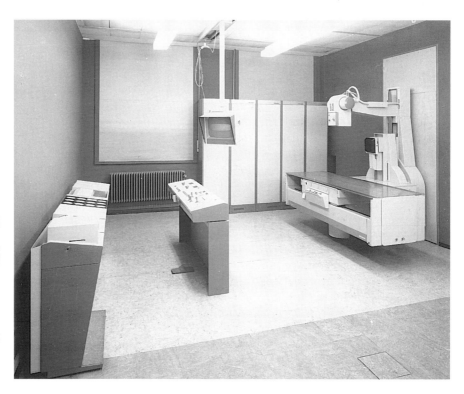

Fig. V, 129. 1975: Fully automatic, remote-controlled radiography and fluoroscopy SIREMAT unit [P16]. This was a cassette-less system based on magazine films for direct radiographs, spot-films, and spot-films of the image intensifier. The processed film was transported to the back of the control console so that the radiologist could assess the images immediately after the procedure.

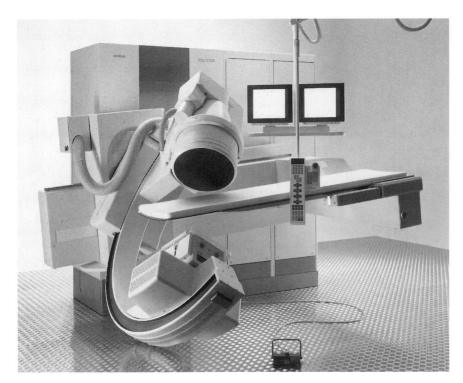

Fig. V, 130. 1991: POLY-STAR universal tilting table based on the C-arm design for diagnostic and interventional procedures. Fluoroscopic and instant images are provided by the 40-cm image intensifier and the digital imaging system FLUOROSPOT H, using high-resolution monitors and reference images.

and then back to the radiologist (behind the remote-control console). High investment costs, including the film transport, prevented the widespread use of this system, particularly because the number of gastrointestinal examinations was decreasing.

The idea of E. Pohl to let the beam rotate around the patient could not be implemented with remote-controlled tilting tables. Angiography taught the appreciation of the usefulness of the free projection which the C-arm permitted. In addition, radiologists started to perform internal interventions as well. Image intensifiers with a 40 cm diameter and instantaneous digital images became possible. The combination of all these features led to the creation of a new type of unit in 1991 – the POLYSTAR (s. Fig. V, 130).

Urology

Urological examinations required the development of specialized units better suited to the special demands of this discipline. Such specialized units have held their place to this day. Fig. V, 131 shows how the conditions of urological examinations are taken into account: using leg supports, as the patient is usually lying at the end of the table in a tilted position, overtable tube, cassette

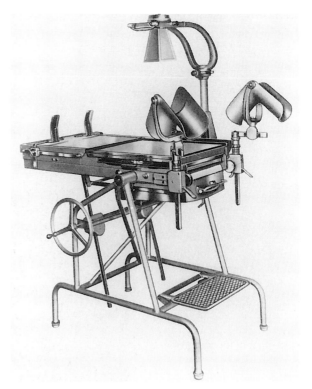

Fig. V, 131. ca. 1960: Table for urological examinations. Liebel-Flarsheim [5] built a table with an integrated Bucky tray and manual tilting in the sixties.

tray under the table top with positioning up to the farthest edge, and pelvic Trendelenburg and reversed Trendelenburg positions from the horizontal. A combination of a urological table with a floor-to-ceiling stand was introduced in the mid fifties. The X-ray tube was given a multi-leaf collimator. A fluorescent screen or a cassette was positioned on the patient.

In 1977, the UROSKOP B met all the requirements – even zonography was possible. Furthermore, the footboard was removable and foot supports could be attached instead. Fluoroscopy was performed at a reduced dose rate and without the need for adaptation to a dark environment due to an image-intensifier television system. The physician could also activate the operating controls by foot-switch. Surfaces were designed for easy cleaning.

For renal stone surgery, the RENODOR was used for intraoperative radiography. However, this required special generators and tubes such as the one in the STATUS X (s. Fig. V, 57).

In the eighties, lithotripsy, using a biplanar X-ray television system for renal stone localization and patient positioning, became widespread. These systems fragment stones in the kidney using extracorporeal shock-waves (Krestel, 1990) [34]. The LITHOSTAR Multiline (Fig. V, 132), introduced in 1993, is a multipurpose urological system for radiological diagnostics, interventions, and shock wave treatment.

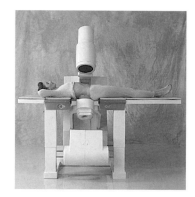

Fig. V, 132. 1994: LITHOSTAR Multiline 15° tilting table for urological diagnostics, interventions and lithotripsy. The C-arm with tube and image intensifier TV system can be moved along the length of the patient.

Paediatrics

X-ray equipment suitable for the examination of children was developed. Positioning aids for chest radiography (Fig. V, 133) were introduced in 1950. By 1964, the THORAKOMAT paediatric chest unit (Fig. V, 134) was available, protecting the technician from radiation exposure. By 1968, it was possible to trigger chest radiographs with the RESPIRAMAT in the correct respiratory phase. This improved the image quality for the examination of infants.

The seventies offered a comprehensive programme of X-ray systems for children. The INFANTOSKOP (Fig. V, 135) is just one example of such a universal unit for fluoroscopy and radiography, with greatly reduced radiation exposure offered by many manufacturers (Gajewski and Schuster, 1968) [12, 13]. Since the onset of

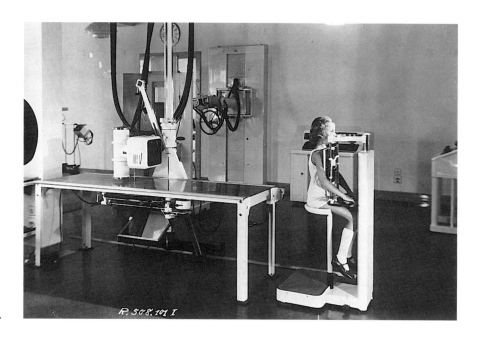

Fig. V, 133. 1950: THORAFIX, a stand for pediatric chest radiographs.

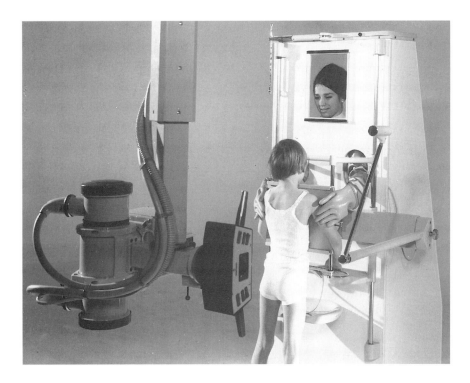

Fig. V, 134. 1964: THORACOMAT paediatric chest stand. To avoid retakes, radiographs were taken with an automatic exposure control system. To reduce radiation exposure, the radiation sensor was placed behind the cassette.

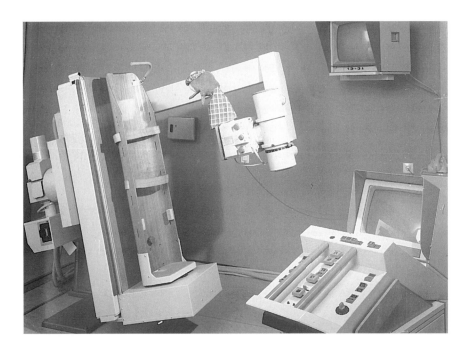

Fig. V, 135. 1973: INFANTOSKOP multipurpose paediatric radiography and fluoroscopy table. Remote-controlled, detachable cradle or table top, image intensifier, TV and 100 mm camera (after 1976).

digital images in the nineties, radiation exposure has been reduced still further (Gindl et al, 1993; Hruby et al, 1993; Krampla et al, 1993) [16, 24, 33].

For our children, though, health services were not yet prepared to commit themselves to the acquisition of special production units for babies, infants, and school children, including up to 18-year-old adults. Consequently, the X-ray equipment industry could do no better than to supply add-on devices for use with tilting tables for the examination of children on units designed for adult examinations. Since children have no political lobby, there was not enough business volume to justify serious interest on the part of industry to further supply special paediatric units. Today, tilting tables with C-arms such as the POLYSTAR (s. Fig. V, 130), equipped with dose-saving digital imaging systems are emerging. Providing excellent access to the patient, they are, again, useful in paediatric radiology.

General angiography – vascular imaging in special procedure rooms

All pioneering activities had to begin with X-ray equipment unsuited to the purpose at hand. In the case of vascular imaging, fluoroscopy took on a new meaning: It furnished the means to navigate the guide wire and the catheter tip under observation and to control its position at any time. Increasingly finer catheters, up to the tracker catheter, did in fact obtain the desired diagnostic information, but at the cost of ever longer fluoroscopy times. The necessary reduction in radiation exposure became possible with the introduction of low-frequency, pulsed fluoroscopy, made possible only with the introduction of digitally stored images. Since 1990, monitors have operated at an image refresh rate of 100 Hz, producing a high-contrast, flicker-free image display. This represented the most significant contribution to image viewing since the introduction of the image-intensifier television system. Documentation onto individual cassettes, cassette changers, rollfilm, and then cut film had always been under the influence of the film and its processing. The frame rate of 6–12 images per second was the upper limit due to a number of mechanical transport reasons.

The historical evolution of the film changer goes back to 1908, as described in the Cardiology section. In Sweden, Georg Schoenander designed a cassette changer according to Lind-Axén's idea which operated at one image per second. In 1954, Buchtala developed a rollfilm changer based on an RGS patent [P 3] of 1910, and so did Gidlund (1956) [15] and Magni. Sjoegren [46] and Fredzell (1953) (s. Fig. V, 139) of the Schoenander company built the AOT cut film changer (six frames per second) in 1953. The PUCK cut-film changer designed for two frames per second was introduced by Elema-Schoenander in 1959 as an alternative to the AOT.

Fluoroscopy was, in fact, rather complicated, as Fig. V, 136 from 1949 indicates (Janker, 1949, 1950) [26]. In the sixties, the image intensifier brought some simplification (Fig. V, 137) and the television system became standard shortly

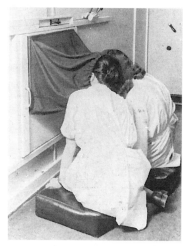

Fig. V, 136. 1949: Position of physician and technician during monitoring of an angiocardiogram. A fluorescent screen was built in beneath the table top, with lead glass of 2 mm lead equivalent, to protect the staff from radiation. Black fabric was used to keep the light out. Two people could monitor the scene. This is a type of KRYPTOSKOP – this system had a CHF Mueller oil ROTALIX Roe 30 X-ray tube with a focal spot of 1.2. This 35 × 35 cm fluorescent screen dated from 1937 and images were recorded via this screen with an Askania camera according to Janker [26].

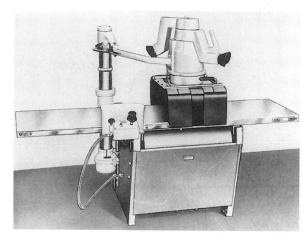

Fig. V, 137. 1960: KOORDINAT catheterisation table. Floating table top, X-ray tube under the table and image intensifier above the table with two optical viewing devices and a lead rubber protection around the patient. Manufactured by Elema [5].

after. Until the mid-seventies, examinations took place in two planes (Fig. V, 138) with image intensifier, television, AOT changer, 35 mm cine film and/or 70 mm rollfilm, and later, 100 mm cut film. But the orthogonal projection in two planes was not able to produce an optimal view of the vascular system and its pathology: the free selection of projections was still desired. Georg Fredzell (Fig. V, 139) and his team of engineers at Elema picked up B. Nordenstroem's and L. Holmstroem's (1980) [40] idea of the BINO C-arm system – an experimental unit built in 1970. A C-arm, on which the X-ray tube and image intensifier–PUCK revolver was mounted. This revolver allowed the image receptor system to be changed quickly and by remote control from television to the film changer. Figure V, 140 shows the result – ANGIOSKOP – introduced in 1977.

The availability of image intensifiers with a field diameter of 40 cm and digital imaging systems with a real 1024 × 1024 matrix (POLYTRON since 1987, see Fig. V, 180) has made possible a resolution capability almost equivalent to that of film. Interventional techniques require an instant image, which a cut-film changer or spot-film camera cannot provide, the best choice being a really good digital imaging system.

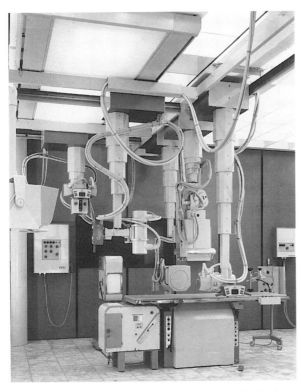

Fig. V, 138. 1969: Special procedures room for biplane angiography. KOORDINAT table, AOT film changer for 6 frames per second, image intensifier TV system with cine camera, and ceiling-mounted, three-dimensional telescopes for tubes and image intensifiers.

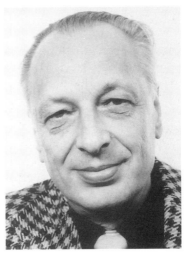

Fig. V, 139. Georg Fredzell (born 1919), engineer and manager of Siemens Elema in Sweden. Angiography was his speciality, especially the AOT cut-film changer and the C-arm devised by Nordenstroem and Holmstroem [40]. Multidirectional projections are very important for diagnostic and interventional procedures. He and his engineering team introduced the ANGIOSKOP (Fig. V, 140). Today, the C-arm design is the preferred system for angiographic and internal procedures.

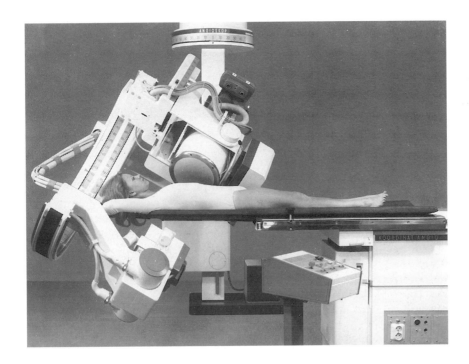

Fig. V, 140. 1977: A universal special procedures room with the ANGIOSKOP. The C-arm design provided an isocentre for all examinations. Its height and the table height could be altered to a convenient position for the examining physician. The image receptor above the patient was designed with a revolving image intensifier with cine or 100 mm cameras and a PUCK film changer. The table top of the KOORDINAT was made of carbon fibre so that radiation exposure to the patient was minimized. This system was the first to allow multidirectional beam projections through an isocentre.

Angiography had become a useful technique for preoperative diagnostics of the arterial blood supply to a tumour. Embolization through the vessels to supplement surgery at first did not produce the long-term benefits hoped for, but is now being used preoperatively again, in support of surgery. Since the advent of computer tomography, nuclear medicine, ultrasonography and magnetic resonance imaging, angiography has been entirely replaced as a method of tumour diagnosis.

Peripheral angiography

This method of examination gained rapid favour. As a rule, it required a maximum of only two images per second, performed originally on Bucky or tilting tables (s. Fig. V, 128) with cassette changers [P 13]. Later on, the PUCK film changer (Roth et al, 1972) [43] beneath the table top of R/F tables were used with an automatic stepping device.

The generator was connected to a kilovoltage reduction device – a stepwise adaptation of tube voltage to the anatomy of the leg in every position. Other methods employ milliamperage reduction. The use of a suitable automatic exposure control system eliminated the need for both techniques. Control over table position and film changer made it possible to program the examination sequence individually, as indicated. Since 1992, peripheral angiography in

fully digital form has also been possible with PERIVISION (s. Fig. III, 113).

Neuroradiology and cerebral angiography

Myelograms (Wellauer, 1961; Valentino, 1965) [50, 53], performed on tilting tables with a 45° Trendelenburg position, have now been largely discontinued in favour of computer tomography and magnetic resonance imaging.

Pneumencephalographies were very painful for the patient and, not infrequently, resulted in death. They required special equipment (Piepgras et al, 1970) [41], such as the MIMER (s. Figs. IV, 36 and IV, 37). With the introduction of computer tomography in the mid-seventies, this technique disappeared for good.

Cerebral angiographies were usually performed in two planes, partly using rollfilm changers, ODELKA image intensifier cameras (Fig. V, 141), or the MIMER. A simpler cerebral angiographic procedure, however, employed two ceiling stands for the X-ray tube and the mutileaf collimator, together with two AOT cut-film changers (s. Fig. V, 138) or, later, PUCK cut-film changers. The patient lay on the KOORDINAT table which had a floating table top. The angiographic examination of cerebral vessels had to be performed partly under anaesthesia, requiring appropriate access to the patient. This is a prominent feature of the neuroradiologic angiography system, particularly since all other angiographies are

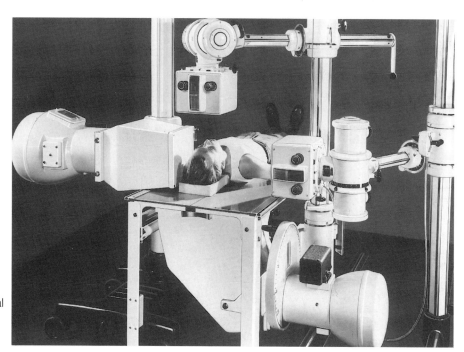

Fig. V, 141. 1954: Special procedures room for cerebral angiography in two planes. Two ODELKA cameras served as image receptors.

performed without general anaesthesia. By the middle of the seventies, it was at last possible to combine fluoroscopy with PUCK film changer series (see Fig. V, 140). The C-arm supported the X-ray tube, which had exceptionally small focal spots, permitting an excellent display of even the fine vascular tree of the brain.

Opposite the tube on the C-arm was a 'revolver' construction with the image intensifier and the PUCK. This allowed positioning the patient's head at the isocentre and any necessary projection could be set up quickly and reproducibly. This system also provided for easy access to the patient by the anaesthetist. This access is an important medical prerequisite, often underestimated or even forgotten in the early days. Changing from fluoroscopy to radiography required only rotating the PUCK film changer to the image-intensifier position. The injection of contrast medium and the exposure series for documentation could then begin. But much time was lost during the examination until the film was developed and positioned correctly on the viewing box, all of which was necessary before deciding how to continue.

In neuroradiology too, three parallel tendencies could be seen in the second half of the eighties: catheter material and guide wires were made still finer in order to be able to penetrate into even tinier vessels. The high-resolution television and digital system (POLYTRON) produced DSA images with a detail sharpness never seen before, so that the resolving power was sufficient to diagnose therapeutically relevant vascular structures (Becker and Brassel, 1991) [2]. Finally, interventional techniques and materials – such as balloons, coils and embolization material – also became increasingly finer. As an alternative to surgery, in special cases of certain arteriovenous malformations and aneurysms, it was now possible to help the patient faster and without undue stress, by intervention. For this purpose, however, an instantaneous digital image of highest quality was needed – and also available. Here again, as in cardiology, a biplane system such as the NEUROSTAR (Figs. V, 142 and 5.143) made a reduction in examination time possible, providing a shorter time for the catheter to be in the vessel. Diagnosis in neuroradiology is no longer based on the angiographic image series alone, but also uses additional dynamic information available from angiography (Fig. V, 143, DYNAVISION). Stereo radiography has been in and out of fashion since 1896 – also in cerebral angiography. However, the method remained limited to only a few centres and never

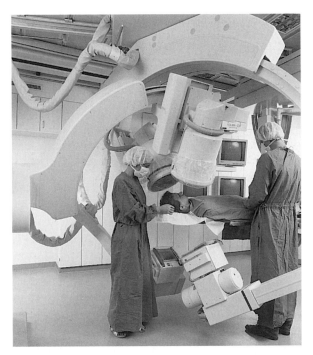

Fig. V, 142. 1991: Special procedures room for biplane neuroradiology with the NEUROSTAR system and the POLYTRON digital imaging system for diagnostics and interventions. The system provides good access for the anesthesist.

gained favour, although anyone seeing stereo images is enthusiastic about it. Pairs of stereo images can now be acquired again with the NEUROSTAR.

In addition, SUPERVISION was introduced, reducing the radiation dose by a factor of two (Fig. V, 144). Today, angiography is clearly no longer the first method of choice for diagnosis. Instead, computer tomography and magnetic resonance imaging – and, with the carotid artery, even ultrasonography – are now preferred. Nowadays, angiography is called for only when CT or MRI fails to give an unequivocal diagnosis; however, it is employed when intervention or surgery offers chances of success.

Stereotaxy serves to localize lesions in the brain. It is also performed with CT/MRI. Radiosurgery (GAMMAKNIFE by Leksell) and surgical intervention to treat disorders in the brain rely on function diagnosis and the superimposition of morphological and functional images for correct localization ('image fusion'). Following three decades of successful advances in the field of cardiac and circulatory diseases, the age of the refined diagnosis and therapy of lesions in the human brain may well be dawning.

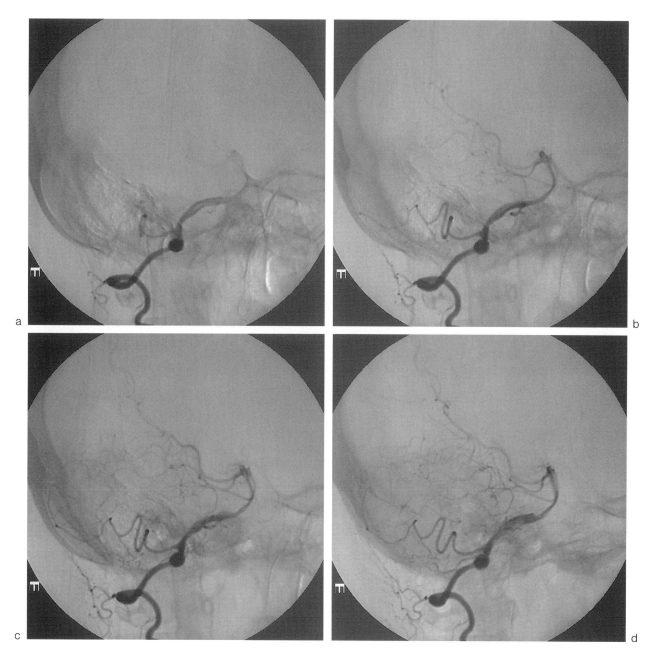

Fig. V, 143. 1993: Rotational angiography with digital subtraction on the POLYTRON in DYNAVISION mode (Siemens). The C-arm first acquires the mask images in different positions, then contrast medium is injected and the C-arm moves back, subtracting the images showing vessels filled with the contrast medium. Images are displayed with or without landmarks. Only one injection is necessary to get several different views of the vessel, which reduces the dose and saves contrast medium.

Cardiology – angiocardiography

Not only the motion blurring of X-ray images resulting from long exposure times complicated the evaluation of the cardiac shadow by the physician, but also the exact time of the exposure release between the systole and the diastole. Thus, even in 1908, the first patent for a cassette changer device was filed (Fig. V, 145) [P 2]. It already claimed turning off X-radiation during cassette transport. A second patent, which essentially improved cassette guidance to reduce wear, and thus obtained a greater frame rate [P 5], followed in 1911. F. Dessauer (s. Fig. I, 29) described the nature of the problem in his patent [P 6] in the following way: *'Such apparatus has*

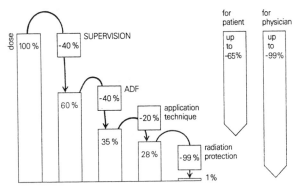

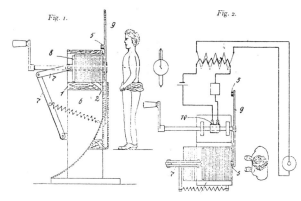

Fig. V, 144. 1992: The Siemens CARE package (Combined Applications to Reduce Exposure in angiography) reduces the dose to the patient by up to 65% and the dose to the physician and medical staff by up to 99%. The reduction in radiation exposure in fluoroscopy via SUPERVISION means reducing fluoroscopy dose to the patient without compromising the image-quality standard. ADF = Adaptive Dose Filter, a programmable filter consisting of 0.1 mm beam hardening copper. Application technique = automatic brightness control via the VIDOMATIC and setting appropriate digital values via the DIGIMATIC for good image quality and collimation down to the smallest possible field size. For the medical staff, additional protective measures are available to reduce the dose they are exposed to.

Fig. V, 145. Sketch of RGS 1908 patent [P2]. Fig. 1 shows an apparatus for acquiring cine images. The photographic plates are in a cassette with lead protection on the back cover. Each cassette is brought in front, exposed and released to fall down a slope, in a rapid sequence. During cassette changing, the radiation is turned off. Figure 2 shows the schematic of the inductor and the cassette changer from a bird's-eye view. RGS patented the transport mechanism for the cassettes and the interruption of the current for the X-ray tube, a radiation protection measure.

to perform movements of a mass equivalent to one or more film cassettes in a special pattern. The cassette has to be set in motion quickly. It then has to be brought to a complete halt, after which it must execute an equally quick movement once again.' To prevent motion blurring of the image, this requires two accelerations and one rest position. Figure V, 146, from the year 1914, illustrates Dessauer's changer in operation during an examination of the heart.

In 1910, RGS patented a rollfilm changer [P 3], with which the film remained still during exposure and was pressed between intensifying screens (Fig. V, 147). This rollfilm changer, with a film strip that moved step-wise, incorporated a device that held the film between a fixed and a movable plate during the X-ray exposure and then released the film for transport. The pressure plates were covered with an intensifying screen. Franz M. Groedel (1881–1951) (s.

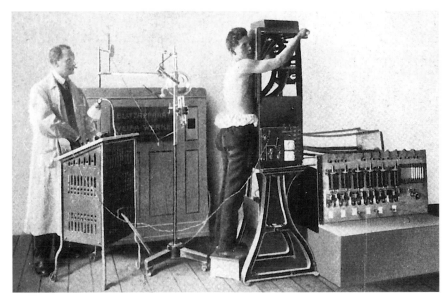

Fig. V, 146. Cassette changer for radiographs of the heart, according to the patent [P6], 1911/14.

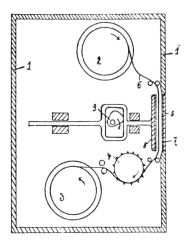

Fig. V, 147. Sketch of a roll film changer with fixed screens on the pressure plates, from an RGS 1910 patent [P3].

Fig. II, 37) not only proposed a diaphragm for the radiograph of the apex of the lung in 1908 (s. Fig. V, 79) but is also well remembered as the father of the 'air gap' technique for chest radiography. He was also very actively concerned with cinematography of the heart (Goerke, 1980) [17]. His X-ray cinematographs were based on the use of rollfilm and the RGS patent [P 3] of 1910.

Siemens designed a pulsed cine radiography unit with a grid-controlled X-ray tube in 1937 (Fig. V, 148). R. Janker (1894–1964) (s. Fig. II, 100) concentrated, among other things, on the photography of the fluorescent screen image

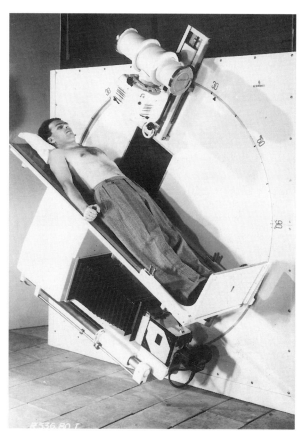

Fig. V, 149. 1951: Ring stand for cinematography according to R. Janker (s. Fig. III, 100). Cine images were exposed from the fluorescent screen on the Askania camera, applying an angled cone (manufactured by SRW).

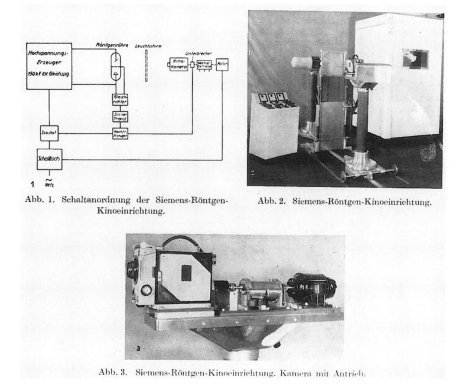

Abb. 1. Schaltanordnung der Siemens-Röntgen-Kinoeinrichtung.

Abb. 2. Siemens-Röntgen-Kinoeinrichtung.

Abb. 3. Siemens-Röntgen-Kinoeinrichtung. Kamera mit Antrieb.

Fig. V, 148. 1937: Pulsed cine radiography with a PANTIX grid-controlled X-ray tube from Siemens.

(Janker, 1937, 1939) [27], using various X-ray systems built by Philips and Siemens for his experiments. He had the optical image intensifier of De Oude Delft modified as CINELIX (s. Fig. V, 165). By 1951–52, a ring stand (Fig. V, 149) or a tilting table was used for cineradiography of the heart (Bischoff and Gellinek, 1965) [5].

In the 1950s, the AOT cutfilm changer was also employed in the biplane version. Figures V, 150a and b were taken at Krankenhaus St. Marien (St Mary's Hospital) in Erlangen in 1959 and show a

special procedure room for angiocardiography with the SIRESKOP table using a fluorescent screen for fluoroscopy, and a biplane AOT.

The high speeds of oscillating heart movements (Berger, 1961) [3], up to 200 mm/s, led to the demand for shorter exposure times and higher frame rates. Moreover, the position of the heart within the thorax required a deviation from pure anteroposterior and lateral projections of the X-ray beam. From the technical side, the first design consisted of a cradle in which the patient was placed. The patient could

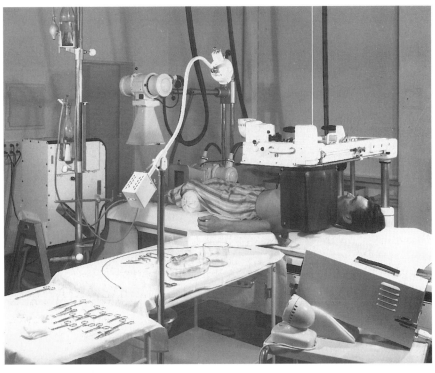

Fig. V, 150a, b. 1959: Special procedures room for angiocardiological procedures with AOT film changers on a SIRESKOP in the St Marien Hospital in Erlangen.

Fig. V, 150a. Position for fluoroscopy with the fluorescent screen.

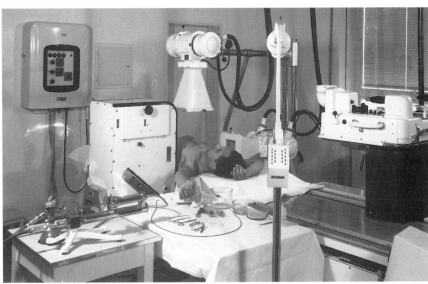

Fig. V, 150b. Exposure position with biplane AOT film changers.

then be turned about his longitudinal axis in the anteroposterior and lateral beam. A caudocranial swivel of the X-ray tube was then introduced in addition as shown in Fig. III, 82. The swivelling, U-shaped tube image-intensifier stand CARDOSKOP U was derived from a therapy simulator. For the first time, a true, free projection of all coronary vessels could be achieved by positioning the patients heart at the system isocentre and rotating the table in a horizontal plane. Also, 16 mm cine film with up to 400 frames per second was replaced by standard 35 mm cine film (ARRIFLEX), with 150 frames per second. Such oblique projections, however, due to the much thicker volume, required increased X-ray output and more energy. Siemens used the proven technology of grid-controlled X-ray tubes and Philips designed a switch with high voltage control tetrodes to produce X-ray pulses of 1–10 ms. This was the age when the dose rate looked like the profile of a church: a huge peak at the beginning of each pulse. This finally ended with the appearance of the PANDOROS OPTIMATIC generator (s. Fig. V, 45). The automation of fluoroscopy and cine mode with the image intensifier was used fully in the interest of a fast and safe procedure.

In 1911, RGS patented an idea for documenting the exposure time between systole and diastole on the film [P 4]. Later, it became possible to record physiological parameters before, after and – in any case, during – cine runs with correlation marks on each single cine image and the

ECG recording (Bergmans et al, 1972; Hettler, 1965, 1966) [4, 21, 22]. The CINECHRONO-CARD (Bühlmeyer et al, 1972) [6; P 14, P 15] was such a device. It helped to correlate cardiac motion with the ECG. By the mid-seventies, there was a veritable explosion in the number of cardiac procedures, now that automation had become well advanced. Preprogrammed settings (Schmitmann and Ammann, 1973) [44] now required only the positioning of the X-ray beam direction and releasing the cine run.

The medical team was now able to concentrate entirely on the patient and the examination it-

Fig. V, 152a, b. 1991: HICOR digital angiocardiography system.

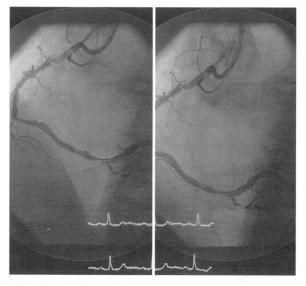

Fig. V, 152a. HICOR fluoroscopy and digital cine radiography images are displayed on a high-resolution, high-brightness monitor using split screen technology. It also can be used for comparisons of images before and after coronary dilatation, indicating the ECG phase of each corresponding image.

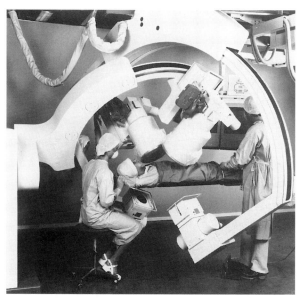

Fig. V, 151. 1985: Special procedures room for biplane angiocardiography and percutaneous transluminal coronary angioplasty (PTCA) with the BICOR.

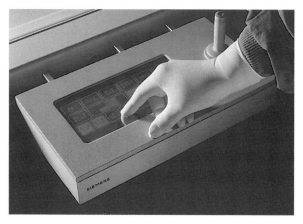

Fig. V, 152b. The touch screen control panel is mounted at the bedside of the KOORDINAT examination table.

self. Research was conducted in videodensitometry and cinedensitometry – the relative determination of contrast medium concentration in blood vessels. The determination of the volume of the heart with the VOLUMAT, though, did not become routine.

The problem remained of how to examine the patient while at rest. G. Fredzell (s. Fig. V, 139) offered the answer in 1975 with the development of the C-arm stand (s. Fig. V, 140, ANGIOSKOP), which was well accepted by the end of the seventies. This allowed all free projections finally even in two planes (BICOR, Fig. V, 151) which saved contrast medium: two different views could be obtained with only one injection. It also considerably reduced the examination time. In 1985, Angiotec showed it was possible to greatly reduce radiation exposure during fluoroscopy of fast moving objects. This was achieved by combining pulsed fluoroscopy with 'gap filling' – the repeated fill-in of digital images. The nineties have witnessed the introduction of digital and flicker-free monitor images (HICOR, Fig. V, 152). Quantitative information is now immediately available to help the user decide faster and with greater confidence how to proceed further.

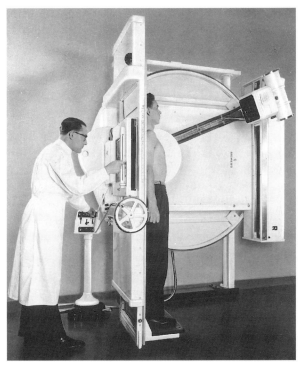

Fig. V, 154. 1951: Linear tomography in any patient position, with the UNIVERSAL PLANIGRAPH. The patient could be positioned using fluoroscopy and a fluorescent screen [P11, P12].

Conventional tomography

The technological evolution (Grossmann, 1935; Kieffer, 1939; Meiler, 1970; Heckmann, 1984) [19, 20, 29, 37; P9, P10] can be seen in Figs. V, 153–V, 156. Automatic exposure control systems for tomograms are discussed in the section on generators.

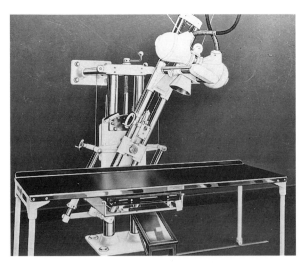

Fig. V, 153. 1938: The Sanitas company's tomography system.

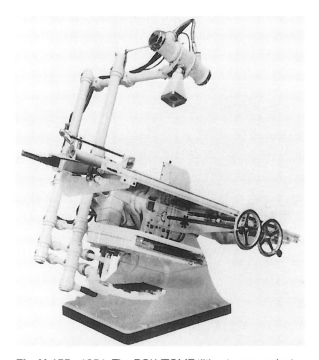

Fig. V, 155. 1951: The POLYTOME tilting tomography table with two-dimensional tomography: linear, circular, elliptical, and hypocycloidal. The X-ray tube and the cassette tray were coupled with a mechanical parallelogram connection and moved on the surface of a sphere (manufactured by Massiot) [5].

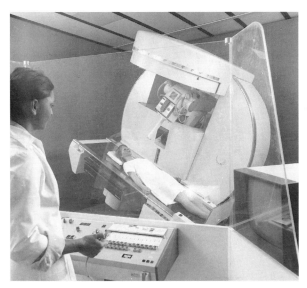

Fig. V, 156. OPTIPLANIMAT manufactured from 1975 to 1980. A universal tomography unit with image intensifier for positioning under fluoroscopy. Linear and two-dimensional movements, including spiral motion, could be performed in any tilting position.

Transverse axial tomography (Figs. V, 157 and V, 158) (Kotoulas and Sinis, 1970) [31] had been in use since 1949. Sir Godfrey Newbold Hounsfield (s. Fig. IV, 16) developed the computer tomograph, which replaced multidirectional and transverse tomography, but not simple linear tomography.

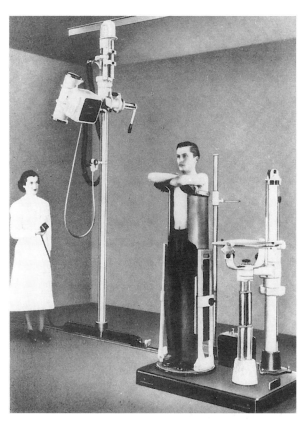

Fig. V, 158. 1949: Transverse tomography unit in operation. The patient and cassette tray rotate synchronously in opposite directions. Several companies such as SRW, Zuder in Italy and CGR manufactured them at that time.

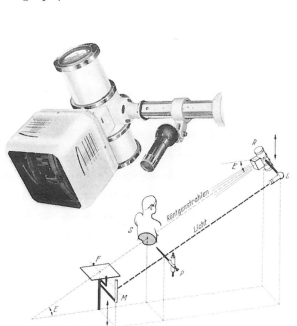

Fig. V, 157. 1949: TRANSVERSAL PLANIGRAPH with X-ray tube and multileaf collimator with aiming device. The picture shows the principle of transverse tomography positioning of focus, patient and film cassette.

The digital radiology department: from dream to vision to reality

Digital technology matured in the eighties. Image quality on monitors and speed of operation were the two major obstructions to introducing networking in a radiology department. Many Newport Beach and CAR (Computer Assisted Radiology) symposia passed with discussions about dreams, visions and trials.

W. Hruby's vision [24a, 25] became reality with the Siemens SIENET system in the Danube Hospital, a community hospital in Vienna, Austria, in April 1992 (Figs. V, 159 and V, 160). Around the same time, F. Goeringer and his team of the American Armed Forces began to implement the first Medical Diagnostic Imaging Support system (MDIS) installation in Madigan, USA, designed by Loral and Siemens Gammasonics. Danish pioneers J. Joergensen in Aarhus as well as F. E. Lindhardt and J. Dalgaard in Viborg implemented SIENET in 1992.

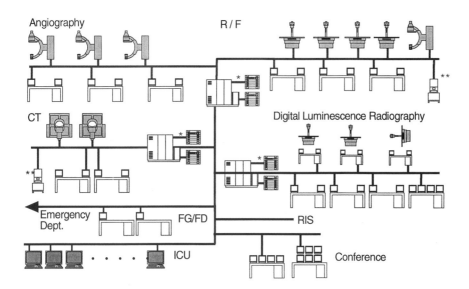

Fig. V, 159. 1992: The digital radiology department at the Danube Hospital of the Social Medicine Centre East (SMZ Ost), a community hospital in Vienna, Austria. All modalities acquire digital images and are networked via the SIENET system. * = Storage and digital archiving; ** = laser camera; R/F = radiography and fluoroscopy system; FG/FD = frame grabber for ultrasound modalities and film digitizer; ICU = intensive care unit where DIGISCAN images are acquired, read in the radiology department and displayed with the report on the monitors in the ICU. RIS = Roentgen Information System and link to the hospital information system.

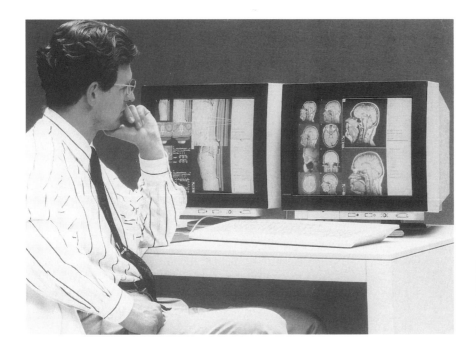

Fig. V, 160. 1992: Soft copy reporting on SIMOMED flikker-free monitors with a brightness of 500 cd/m^2 or 170 foot lamberts, in the SMZ Ost.

Economic pressures became increasingly apparent in the nineties. Gradually, less invasive therapy by interventional techniques began to gain favour over surgery – without doubt compelled by cost factors. This posed new demands, including better and faster access to images (Hruby et al, 1992, 1993, 1994; Krampla et al, 1993; Mathiaschitz et al, 1993; Wirsz E, 1994; Wirsz N, 1994; Grassmann, 1994) [18a, 24a, 24, 25, 33, 36, 54, 55]. From the standpoint of the engineer, this meant managing digital images between acquisition, archive, and work stations for diagnosis, conference and viewing. The result was a reduction in the amount of films, chemicals, and water consumption for the processor, archive costs, and the loss of time which these involve.

Once again, human intellect had succeeded under pressure in developing innovations for the benefit of everyone – patients, clinics, taxpayers, and our environment.

Patents

P 1   DP 156 389 vom 3. April 1902, Siemens & Halske, Berlin: Verfahren und Apparat zum Durchleuchten von Körperteilen mittels Röntgenstrahlen (Kompression von Weichteilen).

P 2   DP 215 648 vom 22. April 1908, Reiniger, Gebbert und Schall, Erlangen: Kinematograhischer Aufnahmeapparat für Röntgenbilder.

P 3   DP 243 256 vom 6. Nov. 1910, Reiniger, Gebbert und Schall, Erlangen: Vorrichtung zur Aufnahme von Röntgenreihenbildern mit schrittweise fortschaltbarem Bildband, das während der Aufnahme in einem Bildfenster zwischen gegeneinander verschiebbare Platten festgeklemmt und von diesen während der Fortschaltung freigegeben wird.

P 4   DP 255 574 vom 10. Jan. 1911, Reiniger, Gebbert und Schall, Erlangen: Verfahren und Einrichtung zur Röntgenaufnahme sich bewegender Körper zur Bestimmung ihrer Bewegungsphase zur Zeit der Aufnahme.

P 5   DP 242 443 vom 23. April 1911, Reiniger-Gebbert und Schall, Erlangen: Verfahren und Vorrichtung zur kinematographischen Aufnahme von Röntgenbildern.

P 6   DP 248 973 vom 10. Dez. 1911, VEIFA-Werke und Friedrich Dessauer, Frankfurt a. M.: Maschine zum raschen Wechseln von lichtempfindlichen Platten oder Films, hauptsächlich für Reihenaufnahmen mit Röntgenstrahlen.

P 7   DP 284 371 vom 9. Feb. 1913, Dr. Gustav Bucky, Berlin: Verfahren zum Erzeugen von Röntgenbildern unter Vermeidung der bildverschleiernden Wirkung der sekundären Röntgenstrahlen.

P 8   USP 1 471 081 vom 28. Sept. 1921, H.F. Waite, USA: Vibrating Bucky Diaphragm for Scattered X-ray Radiation.

P 9   USP 652 005 vom 14. Aug. 1936, Heinrich Kunz, SRW Erlangen: Einrichtung zur Erzeugung von Körperschnittbildern mittels Röntgenstrahlen.

P 10   DP 707 129 vom 17. Juni 1937, Dipl.-Ing. Herbert Graf, Erlangen: Einrichtung zur Erzeugung von Körperschichtbildern mittels Röntgenstrahlen. (SRW, Schichtgerät mit Maßraster).

P 11   DP 818 990 vom 2. Okt. 1948, Josef Gerneth, Erlangen: Gerät zur Herstellung von Körperschnitt- bzw. Körperschichtbildern mittels Röntgenstrahlen (SRW-Horizontal-Planigraph).

P 12   DP 818 675 vom 26. April 1949, Josef Gerneth, Erlangen: Elektromedizinisches Gerät, insbesondere Röntgenuntersuchungsgerät (Für SRW-Universal-Planigraph).

P 13   DP 932 340 vom 17. Juli 1953, Josef Gerneth, Erlangen: Röntgenuntersuchungsgerät mit einer Einrichtung für Röntgen-Serienaufnahmen (SRW, für Extremitätenarteriographie, Realisierungsvorschlag auch mit Leuchtschirm).

P 14   DP 202 6504 (Auslegeschrift) vom 30.Mai 1970, Dipl.-Ing. Herbert Lutz und vier Miterfinder Marhoff, Pfeiler, Brunn, Goering, Siemens Berlin/München: Medizinische Untersuchungseinrichtung, bestehend aus einem Röntgenuntersuchungsgerät und einem Gerät zur Aufzeichnung physiologischer Meßgrößen.

P 15   DP 202 8515 vom 15. Juni 1970, Dipl.-Ing. Herbert Lutz, Seukendorf und vier Miterfinder Marhoff, Pfeiler, Brunn, Goering, Siemens Berlin/München: Einrichtung zur Aufzeichnung eines Zeitmaßstabes auf dem Registrierstreifen eines Gerätes zur Darstellung physiologischer Meßgrößen.

P 16   DP 23 34 250 vom 5. Juli 1973, Ing. (grad) Kurt Künne; Alfred Hahn; Georg Vogel; Ing. (grad.) Heinz Wons; Siemens Berlin/München: Röntgenuntersuchungsgerät (vollautom. Magazintechnik).

References

1. Barth, V., K. Deininger, H. v. Babo: Erste Erfahrungen mit einem neuen Mammographiefilm für 90 Sekunden Maschinenverarbeitung. Röntgen-Bl., 25. Jg., 4 (1972) 150–160
2. Becker, H., F. Brassel: 2 Ebenen DSA für die diagnostische und interventionelle Neuroradiologie. Klin. Neuroradiol. 1 (1991) 229–236
3. Berger, A.: Zum Problem der Bewegungsunschärfe im Röntgenbild der Lunge und des Herzens. Röntgen-Bl. 14 (1961), 369
4. Bergmans, R. F., W. Pouwelse, G.P.M. Vijverberg: Die Synchronaufzeichnung von physiologischen Kurven im Röntgenkinobild – ein neues Verfahren. Röntgen-Bl. 1 (1972) 1–4
5. Bischoff, K., W. Gellinek: Geräte für die Anwendung ionisierender Strahlen (mit 345 Abbildungen), 121–323. In: Vieten, H. (Herausgeber): Physikalische Grundlagen und Technik Teil 2, Springer Verlag 1965. Gesamtwerk Diethelm, L., O. Olsson, F. Strand, H. Vieten, A. Zuppinger (Herausgeber): Handbuch der Medizinischen Radiologie. Band I, Teil 2, Springer-Verlag 1965
6. Bühlmeyer, K., H. Lutz, K. Brunn, W. Maass: Zuordnung physiologischer Daten zu gespeicherten Röntgenbildern. Röntgen-Bl. 1 (1972) 5–9
7. Chérigié, E.: La télévision technique actuelle du radiodiagnostic. Ann. Radiol. 5/6, Editorial 1960
8. Fassbender, C.W.: Zur ferngesteuerten Untersuchungstechnik – Erfahrungen mit ferngesteuerten Untersuchungsgeräten herkömmlicher Bauart. Röntgen-Bl. 5 (1970) 203–212
9. Feddema, J.: Considerations on Remotely Controlled Examinations and the Development of the Diagnost 100. Röntgen-Bl. 7 (1970) 331–339
10. Fehr, W.: Über ein neues Diagnostikgerät mit universeller Anwendung. Fortschr. Röntgenstr., Beil. zu Bd. 79 (1953) 36–37
11. Finkenzeller, J., H. Schwesig: Das neue Untersuchungsgerät Orbiskop und seine technischen Besonderheiten. Röntgen-Bl. 5 (1970) 221–226
12. Gajewski, H., W. Schuster: Bildverstärkerphotographie mit 70-mm-Kameras in der pädiatrischen Röntgendiagnostik. Dtsch. med. Wschr. 93 (1968) 2201–2203
13. Gajewski, H., W. Schuster: Bildverstärkerphotographie mit 70-mm-Kameras in der pädiatrischen Röntgendiagnostik. Dtsch. med. Wschr. 46 (1968) 2201–2203

14. Gajewski, H.: Röntgenuntersuchungsgeräte mit frei wählbarer Kombination der Patientenlage und der Projektionsrichtung (Eine Übersicht über die technische Entwicklung mit zehn Literaturstellen aus den Jahren 1934–1968). Röntgen-Bl. 5 (1970) 213–220

15. Gidlund, A.: Development of Apparatus and Methods for Roentgenstudies in Haemodynamics. Acta Radiol. Suppl. Vol. 130 (1956)

16. Gindl, K., A. Bach, G. Alth, H. Mosser, W. Hruby: Strahlenhygiene durch digitale Radiographie am Beispiel der Mictionscystourethrographie in der pädiatrischen Radiologie. Österr. Krankenhaus-Zeitung, Sonderfolge Radiologie (1993), 22

17. Goerke, H.: Fünfundsiebzig Jahre Deutsche Röntgengesellschaft. G. Thieme Verlag Stuttgart, New York 1980

18a. Graßmann, P., C. F. C. Greinacher, W. Maly: Wirtschaftlichkeit und Patientennutzen digitaler Bildmanagementsysteme für die Radiologie. Akt. Radiol. 4(1994), 198–206

18. Grigg, E.R.N.: The Trail of the Invisible Light. Charles C. Thomas Publisher Springfield, USA, 1965.

19. Großmann, G.: Tomographie I und II. Fortschr. Röntgenstr. 51 (1935) 61 und 191

20. Heckmann, K.: Die Entwicklung der Schlitzaufnahmen. Röntgen-Bl. 37 (1984) 29–39

21. Hettler, M. G.: Die kinematographische Funktionsanalyse mit filmsynchroner Kreislaufregistrierung. Fortschr. Röntgenstr. 102 (1965) 156

22. Hettler, M. G.: Über eine universell verwendbare elektronische Angiographiesteuerapparatur. Fortschr. Röntgenstr. 104 (1966) 463

23. Hoxter, E.A., A. Schenz: Röntgenaufnahmetechnik – Grundlagen und Anwendungen. Verlag Siemens Aktiengesellschaft Berlin und München, 1991, 14. Auflage

24a. Hruby, W., H. Mosser, M. Urban, W. Krampla, M. Ammann, R. Mayrhofer, K. Kaissas: Klinische Erfahrungen mit PACS: Digitale Radiologie. Radiologe 34 (1994) 291–299

24. Hruby, W., H. Mosser, M. Urban, M. Wassipaul, K. Gindl, E. Kucera, K. Kaissas: Digitale Radiologie – Klinische Realität. Österr. Krankenhaus-Zeitung, Sonderfolge Radiologie (1993), 3

25. Hruby, W. et. al.: Datenvernetzung in einem neu errichteten Röntgeninstitut am Beispiel des Donauspitals Wien. Röntgenpraxis 45 (1992) 103–110

26. Janker, R.: Apparatur und Technik der Röntgenkinematographie zur Darstellung der Herzbinnenräume und der großen Gefäße (Angiokardio-Kinematographie). Fortschr. Röntgenstr. 72 (1949/50) 513–520

27. Janker, R.: Die Photographie des Leuchtschirmbildes (Einzelbild und Röntgenkinematographie. Röntgenpraxis 9 (1937) 58; Röntgenpraxis 11 (1939) 271

28. Jutras, A., G. Ducket: Roentgen diagnosis by remote control tuberfluoroscopy and cineradiography. Medica Mundi 4, No. 3 (1958) 77–82

29. Kieffer, J.: Analysis of laminagraphic motions and their values. Radiology 33 (1939) 560

30. Köhler, R.: Vergleichende Untersuchung über Strahlenexposition im röntgendiagnostischen Routinebetrieb mit konventioneller bzw. Bildverstärker-Fernsehkette-Durchleuchtung. Röntgen-Bl. 11 (1970) 543–553

31. Kotoulas K., G. Sinis: Theoretische Untersuchung der Projektionsbewegungsbedingungen der transversalen Tomographie. Röntgen-Bl. 1 (1970) 15–19

32. Kraemer, E.: Erfahrungsbericht mit einem ferngesteuerten, universellen Röntgenuntersuchungsgerät in einer freien Röntgenpraxis (Zweijahresbericht). Röntgen-Bl. 7 (1970) 288–297

33. Krampla, W., G. Oberhauser, H. Mosser, W. Hruby: Klinische Erfahrungen im digitalen Röntgeninstitut. Österr. Krankenhaus-Zeitung, Sonderfolge Radiologie (1993), 28

34. Krestel, E. (Ed.): Imaging Systems for Medical Diagnostics. Published by Siemens Aktiengesellschaft Berlin und München, 1990, 2. Auflage

35. Lohmann, Th.: Ferngesteuerte Untersuchungsgeräte. Röntgen-Bl. 5 (1970) 190–196

36. Mathiaschitz, U., H. Mosser, K. Gindl, A. Tekusch, J. Malcher, W. Hruby: Digitale Fluoroskopie in einem PACS-Netz. Österr. Krankenhaus-Zeitung, Sonderfolge Radiologie (1993), 11

37. Meiler, J.: Die Abhängigkeit der Schichtdicke von Verwischungsfigur, Pendelwinkel und Detailgröße bei Schichtaufnahmen. Röntgen-Bl. 9 (1970) 389–399

38. Morel, J.K.: Über ein universell verwendbares Röntgen-Untersuchungsgerät mit großer Beweglichkeit. Röntgen-Bl. 21 (1968) 271–275

39. Mosser, H., M. Wassipaul, G. Pärtan, M. Urban, W. Hruby: Digitale Mammographie am Monitor eines radiologischen Befundarbeitsplatzes vs. Film-Folien-Mammographie. Österr. Krankenhaus-Zeitung, Sonderfolge Radiologie (1993), 18

40. Nordenström, B., L. Holmström: Versatile Single and Biplane Systems for Radiological Procedures, Percutaneous Biopsy and Therapeutic Vascular Occlusion. Internation. Symposium, München. In: Anacker, H. et al: Georg Thieme Verlag, Stuttgart (1980) 90–96

41. Piepgras, U.; F. Heuck, F. Pampus: Ein Universalarbeitsplatz für die Neuroradiologie (Erfahrungen mit einem Spezialgerät für die Röntgendiagnostik des Schädels und der Wirbelsäule). Röntgen-Bl. 1 (1970) 1–14

42. Rackwitz, K.: Bildverstärkeraufnahmen im Operationssaal und bei der Notversorgung. Röntgen-Bl. 8 (1972) 382–386

43. Roth, F.-J., H.-J. Encke, H. Lohölter: Erfahrungen mit dem neuen Serienangiographiegerät „PUCK". Röntgen-Bl. 12 (1972) 557–561

44. Schmitmann, H., E. Ammann: PANDOROS OPTIMATIC – ein Röntgengenerator mit neuen Möglichkeiten. Electromedica 41 (1973) 177–181

45. Schorr, H.: Das Orbiskop im praktischen klinischen Gebrauch. Röntgen-Bl. 5 (1970) 227–229

46. Sjögren, S.E., G. Fredzell: Apparatus for Serial Angiography. Acta Radiol. 40 (1953) 361–368

47. Sommer, E.: Röntgen-Taschenbuch, II. Band, Otto Nemnich Verlag Leipzig 1909

48. Stieve, F.E.: Die Technik der Röntgenuntersuchung an Durchleuchtungsgeräten; Klinische Forderungen an die Gerätekonstruktion. Röntgen-Bl. 7 (1970) 310–330

49. Strnad, F.: Das neuartige Röntgen-Untersuchungsgerät Müller UGX und seine universelle Verwendbarkeit. Röntgenstrahlen. Geschichte und Gegenwart. C.H.F. Müller AG (1955) 14

50. Valentino, V.: Myelography. Charles C. Thomas Publisher, Springfield, Ill., 1965

51. Van Der Plaats, G.J.: Fernbedienung und Fernsteuerung. Röntgen-Bl. 5 (1970) 197–202

52. Verse, H., K. Weigel: Eine gerätetechnische Betrachtung zur Röntgendiagnostik. Fortschr. Röntgenstr. 80 (1954) 520–524

53. Wellauer, J.: Die Myelograhie mit positiven Kontrastmitteln. Georg Thieme Verlag, Stuttgart, 1961

54. Wirsz, E.: Analysis of picture archive and communication systems architectures; expert configurations, modeling simulation, validation and verification. Dissertation, Graduate School of the Illinois Institute of Technology, Chicago, 1994

55. Wirsz, N.: Interfacing picture archive and communications systems with radiology information systems and hospital information systems. Dissertation, Graduate School of the Illinois Institute of Technology, Chicago, 1994

Fluoroscopy and recording of digital and image-intensifier images

E. Ammann, G. Rosenbusch, M. Oudkerk

Fluoroscopy with fluorescent screens

Fluoroscopy is used in medical diagnostics in connection with a number of examination techniques for orientation and evaluation of organ functions. The image obtained from fluoroscopy is visible on the fluorescent screen and can be viewed from different directions (Fig. V, 161).

From the innovations in patient positioning (Fig. V, 162) it can be seen that the fluorescent screen was soon coupled to the X-ray tube holder. The physician could move both together longitudinally and transversely to the patient. Here as well the radiologist was able to take advantage of measures contributing to improved image quality, i.e. collimating the primary X-ray beam to the size of the fluorescent screen or even smaller, together with compression of the irradiated patient volume.

Due to very low luminance of the screen, about $1.7 \, \text{cd/m}^2$ or (6 foot lamberts), it was necessary to

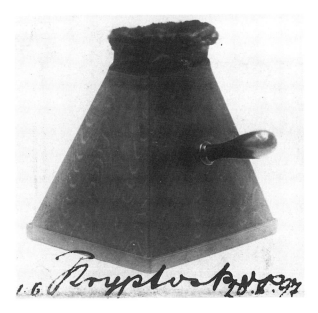

Fig. V, 161a. 1897: KRYPTOSKOP. The bottom of the device contained a fluorescent screen.

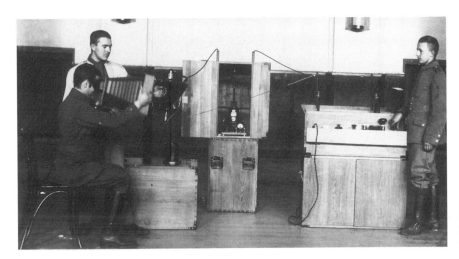

Fig. V, 161b. Fluoroscopy of a soldier's hand in a military X-ray unit during the First World War (1914–18).

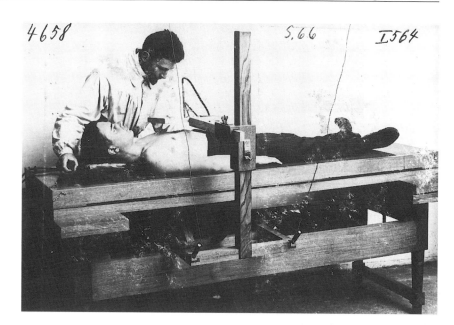

Fig. V, 162. 1909: Fluoroscopy on a recumbent patient.

fluoroscope in a fully darkened room. For this reason there was not only danger from a continuously emitting X-ray tube, but also, during the early decades, of electric shocks from high voltage which was led in the open from the inductor to the X-ray tube. In 1932, H.F. Waite [P 3] patented an arrangement which made it no longer necessary to examine the patient in a darkened room. However, his idea was not widely used.

Only with the introduction of insulated high-voltage cables and radiation-protective tube housing assemblies in the 1930s could this hazard for both physician and patient be eliminated. Lesions, however, were always documented onto film plates and later onto film. For this reason fluoroscopy served essentially for orientation and localization. From this the spot-film device evolved. It was able to park a film cassette alongside the fluorescent screen where there was no danger of exposure due to radiation. Figure V, 163 shows a tilting table with spot-film device. At the right, next to the large fluorescent screen, the cassette was moved to the park position. When the lesion was clearly visible on the fluorescent screen, the physician moved the cassette to the left into position between the patient and the fluorescent screen. The lesion was then documented onto the film.

With the introduction of the high-vacuum tube by Coolidge (1913), it was now possible to set the tube voltage and tube current independently, even for fluoroscopy. The transition phase from fluoroscopy to radiography and back soon became the focus of particular attention: Fluoroscopy required the movement of the X-

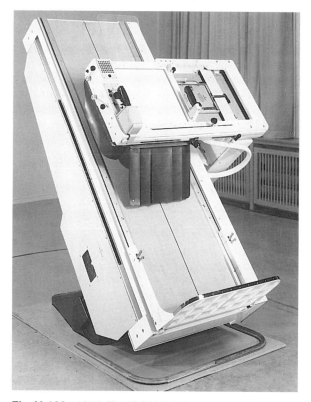

Fig. V, 163. 1958: The ISOSKOP tilting table with fluorescent screen and spot-film device.

ray tube, fluorescent screen, table top, patient and continuous radiation with a low dose rate. For radiography, however, everything had to be firmly fixed, 'braked', and the radiation available for a short exposure time.

Physicians examined the movements of organs such as cardiac motion under fluoroscopic observation. Above all, surgeons made use of fluoroscopy to search for foreign bodies and to reposition broken bones. Thus for example it was reported in 'The Doctors Mayo' (Clapesattle, 1941) [9]:

Just two months after Roentgen's announcement an X-ray machine made its appearance in Rochester. Dr. J. Grosvenor Cross . . . bought one for his office in February 1896. For a time it was merely a new toy, but in August he demonstrated his pictures and their uses at the annual meeting of the Southern Minnesota Medical Association, and early in 1897 he repeated the demonstration for the Olmsted County Society.

A week later the Mayo brothers had an occasion to test the machine for themselves. A little boy who had swallowed a vest buckle was brought to the office. It would help in deciding how best to remove it if the doctors could know just where in the esophagus it was lodged, whether it was open or closed, and if open in what direction its prongs were pointing, so they went over to see whether Cross's X-ray machine could tell them.

Dr. Cross made two pictures, one of which showed the buckle in remarkably clear outline, with the prongs pointing upward, so that drawing it out through the mouth would punch them into the esophagus walls. Consequently Dr. Charlie made an incision into the esophagus and pulled the buckle out blunt end first. His subsequent report of the case, written

quite uncharacteristically without any refence to Dr. Cross's part in it, was one of the first on the use of the skiagraph, as an X-ray picture was called, to appear in the Northwest.'

The diagram (Fig. V, 164) (Gebauer et al, 1974) [24] shows the fluorescent screen brightness as a function of dose rate. The use of modern image intensifier and television technology reduces the dose rate, at the same time improving the image brightness by roughly 10^5 and the discriminating sensitivity of the eye by a factor of 30.

X-ray image intensifiers

The country physician Helge Christensen experimented with optical systems at the end of the 1930s and designed a device with which images could be photographed from the fluorescent screen onto 25-mm roll film. He employed this device for 15 years in clinical routine. A. Bouwers (s. Fig. V, 14) continued these experiments in 1941, after joining De Oude Delft, using a 40-cm input screen and 70-mm roll film in 1945. In Germany, R. Janker (s. Fig. III, 100) performed examinations with such an apparatus called the ODELKA. The advantage of this apparatus was that it was able to take a large number of

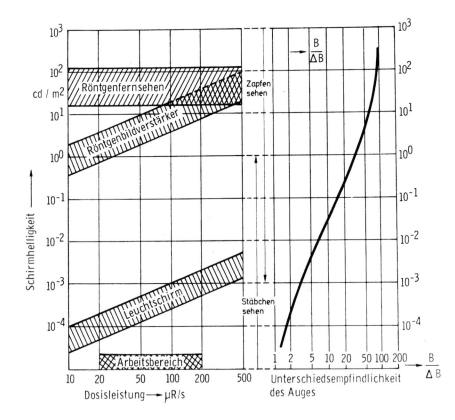

Fig. V, 164. The diagram shows the luminous intensity in cd/m^2 as a function of the dose rate in R/s and the sensitivity of the eye's cones and rods. Roentgenfernsehen = television; Roentgenbildverstaerker = image intensifier; Leuchtschirm = fluorescent screen; Arbeitsbereich = working range; Zapfen sehen = cone vision; Staebchen sehen = rod vision. The luminous intensity of a fluorescent screen is approximately that of a clear, moonlit night. The sensitivity of the rod vision depends on the period of adaptation. It increases by a factor of 100 within the first 20 minutes of adaptation to the dark. The difference between the illumination of the surrounding area B and the deviation ΔB is given at an angle of vision of 0.5°. The television system can compensate for different intensities of the image intensifier [24].

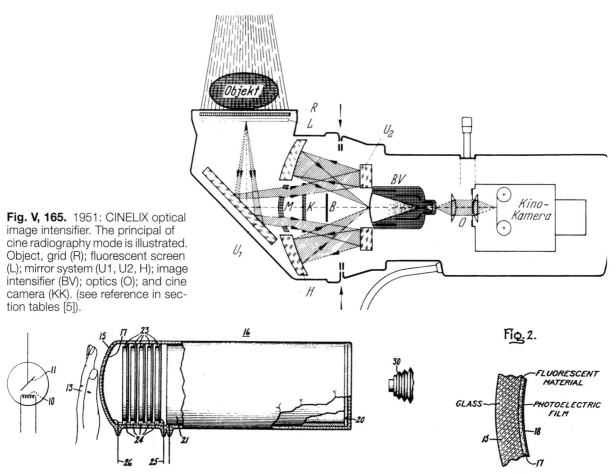

Fig. V, 165. 1951: CINELIX optical image intensifier. The principal of cine radiography mode is illustrated. Object, grid (R); fluorescent screen (L); mirror system (U1, U2, H); image intensifier (BV); optics (O); and cine camera (KK). (see reference in section tables [5]).

Fig. V, 166. I. Langmuir at GE filed a patent [P4] for an image intensifier on 3 November 1937. Figure 1 of the patent is an application schematic and Fig. 2 is an important detail of the input screen. The input glass wall (15) is coated with a fluorescent material (17) (calcium tungstate) and with a film (18) of photoelectric active material (slightly oxidized silver activated with an alkali metal, preferably caesium). This emits electrons only when excited by light from the fluorescent screen. Radiation transmitted through the object falls on the end wall (15) of an evacuated transparent envelope (16). The electron pattern corresponds closely to that of the image itself. The electrons may be focussed electron-optically (23) to impinge on another fluorescent screen (20) where they will produce a secondary visible image. Greater intensity of this image can be achieved by accelerating the electrons to a higher velocity via high voltage applied between the electrodes (25, 26). A patent on this idea by W.D. Coolidge at GE was filed earlier, known to Langmuir and granted 16 May 1939. The visible X-ray image can be recorded from the output screen (20) with a camera (30).

images in rapid succession because there was no longer a change of cassettes. As early as 1937, Janker used a grid-controlled PANTIX tube to produce the first high-frequency cine film. This radiographic technique remained in use into the 1960s. For example there is the familiar CINELIX 12.5-inch image intensifier with 35-mm cine radiography at 50 frames per second (Fig. V, 165). Using a light distributor, a television camera could be connected. The ODELKA was employed primarily for mass fluorography of the lungs and heart (s. Figs. V, 113, V, 114, V, 141 and V, 149).

From as long ago as 1937 there existed a patent [P4] from I. Langmuir for the electron-optical intensification of a fluoroscopy image (Fig. V, 166).

But it was only in 1948 that J.W. Coltman (Fig. V, 167), an engineer at Westinghouse, was able to introduce the first X-ray image intensifier in electron-optical design (Coltman, 1948) [10]. Finally in 1953 this new image intensifier was ready for use in a clinical environment. This was the Westinghouse FLUOREX unit, the first tilting table equipped with an image intensifier on the market. The 5-inch FLUOREX image intensifier had a gain of 1:200 and a field size reduction of 5:1. With both eyes the operator could view the output screen using a mirror or an optical system (s. Figs. V, 104, V, 137 and V, 169 to V, 171). The resolving power was 50 copper wires per inch, that is, about two wires per millimeter. The accelerating voltage was

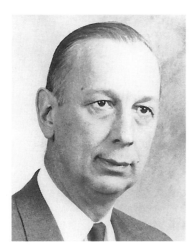

Fig. V, 167. John W. Coltman, PhD (born 1919), who worked for Westinghouse in Pittsburgh, designed the first X-ray image intensifier in 1948. First clinical trials were done at the Johns Hopkins Hospital in Baltimore and the Temple University in Philadelphia in 1950. About 250 Westinghouse FLUOREX systems were installed between 1953 and 1958 [12].

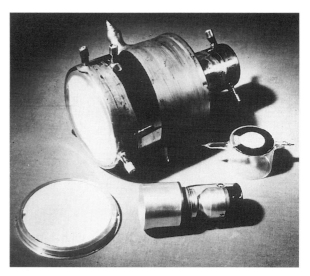

Fig. V, 168. 1952: Image intensifier tube with 90 mm diameter input screen (manufactured by Siemens).

25 kV, the viewing screen had a diameter of 1 inch, and its weight was 40 pounds. At that time only one of every two image intensifiers produced could be used. This is an indication of the enormous difficulties in the manufacturing process of image intensifiers, which even now is a formidable challenge.

Research in the area of image intensifiers played an important role in Europe during the post-war years. This is seen in the work of Philips and Siemens which began experiments with electron-optical image intensifiers at almost the same time. By 1950, Philips was able to produce an image intensifier with a field diameter of 13 cm which was available in serial production by 1952. Siemens began with its first laboratory experiments in 1947 and, by 1950, offered a 9-cm image intensifier (Fenner *et al*, 1952; Teves *et al*, 1952) [15, 78] (Fig. V, 168) with which R. Janker performed cine radiography. At the 1952 Roentgen congresses in Wiesbaden (Germany) and Utrecht (Netherland) Janker demonstrated the first German cine film, showing the peristalsis and pyloric function of the stomach. E. Fenner and O. Schott (Fenner and Schott, 1954) [17] reported on the possibilities and limits of image intensification in 1954.

The second half of the 1950s witnessed the extended use of the X-ray image intensifier. However, the spot-film device with fluorescent screen was still state-of-the-art, as can be seen in Fig. V, 169 from the year 1956. The image intensifier with its viewing system was mounted on an adapter plate. This arrangement permitted the possibility of use with the fluorescent screen on the SIRESKOP spot-film device. In the meantime, im-

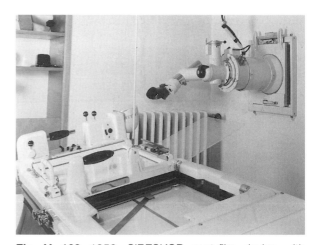

Fig. V, 169. 1956: SIRESKOP spot-film device with adapter plate to exchange the fluorescent screen with an image intensifier and optical viewing device.

age intensifiers with larger diameters and light distributors (Fig. V, 170) were now on the market. The light distributor comprised a mirror system which distributed the image from the output screen of the image intensifier in two or even three directions. One could view the fluoroscopic image without having to remove the camera. Figure V, 171 from 1961 gives an impression of how important the television camera was to be on the image intensifier. Although viewing the fluoroscopy image no longer demanded a fully darkened room, the physician still had to adapt to the thoroughly uncomfortable spot-film position required by the examination technique employed.

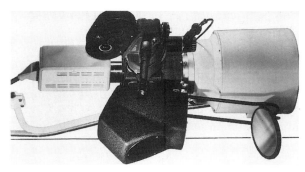

Fig. V, 170. 1959: Westinghouse image intensifier with mirror optics.

The image intensifier in the 1960s and 1970s

The X-ray image intensifier underwent further development and became an independent image receptor system. The year 1964 saw the introduction of the so-called SIRECON Duplex, with two input field sizes containing a zoom switch-over between 25-cm and 15-cm field diameters. The resolution capability rapidly improved. Thus, the 25-cm input screen had a resolution of 1.6 line pairs per millimeter and the 15-cm input screen of 2 line pairs per millimeter. In 1967 Fenner [18] reported on the characteristic values of image intensifiers. Comparisons in fluoroscopic and radiographic mode between the SIRECON Duplex and the CINELIX showed that electron-optical image intensifiers were not always superior to the optical CINELIX design. In fact its contrast was actually better, but for the same optical film density its dose require-

ment was a factor of 2.5 higher (Denecke and Fenner, 1965) [11].

M. Pfeiler (Pfeiler et al, 1966) [59] made use of the modulation transfer function (MTF) for the evaluation of the X-ray–television system. He pointed out that both the spatial frequency and the temporal frequency are of interest here.

'The image at the output of the television system should represent an equivalent copy of the intensity distribution of the radiation relief. This means that the spatial MTF must be determined by the highest spatial frequency and the temporal MTF by the highest temporal frequency. The study presented here is limited to the determination of spectral components as a function of spatial frequency. . . . The spectra determined give an overview, comparing the spatial MTF of X-ray–television systems, of the suitability of these systems with regard to diagnostic indication and furnish useful information for matching the transfer system to the radiation relief.'

On the same subject it is worth mentioning publications of K. Rossmann (Rossmann 1968; Rossmann and Moseley, 1969) [64, 65] and M.C. Ziskin (Ziskin and Revesz, 1969, 1970; Ziskin et al, 1971) [83, 84]. Pfeiler (1969) [61] demonstrated that system-theory applies to transmission systems for X-ray images. On the basis of an X-ray image example, he could illustrate how procedures originating in the system theory of electrical transmission technology and general terms can also be applied for the transmission of images. Fenner (1967) [19] summarized the characteristic values and the use of electron-optical image intensifiers in roentgen diagnostics.

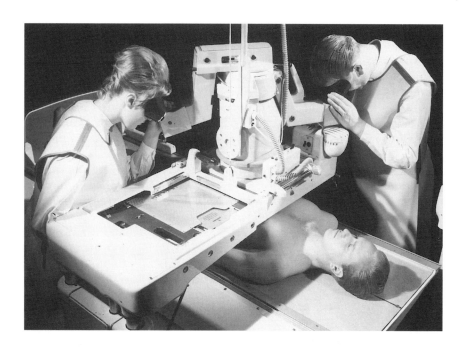

Fig. V, 171. 1961: Clinical operation of an image intensifier, with optics for two people, on a SIRESKOP spot-film device.

The effect of focal spot size was studied in detail with regard to its meaning for the fluoroscopy image and also for image intensifier radiography (Meiler, 1968) [51]. It was found that the unit geometry and the use of image magnification greatly influenced detail recognition. Comparing the 2.0 focus with the 0.3 focus at normal distances had no significant effect on image quality.

At the ICR in Tokyo in 1969, Philips exhibited a prototype version of a 5-inch image intensifier tube with a caesium iodide input screen instead of the usual zinc–cadmium sulphide. This CsI coating produced a brighter, better defined, and higher-contrast image. Physicians had to wait nearly another 2 years, however, before the first commercially produced 25-cm image intensifier tube with CsI coating was delivered by Siemens. This input screen had 2.5 times higher quantum absorption at 34 keV, compared with the earlier zinc–cadmium sulphide screen. Its resolving power was 3.6 line pairs per millimeter at 17-cm zoom and 2.4 at the 25-cm field.

G. Schwierz (Schwierz, 1972) [68] was awarded his doctorate in 1972 for the calculation of the electron-optical characteristics of image intensifiers. This represented a very important contribution to their design. F.W. Hofmann (1972) [33] wrote:

'The imaging quality of image intensifiers has been enormously improved by the introduction of cesium iodide screens and by new electron optics calculations. The resolution limit, which, by experience, corresponds to the spatial frequency at a modulation transfer function of 0.04, is 4.4 periods per millimeter for the 17 H image intensifier. For the 25/15 H image intensifier, it is 2.5 periods per millimeter for the 25 cm and 3.6 periods per millimeter for the 15 cm field diameter. Moreover, the effective absorption of the X-ray quanta is at least twice as high as with image intensifiers of previous designs. The image quality of a photograph from the image intensifier output screen is now comparable with that of a direct radiograph with a film screen combination, even though the required dose is lower by a factor of 5–10. This clearly points the way to the increased use of indirect radiography.'

With the so-called metal window tube, first manufactured in 1974, which had a thin 0.8 mm aluminium input window instead of glass, a resolving power of 5 line pairs per millimeter was achieved. W. Kuehl and H.J. Schrijvers (Kuehl and Schrijvers, 1977) [47] reported in 1977 on the titanium input screen and a fibre-optical output screen. They called attention to problems with the electron optics and with the size and design of the 14-inch image intensifier tube.

The image intensifier in the 1980s and 1990s

At the ICR in Brussels in 1981, Siemens exhibited an image intensifier of 57-cm diameter, which reduced the dose level for chest radiographs (s. Fig. V, 112). From the middle of the 1980s, 40-cm image intensifier tubes were used not only in gastro-intestinal examinations, but also gained favour in angiography of the thoracic, abdominal, and peripheral vascular systems. Thomson developed a new input screen coating with 170 mg caesium iodide per cm^2, which improved quantum absorption. Siemens then introduced the metal-ceramic design at the beginning of the 1990s which greatly improved rotational accuracy.

Television in medical roentgen diagnostics

The years 1915–1958

Already in 1915 Dauvillier was concerned with the problem of how to utilize the principle of television in radiographic diagnoses [P 1]. Using a Nipkow disk he fluoroscoped the object line-by-line with a narrow beam collimation. By 1929 he had obtained an image of 100 elements, and reported as follows:

'The fluoroscopy image can be displayed with any desired brightness (complete visibility of all details). It can be displayed in all desired sizes, in positive and in negative, and it can be projected. The image is free of any fogging, such as scattered radiation produces. The radiation exposure to the examiner and the patient is one ten-thousandth of the primary intensity, solving the problem of protective measures entirely.'

In spite of this optimistic account, practical application was clearly far less satisfactory. R. Janker and E. Kaeser [P 2] tried to apply a new ionization chamber for television recording of fluoroscopic images in 1932. H. Lorenz (1940) [50] concluded as late as 1940 that *'...neither the energy nor the gain of the television chain are adequate to produce a roentgen TV image which is equivalent to a fluoroscopic image. The roentgen TV image may be brighter than the fluoroscopic image but spatial resolution is far inferior.'*

Many experiments (Moon, 1948, 1950; Rose, 1948; Sturm and Morgan, 1949; Nell and Heller, 1951; Keller and Ploke, 1955; Janker, 1956; Morgan and Sturm, 1961) [53, 54, 63, 77, 38, 56, 55, 42] did not bring the expected success in the 15 years to come.

Janker (1967) [39] coupled the image intensifier with the SUPERORTHICON in 1955, H. Stauffer and co-workers (Stauffer *et al*, 1955)

[72] and M. Noix (1962) [57] did the same with the VIDICON. Thereafter, the VIDICON gained steadily in favour, at first with fluoroscopy in surgery (Wallmann and Wickbom, 1959) [79] and then in internal medicine (Stevenson, 1961) [75]. L. Heijne (1967) [30] had reported on the LEAD OXIDE VIDICON in 1956. This in turn led to the PLUMBICON television pickup tube. Electronic control systems followed the introduction of television technology in radiology. In 1957, K. Bischoff and O. Schott (1957) [3] described a system for the contrast enhancement of fine details. In 1958, H. Wallmann and I. Wickbom (Wallmann and Wickbom, 1959) [79] introduced electronic image storage with the TONO-TRON. In the same year T. Schut and W. Oosterkamp (1959) [67] demonstrated the possibility of magnetically storing single-frame images. Following on the heels of this, still in the same year, A. Jutras (1964) [41] was able to store fluoroscopic scenes on magnetic tape. A. Gebauer, J. Lissner and O. Schott gave a detailed account of the historic evolution in their book 'Das Roentgenfernsehen' (X-ray television) (Gebauer et al, 1974) [24]. In the preface to the first edition of 1965, they wrote:

'Within a very short time, X-ray television has become a widely discussed topic. It is not only a question of new apparatus and technology, but also of the changes which these prompt in methods of roentgen diagnostics. Moreover, these discussions point the way to the decisive question of the clinical-radiological value which can be assigned to X-ray television. . . . This book has appeared at the present time, because X-ray television has now reached a stage beyond the 'growing pains'. Working with the method under actual conditions of practice can now begin on a broad basis.'

The book (Gebauer et al, 1974) [24] contains a technical section with an excellent account of the fundamentals, and a detailed clinical section with a comprehensive source of literature; the second edition includes 580 references.

Visual characteristics and brightness

Spatial resolution in fluoroscopy (Fig. V, 172) is limited by the television system although it is still better than that of a fluorescent screen, as Fig. V, 172 demonstrates. However, television was able substantially to increase the screen brightness, above all in relation to the dose rate applied for the various fluoroscopic and radiographic examination techniques. Comparing the average luminance between the fluorescent screen and

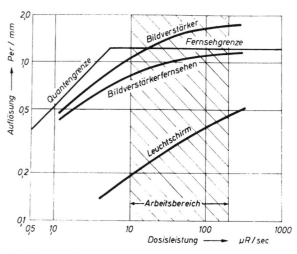

Fig. V, 172. Spatial resolution in periods/mm as a function of dose rate in R/s. Indicated is the working range (A), the fluorescent screen (L) and the image intensifier and TV system (B). The boundaries Q and F are shown for the quanta and the TV system at the time [24].

television, the luminance which the radiologist sees on the fluorescent screen corresponds roughly to that of an illuminated moon landscape (Frik, 1959) [20]. At such a low brightness level, visual perception depends on the rods of the eye and is therefore at a great disadvantage in comparison with viewing by daylight with the cones of the eye (Schober, 1964) [66]. Viewing with the rods of the eye requires a long period of visual adaptation. Especially during the first 20 min, the sensitivity of the eye increases by a factor of 100. In spite of this, sharpness (Siedentopf et al, 1941) [71] and speed (Zimmermann, 1936) [82] of visual perception remain very reduced.

Television from the 1960s to the present

K. Bischoff [4] wrote in 1961 on the meaning of television for broadening the use of fluoroscopy in medical diagnostics. In 1964, he posed the question of whether a significant increase of reliability of the diagnosis could be expected using fluoroscopy as a result of further developments in the television system (Bischoff, 1964) [5]:

'Even if there are only limited possibilities with television to improve system resolution beyond 1 period per millimeter, there is much to be gained. Zooming and reduced frame rate can still contribute to considerable improvements in object resolution. This is especially true for those image regions with low input dose and contrast levels. . . . Television satisfies all the con-

ditions for fluoroscopy of motion and promises especially high diagnostic reliability, even in the thorax.'

The use of television technology with spot-film devices (Fig. V, 173) had become routine in internal medicine by 1962. This had a dramatic effect on the design of tables and stands and the working procedure of the medical team. A 70-mm camera was connected to the light distributor in 1963, permitting the documentation of images from the image intensifier as well. In the same year it became possible to record onto magnetic tape.

From the field of photography the technique of fine contrast enhancement is familiar. K. Bischoff [P 5] carried this idea over to fluoroscopy in his patent of 1960. He proposed using two television cameras, one focused and one defocused. With this arrangement a mixed signal was generated, the difference signal which then displayed the details not seen with the defocused camera. However, it could not be incorporated into an X-ray system. Consequently, J. Haendle [P 6] patented a design based on television technology in 1963. The TRANSICON used this idea and selectable edge enhancement for fluoroscopy was available from 1968.

J. Haendle and H. Horbaschek [28] reported in 1976 on the initial results of using a high-resolution television system in a laboratory version. This permitted an increase in the number of lines at 50 Hz from 625 to 1249. The improvement in quality of the fluoroscopic image was comparable with that seen in image intensifier radiography with the introduction of the high-resolution image intensifier. This television system came to be regarded as the standard of quality.

Experiments began in the 1970s with optical sensors in semiconductor technology, producing a digital output signal, as a replacement for the television camera. These were given the name 'charge-coupled devices' or CCD cameras. In spite of their promise it took many years until they were able to satisfy the demands of image quality for medical purposes. Finally in 1991, the first CCD camera replaced conventional television, e.g. on the mobile SIREMOBIL 2000 C-arm system.

Digital technology in medical roentgen diagnostics, especially in interventional angiography, led in turn to fully new black-and-white monitors. The brightness level increased at high contrast to more than three times the level of earlier monitors and cathodes of longer lifespan were introduced. The SIMOMED monitor of 1992 achieved a luminance of 500 cd/m², corresponding to 170 foot lamberts. Furthermore the image was now flicker-free, greatly reducing optical fatigue for the physician. The image quality of classical chest and bone examinations is good enough to diagnose lesions.

X-ray image intensifiers in surgery

The combination of surgery and radiology was in great demand in the operating theatre. Initially, however, it was not possible because of the light levels. The KRYPTOSKOP (Fig. V, 174) was one – however inconvenient – solution for the physician. In 1956, Philips went a completely new way with its BV 20 (Fig. V, 175). X-ray tube and image intensifier were mounted on a C-arm. This design permitted fluoroscopy and radiography in all projections, e.g. of a broken bone, on a patient at rest in the operating room. Especially in orthopaedic surgery, physicians were now grateful to be able to view fluoroscopic images in an illuminated environment. These C-arm stands, both as mobile units and as ceiling-mounted versions (s. Fig. V, 105) installed in the operating room, proved to be of great value. By the end of the 1950s, 14-cm image intensifiers with a resolution of 2 line pairs per millimeter were available. L. Koslowski [44] reported in 1960 on his experience with new image intensifiers, with emphasis on the surgical environment. He wrote:

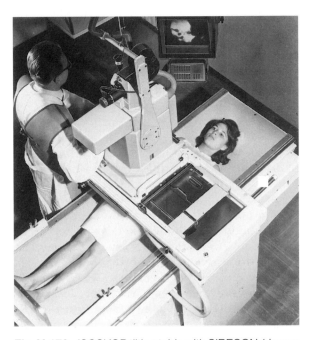

Fig. V, 173. ISOSKOP tilting table with SIRECON 1 image intensifier system with cine camera and TV monitor in 1993 (manufactured from 1962 to 1966 by Siemens).

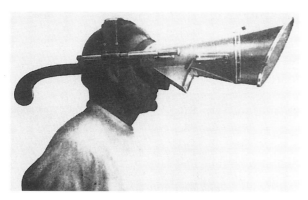

Fig. V, 174. Fluoroscopy during surgery was done with a KRYPTOSKOP manufactured by Patzer in Hermsdorf, Thuringia. The surgeon saw the roentgen image on a fluorescent screen in the horizontal direction and, looking down, he or she could see the surgical field.

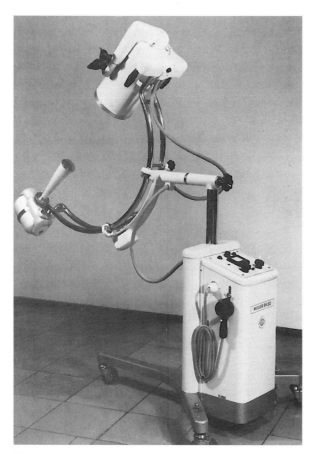

Fig. V, 175. The first image intensifier unit BV 20 for surgical fluoroscopy designed by CHF Mueller in 1956 (see reference in section tables [5]).

'The use of image intensifiers makes a number of surgical procedures possible. Especially with fractures and not the least with their bloodless repositioning, the procedure is now simpler. Savings in radiation dose, time, and number of radiographs are enormous. Operating the image intensifier requires practice and experience, especially concerning its use in the operating room. For this reason both physicians and assisting personnel must be familiar with positioning the unit for typical procedures and with operation of the equipment. In searching for foreign bodies, image intensifiers are superior to earlier acoustic locating devices. The respect of surgeons for the danger of radiation-induced effects in the operating and plaster room has declined further since the introduction of image intensifiers. Nevertheless, it is still essential that fluoroscopy be restricted to the minimum necessary time and radiation dose. The application of image intensifiers during surgery presents a problem in ensuring asepsis and requires careful observation. In order to realize fully the advantages of this new technique, it is necessary to plan carefully the application of image intensifier fluoroscopy in advance and consider surgical measures. This includes partial adaptation, optimal positioning of the stand, setting of technique factors, and efficient task distribution among the surgical team.'

It was only with the introduction of television to Philips' BV 20 in 1962 that increased utilization of fluoroscopy in the operating room significantly. A ceiling-mounted system (s. Fig. V, 105) permitted movement to any desired position in the operating room, which represented a gain in freedom of movement about the floor and thus an advantage for the medical team. The years following saw the introduction of image data storage, electronically controlled exposure techniques, and subtraction of images, including roadmapping (s. Fig. V, 181).

Storage technology and spot-filming with the image intensifier

After T. Schut and W. Oosterkamp (1959) [67] had reported on the magnetic storage of single-frame images in 1958 and A. Jutras (1964) [41] on fluoroscopic scenes onto magnetic tape, storage onto magnetic tape became a reality in the early 1960s (Figs. V, 176 and V, 177). H. Haslauer and K. Steiner (1964) [29] reported on the application of tape recording to fluoroscopy examinations, emphasizing functional studies. Important phases of functions could now be reviewed and studied repeatedly without radiation (Herrschaft, 1972) [31]. In order to render

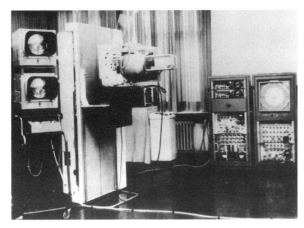

Fig. V, 176. 1961: Electronic roentgen image storage system built by SRW.

image details more visible, F. Groh (1967) [25] built a subtraction unit in 1965. A review article on the status of television single-frame image storage in internal and angiographic roentgen diagnostics appeared in 1974 (Haendle *et al*, 1974) [27].

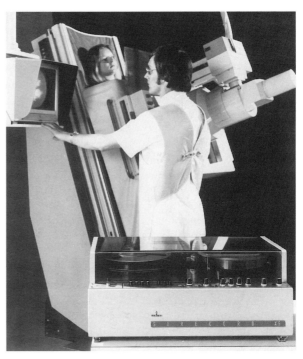

Fig. V, 177. 1973: Electronic storage of fluoroscopy scenes and spot-film exposures with the MEMOSKOP and SIRECORD XS tape recorder.

Cine radiography with the image intensifier

As mentioned above, Janker began with cine radiography in 1937. In 1949, he used the SUPERIONOSCOP and the first 9-cm image intensifier in 1950. By 1955 his equipment also included a 16-mm ARRIFLEX cine camera; 35-mm cine film became the standard in the 1960s. The components of the SIRECON image intensifier system can be seen in Fig. V, 178. The display of cardiac vessels filled with contrast medium

was, however, not the only information of relevance. Correlation with the ECG also yielded important information. This problem was solved in 1970 when H. Lutz and co-workers developed the CINECHRONOCARD, a time-synchronized marking of ECG and cine film.

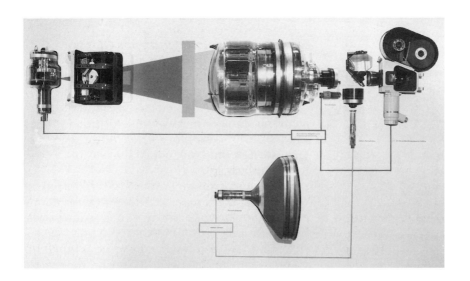

Fig. V, 178. 1966: Components of the SIRECON image intensifier system. These were displayed at the German Roentgen Congress in Berlin, 18–21 May 1966. From left to right: X-ray tube; automatic multileaf collimator system; image intensifier tube with the light distribution system to the photomultiplier for automatic brightness control; TV camera with the monitor and cine camera on the right.

Spot-filming of single-frames from the image intensifier

H.M. Stauffer (Stauffer *et al*, 1955; Stauffer, 1958) [72, 73] reported as early as 1958 on 'spot photofluorography' using the image intensifier and the Polaroid principle. Around 1955 the cost effectiveness of photofluorography was a topic of interest (Feindt, 1955) [14]. Janker [37] reported in 1956 on his experience with the Philips 5-inch image intensifier. F.E. Stieve [76] summarized the clinical requirements based on 10 years of experience with the image intensifier system in 1972. This publication represents a gold-mine for references to this issue. In time, other publications continued in the spirit of this article. H. Woeke (1972) [81] reported on the technical possibilities of the image intensifier spot-filming system. R. Balfanz (1972) [1] dealt with cameras for spot-filming and serialography. J. Becker (1972) [2] discussed matching the camera to the image intensifier. Finally L. Widenmann (1972) [80] contributed an account of image intensifer spot filming techniques, in which she also discussed factors influencing image quality such as tube voltage, narrow collimation of the radiation field, preventing direct primary radiation on the image intensifier, and setting correct dose values.

J. Feddema [13] reported in 1962 on 70-mm roll-film radiography using a 9-inch image intensifier with a remote-controlled ring stand. H. Gajewski and W. Schuster (1968) [22] emphasized especially dose reduction for examinations in paediatric radiology made possible by the image intensifier–television system together with a 70-mm camera. With the MEMOSPOT, fluoroscopic images could be stored and displayed on the monitor immediately after exposure. The year 1970 witnessed contributions to image quality (Feleus and Vijverberg, 1970) [15] and the optimization of exposure conditions (Gajewski and Kuhn, 1970) [23]. M. Pfeiler and G. Linke [60] reported again in 1972 on the applications of 70-mm technique, now requiring only 100 microroentgens per image. Shortened exposure time and matched tube voltage even improved image quality. In paediatrics, only 50 microroentgens per image were needed. The effect of the caesium iodide image intensifier on image quality (Fuchs and Hofmann, 1971; Gudden *et al*, 1972) [21, 26] represented yet another step toward the acceptance of television fluoroscopy and indirect radiography.

E. Chérigié [8] posed the question in 1972 of what the future held for the 70-mm technique. With systems of good quality – including the image intensifier, automatic exposure control, film, and film processing – the many advantages weighed in favour of such a system by comparison with cassette radiography. In addition to a reduction in the radiation level, motion blurring in the image was less pronounced. Moreover the sheer weight of the documented patient history, and along with it the archiving volume, was much less. Chérigié offered the opinion that in the future image intensifier spot-filming would replace 40-50% of conventional radiographs. Today, in retrospect, we know that clinical acceptance of this film had been very slow and that physicians did not make full use of the – rightly – cited advantages. Nevertheless, this technique found its way partly into angiography (Hom and Kaude, 1972) [34]. A number of companies produced 70-mm (Bouglé and Lohmann, 1972) [6] and 105-mm roll-film cameras as well as 100-mm cut-film cameras on the strength of Chérigié's optimism.

100-mm cut-film

The 100-mm cut-film camera offered two advantages: The format with clinical image information became larger, and the film was not rolled. The frame rate was initially limited to 2 frames per second, but this was later increased to 6 frames per second. This was sufficient for most examinations in internal medicine and angiography. Higher frame rates, when required, could be obtained by connecting a cine camera to the light distributor in place of the cut-film camera. Furthermore the operation became so simple that only a single function key was required to select technique factors and camera parameters. With regard to 100-mm technique with a 30-cm large-format image intensifier (Lissner et al, 1976) [49], it is well worth again emphasizing the dose reduction: Radiographs made with it reduced radiation exposure by a factor of two compared with special screens and by a factor of four compared with universal screens. Today the quality of 100-mm radiographic images is as good as that obtained with direct radiography. Even the evaluation of these 100-mm images does not necessarily require a magnifying glass. On the other hand, there had been reports of difficulties in adapting to this format, especially from hospitals, due to the unusual format size. Savings in terms of film costs are substantial. But savings in terms of archiving space and archiving methods can be realized only through full commitment to this format. By 1976 a further decrease in dose (Hofmann, 1976) [32] to 75 microroentgens per image was recommended. This represented a substantial difference, compared with the 100 to 200 microroentgens per image with rare-earth screens. This again, meant shorter exposure times and reduced motion blurring. Image series with up to 6 frames per second also permitted the documentation of dynamic studies, with the exception of the heart.

Digital radiography with the X-ray image intensifier

Digital subtraction angiography (DSA)

In 1980 Philips introduced the first digital subtraction angiography system, the DVI (Digital Vascular Imaging) to the market (Kruger et al, 1979) [46]. This system ushered in the digital age of conventional radiology. It made use of image intensifier and television technology and converted its analogue signal to digital format. In this way the image information could be further processed digitally. The result was then displayed in analogue form on the monitor screen. The technique of hybrid subtraction (Brody, 1981; Lehmann et al, 1981; Keyes et al, 1982) [48, 7, 43] is a subtraction of two radiographic images each taken with a different tube voltage. It was first reported in 1981. But the method did not establish itself in routine examinations. A number of DSA systems (Seyferth et al, 1982) [69] appeared in 1982 (Fig. V, 179). Around the middle of the 1980s the Roadmap technique (Seyferth and Polster, 1985) [70] – a form of DSA application in fluoroscopy mode – began to take hold. In 1986 Siemens improved the image matrix standard (Rath, 1984) [62] from 512×512 to 1024×1024. For years, the POLYTRON (Fig. V, 180) remained the only production system on the market with a true 1024×1024 image matrix. The image quality was now almost equal to that of film changers for therapeutically relevant vessels.

The DSA technique was also applied in the operating room (Fig. V, 181).

Digital cine radiography

Angiocardiography requires frame rates of at least 30 frames per second and demands good

Fig. V, 179a, b. Digital subtraction angiography (DSA) with the ANGIOTRON. It was the first system to use an organ-programmed technique and the automatic exposure control system IONTOMAT.

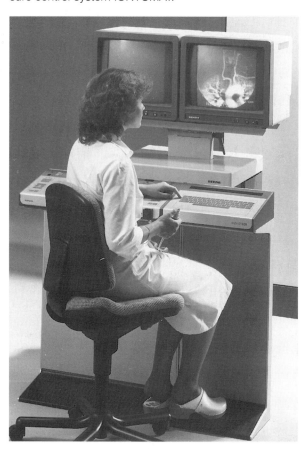

Fig. V, 179a. Alphanumeric input for information to be shown on each image in 1982.

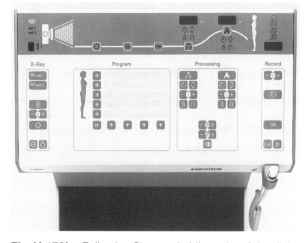

Fig. V, 179b. Following Siemens' philosophy of simplicity in operating control functions: automatic DSA control with the DIGIMATIC in 1981.

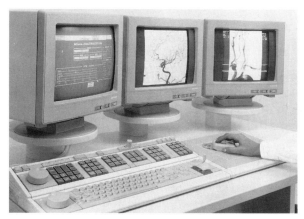

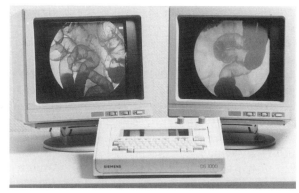

Fig. V, 182. Digital radiography system DS 1000 of 1988 (Siemens).

Fig. V, 180. The first DSA system with a real 1024 matrix in acquisition, processing, and display: the POLYTRON in 1987.

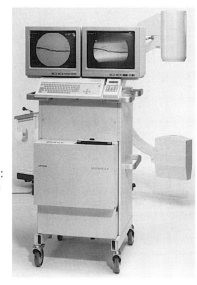

Fig. V, 181. 1990: The mobile C-arm unit with digital imaging SIRE-MOBIL 4, with subtraction capability on the MEMOSKOP Sub 100.

spatial resolution for coronary arteries. The Philips DCI and Siemens DIGITRON offered the earliest digital cine radiography systems for routine applications which, however, still required 35-mm cine film for documentation. First results obtained with the HICOR in 1990 (O'Neil, 1992; Meinertz, 1993) [58, 52] showed that for the first time digital angiocardiography now offered serious competition for cine film. Application software and expert systems will be on hand for the support of the physician.

Digital radiography

Some DSA systems were capable of generating unsubtracted single-frame images but the system was too expensive because subsystems for subtraction were not used, which led to the appearance of digital systems designed specifically for spot-film radiography replacing 70-mm and 100/105-mm cameras. INFICON, DS 1000 (Fig. V, 182), DSI, and FLUOROSPOT H are a few examples of such product names. Digital radiograms proved of great advantage when acquired, diagnosed, and distributed within a digitally networked hospital (Hruby et al, 1992, 1993; Krampla et al, 1993) [36, 35, 45] (see also section tables: 'The digital radiology department').

For digital cassette radiography, the film-screen system was replaced by a storage phosphor system. This permitted the continued use of all existing cassette trays while still obtaining a digital radiogram using digital luminescence radiography. Fuji introduced this method as a product and most companies were compelled to obtain their key components and licensing rights. The superiority of this technique with regard to radiation hygiene is demonstrated by figure V, 100. The technique gained enormous popularity in intensive care units and in wards. Moreover the diagnosis of the radiologist is available to the attending physicians and surgeons much faster in a digitally networked hospital (Hruby et al, 1992, 1993; Krampla et al, 1993) [36, 35, 45].

Automation in fluoroscopy

Attempts to automatically control the tube voltage (kV) and tube current (mA) go back as far as the 1960s. The so-called anti-isowatt circuit introduced by SRW meant that the physician only had to turn on radiation in order to obtain an immediate, high-contrast, low-dose image on the television monitor screen. In the 1970s with the VIDOMATIC it became possible to refer to information from fluoroscopy and automatically set the tube voltage for 70-mm or 100-mm indirect radiography (SIRCAMATIC). Spot-filming was then controlled by the automatic exposure control system and provided reproducibly high image quality (Joetten, 1972; Steiner et al, 1973) [40, 74]. For cine radiography, the CINEMATIC, which grouped numerous setting parameters together into organ programmes, greatly simplified operation and eliminated faulty settings.

Since 1982 in digital subtraction angiography all radiographic parameters and also the iris diaphragm of the television camera can be set automatically in accordance with the frame rate, focal spot, and dose per image. The VIDOMATIC made this possible by acquiring all necessary information during fluoroscopy of the patient and transmitting this information to the DIGIMATIC. Recording the DSA series could, therefore, start immediately after positioning with fluoroscopy.

In 1986 the POLYMATIC controlled all parameters automatically for any examination mode using fluoroscopy before recording an image or a series of images.

To further reduce the level of radiation exposure during fluoroscopy, an idea going back more than 10 years, that of pulsed fluoroscopy, was revived in 1987. Frame rates of 25 frames per second or less are perceived as flickering, which is highly disturbing. But a continuously moving fluoroscopic image requires more than 25 frames per second. Digital memory technology, however, permitted the storing of individual fluoroscopy images and the repeated replaying of them on the television monitor screen, without radiation ('gap filling'). Flickering was no longer perceived. In angiocardiography this led to even better defined fluoroscopic images, with less radiation exposure to the patient and the medical team. This was a matter of great importance in connection with the marked increase in the number of interventional procedures now performed.

SUPERVISION (s. Fig. V, 144) has been applied for interventions in the cerebral region since 1992, reducing radiation exposure certainly by a factor of two using TV techniques. Making use of all available technical means and innovations in the interest of minimizing dose, physicians and patients should accept such solutions. Experience indicates that simplification of controls and reducing radiation exposure in fact usually lead to improved image quality.

Diagnosis

Figure V, 183 makes clear that the information content of a radiogram must be compressed for the clinician or surgeon (Gebauer et al, 1974) [24]. A reporting system (Fig. V, 184) was developed in the middle of the 1970s to support the radiologist in formulating the diagnosis and generating the report. However, this was not really a success because of inconvenient system operation, even though translated into several languages. Soft copy reporting (Hruby et al, 1992, 1993; Krampla et al, 1993) [36, 35, 45]

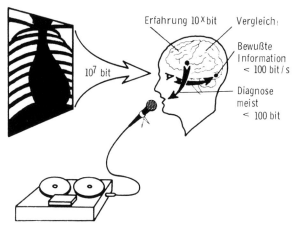

Fig. V, 183. Reducing information during the process of diagnosis: an X-ray image contains about 10^7 bit of information. With experience, the physician can select and combine the information down to a density of about some 100 bits, this being the only diagnostic information with therapeutic relevance [24].

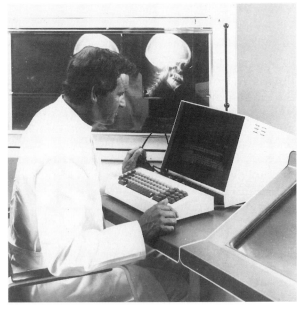

Fig. V, 184. 1975: The reporting workstation SIREP.

(s. Fig. V, 160) was introduced to daily routine in 1992.

Digital memories have successfully replaced the magnetic tape of the Dictaphone, permitting rapid access for the clinician to the diagnosis. High expectations of the early 1980s for speech recognition have so far not been fulfilled – but it is coming, as we have seen successful results in clinical routine in 1993.

Patents

P 1   FP 521 746 vom 12. Aug. 1915, A. Dauvillier: Röntgenfernsehen.

P 2   J 45552 IX 57a von 1932, R. Janker und E. Kaeser: Ionisationskammer, geeignet für Verwendung des Fernsehproblems zur Röntgenkinematographie oder Fernröntgenuntersuchung.

P 3   USP 1 936 342 vom 22. Juni 1932, H. F. Waite, USA: Daylight Fluoroscope.

P 4   USP 2 198 479 vom 3. Nov. 1937 (filed), Irving Langmuir (GE): Image Reproduction (Röntgenbildverstärker).

P 5   DP 1 123 410 vom 19. Aug. 1960, Dipl.-Ing. Kurt Bischoff, SRW Erlangen: Vorrichtung zur Verstärkung der Feinkontraste von Röntgendurchleuchtungsbildern.

P 6   DP 1 224 352 vom 17. Dez. 1963, Dipl.-Ing. Jörg Haendle, SRW Erlangen: Röntgenfernseheinrichtung mit einer Vorrichtung zur Verstärkung der Feinkontraste von Röntgendurchleuchtungsbildern mit fernsehtechnischen Mitteln.

References

1. Balfanz, R.: Kameras für Einzel- und Serienaufnahmen vom Röntgenbildverstärker. Röntgen-Bl. 7 (1972) 304–310
2. Becker, J.: Optische Anpassung der Kameras an den Bildverstärker. Röntgen-Bl. 7 (1972) 311–314
3. Bischoff, K., O, Schott: Eine neue Kontrastverstärkungseinrichtung für Röntgenaufnahmen. Fortschr. Röntgenstr. 87 (1957) 239–248
4. Bischoff, K.: Die Bedeutung des Röntgenfernsehens für eine Erweiterung des Durchleuchtungseinsatzes in der medizinischen Diagnostik. Fortschr. Röntgenstr. 95 (1961) 104–123
5. Bischoff, K.: Ist noch eine wesentliche Steigerung der diagnostischen Befundsicherheit bei der Durchleuchtung durch eine Weiterentwicklung der Fernsehverfahren zu erwarten? Radiologe 4 (1964) 136–141
6. Bouglé, J., Th. Lohmann: Eine neue 70-mm-Fotokamera für Bildverstärkeraufnahmen. Röntgen-Bl. 12 (1972) 575–577
7. Brody, W. R.: Hybrid substraction for improved arteriography. Radiology 141 (1981) 828–831
8. Chérigié, E.: Die 70-mm-Aufnahme vom Bildverstärker und ihre Zukunftsaussichten. Röntgen-Bl. 6 (1972) 275–291
9. Clapesattle, H.: The Doctors Mayo. The University of Minnesota Press, Minneapolis 1941
10. Coltman, J. W.: Fluoroscopy image brightening by electronic means. Radiology 51 (1948) 359–367
11. Denecke, R., E. Fenner: Die Röntgen-Bildverstärker-Röhre SIRECON duplex 25/15. Röntgen-Bl. 2 (1965) 85–89
12. Donner, M.: John W. Coltman, PhD. Röntgen-Bl. 10 (1970) 445–446
13. Feddema, J.: 70 mm fluorography with a 9„ image intensifier mounted on a remotely controlled Ring Stand. Medica Mundi 8, 1 (1962) 7–13
14. Feindt, H.-R.: Wirtschaftlichkeit des Schirmbildverfahrens in der röntgendiagnostischen Routinearbeit. Das Krankenhaus, Wien, 2, 1955
15. Feleus, R., G. Vijverberg: Bildqualität bei 70-mm-Bildverstärkeraufnahmen. Röntgen-Bl. 3 (1970) 125–129
16. Fenner, E., K. Gabbert, Th. Zimmer: Die Lichtverstärkung von Leuchtschirmbildern in der medizinischen Diagnostik. Fortschr. Röntgenstr. 77 (1952) 459–468
17. Fenner, E., O. Schott: Möglichkeiten und Grenzen der Bildverstärkung. Zeitschr. für angew. Physik 6. Band z.H. (1954) 88–95
18. Fenner, E.: Elektronenoptischer Röntgenbildverstärker – Kennwerte und Einsatz in der Röntgendiagnostik. Siemens-Zeitschrift 41 (1967) 749–755
19. Fenner, E.: Elektronenoptischer Röntgenbildverstärker – Kennwerte und Einsatz in der Röntgendiagnostik. Siemens-Zeitschrift 41 (1967) 749–755
20. Frik, W.: Detailerkennbarkeit und Dosis bei der Röntgendurchleuchtung. Hüthig, Heidelberg 1959
21. Fuchs, H., F. W. Hofmann: Ein Röntgenbildverstärker mit verbesserter Bildqualität – Ergebnisse der praktischen Erprobung mit der 70 mm Kamera. Electromedica 39 (1971) 94
22. Gajewski, H., W. Schuster: Bildverstärkerphotographie mit 70-mm- Kameras in der pädiatrischen Röntgendiagnostik. Dtsch. med. Wschr. 46 (1968) 2201–2203
23. Gajewski, H., H. Kuhn: Optimierung der Aufnahmebedingungen an Magen-Untersuchungsgeräten. Röntgen-Bl. 7 (1970) 298–309
24. Gebauer, A., J. Lissner, O. Schott: Das Röntgenfernsehen. Technische Grundlagen und klinisch-röntgenologische Anwendung. 2. neubearb. und erweiterte Auflage, Georg Thieme Verlag, Stuttgart, 1974
25. Groh, F.: Ein elektronisches Subtraktionsgerät. Röntgenpraxis 20 (1967) 43–51
26. Gudden, F., F. W. Hofmann, P. Marhoff: X-ray Image Intensifiers and their Use for TV-Fluoroscopy, Electronic and Photographic Image Recording. Medical Progress through Technology 1 (1972) 3
27. Haendle, H., J. Haendle, J. Lissner, K. J. Pfeifer: Stand der Fernseh-Einzelbildspeicherung in der internen bzw. angiographischen Röntgendiagnostik. Röntgenpraxis 27 (1974) 209
28. Haendle, J., H. Horbaschek: Die hochauflösende Röntgenfernsehkette. Röntgenpraxis 29, 5 (1976) 1–11
29. Haslauer, H., K. Steiner: Der Röntgenbandspeicher in der radiologischen Funktionsdiagnostik. SRW Nachrichten 23 (1964) 11–15

30. Heijne, L.: Das Blei-Oxid-Vidikon. Acta electron. 2 (1967) 124–131

31. Herrschaft, H.: Die kontinuierliche Fernseh-Bandaufzeichnung bei der Gesamtspinalkanal-Myelographie. Röntgen-Bl. 1 (1972) 10–21

32. Hofmann, F. W.: Röntgenbildverstärker mit Caesiumjodid-Eingangsschirm - ihre Bedeutung für das Röntgenfernsehen und für die Indirektaufnahmetechnik. Radiologische Praxis 1, 2 (1976) 60–65

33. Hofmann, F. W.: Röntgenbildverstärker mit verbesserter Bildqualität. Röntgen-Bl. 25, 5 (1972) 198–205

34. Hom, T., J. Kaude: Aufnahmen vom Bildverstärker – Die Angiographie im Rahmen der klinischen Indikation. Röntgen-Bl. 9 (1972) 404–41#

35. Hruby, W., H. Mosser, M. Urban, M. Wassipaul, K. Gindl, E. Kucera, K. Kaissas: Digitale Radiologie – Klinische Realität. Österr. Krankenhaus-Zeitung, Sonderfolge Radiologie (1993), 3

36. Hruby, W. et al.: Datenvernetzung in einem neu errichteten Röntgeninstitut am Beispiel des Donauspitals Wien. Röntgenpraxis 45 (1992) 103–110

37. Janker, R.: Experience with the Philips 5" image intensifier in radiologic practice and scientific work. Medica Mundi 2 (1956) 22

38. Janker, R.: Fernsehen in der Röntgendiagnostik. Röntgen-Bl. 9 (1956) 118-126

39. Janker, R.: Weitere Fortschritte des Röntgen-Fernsehens. Röntgen-Bl. 10 (1967) 174–179

40. Jötten, G.: Zur Belichtungsautomatik beim Bildverstärkeraufnahmeverfahren. Röntgen-Bl. 7 (1972) 315–321

41. Jutras, A.: Teleroentgen diagnosis by means of video tape recording. Am. J. Roentgenol. 82 (1964) 1099–1102

42. Keller, M., M. Ploke: Sichtbarmachung von Röntgenbildern mittels einer auf Röntgenstrahlen ansprechenden Fernsehaufnahmeröhre. Zeitschr. für angew. Physik 7 (1955) 562–571

43. Keyes, G. S., S. J. Riederer, B. F. Belanger, W. R. Brody: Hybrid subtraction in digital fluorography. SPIE 347, Application of optical instrumentation in medicine X (1982) 34–41

44. Koslowski, L.: Erfahrungen mit neuen Röntgen-Bildverstärkern. Der Chirurg 1 (1960) 10–13

45. Krampla, W., G. Oberhauser, H. Mosser, W. Hruby: Klinische Erfahrungen im digitalen Röntgeninstitut. Österr. Krankenhaus-Zeitung, Sonderfolge Radiologie (1993), 28

46. Kruger, R. A., Ch. A. Mistretta, et al.: Computerized fluoroscopy in real time for noninvasive visualization of the cardiovascular system. Diagn. Radiol. 130 (1979) 49–57

47. Kühl, W., J. E. Schrijvers: A new 14 inch X-ray image intensifier tube. Medica Mundi 22 (1977), 9

48. Lehmann, L. A., R. E. Alvarez, A. Macovski, W. Brody: Generalized image combinations in dual kVp digital radiography. Med. Phys. 8 (1981) 659–667

49. Lissner, J., V. Remplick, U. Scherer, O. Kotschak, M. Schätzl: Erfahrung in der klinischen Praxis mit einem 30-cm-Bildverstärker unter besonderer Berücksichtigung der 100 mm Aufnahmetechnik. Fortschr. Röntgenstr. 125, 6 (1976) 551–555

50. Lorenz, H.: Zur Frage der „Tageslichtdurchleuchtung". Die Verbesserung der medizinischen Röntgendurchleuchtung mit Mitteln der Fernsehtechnik. Jb. elektr. Fernmeldewes. 4 (1940), 373

51. Meiler, J.: Die Bedeutung der Brennfleckgröße für das Durchleuchtungsbild und die Bildverstärkeraufnahme. Röntgen-Bl. 21, 6 (1968) 257–270

52. Meinertz, T. W.: HICOR – Angiographie gegen den Herzinfarkt. Siemens Zeitschrift 1 (1993) 14–18

53. Moon, R.: Amplification of the fluoroscopic image by means of scanning X-ray tube. Am. J. Roentgenol. 59 (1948) 886–888

54. Moon, R.: Amplifying and intensifying fluoroscopic image. Science 112 (1950) 389–395

55. Morgan, R. H., R. E. Sturm: The Johns Hopkins fluoroscopic screen intensifier. Radiology 57 (1961) 556–559

56. Nell, W., S. Heller: Die Röntgendurchleuchtung bei Tageslicht und ihre Anwendung in der Chirurgie. Chirurg 22 (1951) 118–120

57. Noix, M.: La télévision radiologique. Ses problemes physiques, physiologiques, pathologiques. Doin, Paris, 1962

58. O'Neil, W.: Defending the Heart. Siemens Review 59, 6 (1992) 10–14

59. Pfeiler, M., K. H. Reiß, O. Schott: Die Intensitätsverteilung im Strahlenrelief als Eingangsgröße beim Röntgenfernsehen. Elektromedizin 11, 4 (1966) 17–28

60. Pfeiler, M., G. Linke: Bessere Indirektaufnahmen durch hochauflösende Röntgenbildverstärker. Elektromedica 40 (1972), 139

61. Pfeiler, M.: Systemtheoretische Betrachtungen zur Röntgenbildübertragung. Elektromedizin 14, 1 (1969) 8–14

62. Rath, M., J. Lissner, R. Rienmüller, J. Haendle: Digitale Radiographie-Gerätetechnik und erste klinische Ergebnisse der digitalen Angiographie mit einem elektronischen Universalarbeitsplatz. Fortschr. Röntgenstr. 140, 3 (1984) 243–250

63. Rose, A.: The sensitivity performance of the human eye on an absolute scale. J. Opt. Soc. Am. 38 (1948) 196–208

64. Rossmann, K., R. D. Moseley: Measurement of the input to radiographic imaging systems. Radiology 92 (1969) 265–271

65. Rossmann, K.: The spatial frequency spectrum: A means for studying the quality of radiographic imaging systems. Radiology 90 (1968) 1–13

66. Schober, H.: Das Sehen. Band 22. VEB Fachbuchverlag, Leipzig, 1964

67. Schut, T. G., W. J. Oosterkamp: The application of electronic memories in radiology. Medica Mundi 5 (1959) 85–88

68. Schwierz, G.: Berechnung elektronenoptischer Kenngrößen von Röntgenbildverstärkern. Dissertation, Universität Erlangen, 1972

69. Seyferth, W., P. Marhoff, E. Zeitler: Digitale Subtraktionsangiographie: Diagnostischer Stellenwert und Risiko. Electromedica 50 (1982) 60–80

70. Seyferth, W., W. Polster: Pfadfindertechnik: Eine Ergänzung der Digitalen Subtraktionsangiographie im fluoroskopischen Betrieb. Electromedica 53 (1985) 39

71. Siedentopf, H., E. J. Meyer, J. Wempe: Neue Sehschärfemessungen. Z. Instrumentenk. 51 (1941) 372

72. Stauffer, H., M. J. Oppenheimer, G. H. Stewart III, A. W. Blackstone: Practical Image amplifier technics, fluoroscopy, cinefluoroscopy, spot-film radiography

and use with closed circuit television. Radiology 65 (1955) 784

73. Stauffer, H. M.: „Spot" photofluorography with image intensifier and new polaroid projection film. Am. J. Roentgenol. 79 (1958) 887

74. Steiner, K., B. Brundin, W. Sladek: Das OPTIMATIC-System. Electromedica 41 (1973) 182–187

75. Stevenson, J. J.: Television techniques with the 5 inch, 7 inch and 9 inch image intensifiers. Br. J. Radiol. 34 (1961) 273–285

76. Stieve, F. E.: Das Aufnahmesystem vom Ausgangsschirm des Bildverstärkers; Klinische Forderungen (aus 10 Jahren Erfahrung). Röntgen-Bl. 6 (1972) 244–274

77. Sturm, R. E., R. H. Morgan: Screen intensification systems and their limitations. Am. J. Roentgenol. 62 (1949) 617–634

78. Teves, M. C., T. Tol, W. J. Oosterkamp: Die Röntgen-Bildverstärkerröhre. Verh. Dtsch. Röntgenges. 34 (1952), 26. Bericht 33. Tagung 1951, Beih. zu Fortschr. Röntgenstr. 76 (1952)

79. Wallmann, H., I. Wickbom: Roentgen-television equipment for use in surgery. Acta Radiol. Stockholm 51 (1959) 297–304

80. Widenmann, L.: Zur Aufnahmetechnik vom Bildverstärker. Röntgen-Bl. 9 (1972) 393–403

81. Woelke, H.: Das Aufnahmesystem vom Bildverstärker (Technische Möglichkeiten). Röntgen-Bl. 7 (1972) 297–303

82. Zimmermann, K. F.: Lichttechnische Untersuchungen über Lichtbildprojektion. Dissertation, Karlsruhe, 1936

83. Ziskin, M. C., G. Revesz: Mathematical Analysis of imaging systems. Temple Univ. Philadelphia, Progress Report, June 1969 and May 1970

84. Ziskin, M. C., G. Revesz, H. L. Kundel: Spatial frequency spectra of radiographic images (Ortsfrequenzsspektren von Röntgenbildern). Radiology 98 (1971) 507–515

Roentgen photography

G. Rosenbusch, E. Ammann, M. Oudkerk

In his first publication on the new rays, Roentgen established that fluorescence of bariumplatin-cyanide was not the only recognizable effect of X-rays, and continued: *'It is a fact that in many respects photographic dry plates have proved themselves sensitive to X-rays. It is possible to document many phenomena, so that it is easier to exclude mistakes. Whenever possible I have checked every important observation I saw on the fluorescence screen on a photograph.'*

These observations testified to the dedication of the experimental physicist Roentgen, who had a desire to record and prove. But documentation of phenomena was only possible because during those last few decades photography had seen an impressive development. The desire to record visible images not only artistically but also technically had already existed for some time.

Photography's history

As far back as the sixteenth century the camera obscura was built to observe solar eclipses. A small hole in one wall of a box projected a reversed picture onto the opposite wall. It took, however, a long time to attain fixation of an image. The principle to record must have been known for some thousand years and was also mentioned in Leonardo da Vinci's manuscripts (Encyclopaedia Britannica, 1975) [17].

The blackening of silver salt was known in Europe by the sixteenth century, but was considered to be based on heat. Not until the eighteenth century did investigators understand that it was based on the influence of light. In 1826 the Frenchman Joseph-Nicéphore Niepce succeeded in producing a photograph, not with a silver-salt solution but an asphalt solution exposed to sunlight (heliography).

Louis-Jacques-Mandé Daguerre, a French painter who copied images of his scenic paintings in the camera obscura, showed an interest in Niepce's work. Their collaboration ended in 1833 when Niepce died. In 1839 Daguerre described the method he used, and which was named after him. It was based on the properties of silver iodide, which after exposure to light attracted mercury vapours and therefore turned mat. With this method a silver-plated copper plate was treated with iodine vapour and formed silver iodide. After exposing the plate to light, it was exposed to mercury vapour. Amalgam developed in places that had been exposed by light. During fixation with sodium thiosulphate the non-exposed silver iodide was dissolved. The photograph was very pale.

Almost at the same time in England Thomas Wedgwood and William Henry Fox Talbot were experimenting with a different method to fix an image. Although Wedgwood succeeded in producing silhouettes of objects by using paper or leather drenched in silver salt, he failed to make them last. Talbot, however, made paper photosensitive by drenching it alternately in sodium chloride and silver salt solutions. Exposure to light changed silver salt into silver, which turned black. Parts that were not exposed to light were washed out with a concentrated sodium-chloride solution. In this way a negative was made, and could be used to produce many positive photographs. Later, sodium thiosulphate was used as a wash-out agent.

The Daguerre method was adopted and improved in many countries and the exposure time was reduced from several minutes to 20–40 s. Apart from photographs of landscapes and buildings it also became possible to take portraits.

But Talbot did not remain inactive. He increased the photosensitivity of his paper. He thought that it was not necessary to see immediate effect. With a much shorter exposure to light, a 'latent' image would be generated that would emerge under the influence of chemicals, 'develop' so to speak.

Scott Archer applied a colloid coating to glass plates (a solution of gun cotton, alcohol and ether) which, immediately before the exposure had to be made photosensitive, by using a liquid silver-salt solution (silver bath). This was called the wet colloidin method. Later the plate could also be stored for a few days.

Richard L. Maddox developed the silver-bromide gelatin plate in 1871 which meant a considerable step ahead. Gelatin was dissolved with potassium bromide in water, silver nitrate was added so that silver bromide was formed and finely dispersed throughout the gelatin. Either through boiling or by addition of ammonia, the photosensitivity of the solution was increased. The gelatin emulsion congealed as it cooled and was then pulverized. Soluble salts were washed out with water and the emulsion heated again and when liquidized coated on the glass plate. After congealing and drying, the dry gelatin plates were ready for use. As a developer or, 'evoker', hydroquinone and other derivatives of benzene were used to fix the sodium thiosulphate.

By 1879 the American George Eastman (Fig. V, 185) had already built a machine to coat plates. It is remarkable that Eastman had also developed a paper as carrier, which could be removed after

exposure and development, so that a transparent film (emulsion skin) remained from which prints could be made.

In 1889 Eastman succeeded in producing a photosensitive emulsion with a flexible transparent base made of nitrocellulose (gun cotton) (Meyers, 1909; Fuchs, 1956; Callear, 1970; Carroll, 1990) [32, 10, 19, 9].

This then was the situation of photography at the time Roentgen discovered X-rays. Roentgen himself used dry plates and not so many films in his experiments (Fig. V, 186), as was mentioned in the introduction.

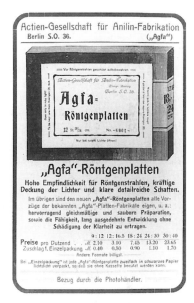

Fig. V, 186.
Advertisement for Roentgen plates in 1909 (Roentgentaschenbuch).

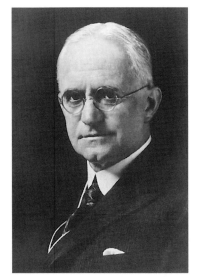

Fig. V, 185.
George Eastman (1845–1932). American inventor and entrepreneur. Perfected the production process of dry plates for photography. Produced a flexible transparent film base. Founder of Kodak, Eastman was a caring person and benefactor.

Roentgen photography in the early years

E. Sommer [36] described the goal of Roentgen photography in 1908 as follows:

'If we want to keep radiographs for a long period of time we must project these images not onto a screen, but onto an especially prepared, highly photosensitive photographic plate which after radiation exposure must be developed and fixed according to the principles of photography.'

In 1898, Gocht [20] wrote from his own experience that the treatment of photographic dry plates up to the developing process, just as in photography, played an important role. Although the plates were securely packed in their boxes and covers against sunlight by the factory, one should always store them in a dark and dry environment. Unused plates had to be protected, particularly against X-rays, and should under no circumstance remain in the same room where the roentgen equipment was, even not in a metal-lined closet. For economic reasons it would be an advantage if there were as many different plate sizes as possible in stock, so that they were always *'adjustable to the size of the object to be photographed. . . . Because radiographs are normally taken by artificial light or daylight, the plates have to be placed in a lightproof wrapping.'*

Various procedures were possible, and Gocht only stated what had proved itself in practice: unsized paper, lightproof black lining, and cassettes, the latter for really large plates, and for all radiographs, where plates that were only wrapped would be too heavily stressed and could break if not supported.

Smaller plates for smaller parts of the body, e.g. foot, elbow, etc., were wrapped in double layers of black paper; in these instances the black material that was utilized for larger plates and could also be used because it was easier to wrap.

For Gocht the lids of cassettes, black cardboard or pressed-silk paper were important. They were thicker than double-black paper, so that the object (hand, elbow, etc.) did not lie too close to the coated side of the plate and as a result the image would not come out so well. The more details that were required, the thinner and more flexible the plate wrappings had to be.

Gocht (1914) [21] wrote about cassettes in 1914:

'Nowadays they are really usable and of neat manufacture. The bottom is perfectly flat and so strong that even with the heaviest load it is guaranteed that the dry plate lying on top of it does not break. The lid is absolutely lightproof, so that one can take the photographs in broad daylight without a problem. When the plates are wrapped in paper or material then daylight should be tempered or the radiographs should be taken by electric or paraffin light. The best thing to do is to buy one sized 24:30, and a second one sized 40:50 cm. . . . We load the plates in complete darkness.'

As to plates or screens, Gocht answered clearly: *'In all cases we will rely on photographic plates for their greater accuracy and objectivity.'* When it was necessary to keep the image on the screen *'. . . then one lays a transparent piece of paper over the celluloid plate and copies the image with a pencil'* (Fig. V, 187). *'If electric light is available, one begins the development process in the dark; if one has to work in gas or paraffin light, then first turn the light low'* (Figs. V, 188 and V, 189).

For development, Gocht preferred earthenware dishes (basins) because they were cheaper, extremely strong and did not chip on touch; they were easier to clean than glass

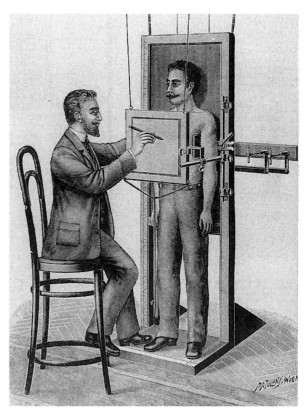

Fig. V, 187. Vertical ORTHODIAGRAPH designed by Dr. Kienboeck (s. Fig. II, 4) in 1911 (manufactured by RGS).

dishes. The most important thing with the developer was not its nature, but the proportions of its mixture. Before putting the plate into the dish with developer it was advisable to dip the plate into water first, so that the developer could wash the plate better. As it was often difficult to lift the larger plates (size 40:50), because they tended to lie flat on the bottom of the dish, he advised the placing of a piece of gauze bandage with the edges sticking out from under the plate, with which it could be lifted out of the basin.

The development had to be continued for some time until the plate had become completely opaque. Places where the rays had been most intense had to be completely blackened on examination, or well covered, as was the term in those days. Because the developer had to be in constant motion for an even development, seesaws were designed to make the bathing procedure of the plates easier (Cowl 1898–1899) [11]. This really was an improvement, as development of a pelvis radiograph of an adult in a seesaw bath took 20–25 min.

When the plate was still wet, the *'caring roentgenologist'* looked at them carefully, said Harras [24] in 1909, for small details were often more

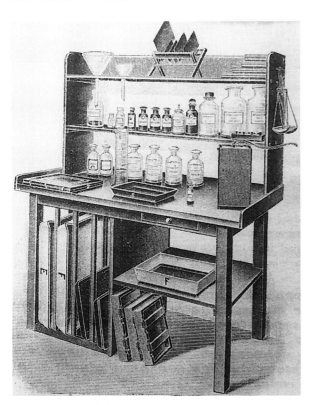

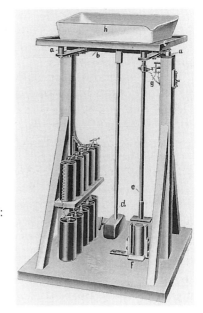

Fig. V, 190. 1909: Developer bath devised by Gocht (s. Fig. I, 23). An electromagnetic system generates an oscillating motion [21].

Fig. V, 188. 1911: Dark-room table. Shelves for pots, bottles, funnels and lamps (RGS).

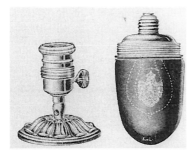

Fig. V, 189. 1907: Dark room lamp (manufactured by RGS).

explicit on the wet plate than on the dry. *'The real study of the negative was performed after drying, when it was held against a diffuse light. . . . Contrary to photography the negative is everything to roentgenology and the positive very little. . . . Therefore copying is of minor importance.'*

Gocht recommended that if the plate were developed too long and the bones hardly recognizable, then it should remain for 12–24 h in a sodium fixation bath. If the plate were not 'covered' enough, and the differences between the bones and soft parts indistinct, they could be intensified by using a watery sublimate solution 1:16 and an ammonia solution 1:10. When the plate was taken from the sublimate solution it had to be rinsed with running water for 15 minutes otherwise stains would occur.

In the two decades following Roentgen's discovery, textbooks on roentgenology gave many recipes for both developer and fixation baths, as well as finishing operations e.g. *'intensifying'* or *'weakening.'* (Albers-Schoenberg, 1903, 1919; Bauer, 1914) [2, 3, 5].

In 1909, R. Grashey [22] studied reasons for inferior images and methods that avoided them:

'If one traces the cause why suddenly the images do not turn out well, one must keep to a certain scheme. The many factors involved in the process of making an image should be taken into consideration, and verified in sequential order. One has to separate the equipment part from the photographic part.'

Grashey complained: *'Many physicians who do not make many radiographs simply send the plates to the photographer because it is easier, takes less time, and because they feel insecure about the photographic technique. I would most strongly advise against this type of simplification of the work.'* One had to pay the penalty in many respects.

'Anyone occupied in amateur photography has an advantage in roentgen technique. Those who employ assistants should send them to a professional photographer to learn and use all skills of the profession; in course of time this pays off. He will learn, for instance, how to manage the developer economically. The developer deteriorates when exposed to air; thus immediately after developing a plate the developer should be poured back into a glass container where, because of the smaller surface area, less liquid is exposed to air. If the developer is poured too quickly onto the dry plate, air bubbles will occur, which disturb the image and could be thought of as plate errors. By using equal measures of used and fresh developer one

can work more economically. There are many of these little but important things. Those who know and practise them have a not unimportant advantage over skilful but self-taught persons.'

The remark from E. Sommer (1908) [36] completed the quotation from Grashey:

'The basic requirement for a good result in roentgen technique depends on having good equipment, but more so on being in control of all technical factors. In addition, a thorough understanding of the internal processes of the roentgen apparatus, the construction of its essential components and operation, at least an elementary knowledge of additional photographic methods, developing and fixation, are necessary.'

The prepared plates were especially protected from damage in case they were passed from hand to hand during demonstrations. The coated side was covered with varnish or *'with a clean glass plate and both plates sealed together around the edges.'* (Figs. V, 191 and V, 192).

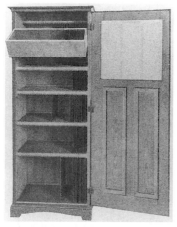

Fig. V, 191. Cabinet for storing X-ray plates.

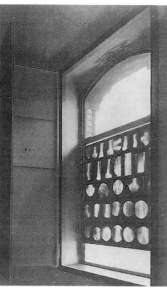

Fig. V, 192. 1909: Window, modified for viewing radiographs (by Albers-Schoenberg).

From a photographic point of view that was the situation from a few years before the turn of the century until between one and two decades afterwards. It was also described by Dessauer and Wiesner (1903) [13] (s. Fig. I, 29), Albers-Schoenberg [2, 3] (s. Fig. I, 22) in 1903 and 1919, Grigg (1965) [23], Harras (1909) [24], Koehler (1913, 1919, 1937, 1954) [26, 27, 28, 29] (s. Fig. II, 1) and Rieder and Rosenthal (1907) [33] (s. Fig. III, 9).

How could exposure time be reduced?

Doubling the photosensitive coating

In his textbook on roentgenology, Gocht (1898) [20] recommended these exposure times: for the hand 10 s – 1 min; for the forearm and foot 30 s – 2 min; for the upper arm, lower leg and, knee 1 – 3 min; for the shoulder joint and thigh 3 – 5 min; for the head, chest, abdomen, and pelvis 2 – 10 min.

It is obvious that he tried to reduce the exposure time in the interest of the image, the patient, and the experimentalists and equipment. Only with really excellent roentgen material could he have made instantaneous radiographs of hands and pelvises of adults in 5 min. Nowadays the tube plays the most important role, but because the early tubes were not of constant quality and differed widely, it was difficult to provide certain, fixed exposure times. The interest in reducing the exposure time was therefore directed at the photographic part of the process.

As far as the photographic material was concerned, *'a higher degree of photosensitivity of the layer'* was not found. As early as 1896 Dr Carl Schleussner, a German photographic-material manufacturer produced, at Roentgen's request, a plate with a stronger silver-bromide emulsion. In Europe and America this plate was popular because of the increased photographic density; in cases where a 1-h exposure time was normal, the Schleussner plate took only 20 min.

Increasing the sensitivity by using a thicker layer of emulsion did not work because the desired result did not ensue and the procedure prolonged the development period. Heating the plates before the exposure and development was not successful either. But in 1897 Max Levy [30] recommended coating both sides of the plates with photosensitive emulsion (Fig. V, 193):

Fig. V, 193.
Microcut of a dou-
ble-coated X-ray
film (Poppe, 1961).
A = type to be used
without screens;
B = type for film
screen
combination;
a = base;
b = emulsion;
c = layer between base and emulsion;
d = protective layer.

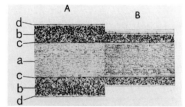

*'The roentgen rays . . . freely pass the front photosen-
sitive coating, penetrate the extremely thin and non-
transparent glass, and generate on the back coating
an almost equally strong negative as on the front
one. The lights and shadows cover each other and produce a substantial intensifying effect.'*

He was said to be able to intensify plates three
times, and films even four times. Levy prophesied
that in the future more celluloid films would be
used. The films will then be unbreakable, light-
weight, and simple to store, moreover they will
be pliable to the body if necessary. It is the task
of the technique *'to improve the carrier and to lower
the price'.*

To develop these double-coated plates on both
sides, Levy designed longitudinal clamps that allowed the plate to be turned around without
breaking (Fig. V, 194). For his double-coated
films he adapted the clamps, providing corner
holes to keep the films in place better. Gocht
(1898) [20] mentioned in 1898 that the film cor-
ners could be folded so that it was easier to
handle them in the developer or fixing solution. The sensitivity and contrast factor of the
photographic material was low, so that contrast

accentuation using copying and miniaturization
on steep-acting photographic paper was undertaken (Borcke, 1970) [7].

Conversion of X-rays to light

Roentgen not only discovered the fluorescent
property of barium-platincyanide, but of other
substances such as fluorspar.

In his provisional report Roentgen left the
question open of whether the chemical effect
on silver salts on the plate was produced directly
by X-rays, or indirectly using the fluorescent
property of glass plates, or even the gelatin
layer, because films were also exposed. The possibility that fluorescence was released by roentgen rays became a field of research immediately
after Roentgen's work was published. But it soon
appeared that fluorescence to expose plates did
not play a role in Roentgen's experiments.

Rumour has it that Thomas Alva Edison in the
USA had experimented with about 8500 different substances for the 'new light bulb' within a
year of the discovery of X-rays becoming known
to him. He described 1800 substances to be fluorescent, of which calcium tungstate showed an
intensity six times greater than barium platincyanide (Fuchs, 1956) [19]. In February 1896, Edison sent a few fluorescent screens to the New York
physicist Michael Pupin, who within the same
month had made a radiograph of a hand in a
few seconds using a fluorescent screen and a
photographic plate. The result was better than
expected.

At the same time, Winkelmann and Straubel in
Jena used fluorspar as a fluorescent substance for
radiographs (Gocht, 1898) [20]. Calcium tungstate prevailed in the course of time because it
was less expensive, could be produced artificially, was pulverizable to a fine grain without los-
ing its fluorescent quality, and in addition, radiated blue light to which the plates were extremely sensitive.

The principle of fluorescence was that the
screen with its fluorescent substance was placed
with the coated side towards the dry plate. Roentgen rays passed without hindrance, triggering
fluorescence, which activated a chemical reaction in the photosensitive coating. Therefore
roentgen rays became more effective in exposing dry plates; for in the meantime it became apparent that compared to ordinary light the roentgen rays had little direct influence on the photosensitive coating, and largely left plates and films
unaffected.

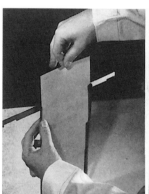
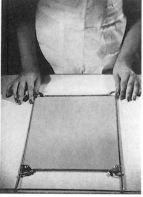

Fig. V, 194. Mounting a film in a rack. Frame with groove
(left) and frame with clamps (right) (Poppe, 1961).

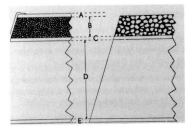

Fig. V, 195. Composition of the layers in an intensifying screen (Poppe, 1961). D = base; C = reflective layer; B = X-ray luminescent material; A, E = protective layer.

Some reports on the use of fluorescent substances were very optimistic, such as Max Levy's in 1897 [30]. According to him the exposure time could be reduced four to five times. In 1897 Levy also took radiographs with his double-coated dry plates and films by using intensifying screens on both sides of the photographic coating (Fig. V, 195). This principle proved its usefulness. According to Levy's records he succeeded in reducing the exposure time to 1/12th of the then prevailing time. It was generally admitted that the image had worsened with the intensifying screen because fine details were lost. This was caused by the relatively large grains of the fluorescent substance each acting as a separate light source. A very coarse-grained image was the result. For the time being the intensifying screen would only be useful for radiographs of fatty parts of the bodies of restless patients, or in cases where only a broad anatomical outline was required (Gocht, 1898) [20].

In 1899, Alban Koehler had such poor results with his first intensifying screens that for some years he did not want to hear a word about them. In the period from 1905 to 1907 the quality of radiographs improved because intensifying screens were increasingly more finely grained. They were used systematically and effectively after 1909 (Stürmer, 1962) [37].

In 1913, Koehler [26] saw the advantages of the use of intensifying screens, '...in all radiographs that have to be taken in the shortest possible exposure time, and where fine details do not matter but size and contours of organs do, that means mainly in radiographs of the heart, stomach, intestines. . . . In large survey radiographs to determine gravidity.'

In the year 1930 the best effect of intensifying screens amounted to a factor of 5 (Bauer, 1940) [6].

Roentgen films – belated acceptance?

Even though photographic films as well as dry plates existed at the time of the discovery of X-rays, the plates remained in general use well into the 1920s. One reason was that gelatin and celluloid films curled up and broke easily in those days; another cause was that photographers influenced roentgen diagnostics tremendously, and often even took their own radiographs. Films had a shelf-life of only 1–2 months around 1914; moreover they were more expensive than plates. It is noteworthy that in 1896 not only were plates double coated but films also, as mentioned above. The Schleussner factory was particularly interested in the photographic importance for roentgenology, and developed dry plates and films to meet the needs of radiography. Therefore, many opted '...*for very large objects and where it is important to reduce exposure for special reasons, and where the beauty of the image is not of great consequence, films with front and back coating, so-called roentgen films. They provided shorter exposure times than roentgen plates, while the light absorption of the glass is omitted, moreover, they give sharper copies than glass plates with front and back coating because the space between the coatings is narrower*' (Dumstrey and Metzner, 1897) [14].

Although in the meantime, containers for developer, washing and fixation of the dry plates were available, handling the plates was still problematic (s. Fig. V, 196).

During the First World War (1914–1918) the demand grew for quickly available radiographs and also for unbreakable photographic material. Archiving the plates was another problem. Because nitrocellulose as a base for roentgen films was highly flammable, other suitable materials such as cellulose acetate were developed.

Further developments concerned more sensitive emulsions and blue toning of the transparent base at the beginning of the thirties. Finally, from

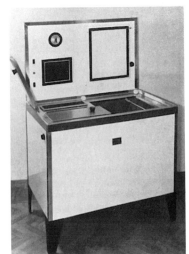

Fig. V, 196. Small film processing unit for a dark room (Poppe, 1961).

1897 to 1970, the sensitivity of roentgen films increased 100 times, and in ordinary photography about 300 times (Borcke, 1970) [7] (s. Fig. V, 205). The increase of film sensitivity corresponded to reduction of the radiation dose. Since 1930, using the maximum film sensitivity, improvements have been made in developing techniques using sensitometer strips to check the developing process.

Requirements for the composition of intensifying screens were specified. Thus the fluorescent substance had to be pure and fine-grained, it had to fluoresce brightly and uniformly and have only minimal afterglow or phosphorescence (Fuchs, 1956) [19].

To increase the definition of intensifying screens, J.H. Hartmann, who worked firstly at Veifa AG in Frankfurt and later at Phoenix AG in Rudolstadt, hit upon the idea in 1929/30 of colouring the binder for the pulverized calcium tongstate ($CaWO_4$).

He initially used eosin for this and later the less light-sensitive zapon true scarlet ('Rubra' screen). Use of an absorbing background brought a further improvement: black cardboard backing in combination with thin $CaWO_4$ layers. Other studies concerned the binders which were produced from cellulose and gelatin (Grigg, 1965) [23]. The 'Ilford SX screen' using zinc sulphate came onto the market in 1933. Its intensification was certainly higher but its definition lower so that this screen was used only for certain clinical indications, such as in exposures in pregnancy.

Cassette and film formats of 13 × 18, 18 × 24, 24 × 30 and 30 × 40 cm, which are still customary in Europe, were already included in the 1911 catalogue of the Veifa Werke (Aschaffenburg). This catalogue also included the 19 × 12 and 40 × 50 cm formats.

'Light boxes' for viewing and studying the finished negatives were offered in this catalogue up to the plate size of 24 × 30 or 40 × 50 cm (Fig. V, 197). These light boxes were equipped with two or four bulbs. The brightness of these boxes was *'controllable to the finest degree'*. Even today an essential feature of a light box is that its brightness and shutters are adjustable.

Screenless films are used only rarely. Cassettes have become more and more popular since they have intensifying screens at the front and back. Apart from being completely lightproof, permitting simple handling and having complete and uniform contact between film and screen are also required. This avoids loss of definition due to lack of contact. The front cover must be

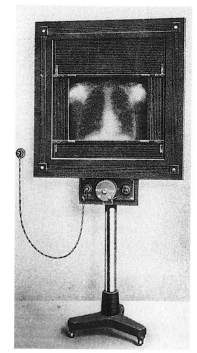

Fig. V, 197. This lightbox with shutters to block out light has been available from Siemens since 1907.

permeable to X-rays, and the back must be radiopaque. Cassettes were first produced from wood and the back was lined with a lead plate 0.5 mm.

State thickness thick. Today cassettes are made from plastic.

Intensifying screens, foam plastic and lead lining are glued in and must adhere securely during the life of the cassette. The hinge must open at least 180° in order to be able to insert the film without special precaution. There must always be a window for the identifying label. The weight of the cassettes should be as low as possible in the interest of easy handling and perfect operation of the spot-film devices.

Image Quality –
subjective and objective

The investigations by Heinrich Franke, John Eggert (1923, 1951) [15, 16], R. Glocker and Willem Bronkhorst (Bronkhorst et al, 1927) [8] had provided roentgenology with a profound scientific basis (Ackermann et al, 1968) [1]. W. Bronkhorst [8] wrote in 1927 the introduction of his work 'Kontrast und Schärfe im Röntgenbilde':

'For thirty years we have been using roentgenography in medicine. That the phase of its technical basis is still almost entirely in the first stage of the empiric is strange. Contrary to roentgen therapy, which was from the start based on experimental–physical assumptions, roentgen diagnostics is, up to now, almost de-

prived of every experimental base. . . . Still there has been some change these last few years.'

Investigations of these researchers proved that the quality of roentgen images depended primarily upon two characteristics: spatial resolution and contrast.

The poor sharpness of a radiograph can be caused by geometric blurring, film and screen blurring, or kinetic blurring. In practice the cause had to be identified and the proper remedy applied.

Contrast is the differences of optical density in a radiograph. If it is physically defined or measurable it is called objective contrast. But if the contrast is caused by our physiological or subjective perception it is called subjective contrast.

The contrast range is defined as the largest difference of optical density between the darkest and brightest spot in a radiograph. The object itself, tube voltage, radiation intensity, scattered radiation, film screen combination, developer, and so on all influence contrast. In order to judge image quality, test objects were developed with which the various factors and variables could partly or completely be determined in an objective way. Characteristics of images are deducible from the so-called modulation transfer function. Distortion and noise are two other characteristics. Other criteria should be used to judge them (Frommhold et al, 1979; Angerstein, 1988) [18, 4]. An optical density diagram was introduced to characterize the film. The roentgen film should have a curve with a rather steep slope, between 68 and 76 degrees because the relief of the radiation image in roentgen diagnostics contains only a relatively small contrast, corresponding to a large object volume.

Since 1964 a polyester sheet has served as the basis for the light-sensitive emulsion layer. These films were simpler to handle and faster to process. Present-day roentgen films consist of seven layers. On each side of the polyester base is one adherent layer, one emulsion layer and one external protective layer (s. Fig. V, 193).

The light-sensitive emulsion layer is composed mainly of silver bromide and a little silver iodide, while the adherent layer serves to fix the emulsion layer to the base and the protective layer hardens on drying so that the film is protected from outside damage. For some special research purposes films are manufactured with the layers on one side only (Ackermann et al, 1968) [1].

From this description the production of films seems simple, but in reality it is a very complex procedure. With newly gained insight in the different processes of radiography, further improvements can be expected.

Today the mechanism of generating an image can be described as follows:
- Film production
  - $KBr + AgNO_3 \rightarrow AgBr + KNO_3$
  - Heating Increases the sensitivity of the emulsion
  - Rinsing KNO_3 washed away
  - AgBr again heated and mixed with gelatin
  - Application of emulsion on film base, after application of adherent layer
  - Protective layer on light sensitive layer
- Generation of the latent image
  - $AgBr + roentgen\ rays \rightarrow Ag + \frac{1}{2} Br_2$
  - Exposure leads to colloidal silver distributed in silver bromide.
- Development of latent image into a radiograph
  - Reduction of silver ions into silver atoms
  - Additional enrichment of finely dispersed silver (increased absorption of light) in exposed areas.
- Fixation
  - Non-exposed silver bromide is converted to complex salts and dissolved out by the fixer.

Since manual film processing is highly labour intensive with fluctuations in quality, the desire for mechanical, standardized processing of the exposed films arose (Fig. V, 198). The development process was controlled 'by sight' and therefore prolonged or interrupted according to the subjective, optical impression. One spoke of 'tormenting' an underexposed negative and of the underdevelopment of an overexposed film. The use of automatic exposure control resulted in uniform exposure, so that overexposed or underexposed films became increasingly rare. In 1942 the Paco company presented the first automatic film processor (Fig. V, 199). It was still very bulky and required much space. In this frame or rack film processor the films were transported at fixed intervals in frames or racks. The films in the frames remained for a preset time in the processing baths (developing, washing, fixing, washing) and the drier. Thermostats ensured constant temperature. Naturally the processing baths required constant control to renew the developer and fixer once a certain area of film had been processed. A further development was the film processor which no longer required a frame or rack. The film was transported by rollers (Frommhold et al, 1979) [18].

Nowadays film processing machines are compact, reliable, and produce results of constant

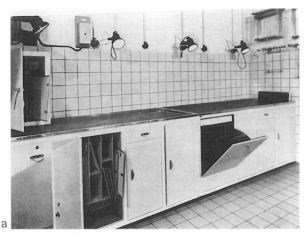

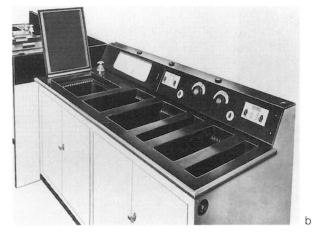

a   b

Fig. V, 198a, b. Dry table (a) and larger processing system (b) made of plastic (Poppe, 1961).

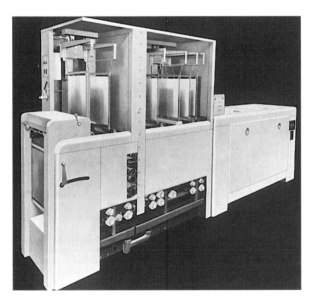

Fig. V, 199. Automatic film processor by Pako (Poppe, 1961). The film was processed at fixed intervals.

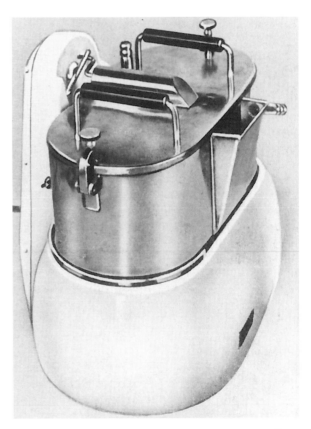

Fig. V, 200. Film processor for mass fluorography films. Developer tank (top) and motor drive (bottom) (Poppe 1961).

quality. Temperature and regeneration of chemicals are usually electronically controlled and can be adjusted to match requirements. Maintenance of the machine is simple: Just taking out the rollers or other parts to clean. The speed is adjustable from 30 s up to some minutes. A film transport of 100–350 films per hour is possible. The film is loaded into the machine in the dark room. After being processed and dried in the machine, it is ready for viewing and reporting.

Special film processing machines were designed for films used in mass fluorography and in cine cameras (Figs. V, 200 and V, 201).

Another step forward is the daylight processor. Cassettes with exposed films are placed in the daylight system which empties the cassette and processes the film. The empty cassette is again loaded in an automatic film feeder in broad daylight. The dark room has, therefore, lost a lot of

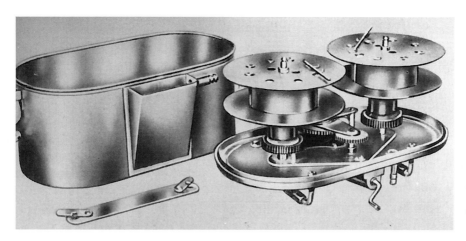

Fig. V, 201. Film processor for mass fluorography films showing an open system with film spools upside down (Poppe, 1961).

its significance, although it is far from being abandoned.

Different systems were designed to recover the silver released during film processing. Only a small part of the bromine silver of the light-sensitive film emulsion is reduced to image silver in processing. The fixing bath dissolves out the remaining silver content. In the 1950s, 1 m² X-ray film produced between 15 and 30 g of silver depending upon the nature of the film. Two methods have become established to recover this released silver: filling with substances such as ammonium thiosulphate or sodium sulphate, and electrolysis which has the advantage that the silver is regained in metal form.

Since 1970, in the field of intensifying screens, fluorescent substances on the basis of rare earths have been produced: the green-fluorescent gadolinium oxysulphide, the blue-fluorescent lanthanum oxybromide and red fluorescent yttrium oxysulphide. Unlike calcium tungstate, zinc sulphide or barium lead sulphate, they require a radiation dose of only a quarter. Films must be matched to the colour of the light emitted by the intensifying screens (Degenhardt, 1983; Haus and Cullinan, 1989) [12, 25].

The production of radiographs by non-photochemical methods was also attempted. Already one decade after Roentgen's discovery, the Italian A. Righi (1907) [34] experimented with electroradiographic exposures, electron radiography, in which the gases were ionized.

The first electrophotographic copies of documents were produced in 1938 (Figs. V, 202 and V, 203). This initiated intensive development work on electrostatic image production. The use of selenium produced a turning point and this process was available in 1950, initially for material testing (McMaster and Schaffert, 1950) [31] and since 1954 for radiology as well.

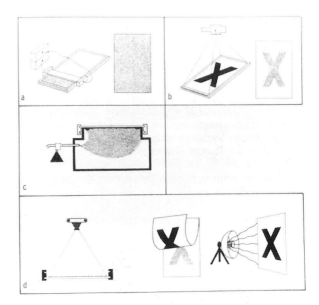

Fig. V, 202a–d. The principle of xeroradiography. (a) Electrostatic charging of a selenium layer; (b) X-ray exposure partially discharges the radiation-sensitive selenium layer which now carries the latent image. (c) Applied powder makes the latent image visible by transferring this image onto the paper (d) followed by a fixing process.

A thin layer of selenium applied to a carrier is charged positively by corona discharge. The selenium plate is inserted in a charging device for this purpose. After charging at 600–1200 V, the selenium plate is inserted in the cassette. The plate is partially discharged by the incident X-rays. It contains the latent image and is dusted with powder in a chamber. The powder is distributed over the selenium plate depending upon the charge. Subsequently, the image, that is the powder coating corresponding to the image, is transferred to paper. It is fixed on the paper by heat. The selenium plate is cleaned, heated, charged up anew and is available in a cassette for the next exposure. The

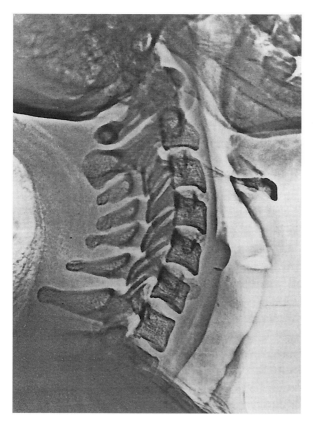

Fig. V, 203. Lateral xeroradiogram of the neck (by Dr J. N. Wolfe, Hutzel-Hospital, Detroit, Med. Roentgenb., Thieme, 1979).

image can be influenced by changing the exposure data, the tube voltage and the processing method. A tube voltage between 40 and 50 kV is the most favourable. The processing method can be chosen so that the image is reproduced as positive or negative. Like intensifying screens, selenium plates can be used many times.

In comparison to a film screen radiograph, the high dose and thus excessive radiation exposure to the patient is a severe disadvantage. Soft tissues or peripheral extremities such as hands and feet were preferred objects for this technique because of the low kV applied. A larger contrast range could be achieved here, i.e. bone and soft tissue structures could be assessed well on one exposure, which was not the case in customary radiographs and for which sometimes two exposures were necessary under different exposure conditions. In addition, this method was used in mammography (Wolfe, 1968) [38], for displaying soft tissue of the neck, in particular of the larynx, but also of the bronchial system. Xeroradiography is scarcely ever practised today (Schertel, 1976) [35].

Film with all its advantages and disadvantages was enriched by computers and microelectronics: digitally acquired images are immediately available on the monitor for diagnosis and can be digitally stored inexpensively. Laser cameras can now generate any number of films of identical quality. Thus the most important images are available in outstanding quality for teaching and publication without the clinician or surgeon having to give away the originals. Digital networking ensures improved communication between specialists. Soft tissue and bone structures can be enhanced, again without X-rays, by postprocessing digital images. The diagnosis can in this way be made more accurately and faster – especially if specialists can be consulted. We still have the unique features of the film, but the digital image has developed to become a new standard. It is always accessible everywhere for everyone authorized to view it. Valuable resources such as water and chemicals can be saved.

References

1. Ackermann, L., H. Mergler, H. Schleussner: Dokumentation des Strahlungs- bzw. Dosisbildes. Hdb. Med. Radiologie, Bd. 1, T1. Springer, 1968
2. Albers-Schönberg, H.: Die Röntgentechnik. Hamburg 1903
3. Albers-Schönberg, H.: Die Röntgentechnik. Hamburg 1919
4. Angerstein, W.: Lexikon der radiologischen Technik in der Medizin. 4. Aufl. Leipzig 1988
5. Bauer, H.: Einiges über Entwickler für Röntgenplatten. Röntgen-Taschenbuch. Bd. 6. Leipzig 1914
6. Bauer, K.: ABC der Röntgentechnik. Leipzig 1940
7. Borcke, E.: 75 Jahre Röntgenstrahlen und Röntgenphotographie. Röntgenpraxis 23 (1970) 277–291
8. Bronkhorst, W.: Kontrast und Schärfe im Röntgenbilde. Leipzig 1927
9. Callear, Th .E.: Kodak and Radiography. Med. Radiogr. Photogr. 3 (1970) 79–106
10. Carroll, Q. B.: Fuchs's principles of radiographic exposure, processing and quality control. 4th.ed. Springfield 1990
11. Cowl, W.: Zur Technik. Fortschr. Röntgenstr. 2 (1898–1899) 104–105
12. Degenhardt, H.: Die historische Entwicklung der Leuchtsubstanzen und deren Anwendungen in der Röntgentechnik. Electromedica 51 (1983) 155–159
13. Dessauer, F., B. Wiesner: Leitfaden des Röntgen-Verfahrens. Berlin 1903
14. Dumstrey, F., Metzner: Die Untersuchung mit Röntgenstrahlen. Fortschr. Röntgenstr. 1 (1897–1898) 115–130
15. Eggert, J.: Einführung in die Röntgenphotographie. 7. Aufl. Zürich 1951
16. Eggert, J.: Einführung in die Röntgenphotographie. 2. Aufl. 1923,

17. Encyclopaedia Britannica, 15th ed., vol. 14: Photography. Chicago 1975
18. Frommhold, W., H. Gajewski, H.D. Schoen: Medizinische Röntgentechnik. Bd. 1: Physikalische und technische Grundlagen. Stuttgart 1979
19. Fuchs, A.W.: Evolution of roentgen film. Am. J. Roentgenol. 75 (1956) 30–48
20. Gocht, H.: Lehrbuch der Röntgenuntersuchung. Stuttgart 1898
21. Gocht, H.: Handbuch der Röntgenlehre. 4. Aufl. Stuttgart 1914
22. Grashey, R.: Photographische Notizen. In: Röntgen Taschenbuch, hrsg. von E. Sommer, 1909
23. Grigg, E.R.N.: The trail of the invisible light. Springfield 1965
24. Harras, P.: Vorbereitungen zum Arbeiten im Röntgenlaboratorium. Stuttgart 1909
25. Haus, A.G., J.E. Cullinan: Screen film processing systems for medical radiography. A historical review. Radiographics 9 (1989) 1203–1224
26. Köhler, A.: Über Verstärkungsschirme, ihre richtige und ihre falsche Anwendung. Röntgen Taschenbuch Bd. 5. Leipzig 1913
27. Köhler, A.: Welche Mittel hat man, aus beträchtlich unterbelichteten Röntgenaufnahmen möglichst vollwertige Negative zu erhalten? Röntgen Taschenbuch Bd. 8. Leipzig 1919
28. Köhler, A.: Ärztlicher Röntgenbetrieb um die Jahrhundertwende. Strahlentherapie 60 (1937) 283–289
29. Köhler, A.: Lebenserinnerungen. Frankfurt a.M. 1954
30. Levy, M.: Über Abkürzung der Expositionszeit bei Aufnahmen mit Röntgenstrahlen. Fortschr. Röntgenstr. 1 (1887–1898) 75–82
31. McMaster, R.C., R.M. Schaffert: Xeroradiographie – a basic development in X-ray nondestructive testing. Nondestr. Test 9, Nr. 1 (1950) 11 u. 22
32. Artikel "Photographie", in Meyers Konversationslexicon 6. Aufl. Bd. 15. Leipzig u. Wien 1909
33. Rieder, H., J. Rosenthal (Hrsg): Lehrbuch der Röntgenkunde. Bd. II, 2. Aufl. Leipzig, 1907
34. Righi, A.: Die Bewegung der Ionen bei der elektrischen Entladung. Leipzig 1907
35. Schertel, L, D. Puppe, E. Schnepper, H. Witt, K. zum Winkel: Atlas der Xeroradiographie. Urban & Schwarzenberg, München 1976
36. Sommer, E.: 13 Jahre Röntgenologie, Rückblick und Ausblick. Röntgen Taschenbuch. Leipzig 1908
37. Stürmer, W.: Zur Geschichte der Röntgen Leuchtstoffe. Fortschr. Röntgenstr. 97 (1962) 514
38. Wolfe, J.N.: Xeroradiography of the breast. Radiology 91 (1968) 231

Radiation exposure: changing risk and benefit over time

Th. Schmidt

The first radiation burn, of a hand, was reported hardly a year after the discovery of X-rays. The description originates from O. Leppin in 1896. He used his left hand as the test object for tube testing (see Fig. V, 64). He correlated the diffuse swellings and blisters, except for 'where the ring surrounded the finger', with the exposure to radiation. Further 'remarkable structural changes of the skin' were described in the following years by others, including Albers-Schoenberg in *Fortschritte*.

The nature and extent of the use of X-rays, knowledge about possible radiation effects and the recommendations or legislation to protect the user of X-rays developed in parallel. Table V.6 shows the progress of knowledge about the biological effects of radiation.

Unfortunately, the dosages occurring in the first observations can be reconstructed only with difficulty from the original historical studies. Today, consequences of radiation are classified into deterministic and stochastic effects (Fig. V, 204). An attempt is made in Table V, 7 to classify dose and effect as a function of certain marginal conditions.

Since acute deterministic effects are hardly ever observed today – except for accidents – interest is focused on the stochastic–somatic late effects. The probability of the occurrence of these effects is in dispute. If a threshold for the occurrence of these late effects is not accepted,

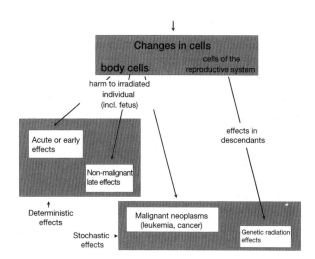

Fig. V, 204. Classification of stochastic and deterministic effects.

Table V, 6. State of knowledge about the effects of radiation

Date c.	Type of radiation effects	Reference
1896	Skin lesions (erythema, ulcer)	Leppin et al.
1903	Skin cancer	First description Frieben, Hesse 1911 (review)
1905	Sterility, Injury to an embryo	Braun and Osgood; Burckhard et al.
1908	Injury to the eye (cataract)	Birch-Hirschfeld
1925	Delayed growth (e.g. breast)	Holfelder et al.
1926	Genetic effects	Muller
1927	Systematic description of the teratogenic effects	Flaskamp
Post-1945	Stochastic-somatic late effects	

Table V, 7. Examples of dose (Sv) and effect

Dose	Effect	Remarks
0.1	probability of death 5 x 10^{-3}due to cancer and leukaemia introduction	homogeneous whole body radiation
< approx. 0.2	no deterministic lesion detectable	
0.2 - 1	first symptoms of acute radiation disease	homogeneous whole body radiation
approx. 4	50 % probability of death	whole body exposure
above 6	100 % probability of death	whole body exposure without medical care
approx. 7	Erythema, epilation	depends upon radiation quality, fractionation, irradiated field etc.
above 10	subcutaneous induration	depends upon radiation quality, fractionation, irradiated field etc.
12	cataract (25 - 50 % of those exposed)	fractionated radiation, partial body
20	radiation ulcer	depending upon radiation, quality, fractionation, irradiated field etc.

The Sievert has been the unit for the equivalent dose since 1985. The old unit was the rem, where 1 Sv = 100 rem. The Sievert honours the radiologist Rolf Sievert of Stockholm, Sweden, 1896-1966.

interest focusses on the dose applied in X-ray diagnostics and must be considered.

Even if the direct relationship between the dose occurring in X-ray diagnostics and the induction of malignant neoplasms cannot be observed directly, on the basis of models, a relationship can be assumed. This relationship will never be directly confirmed epidemiologically (the pulmonary dose in a typical thoracic exposure is only about 0.1 mSv!).

Perhaps new insights into this problem can be expected in the future from experiments in vitro.

Regulations concerning maximum permissible dosages

Recommendations and legal regulations concerning permissible dosages reflect the changing level of knowledge over the past hundred years. Scientists, scientific associations and legislation have made dosage recommendations for employees in the past. The terms used have changed or been adapted to findings in the course of time: tolerance dose, physical effect dose, genetic effect dose, Mutscheller dose, highest permissible dose, maximum permissible dose and limits. Table V, 8 shows these changes as a function of time.

As we can surmise from all the different terms used, the consequences of radiation exposure being prevented or at least minimized depend upon the level of knowledge at the time. The 'Mutscheller dose' (1925), for instance, attempted the exclusion of acute deterministic effects. The 'highest permissible dose' introduced in accordance with Muller's findings was in-

tended to reduce the probability of genetic mutations on doubling the spontaneous mutation rate. Limits valid today are derived from ICRP 26, analogous to the frequency of accidental deaths in industries in which no radiation-related work is performed. This comparison was disputed for various reasons. ICRP 60 has therefore departed from this premise and introduced a very subtly differentiated method for determining limits (ICRP 44, 55 and 60).

Development of radiation exposure in X-ray diagnostics

The radiation exposure of the patient being X-rayed is determined essentially by the sensitivity of the receptor system (e.g. film–screen combination). Gilman-Frost's report of an exposure time of 20 minutes to photograph a forearm fracture on 3 February 1896 indicates the low sensitivity of X-ray plates and X-ray tubes used at the time.

Shortly after the discovery of X-rays, the idea of increasing the 'yield' of the absorption with the aid of fluorescing materials was born, because of long exposure times. Roentgen himself proposed barium platinocyanide and a little later Edison proposed calcium tungstate as the fluorescing material. By around 1900, the necessary dose for generating an X-ray image could thus be reduced to a fifth of the initial figure (Fig. V, 205). The idea of the double-sided coated film to increase sensitivity also originates from the last century (Levy) but these improvements still had considerable disadvantages at this time (graininess, after-glow, etc).

Table V, 8. Development of the dose 'considered permissible' for subjects occupationally exposed to radiation

Year	Relative dose	Comments
1895		
1900	100	Albers-Schönberg: first recommendations on radiation protection
1910		Memorandum of the German Roentgen Society on the use of protective measures against X-rays
1920	2	Tolerance dose 1/10 HED*. Proposed by Sievert. Tolerance dose around 2.5 mSv/day. Proposed by Mutscheller, after questioning radiologists
1930	0,2	Genetic effect dose = 1/10 Mutscheller-dose (German 'Keimschädigungsdosis')
	0,8	NBS Manual 20: 6 mSv/week
1940		
1950	0,4	Maximum permissible dose: 3 mSv/week ICRP** Introduction of values for parts of the body Protection of young people, expectant mothers
	0,1	Maximum permissible dose: 50 mSv/a ICRP
1960		Further differentiation with regard to time of exposure, lifetime dose
1970	0,1	Limit of the effective dose: 50 mSv/a with additional conditions
1980		
1990	0,04	Recommended dose limits 20 mSv/a averaged over 5 years ICRP 60 (with additional conditions and limit values for regions of the body)
1995		

*   HED: Skin entry dose, determined characteristic skin reactions. This unit was partially used for administering dose (therapy) up to 1945 (around 5 Sv = 1 HED).
** ICRP: International Commission on Radiation Protection.

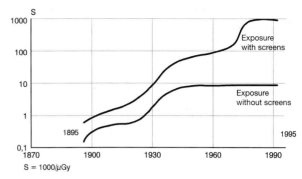

$S = 1000/\mu Gy$

Fig. V, 205. Improvements in the sensitivity of the system from 1895 to today for exposures with and without intensifying screens.

Film–screen combinations in the form known today finally became established in the years between 1920 and 1940. The improvements in the sensitivity of the X-ray film or of the film–screen combination (according to data from Agfa) are shown in Fig. V, 205. As can be seen from the graph, no further increases in sensitivity have been achieved in the film itself in the past 30 years.

It should be emphasized that the search for more sensitive film–screen systems in the first decades of this century was not stimulated by the desire to reduce dosages but solely to minimize motion blurring and thus achieve better image quality.

A glance at historical exposure tables illustrates the progress made. An extract from an exposure table from the year 1913 is given in Table V, 9.

Table V, 9. Extract from an exposure table (1913)

Head (antero-posterior)	8 mA	6 s	50 cm distance
Cervical spine	3.5 mA	6 s	25 cm distance with cylindrical diaphragm
Lungs	32 mA	0.75 s	30 cm distance
Finger	9 mA	1.25 s	25 cm distance

In his book 'X-rays and their Uses' (Teubner 1918), Bucky describes the cassette as *'a lockable container for the photographic plate, which is light-proof on all sides and is manufactured usually of wood in the form of a flat crate, in which, however, the upper cover in contact with the body to be exposed consists of a cardboard sheet, so that the X-rays are not attenuated.'*

Here it should be noted that these values apply mainly to short distances of 60 or 70 cm, since the low output of the X-ray tube could be better used in this way. The voltage is described here as a 'medium hard tube'.

In an exposure table provided by Spiegler in 1928, the milliamperage product for the lungs has been reduced to around a third compared with the value 1913, with a clear reduction of the exposure time. This means that, in this period, tubes became more powerful but the sensitivity of the receptor system could be increased only moderately.

Taking the chest radiograph as an example, the development both for the period since 1900 and also separately for the last 30 years is shown in Figs V, 206 and V, 207. Dose reductions clearly can be achieved with good technical

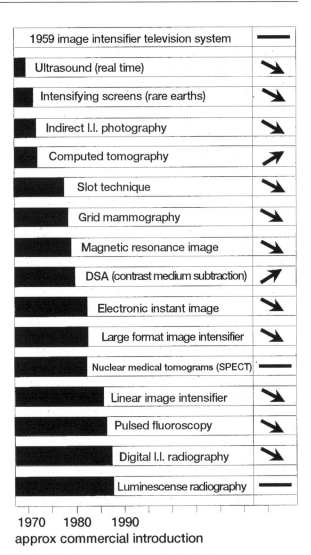

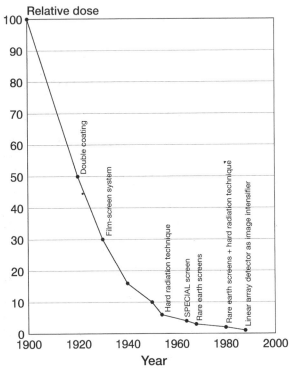

Fig. V, 206. Changes in dose requirements for a chest radiograph since 1900.

Fig. V, 208. Developments in the field of imaging systems since 1960. The effects on the radiation exposure of the population are indicated by arrows. Obviously the different modalities are a substitute for other partially invasive diagnostic methods or therapeutic interventions.

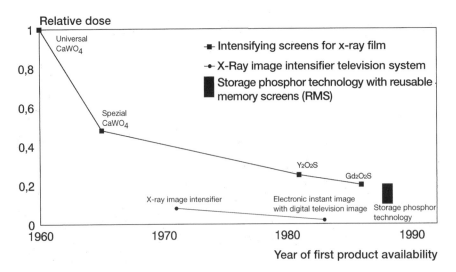

Fig. V, 207. Dose reductions after new technical developments since 1960.

equipment, as can be seen from the graphs. If one considers the innovations in the past 30 years of X-ray diagnostics (Figs V, 207 and V, 208), then most of them have resulted in a reduction in dose. However, it must still be noted that, in some cases, the additional information gained by minimizing the invasiveness of an interventional procedure is accompanied by increased dose levels. A typical example of this is the introduction of computed tomography. CT examinations performed in Germany today, numbering around four million per annum, do not play a significant role in comparison to the total number of X-ray diagnostic procedures (Fig. V, 209). However, these CT examinations account for 30–40 % of the radiation exposure of the population (Fig. V, 210). Perhaps, one day, similar thoughts will have to be formulated for interventional radiological procedures, but the advantage to the patient (no anaesthesia, no surgical risk etc.) implies a certain, inevitable amount of radiation exposure.

As the United Nations (UNSCEAR Report) have ascertained, the development status of a country is linked to the exposure of its population to radiation through medical measures. People living today in highly industrialized countries are exposed to just as much radiation on average through radiological diagnostic procedures as through natural exposure (ambient radiation, incorporation of natural radioactive substances etc.). Higher life expectancy, improved quality of life, the prevention of diseases, less sick leave, etc. are the outcome of a highly developed and efficient healthcare system and the use of efficient medical engineering techniques.

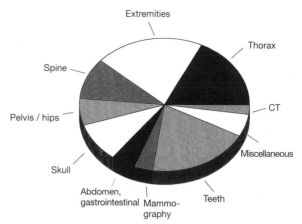

Fig. V, 209. Frequency of X-ray examinations by type of examination (statistics from the German Federal Office for Radiation Protection, 1993).

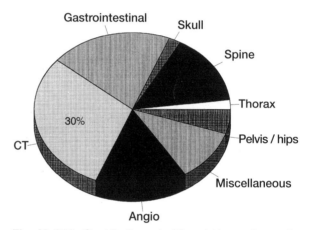

Fig. V, 210. Contribution of different X-ray diagnostic modalities to the exposure of the population because of medical applications of X-rays (estimates on the basis of measurements and censuses).

Epilogue

G. Rosenbusch, M. Oudkerk, E. Ammann

Science and technology have improved the quality of human life throughout the world. The history of science and technology allows us to take part in this development and to understand it. According to Cicero a person who has no knowledge of the things that took place before his birth will remain a child. This book should contribute to the elucidation of the past. Physics and technology began to play an important role in medicine after the year 1895, which is therefore considered a turning point in the history of medicine.

The development of diagnostic radiology began many decades ago, and young radiologists should be aware of how much energy, dedication and ingenuity were needed to achieve what they now take for granted.

Diagnostic radiology – Undiscussed fields

Unfortunately, the history of radiotherapy and nuclear medicine could not be covered in this book. Even principal branches of diagnostic radiology, as applied to obstetrics and gynecology, dentistry and forensic medicine, have only been mentioned in passing so far.

Diagnostic radiology in gynecology and obstetrics

As early as March 1896, the American obstetrician E.P. Davis reported that he had put the skull of an infant into the skeleton of a female pelvis and had obtained a weak shadow of the fetal skull after an exposure time of 1.5 hours. As an experienced obstetrician, he concluded that provided the method improved, it would allow assessment of fetal pathology and detection of multiple pregnancies. Indeed, radiographs were taken throughout the fifties and sixties when atypical positioning of the fetus, anomalies of the female pelvis, hydrocephalus or anencephaly, and multiple pregnancies were suspected (Fig. 1). Frontal

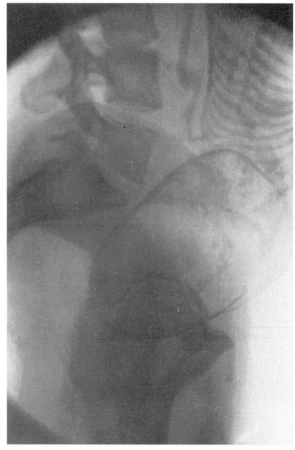

Fig. 1. Gravida at term. Generally narrowed pelvis II. Dextrosinistral projection in supine position, C.v. 8.8 cm (1933).

and axial radiographs were taken to measure the pelvis and to determine the necessity of cesarean section. These measurements could be obtained in various ways, all making adjustments for the magnification of the actual size, generally by adding a radiopaque grid that is included on the obtained radiograph (Fig. 2).

Since hormonal pregnancy tests were not then available (Aschheim-Zondek-test only since 1929), radiographs were taken to decide whether a pregnancy or a tumor is present, but

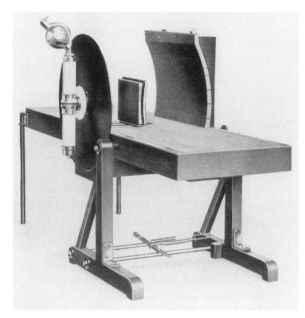

Fig. 2. Table for pelvic measurements after Schubert (1933).

only from approximately the fourth month of pregnancy onwards. It was not until the fourth month that the fetal ossification could have progressed to the stage of radiographically visible skeletal parts. Fetal age could be determined by assessing the maturation of skeleton.

If fetal death was suspected clinically, it could be confirmed by radiographically demonstrated overlapping calvarial bones (Spalding's sign). After intrauterine death, the fetal cranial bones become increasingly indistinct. Even water-soluble contrast media were administered into the amniotic sac after percutaneous puncture of the uterus to diagnose the death of the fetus by the absence of swallowed contrast medium in the gastrointestinal tract.

The placenta was not directly visualized on conventional radiographs. Because of its possible complications, the placenta previa was disclosed by indirect radiographic methods, such as radiographs of the pelvis obtained with the bladder filled with contrast medium. An increased distance between the fetal skull and the bladder indicated the presence of a placenta previa. After angiography became available, it was used but it often required several exposures resulting in a relatively high radiation dose to the fetus.

Ultrasonography was partly developed by obstetricians. It completely changed the diagnostic approach to pregnancy. Today, studies using X-rays are no longer used for assessing the intra-uterine fetus.

Despite sonography and MRI, hysterosalpingography is still used to find the cause of female infertility since it can determine tubal patency and disclose malformations of the genital tract. Hysterosalpingography is no longer used to diagnose tumors of the genital tract, which increasingly are diagnosed, staged and monitored by sonography, CT and MRI. Likewise, pneumoperitoneum and lymphography have been largely superseded.

Dental radiography

Radiographs of the teeth comprise a significant portion of all radiographic examinations, with a proportionate contribution to radiation exposure of the population. The dental radiographs are taken in the dentist's office, which is invariably furnished with a radiographic unit.

The first radiographs of a tooth were taken by Koenig on 2 February 1896. In 1899, T. Sjoegren pointed out that radiography of the teeth requires several modifications of the conventional radiographic technique. Ordinary glass plates were unsuitable since cutting glass to the required size was difficult and intraoral positioning of glass plates inconvenient. To overcome these problems, he cut the film to the appropriate size and wrapped it in lightproof paper. Taking advantage of the film's elasticity, it was shaped for the contour of the jaw. To avoid geometric distortion, the X-ray tube had to be placed in a position that directs the 'light' perpendicular to the film. The exposure time should not exceed 25–30 s and development of the film demanded great care. The radiographs taken by Sjoegren in 1899 are of remarkable good quality.

Otherwise, reports of the use of X-rays in the diagnostic evaluation of teeth are rare before 1900. In 1903, Albers-Schoenberg wrote that the dentists had not yet appreciated the benefits offered by this new method, despite the advances of dentistry in the years before the turn of the century, such as root retractions under cocaine anesthesia and improved restorations of carious cavities. These therapies are contingent radiographic evaluation.

During subsequent decades, special dental units and X-ray tubes were designed to reduce the radiation dose to both patients and dental personnel and to improve the quality of the radiographs (s. Figs. V, 56 and 57).

Today, dental radiology is employed to disclose dental anomalies, to evaluate dental roots and periapical infections, and to detect retained root remnants or foreign bodies. Orthopantomography offers an unobstructed survey view of the entire denture and maxillomandibular region, even in the presence of trauma and deformities, but intraoral radiographs of selected dental regions are still necessary for detailed information.

Forensic radiology

Immediately after X-rays had been discovered, they were used in traumatology, particularly in the evaluation of the skeleton. As knowledge increased, X-rays were used in the assessment of gunshot wounds, to define the passage or the type of bullet. This is still practiced by modern criminologists. From postmortem radiographs, particularly of the skeleton, age and gender of the individual at the time of death or the type of fatal injury can often be deduced. Victims of plane crashes and fires are often so badly mutilated that they cannot be positively identified by inspection. In such cases, comparison with previous skeletal radiographs can be instrumental for proper identification. Dental radiographs can also be helpful.

Recently, abdominal radiography has been used in law enforcement to search suspected drug smugglers for illegal drugs that have been sealed in condoms and swallowed or inserted into orifices.

From radiology to imaging

Progress in the field of diagnostic radiology has been vast and versatile, as described in the preceding chapters. Despite all advancements, radiation exposure has continuously decreased but is, in principle, unavoidable with the use of X-rays.

There are other types of energy that can be used to image internal organs.

Utilization of sound reflection – sonography

The allied forces already used sonar equipment to locate German submarines (U-boats) during the First World War, but it took two decades before ultrasound waves were considered for diagnostic purposes in humans. In 1938, K.T. Dussik, an Austrian neurologist, designed, together with his brother, an apparatus to use ultrasound for diagnostic purposes. As a neurologist, he applied it for the diagnostic evaluation of the brain, but

had disappointing results. It was not until after the Second World War, after sonar and radar equipment had been advanced as part of the war effort, that this technique was developed further for diagnostic applications in medicine. In 1947, the young American D. Howry began his experiments and, in cooperation with W.R. Bliss, he developed a pulse-echo technique. As early as 1952, Howry and Bliss reported their compound-scan technique. J. Holmes and his coworkers carried out investigations of the upper abdomen. The patient's body was submerged in a water-filled bathtub. Later, a semicircular tank with a plastic window pervious to ultrasound was used instead of the bathtub.

Further progress followed rapidly and, since the seventies, ultrasound has conquered many diagnostic territories. The major applications are the abdominal organs, including liver, pancreas, spleen, kidneys, gallbladder and biliary ducts, and the organs of the lesser pelvis, with sonography today generally performed first before other imaging studies. In obstetrics, pregnancy can be confirmed after only a few weeks and its progress easily monitored (Donald and Brown 1958). Obstetrical radiography has become superfluous. In cardiology, ultrasound has become indispensable to assess the heart valves and pericardium. Ultrasound has been found to serve as an addition to the evaluation of joint disorders. In pediatrics, it has lead to a major change in the evaluation of newborns and infants. Ultrasound has also become important as a modality that complements mammography. Many vessels are accessible for Doppler echography. In the diagnosis of the adult brain, ultrasound is no longer of any importance even though the first sonographic equipment was developed for echoencephalography. The cranial bones are too impenetrable for sound waves, and CT and MRI achieve by far superior cerebral imaging.

Compound scanning demanded great technical skill of the operator. Fortunately, the introduction of real-time technology greatly shortened and simplified the performance of sonographic examinations. The design of the transducer, which transmit and receives the sound waves, follows either the mechanical or array principle. The signal processing required for real-time sonography would not be possible without today's computer technology. The transducers are technical masterpieces of the highest precision with the penetration and resolution determined by the desired application. Today, an variety of transducers, each customized for specific application, is available, even for intraoperative and intracavitary examinations.

It is to be regretted that radiologists in many countries were late to recognize ultrasound as a powerful imaging method that could replace or complement radiographic examinations. As a consequence, ultrasound examinations are widely performed by various specialists and often only ultrasound examinations of the abdomen are left for the radiologist. Should these examinations be adopted by internists, surgeons and pediatricians, it would have negative ramifications. It will not only encourage overutilization of ultrasound because of self-referral but also endanger the quality of the examinations because of their performance by clinical specialists with conceivably insufficient knowledge and experience in the field of ultrasound. Referring patients to radiologists for ultrasound examinations would offer the best chance of lowering the number of incorrect or equivocal diagnoses that invariably would have lead to more and essentially unnecessary examinations. Thus, leaving ultrasound examinations under the control of radiologists would ultimately reduce the costs of health care.

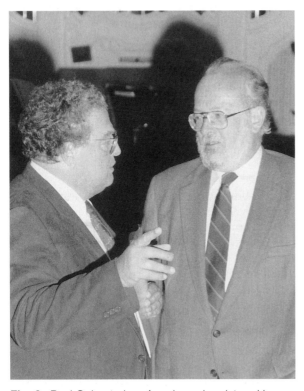

Fig. 3. Paul C. Lauterbur, American chemist and important contributor to imaging with magnetic resonance, in conversation with A. Scharmann in Lennep, Germany, at the awarding of the Roentgen Medal in 1987 (private collection)

Magnetic resonance imaging (MRI)

The CT scanner had hardly begun its triumphant entry in the mid-seventies when the American chemist P.C. Lauterbur (Fig. 3) caused excitement over a new type of imaging. In contrast to the CT scanner, this new method does not use X-rays or other ionizing radiation but is based on nuclear resonance. It had long been known that atomic nuclei have an inherent spin and their own magnetic field. When placed into a strong external magnetic field, they behave like compass needles and align themselves with the magnetic field. They also move around in a certain way at a frequency determined by the strength of the magnetic field and, by means of resonance, a radio frequency pulse of the same frequency will disturb the nuclei, decreasing their longitudinal magnetization and creating a new transversal magnetization. After the radio frequency is switched off, the atomic nuclei reestablish their previous alignment in the external magnetic field and, having their energy level raised by resonance with the radio frequency, release energy in the form of a weak radio signal. The time for the longitudinal magnetization to recover is called the longitudinal relaxation time or T1. The time for the transversal magnetization to disappear is called the transversal relaxation time or T2, and can also be seen as the time for the nuclei to get out of phase. T1 and T2 express tissue properties. Usually the hydrogen nuclei, i.e. protons, are measured since hydrogen is the most abundant element in the human body and relative to other nuclei produce the most intense signals. This is related to the fact that the hydrogen nucleus, comprising only a proton and no neutrons, has a strong magnetic dipole moment responsible for the spin. In principle, only atomic nuclei with an odd number of neutrons and protons have an externally measurable magnetic dipole moment, and are suitable for magnetic resonance imaging. In atoms containing an even number of protons and neutrons, the magnetic dipole moment would be neutralized.

Initially, magnetic resonance was used for the analysis of chemical compounds. The first article on magnetic resonance imaging submitted by Lauterbur to the English scientific magazine 'Nature' was rejected, with the reply stating that it was *'not of sufficient importance for publication in "Nature".'* Lauterbur insisted that his article be published by this particular magazine and asked if it could be reconsidered after revision. This was agreed and in the revised article Lauterbur demonstrated that carcinomatous tissue showed different signal properties compared to normal tissue. The first images of magnetic resonance tomography were published in 1977.

To process the signals coming from the object to be investigated into a two- or three-dimensional image, a gradient magnetic field along three directions is superimposed on the main magnetic field, so that each location in the object experiences has a different magnetic field strength and thus has its specific resonance frequency. All acquired data are integrated into images by the computer by means of very complex equations.

The technical advances have remarkably improved the quality of the images in subsequent years. New pulse sequences and new acquisitions were introduced to reduce the examination times. MRI is a highly sensitive method of differentiating soft-tissue structures. Entirely new diagnostic possibilities have opened up, particularly in the field of neuroradiology and degenerative joint diseases. Neuroradiology, which already had improved on account of CT was further enriched by MRI. Many indications are almost exclusively for MRI. In the diagnosis of skeletal disorders, CT has never played an important role, while MRI already has replaced many methods, for example arthrography or conventional tomography. Progress is so rapid that new indications for MRI are constantly added.

Within certain limits, the magnetic fields do not have any detrimental effects on patients. MRI provides soft-tissue images of high contrast, so that even the grey and white matter of the brain can be distinguished. Moreover, it allows three-dimensional reconstructions, a considerable advantage over CT before the arrival of spiral CT. The MRI images are not based on density differences as in CT, but on the distribution of hydrogen atoms in the tissues, which is relevant for the interpretation of the images. These advantages have to be balanced against the facts that MRI is a very complex and one of the most expensive techniques.

As mentioned earlier, magnetic resonance was initially used for chemical analysis. Today, spectroscopy needed for chemical analysis can be obtained together with the imaging process, so that biochemical processes can be analyzed in normal and diseased tissue. This allows investigations of the exact influence of new pharmaceutical agents at the tissue level. The end is not yet in sight as far as imaging and spectroscopy are concerned.

MRI equipment is susceptible to external magnetic influences but also exposes its environment to a strong magnetic field, potentially disturbing nearby installations. Shielding is therefore of great importance.

While CT represented an extraordinary progress, MRI was something completely new. Harnessing magnetic resonance phenomenon for medical imaging can be considered a major contribution to mankind, comparable to the discovery of X-rays. Radiologists hope that this will be acknowledged by the Nobel Foundation. Awarding the founders of MRI the Nobel Prize would greatly further basic research of medical imaging.

In 1991, approximately 6600 MR installations were in operation worldwide and, if the present trend continues, it has been estimated that western countries will have one MRI installation for approximately 100 000 inhabitants by the end of this century. In the USA and Japan, the ratio of one installation to 80 000 inhabitants has already been reached.

Diagnostic radiologist – new therapeutic radiologist?

The increase in size and scope of radiology eventually led to the separation into diagnostic radiology and therapeutic radiology. Both specialities work with ionizing radiation, with its property of tissue penetration used in diagnostic radiology – to obtain images of internal structures – and its property of energy deposition in therapeutic radiology – to treat neoplasms. Advancing catheterization techniques for therapeutic interventions have added interventional radiology as an additional branch of therapeutic radiology. X-rays and ultrasound have been largely relegated to localizing tools. Interventional methods offer simple, but often preferable alternatives to surgical procedures, since they are less invasive and stressful to the patient and performed at a lower cost. Interventional radiology connects conventional radiology with clinical specialities. As early as 1967, the American radiologist A.R. Margulis stated the concept of a physician who is skilled in radiological techniques and experienced in clinical problems.

As early as the 1920s, attempts had been made to reduce the intussusception (invagination of one segment of the intestine within another) in children with a barium enema and to drain the gallbladder empyema (suppuration) by means of a fluoroscopic guided puncture. However, it took interventional radiology four to five decades to devel-

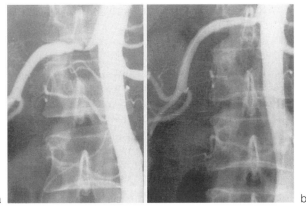

a

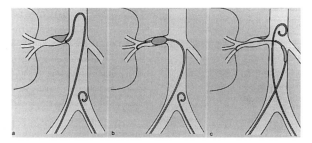

b

Fig. 4a, b. Renal artery stenosis before (**a**) and after (**b**) dilatation (1988).

Fig. 5a-c. Scheme of angioplasty in renal artery stenosis with the transfemoral guide-wire catheter method. **a.** Probing with the sidewinder catheter. **b.** Guide-wire fed through the stenosis, subsequently exchanged for a balloon catheter for dilatation. **c.** Follow-up angiography after removal of balloon catheter (1988).

op into a method accepted in its own right. Today, there are disease processes in almost any organ amenable to interventional radiology, particularly enabled by advancements in the design and manufacturing of catheters and necessary accessories.

Stenotic vessels can be widened by means of a balloon catheter. The catheter and its attached balloon are inserted into the narrowed segment under fluoroscopic guidance and the balloon expanded by inflation to the volume needed to dilate the vascular stenosis.

Catheters and balloons must be available in a variety of sizes and shapes, and the most suitable model selected for the different types of vascular stenoses found in the heart, kidneys (Figs 4 and 5), lower extremities or other parts of the body. Balloon catheters have a very refined double-lumen design with the additional lumen needed for inflating the balloon. The balloon must withstand a high inflation pressure without loosing its shape. Percutaneous transluminal angioplasty

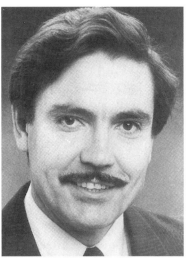

Fig. 7. Andreas Gruentzig (1939-1985). German internist who succeeded to perform percutaneous transluminal dilatation of coronary artery stenosis and other arterial stenoses by means of balloon catheters.

(PTA) or Dotter's method (Ch. Dotter, American radiologist, Fig. 6) has replaced many vascular surgeries. Andreas Gruentzig (Fig. 7) made important contributions to the development of PTA.

In addition to recanalizations, methods of obstruction are used. They are applied to embolize hypervascular tumors, to close arteriovenous fistulae, and to obliterate cysts or veins (e.g. varicocele). Depending on the condition, substances such as Gelfoam, alcohol or even small spirals can be delivered to the desired location via selectively inserted catheters.

Dilatation of the biliary or renal collecting system can be relieved by drainage through a percutaneously inserted catheter, frequently used as a palliative measure. The catheter can often be passed through the site of obstruction, restoring the physiologic route to some degree. Cysts, hemorrhages, effusions, and abscesses can also be drained percutaneously. Cognizance of the ap-

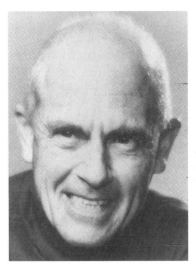

Fig. 6. Charles T. Dotter (1920-1985). American radiologist, one of the spiritual fathers of interventional radiology. He introduced percutaneous transluminal angioplasty (PTA) (1964) and designed devices for interventions.

propriate entry passage is mandatory to avoid unnecessary damage to adjacent organs.

Intravascular and intracardiac objects that have been left behind following pacemaker implantation or angiography and even emboli can be retrieved percutaneously under fluoroscopy with grasping devices attached to the tip of the catheter or a snare-loop catheter. Stones in the bile ducts or renal collecting system can often be extracted percutaneously. Renal and ureteral stones can also be removed by lithotripsy. After stereoscopic localization, extracorporeal sonographic shock waves are aimed at the stone for disintegration, with the produced fragments usually small enough for spontaneous passage.

Interventional radiology is still in its growth phase. To treat stenoses of vessels, biliary ducts, etc. that are recalcitrant to dilatation, intraluminal prostheses (stents) have been designed for percutaneous insertion via a catheter. These prostheses usually consist of a wire mesh that expands to its full diameter after advancement into the luminal obstruction. Furthermore, several mechanical recanalization devices have been designed, such as catheters with a rotational cam or torque-controlled cutter at their tip. In acute intravascular thrombosis, the catheter tip can be placed in front of the thrombus and a thrombolytic agent administered via the catheter. Filters can be percutaneously inserted into the inferior vena cava as prophylactic measure in patients at risk of developing pulmonary emboli. The filter is released after placement in the desired position and its umbrella-like or net-like wire mesh should trap any significant emboli while preserving blood flow. In addition to Charles T. Dotter and Andreas Grüntzig, who have already been mentioned, many others have made major contributions to interventional radiology, including Werner Porstmann, Kurt Amplatz, Cesare Gianturco, Sidney Wallace, H. Joachim Burhenne, Josef Rösch, and Rolf W. Günther.

Percutaneous biopsies have also gained in significance. Under guidance by sonography or CT, lesions in the abdominal or thoracic cavity as well as lymph nodes of the extremities or neck can be punctured and tissue obtained for cytologic or histologic examination. Previously, this often could only accomplished with major operations. Establishing the diagnosis of an unclear finding has become faster and less distressing for the patient and, moreover, less costly.

Requirements in training and continued education

Diagnostic radiology has become a comprehensive and versatile field today. It is comprehensive because it includes the entire patient, involves all clinical specialties and uses a variety of methods. It is versatile because it uses not only X-rays as imaging medium but also ultrasound and magnetic resonance, which are two completely different imaging media. The radiologist has to know the biological effects of radiation, observe proper radiation protection and be familiar with data processing systems, including the use of computers in imaging manipulation. The administration of contrast media requires a basic knowledge of pharmacology. If radiology is to take part in the scientific pursuit of MR spectroscopy, knowing biochemistry is a prerequisite. Thus, the modern radiologist must be a physician with knowledge in physics, biochemistry, pharmacology and engineering, including computer science.

Proficiency in computer science is not only essential for individual examination techniques, such as CT and MRI, but in the future also for image processing, communication and data exchange. This was already mentioned by William Penn in his inaugural address in 1970. Conventional radiographs will decline in importance over the next few years since image interpretation will increasingly take place at the monitor. The image can be manipulated at the monitor for better evaluation of details, for quantitative measurements, or for three-dimensional reconstructions that are valuable for surgical planning. Through networking with the PACS system, examinations can be transmitted and reviewed in various locations at any time, completely eliminating radiographic films. In difficult diagnostic cases, the images can be rapidly and easily transmitted by telephone to a specialist for consultation. Thus, the results of examinations are always available at one's disposal. In the future, storage of radiographic information will largely or exclusively be carried out digitally. It is possible to compress and store data on optical disks, but this technology is still undergoing constant modifications and advancements.

The training of a diagnostic radiologist takes a long time and demands great efforts from both the resident in training and the teaching radiologist. Because of the complexity of radiology, adequate training is only feasible in large clinics or university hospitals that can guarantee involvement of trained personnel (specialized radiolo-

Table 1

Relative costs for examination of patients	Before CT/MR	now
with rectum carcinoma	84.3	18.3
after abdominal trauma	37.0	22.9
with penetrating trauma to the flank	105.9	23.6
with anuria	12.4	6.3
with abdominal aortic aneurysm	25.4	6.3
with obstructive jaundice	37.9	14.6
with focal epilepsy	546.8	98.7
	Before mammography	now
with palpable mammary lesion	31.7	9.9

gists, physicists, biochemists, engineers) in the teaching program and a sufficient number of patients. Radiology departments of such institutions should be responsible for and proficient in all imaging modalities. In addition, it is important that areas of specialization are developed within these departments, preferably according to organ systems or clinical specialties, such as neurology, ENT, lungs, heart, abdomen, skeleton and pediatrics, with integration of the required technologies. The development of organ-related specialization facilitates the communication and cooperation with the clinical specialist. Specialization according to method or equipment is not desirable in diagnostic radiology since it leads to an approach that is to narrow for the complexity encountered in medicine.

Technology – increase or reduction of costs?

In Central Europe, the contribution of high technology medicine adds up to only 1% to the total health care expenses. Though a relatively small amount, it should not rise any further. Certainly, the new imaging technologies of CT, MRI and PET are expensive, but they can provide relevant information unattainable with examinations that are more uncomfortable and often riskier. Their replacement will have a cost saving effect. The new image modalities must be used judicially, guided by strict indications, and properly interpreted, to avoid redundancy and repetition. High technology radiology that is hospital-based and practiced by team-oriented radiologists will produce superb diagnostic work. In addition to internal quality assurance committees, interactions with referring physicians will maintain a high level of quality.

In the U.S.A., the total health care costs amounted to 13.4% of the gross national product in 1992 but was only 7.3% in 1970. The presumed causes of this increase are inflation, population growth, increase proportion of old people in the population, and overutilization technological procedures and laboratory tests, but also more complex disease entities. R.G. Parker has compiled a list of the relative costs of establishing various diagnoses before and after introduction of CT and MRI (Radiology 1993; 189: 363-369) (Table 1).

Self-referral is expensive since often it is overeager and unnecessary. Limiting or prohibiting self-referral would only slightly increase the radiologists' work but provide an incentive for the clinician to be more careful with his request for radiographic studies. The health insurance industry should also discourage self-referral by paying less for studies performed by the referring physician and, furthermore, should ask for regulatory measures. Unnecessary and poor quality radiographic examinations as a result of self-referral would increase radiation exposure and make health care more expensive (Evens 1993).

Final conclusion

Our journey through the history of radiology has consistently demonstrated the interrelationship between medicine and technology and how interdisciplinary discussions have led to improvements and new ideas in both technical and medical fields. Industrial research laboratories supported by large companies are particularly positioned to conceive and implement new ideas. Investing in new developments is of tremendous consequence for the industry to survive the tough competition and of extreme importance for the patients to be guaranteed the best, safest and least demanding diagnostic methods and most effective therapies. Promising methods or techniques that have failed or were soon superseded should not be seen as a waste of resources since the knowledge and experience gained through them might bear fruit later in other ways. To assess the medical merits of equipment and techniques, they should be tested in large institutions. Clinical physicists responsible for quality control should be in every large radiology department. They are the important intermediaries between physicians and representatives of research and industry. Moreover, they should assume new responsibilities in developing criteria that assist in evaluating test results – either by means of quantitative analysis or through training programs and expert systems.

Radiologists and engineers should not consider new methods and techniques as ends in themselves. Technology should serve radiologists to disclose and document diseases. When properly indicated and performed professionally, radiographic examinations subject patients to a relatively low radiation dose. Nevertheless, alternative methods, particularly ultrasound, should be used if they can provide the same or even more information.

The patient should be informed of the purpose of the examination and of the role of the equipment used for the examination. The patient should not be at the mercy of physicians who have become technocrats. Physicians and engineers should work together to make the examinations as comfortable for the patients as possible and, at the same time, as high in quality and diagnostic content as achievable.

List of sources for the illustrations

Fig. I, 1 - I, 9 Deutsches Röntgenmuseum, Remscheid-Lennep

Fig. I, 10 - 12 Walter Friedrich, Leben und Werk. Hrsg. vom Friedensrat der DDR, Berlin (1963), Fig. XXXIII

Fig. I, 13 Deutsches Museum, München

Fig. I, 14 - 16 Deutsches Röntgenmuseum, Remscheid-Lennep

Fig. I, 17 - 20 Siemens Med. Archiv, Erlangen

Fig. I, 21 Private source of the author

Fig. I, 22 - 25 Deutsches Röntgenmuseum, Remscheid-Lennep

Fig. I, 26 Acta Radiologica 34 (1950), 422

Fig. I, 27 Deutsches Röntgenmuseum, Remscheid-Lennep

Fig. I, 28 Siemens Med. Archiv, Erlangen

Fig. I, 29 Deutsches Röntgenmuseum, Remscheid-Lennep

Fig. II, 1 Deutsches Röntgenmuseum, Remscheid-Lennep

Fig. II, 2 Köhler, A.: Lexikon der Grenzen des Normalen und der Anfänge des Pathologischen im Röntgenbilde. Lucas Gräfe und Sillem, Hamburg (1910)

Fig. II, 3 - 4 Deutsches Röntgenmuseum, Remscheid-Lennep

Fig. II, 5 Schinz et al.: Lehrbuch der Röntgendiagnostik. 6. Auflage, Georg Thieme Verlag, Stuttgart (1979) Band II, Teil 1: S. 54-55

Fig. II, 6 Dr. Bosnjakovic-Büscher, Städt. Krankenhaus, Sindelfingen

Fig. II, 7 Private source of the author

Fig. II, 8 Prof. Hauke, Rad. Abt. des Olga Hospitals, Stuttgart

Fig. II, 9 Albers-Schönberg, E.: Eine bisher nicht beschriebene Allgemeinerkrankung des Skelettes im Röntgenbild. Fortschr. Röntgenstr. 11 (1907), Tafel XVII

Fig. II, 10a Albers-Schönberg, E.: Eine seltene bisher nicht bekannte Strukturanomalie des Skelettes. Fortschr. Röntgenstr. 23 (1915/16), Tafel VII

Fig. II, 10b Private source of the author

Fig. II, 11 Sudeck, P.: Über die akute reflektorische Knochenatrophie und Entzündungen und Verletzungen an den Extremitäten und ihre klinischen Erscheidungen. Fortschr. Röntgenstr. 5 (1901/2), Tafel XVI

Fig. II, 12 - 17 Private source of the author

Fig. II, 18 Private source: E. Looser, Zürich

Fig. II, 19 Private source of the author

Fig. II, 20 Siemens Med. Archiv, Erlangen

Fig. II, 21 Am. J. Roentgenol. 36 (1936): 106

Fig. II, 22 Albers-Schönberg, H.: Die Röntgentechnik II. Lucas Gräfe und Sillem, Hamburg (1909) Fig. 119

Fig. II, 23 Albers-Schönberg, H.: Die Röntgentechnik. Lucas Gräfe und Sillem, Hamburg (1903) S. 72, Fig. 33

Fig. II, 24 Siemens Med. Archiv, Erlangen

Fig. II, 25 Groedel, F.M.: Röntgendiagnostik in der inneren Medizin und Grenzgebieten. J.F. Lehmann Verlag, München (1921) S. 43, Fig. 54-57

Fig. II, 26 - 27 Assmann, H.: Klinische Röntgendiagnostik der inneren Erkrankungen. F.C.W. Vogel, Leipzig (1922), Fig. 1, 2 und 14

Fig. II, 28 Assmann, H.: Klinische Röntgendiagnostik der inneren Erkrankungen. 2. Auflage, Gustav Fischer Verlag, Jena (1922), Fig. 2 und 3

Fig. II, 29 Albers-Schönberg, H.: Die Röntgentechnik. Lucas Gräfe und Sillem, Hamburg (1903) S. 227, Fig. 68

Fig. II, 30 Assmann, H.: Klinische Röntgendiagnostik der inneren Erkrankungen. 2. Auflage, Gustav Fischer Verlag, Jena (1922), Fig. 13

Fig. II, 31 Assmann, H.: Erfahrungen über die Röntgenuntersuchung der Lungen. Gustav Fischer

Verlag, Jena (1914) Tafel VIII, Fig. 32

Fig. II, 32 - 33   Rieder H., J. Rosenthal: Lehrbuch der Röntgenkunde. Band I., Johann Ambrosius Barth, Leipzig (1913) Fig. 30 und 40

Fig. II, 34   Assmann, H.: Erfahrungen über die Röntgenuntersuchung der Lungen. Gustav Fischer Verlag, Jena (1914) Tab. XII, Fig. 45

Fig. II, 35 - 36   Schinz, H.R., W. Baensch, E. Friedl: Lehrbuch der Röntgendiagnostik. Thieme Verlag, Leipzig (1928), S. 487, Fig. 787 und 788

Fig. II, 37   Deutsches Röntgenmuseum, Remscheid-Lennep

Fig. II, 38   Groedel, F.M.: Röntgendiagnostik in der inneren Medizin und Grenzgebieten. J.F. Lehmann Verlag, München (1921) S. 386, Fig. 219 bis 221

Fig. II, 39 - 43   Private source of the author

Fig. II, 44   Deutsches Röntgenmuseum, Remscheid-Lennep

Fig. II, 45   Salomon, A.: Beiträge zur Pathologie und Klinik der Mammakarzinome. Arch. klin. chir. 103 (1913) 573

Fig. II, 46   Vogel, W.: Die Röntgendarstellung von Mammatumoren. Arch. klin. Chir. 171 (1931/32) 618-626

Fig. II, 47   Leborgne, R.: Diagnosis of tumors. Am. J. Roentgenol. 65 (1951) 1

Fig. II, 48   Gershon-Cohen: Atlas of Mammography. Springer Verlag, Berlin (1970)

Fig. II, 49   Hicken, N.F.: Mammography: roentgenologic diagnosis of breast tumors by means of contrast media. Surg. Gyn. & Obst. 64 (1937) 593-603

Fig. II, 50   J. Radiol. 66 (1985) 1

Fig. II, 51   Gros, Ch.M.: Les maladies du sein. Masson, Paris (1963), Abb. 168a

Fig. II, 52 - 53   Private source of the author

Fig. II, 54   Dobretsberger, W.: Die isodensische Weichteilaufnahme. Radiologe 5 (1965) 28

Fig. II, 55   Friedrich, M.: Der Einfluß der Streustrahlung auf die Abbildungsqualität bei der Mammographie. Fortschr. Röntgenstr. 123, 6 (1975) 556-566

Fig. II, 56   Friedrich, M.: Neuere Entwicklungstendenzen in der Mammographie Technik: Die Raster Mammographie.

Fortschr. Röntgenstr. 128 (1978) 2

Fig. II, 57 - 62   Private source of the author

Fig. III, 1   Siemens Med. Archiv, Erlangen

Fig. III, 2a,b   Medica Mundi. Philips Zeitschrift, Eindhoven

Fig. III, 2c   Siemens Med. Archiv, Erlangen

Fig. III, 3   Deutsches Röntgenmuseum, Remscheid-Lennep

Fig. III, 4 - III, 7   Private source of the author

Fig. III, 8 - III, 9   Deutsches Röntgenmuseum, Remscheid-Lennep

Fig. III, 10 - 16   Stierlin, E.: Klinische Röntgendiagnostik des Verdauungskanals. F. Bergmann, Wiesbaden (1916)

Fig. III, 17 - 18   Assmann, H.: Klinische Röntgendiagnostik der inneren Erkrankungen. 2. Auflage, F.C.W. Vogel, Leipzig (1922)

Fig. III, 19 - 20   Carman, R.D.: The Roentgen diagnosis of the diseases of the alimentary canal. Second edition, Saunders, Philadelphia (1921)

Fig. III, 21   Berg, H.H.: Röntgenuntersuchungen am Innenrelief des Verdauungskanals. 2. Auflage, Thieme Verlag, Leipzig (1931)

Fig. III, 22   Teschendorf, W.: Lehrbuch der röntgenologischen Differentialdiagnostik der Erkrankungen der Bauchorgane. Thieme Verlag, Leipzig (1937)

Fig. III, 23 - 24   Golden, R.: Radiological examination of the small intestine. Lippincott, Philadelphia (1945)

Fig. III, 25 - 29   Private source of the author

Fig. III, 30a,b, 31   Beck, C.: Die Röntgenuntersuchung der Leber und der Gallenblase. In: Groedel, F.M.: Atlas und Grundriß der Röntgendiagnostik im inneren Medizin. J.F. Lehmann Verlag, München (1909) Fig. 107, 140 und 141

Fig. III, 32 - 33   Deutsches Röntgenmuseum, Remscheid-Lennep

Fig. III, 34   Schinz, H.R. et al.: Lehrbuch der Röntgendiagnostik. 1. Auflage, Thieme Verlag, Leipzig (1928) S. 1070, Fig. 154

Fig. III, 35   Frommhold, W.: Gallensystem. In: Schinz, H.R. et al.: Lehrbuch der Röntgendiagnostik. Band V, 6. Auflage, Georg Thieme Verlag, Stuttgart (1965) S. 390, Abb. 38

Fig. III, 36   Schinz, H.R. et al.: Lehrbuch der Röntgendiagnostik. Band IV, 5. Auflage, Georg Thieme

Verlag, Stuttgart (1952) S. 3508, Fig. 4419

Fig. III, 37 - 40   Frommhold, W.: Gallensystem. In: Schinz, H.R. et al.: Lehrbuch der Röntgendiagnostik. Band V, 6. Auflage, Georg Thieme Verlag, Stuttgart (1965) S. 402, Fig. 56a; S. 406, Fig. 64; S. 406, Fig. 66; S. 408, Fig. 71

Fig. III, 41   Joseph, E.: Die Harnorgane im Röntgenbild. Thieme Verlag, Leipzig (1926)

Fig. III, 42   Voelcker, F., A. von Lichtenberg: Pyelography. Münch. med. Wschr. 53 (1906) 105-106

Fig. III, 43   Joseph, E.: Die Harnorgane im Röntgenbild. Thieme Verlag, Leipzig (1926)

Fig. III, 44 - 45   Schinz, H.R., W. Baensch, E. Friedl: Lehrbuch der Röntgendiagnostik. Thieme Verlag, Leipzig (1928)

Fig. III, 46 - 48   Deutsches Röntgenmuseum, Remscheid-Lennep

Fig. III, 49a,b,c,d   Cocchi, V.: Retropneumoperitoneum und Pneumomediastinum. Georg Thieme Verlag, Stuttgart (1957) S. 13, Fig. 9; S. 25, Fig. 20; S. 29, Fig. 21 und 22

Fig. III, 49e   Rosenstein, P.: Pneumoradiology of kidney position. Z. Urol. 15 (1921) 447-458

Fig. III, 50   Schinz, H.R., W. Baensch, E. Friedl: Lehrbuch der Röntgendiagnostik. Thieme Verlag, Leipzig (1928)

Fig. III, 51a   Deutsches Röntgenmuseum, Remscheid-Lennep

Fig. III, 51b - 52   Boehminghaus, H.: Urologische Diagnostik und Therapie für Ärzte und Studierende. Gustav Fischer Verlag, Jena (1927)

Fig. III, 53   Joseph, E.: Die Harnorgane im Röntgenbild. Thieme Verlag, Leipzig (1926)

Fig. III, 54   Swick, M.: Visualization of the kidney and urinary tract on roentgenograms by means of intravenous administration of a new contrast medium: Uroselectan. Klin. Wschr. 8 (1929) 2087-2089

Fig. III, 55   Löhr, E., P. Mellin, G. Rodeck, J.W. Rohen: Atlas der urologischen Röntgendiagnostik. Schattauer Verlag, Stuttgart, New York (1976)

Fig. III, 56   Rousthöi, P.: Über Angiocardiographie. Vorläufige Mittei-

lung. Acta Radiologica 14 (1933) 419-424 (19)

Fig. III, 57   Radner, S.: Technical equipment for vasal catheterization. Acta Radiologica 31 (1949) 152-154 (26)

Fig. III, 58 - 59   Jönsson, G.: Thoracic aortography by means of a cannula inserted percutaneously into the common carotid artery. Acta Radiologica 31 (1949) 376-386 (28)

Fig. III, 60   Jönsson, G., B. Broden, J. Karnell: Thoracic aortography. Acta Radiologica, Suppl. (1951)

Fig. III, 61   Radner, S.: Vertebral angiography by catheterization. A new method employed in 221 cases. Acta Radiologica, Suppl. 87 (1951)

Fig. III, 62   Private source of the author

Fig. III, 63   Seldinger, S.I.: Catheter replacement of the needle in percutaneous arteriography. A new technique. Acta Radiologica 39 (1953) 368-376 (45)

Fig. III, 64 - 66   Gidlund, A.: Development of apparatus and methods for roentgen studies in haemodynamics. Acta Radiologica 1956, suppl. 130 (60)

Fig. III, 67   Sones, F.M.: Cine-cardio-angiography. Pediatr. Clin. North Am. 5 (1958) 945-979 (64)

Fig. III, 68   Judkins, M.P.: Selective coronary arteriography. Part I. A percutaneous transfemoral technic. Radiology 89 (1967) 815-824 (100)

Fig. III, 69   Silvestre, M.E., F. Abecasis, J.A. Veiga-Pires: Radiology. Elsevier Science Publishers B.V., Excerpta Medica, Amsterdam (1987)

Fig. III, 70   Private source: O. Olsson

Fig. III, 71 - 72   Bierman, H.R., E.R. Miller, R.L. Byron Jr et al.: Intra-arterial catheterization of viscera in man. Am. J. Roentgenol. 66 (1951) 555-568 (17)

Fig. III, 73   Ödman, P.: Percutaneous selective angiography of the main branches of the aorta. Acta Radiologica 45 (1956) 1-14 (20)

Fig. III, 74   Tillander, H.: Selective angiography of the abdominal aorta with a guided catheter. Acta Radiologica 45 (1956) 21-26 (22)

Fig. III, 75   Unpublished

Fig. III, 76   Deutsches Röntgenmuseum, Remscheid-Lennep

Fig. III, 77   Private source of the author

Fig. III, 78   Deutsches Röntgenmuseum, Remscheid-Lennep

Fig. III, 79   Private source of the author

Fig. III, 80   Koch, J.W.: Angiocardiografie in de diagnostiek van longafwijkingen - angiopneumografie. Thesis

Fig. III, 81 - 83   Private source of the author

Fig. III, 84   Heintzen et al.: Z. Elektr. Med. 12, 82 (1967), S. 84, Fig. 1

Fig. III, 85   Heintzen u. Bürsch: Kreislaufmessungen. Band V, 149, Werk Verlag, Banaschewski, München (1965) S. 152, Fig. 3

Fig. III, 86   Heintzen et al.: Com. Biomed. Res. 4, 474 (1971), S. 488, Fig. 2

Fig. III, 87   Brennecke et al.: Proc. Comp. Cardiol., IEEE Computer Society, Long Beach, 255 (1976), Fig. 5 und 11

Fig. III, 88   Heintzen, in: Riemann, H.E, J. Kollath: Digitale Radiographie. Schnetztor Verlag, Konstanz (1985), S. 358, Fig. 7a/c

Fig. III, 89   Private source of the author

Fig. III, 90   Heintzen et al., in: Kaltenbach, M., P. Lichtlen: Coronary Heart Disease. Georg Thieme Verlag, Stuttgart (1978) S. 119, Fig. 4

Fig. III, 91   Private source of the author

Fig. III, 92   Collins, S.M., D.J. Skorton: Cardiac Imaging and Image Processing. McGraw-Hill Comp., New York (1986), S. 268, Fig. 3

Fig. III, 93   Bürsch und Heintzen: Radiol. Clin. N. Amer. 23, 321 (1985): 325, Fig. 3

Fig. III, 94   Bürsch et al.: Radiology 141, 39 (1981): 43, Fig. 5

Fig. III, 95   Bürsch et al.: In: Heintzen, P.H., J. Brennecke: Digital Imaging in Cardiovascular Radiology. Georg Thieme Verlag, Stuttgart (1983), S. 122, Fig. 10

Fig. III, 96   Haschek, E., D.T. Lindenthal: Ein Beitrag zur praktischen Verwertung der Photographie nach Roentgen. Wiener klin. Wschr. 9 (1896) 63

Fig. III, 97   Berberich, J., S. Hirsch: Die röntgenographische Darstellung der Arterien und Venen am Lebenden. Münch. med. Wschr. 49 (1923) 226

Fig. III, 98   Brooks, B.: Intraarterial injection of sodium iodid. JAMA 82 (1924) 1016

Fig. III, 99 - 100   Deutsches Röntgenmuseum, Remscheid-Lennep

Fig. III, 101   Janker, R.: Röntgenologische Funktionsdiagnostik. Verlag Girardet, Wuppertal-Elbersfeld (1954)

Fig. III, 102   Siemens Med. Archiv, Erlangen

Fig. III, 103   Janker, R.: Röntgenologische Funktionsdiagnostik. Verlag Girardet, Wuppertal-Elbersfeld (1954)

Fig. III, 104   Zeitler, E.: Aorto-Arteriographie. In: Angiologie, Begr. v. M. Ratschow, Heberer, G., Rau, G., Schoop, W. 2. Auflage, Thieme Verlag, (1974)

Fig. III, 105 - 106   Janker, R.: Röntgenologische Funktionsdiagnostik. Verlag Girardet, Wuppertal-Elbersfeld (1954)

Fig. III, 107   Zeitler, E.: Aorto-Arteriographie. In: Angiologie, Begr. v. M. Ratschow, Heberer, G., Rau, G., Schoop, W. 2. Auflage, Georg Thieme Verlag, (1974)

Fig. III, 108 - 110   Private source of the author

Fig. III, 111 - 112   Siemens Med. Archiv, Erlangen

Fig. III, 113 - 114   Private source of the author

Fig. III, 115   Schinz, H.R. et al.: Ergebnisse der medizinischen Strahlenforschung. Neue Folge Band I. Georg Thieme Verlag, Stuttgart (1964), S. 258-259, Fig. 11-13

Fig. III, 116 - 117   Private source of the author

Fig. III, 118 - 123   Schinz, H.R. et al.: Radiologische Diagnostik in Klinik und Praxis. 7. Auflage, Georg Thieme Verlag, Stuttgart (1984)

Fig. III, 124 - 125   Private source of the author

Fig. IV, 1 - 2   Siemens Med. Archiv, Erlangen

Fig. IV, 3   Röntgentaschenbuch, hrsg. von E. Sommer, Band VIII, Otto Nemmich, München-Leipzig (1919) S. 104

Fig. IV, 4   Deutsches Röntgenmuseum, Remscheid-Lennep

Fig. IV, 5   Private source of the author

Fig. IV, 6   Stieve, F.E.: Bevorzugte Darstellung einzelner Körperschichten. In: Vieten, H. et al.: Handbuch der Medizinischen Radiologie, Band III. Springer Verlag, Berlin, Heidelberg und New York (1967) 715-1041

Fig. IV, 7   Deutsches Röntgenmuseum, Remscheid-Lennep

Fig. IV, 8 - 12   Stieve, F.E.: Bevorzugte Darstellung einzelner Körperschichten. In: Vieten, H. et al.: Handbuch der Medizinischen Radiologie, Band III. Springer Verlag, Berlin, Heidelberg und New York (1967) 715-1041

Fig. IV, 13 - 15   Gebauer, A. et al.: Das Rönt-
genschichtbild. Georg Thieme
Verlag, Stuttgart (1959), S. 61;
Fig. 98-99; S. 111, Fig. 182-183;
S. 220-221, Fig. 343-345

Fig. IV, 16   Private source: Prof. G. Rosenbusch

Fig. IV, 17 - 18   Electromedica, Zeitschrift
Siemens Erlangen

Fig. IV, 19   Radiology 176 (1990) 181-183

Fig. IV, 20 - 22   Electromedica, Zeitschrift
Siemens Erlangen

Fig. IV, 23 - 24   Deutsches Röntgenmuseum,
Remscheid-Lennep

Fig. IV, 25 - 31   Holfelder, H. et al.: Erg. med.
Strahlenforsch., Band II.
Thieme Verlag, Leipzig (1926)
S. 15, Fig. 8; S. 17, Fig. 11; S. 18,
Fig. 12a; S. 30, Fig. 20; S. 34-35,
Fig. 25, 26c; S. 36, Fig. 27; S. 39,
Fig. 30

Fig. IV, 32   Deutsches Röntgenmuseum,
Remscheid-Lennep

Fig. IV, 33   Poppe, H.: Technik der Rönt-
gendiagnostik. Georg Thieme
Verlag, Stuttgart (1961), S. 45,
Fig. 15a-c

Fig. IV, 34   Deutsches Röntgenmuseum,
Remscheid-Lennep

Fig. IV, 35 - 37   Siemens Med. Archiv, Erlangen

Fig. IV, 38   Deutsches Röntgenmuseum,
Remscheid-Lennep

Fig. IV, 39   Electromedica, Zeitschrift
Siemens Erlangen

Fig. IV, 40 - 41   Krayenbühl, H., M.G. Yasargil:
Die zerebrale Angiographie.
Georg Thieme Verlag, Stuttgart
(1965) S. 4, Fig. 1-2; S. 9, Fig. 7

Fig. IV, 42   Electromedica, Zeitschrift
Siemens Erlangen

Fig. IV, 43   Krayenbühl, H., M.G. Yasargil:
Die zerebrale Angiographie.
Georg Thieme Verlag, Stuttgart
(1965) S. 9, Fig. 7

Fig. IV, 44   Holfelder, H. et al.: Erg. med.
Strahlenforsch., Band II.
Thieme Verlag, Leipzig (1926)
S. 121, Fig. 1

Fig. IV, 45   Peiper, H.: Die Myelographie im
Dienste der Diagnostik von Er-
krankungen des Rückenmarks.
Erg. med. Strahlenforsch. Band
II (1926)

Fig. IV, 46 - 52   Private source of the author

Fig. IV, 53a   Gebauer, A., E. Muntean, E.
Stutz, H. Vieten: Das Röntgen-
schichtverfahren.
Georg Thieme Verlag, Stuttgart
(1959) 6

Fig. IV, 53b - 72   Private source of the author

Fig. IV, 73   Da Vinci, L.: Anatomische
Zeichnungen aus der königli-
chen Bibliothek auf Schloß
Windsor. Prisma Verlag,
Gütersloh (1979)

Fig. IV, 74 - 77   Private source of the author

Fig. V, 1   Deutsches Röntgenmuseum,
München

Fig. V, 2 - 6   Siemens Med. Archiv, Erlangen

Fig. V, 7   Fuchs, F.: Elektrische Strahlen
und ihre Anwendung (Rönt-
gentechnik). Aus: Dannen-
mann, F. Der Werdegang der
Entdeckungen und Erfindungen, Verlag R. Oldenburg,
München und Berlin (1922),
S. 31, Fig. 14.

Fig. V, 8   Patent DP 370022 vom 2. Feb.
1918, Dr. Otto Goetze (Frank-
furt a.M.): Verfahren und
Glühkathodenröntgenröhre
zur Erzeugung scharfer Röntgenbilder.

Fig. V, 9   Private source: Frau Dr.
O. Goetze, Fürth.

Fig. V, 10   Silbermann, K.: Hochleistungsröhren. Röntgen-Bl. (1964)
17. Jg. H 7, S. 290, Fig. 7.

Fig. V, 11a   Patent DP 406067 vom 17. Feb.
1923, Georg Conrad Kucher,
Phönix Röntgenfabriken Rudolstadt: Glühkathoden-Röntgenröhre mit hohem Vakuum

Fig. V, 11b - 12   Siemens Med. Archiv, Erlangen

Fig. V, 13   Dietz, K.: Altes und Neuen über
Röntgenröhren. Sonderdruck
für Siemens-Reiniger-Werke AG
Erlangen aus Röntgenpraxis,
Verlag S. Hirzel, Stuttgart
(1964) S. 30, Fig. 21.

Fig. V, 14   Bouwers, A.: Verleihung der
Röntgenplakette. Röntgen-Bl.
(1963) 16. Jg. H 7, S. 234.

Fig. V, 15   Bouwers, A.: Der Brennfleck
einer Röntgenröhre und seine
Belastbarkeit - Eine Metallröntgenröhre mit drehbarer Anode.
Fortschr. Röntgenstr. (1929) 40:
284-292.

Fig. V, 16   Silbermann, K.: Hochleistungsröhren. Röntgen-Bl. (1964)
17. Jg. H 7, S. 285, Fig. 2.

Fig. V, 17 - 19   Siemens Med. Archiv, Erlangen

Fig. V, 20   Patent DP 1951383 vom 11. Okt.
1969, R. Friedel und W. Wiche
(Siemens): Röntgenröhren-
Drehanode mit einem Ver-
bundkörper aus einem Schwermetallteil und wenigstens einem
Graphitteil und Verfahren zu
ihrer Herstellung.

Fig. V, 21   Siemens Med. Archiv, Erlangen

Fig. V, 22   Dietz, K.: Die Röntgenröhre im diagnostischen Einsatz. Sonderdruck aus Röntgenberichte (1974) Bd. 3, H 1 und 2, S. 13, Fig. 9.

Fig. V, 23   Patent DP 2112672 vom 16. März 1971, K. Dietz, A. Lehnert, K. Silbermann, A. Elsas, G. Appelt: Röntgenröhren-Drehanodenteller.

Fig. V, 24   Patent DE 2852908 vom 7. Dez. 1978, J. Gerkema und E.A. Muijderman: Drehanodenröhre.

Fig. V, 25   Patent DP 2708612 vom 28. Feb. 1977, E. Watanabe, Japan: Vorrichtung zur Gewinnung eines Röntgenstrahlenbildes in einer Querschnittsebene eines Objektes.

Fig. V, 26 - 27   Siemens Med. Archiv, Erlangen

Fig. V, 28a   Fuchs, F.: Elektrische Strahlen und ihre Anwendung (Röntgentechnik). Aus: Dannenmann, F.: Der Werdegang der Entdeckungen und Erfindungen, Verlag R. Oldenburg, München und Berlin (1922) S. 32, Fig. 16.

Fig. V, 28b   Gerthsen, Ch.: Physik. 6. Auflage, Springer Verlag, Berlin (1960), S. 264, Fig. 339.

Fig. V, 29 - 31   Siemens Med. Archiv, Erlangen

Fig. V, 32   Hackl, A.: Röntgenapparate und ihre Schaltungen. Verlag von Hachmeister und Thal, Leipzig (1929). Band VIII von Hachmeister und Thals Schaltungsbücher, S. 17, Fig. 17.

Fig. V, 33   Patent DP 120340 vom 3. Jan. 1899, Dr. Arthur Wehnelt, Charlottenburg: Elektrolytischer Stromunterbrecher.

Fig. V, 34 - 36   Siemens Med. Archiv, Erlangen

Fig. V, 37   Hackl, A.: Röntgenapparate und ihre Schaltungen. Verlag von Hachmeister und Thal, Leipzig (1929). Band VIII von Hachmeister und Thals Schaltungsbücher, S. 25, Fig. 28

Fig. V, 38   Siemens Med. Archiv, Erlangen

Fig. V, 39   Patent DP 292596 vom 29. Juli 1915, Siemens & Halske, Berlin: Einrichtung zum Betrieb von Röntgenröhren mit von Mehrphasenstrom gespeisten Hochspannungstransformatoren.

Fig. V, 40   Siemens Med. Archiv, Erlangen

Fig. V, 41   Patent DP 296464 vom 11. Juni 1916: Siemens & Halske, Berlin: Einrichtung zum Betrieb von Röntgenröhren.

Fig. V, 42 - 43   Siemens Med. Archiv, Erlangen

Fig. V, 44   Patent DP 968848 vom 28. Nov. 1944, Dipl.-Ing. Kurt Bischoff und Ehrhardt Leuteritz, SRW Erlangen: Vorrichtung zur Voreinstellung von Betriebswerten eines Röntgenapparates.

Fig. V, 45   Private source: Dr. Kurt Franke, Erlangen

Fig. V, 46 - 49   Siemens Med. Archiv, Erlangen

Fig. V, 50   Fuchs, F.: Elektrische Strahlen und ihre Anwendung (Röntgentechnik). Aus: Dannenmann, F.: Der Werdegang der Entdeckungen und Erfindungen, Verlag R. Oldenburg, München und Berlin (1922), S. 35, Fig. 19.

Fig. V, 51   Patent 225500 vom 2. März 1909, Siemens & Halske, Berlin: Hochspannungsgleichrichter für Wechselstrom.

Fig. V, 52   Siemens Med. Archiv, Erlangen

Fig. V, 53   Patent 1029948 vom 7. Feb. 1957, Johannes Seidel, SRW Erlangen: Röntgen-Eintankapparat.

Fig. V, 54   Patent 416486 vom 11. Juni 1920 (USA vom 24. Jan. 1919), Intern. General Electric Comp., New York: Röntgenstrahlenapparat mit einer in ein Ölbad eingetauchten Röntgenröhre.

Fig. V, 55 - 61   Siemens Med. Archiv, Erlangen

Fig. V, 62 - 63   Ebersberger, H., K. Morkel: Entwicklung von beweglichen Hochspannungsleitungen und Endverschlüssen für Röntgenanlagen. Sonderdruck Siemens Zeitschrift (1968) 42. Jg., H 11: 920-925.

Fig. V, 64 - 65   Siemens Med. Archiv, Erlangen

Fig. V, 66   Patent DP 250334 vom 8. Mai 1909, VEIFA-Werke und Friedrich Dessauer, Frankfurt a.M.: Verfahren für Momentaufnahmen mit Röntgenstrahlen.

Fig. V, 67   Patent DP 293503 vom 17. Sept. 1915, Siemens & Halske, Berlin: Verfahren und Einrichtung zur Herstellung von kurzzeitigen photographischen Aufnahmen durch Röntgenröhren mit Glühkathode.

Fig. V, 68   Siemens Med. Archiv, Erlangen

Fig. V, 69   Patent 581160 vom 20. Sept. 1928, Dipl.-Ing. Carl Niemann, Erlangen: Einrichtung für

	kurzzeitige Röntgen-aufnahmen.
Fig. V, 70a,b,c	Siemens Med. Archiv, Erlangen
Fig. V, 71 - 72	Bischoff, K., W. Gellinek: Geräte für die Anwendung ionisierender Strahlen. In: Vieten, H.: Physikalische Grundlagen und Technik, Teil 2, Springer Verlag, Heidelberg, New York (1965). Gesamtwerk Diethelm, L. O. Olsson, F. Strand, H. Vieten, A. Zuppinger: Handbuch der medizinischen Radiologie. Band I, Teil 2, Springer Verlag, Heidelberg, New York 1965, S. 126, Fig. 5; S. 132, Fig. 9.
Fig. V, 73 - 75	Siemens Med. Archiv, Erlangen
Fig. V, 76	Patent DP 156389 vom 3. April 1902, Siemens & Halske, Berlin: Verfahren und Apparat zum Durchleuchten von Körperteilen mittels Röntgenstrahlen.
Fig. V, 77	Siemens Med. Archiv, Erlangen
Fig. V, 78	Grigg, E.R.N.: The trail of the invisible light. Charles C. Thomas Publisher Springfield, USA (1965), p. 129.
Fig. V, 79 - 82	Sommer, E.: Röntgentaschenbuch, II. Band, Otto Nemnich Verlag, Leipzig 1909, S. 85, Fig. 40; S. 85, Fig. 41; S. 257, Fig. 94; S. 267, Fig. 106
Fig. V, 83	Bischoff, K., W. Gellinek: Geräte für die Anwendung ionisierender Strahlen. In: Vieten, H.: Physikalische Grundlagen und Technik, Teil 2, Springer Verlag, Heidelberg, New York (1965). Gesamtwerk Diethelm, L. O. Olsson, F. Strand, H. Vieten, A. Zuppinger: Handbuch der medizinischen Radiologie. Band I, Teil 2, Springer Verlag, Heidelberg, New York 1965, S. 250, Fig. 238.
Fig. V, 84	Siemens Med. Archiv, Erlangen
Fig. V, 85	Deutsches Röntgenmuseum, Remscheid-Lennep
Fig. V, 86	Grigg, E.R.N.: The trail of the invisible light. Charles C. Thomas Publisher Springfield, USA (1965), p. 73.
Fig. V, 87 - 96	Siemens Med. Archiv, Erlangen
Fig. V, 97	Bischoff, K., W. Gellinek: Geräte für die Anwendung ionisierender Strahlen. In: Vieten, H.: Physikalische Grundlagen und Technik, Teil 2, Springer Verlag, Heidelberg, New York (1965). Gesamtwerk Diethelm, L. O. Olsson, F. Strand, H. Vieten, A.

	Zuppinger: Handbuch der medizinischen Radiologie. Band I, Teil 2, Springer Verlag, Heidelberg, New York (1965), S. 166, Fig. 61.
Fig. V, 98 - 100	Siemens Med. Archiv, Erlangen
Fig. V, 101	Werbung von Polyphos, München (1906)
Fig. V, 102 - 113	Siemens Med. Archiv, Erlangen
Fig. V, 114	Bischoff, K., W. Gellinek: Geräte für die Anwendung ionisierender Strahlen. In: Vieten, H.: Physikalische Grundlagen und Technik, Teil 2, Springer Verlag, Heidelberg, New York (1965). Gesamtwerk Diethelm, L. O. Olsson, F. Strand, H. Vieten, A. Zuppinger: Handbuch der medizinischen Radiologie. Band I, Teil 2, Springer Verlag, Heidelberg, New York (1965), S. 228, Fig. 186.
Fig. V, 115 - 117	Siemens Med. Archiv, Erlangen
Fig. V, 118	Goerke, H.: Fünfundsiebzig Jahre Deutsche Röntgengesellschaft. Georg Thieme Verlag, Stuttgart, New York (1980) S. 119
Fig. V, 119 - 123	Siemens Med. Archiv, Erlangen
Fig. V, 124	Grashey, R.: Röntgentechnik. Thieme Verlag, (1941) (Pohls Omniskop).
Fig. V, 125 - 126	Siemens Med. Archiv, Erlangen
Fig. V, 127	Bischoff, K., W. Gellinek: Geräte für die Anwendung ionisierender Strahlen. In: Vieten, H.: Physikalische Grundlagen und Technik, Teil 2, Springer Verlag, Heidelberg, New York (1965). Gesamtwerk Diethelm, L. O. Olsson, F. Strand, H. Vieten, A. Zuppinger: Handbuch der medizinischen Radiologie. Band I, Teil 2, Springer Verlag, Heidelberg, New York (1965), S. 130, Fig. 8b.
Fig. V, 128 - 130	Siemens Med. Archiv, Erlangen
Fig. V, 131	Bischoff, K., W. Gellinek: Geräte für die Anwendung ionisierender Strahlen. In: Vieten, H.: Physikalische Grundlagen und Technik, Teil 2, Springer Verlag, Heidelberg, New York (1965). Gesamtwerk Diethelm, L. O. Olsson, F. Strand, H. Vieten, A. Zuppinger: Handbuch der medizinischen Radiologie. Band I, Teil 2, Springer Verlag, Heidelberg, New York (1965), S. 234, Fig. 203.
Fig. V, 132 - 135	Siemens Med. Archiv, Erlangen

Fig. V, 136 — Janker, R.: Apparatur und Technik der Röntgenkinematographie zur Darstellung der Herzbinnenräume und der großen Gefäße. Fortschr. Röntgenstr. 72 (1949) S. 516

Fig. V, 137 — Bischoff, K., W. Gellinek: Geräte für die Anwendung ionisierender Strahlen. In: Vieten, H.: Physikalische Grundlagen und Technik, Teil 2, Springer Verlag, Heidelberg, New York (1965). Gesamtwerk Diethelm, L. O. Olsson, F. Strand, H. Vieten, A. Zuppinger: Handbuch der medizinischen Radiologie. Band I, Teil 2, Springer Verlag, Heidelberg, New York (1965), S. 182, Fig. 85.

Fig. V, 138 — Siemens Med. Archiv, Erlangen

Fig. V, 139 — Private source: Siemens Elema, Stockholm

Fig. V, 140 - 142 — Siemens Med. Archiv, Erlangen

Fig. V, 143 — Prof. Kühne, Alfried Krupp von Bohlen und Halbach Krankenhaus, Essen

Fig. V, 144 — Siemens Med. Archiv, Erlangen

Fig. V, 145 — Patent DP 215648 vom 22. April 1908, Reiniger, Gebbert und Schall, Erlangen: Kinematographischer Aufnahmeapparat für Röntgenbilder.

Fig. V, 146 — Siemens Med. Archiv, Erlangen

Fig. V, 147 — DP 243256 vom 6. Nov. 1910, Reiniger, Gebbert und Schall, Erlangen: Vorrichtung zur Aufnahme von Röntgenreihenbildern mit schrittweise fortschaltbarem Bildband, das während der Aufnahme in einem Bildfenster zwischen gegeneinander verschiebbare Platten festgeklemmt und von diesen während der Fortschaltung freigegeben wird.

Fig. V, 148 - 154 — Siemens Med. Archiv, Erlangen

Fig. V, 155 — Bischoff, K., W. Gellinek: Geräte für die Anwendung ionisierender Strahlen. In: Vieten, H.: Physikalische Grundlagen und Technik, Teil 2, Springer Verlag, Heidelberg, New York (1965). Gesamtwerk Diethelm, L. O. Olsson, F. Strand, H. Vieten, A. Zuppinger: Handbuch der medizinischen Radiologie. Band I, Teil 2, Springer Verlag, Heidelberg, New York (1965), S. 208, Fig. 144.

Fig. V, 156 - 163 — Siemens Med. Archiv, Erlangen

Fig. V, 164 — Gebauer, A., J. Lissner, O. Schott: Das Röntgenfernsehen. Technische Grundlagen und klinisch-röntgenologische Anwendung. 2. Neubearb. und erweiterte Auflage, Georg Thieme Verlag, Stuttgart (1974)

Fig. V, 165 — Bischoff, K., W. Gellinek: Geräte für die Anwendung ionisierender Strahlen. In: Vieten, H.: Physikalische Grundlagen und Technik, Teil 2, Springer Verlag, Heidelberg, New York (1965). Gesamtwerk Diethelm, L. O. Olsson, F. Strand, H. Vieten, A. Zuppinger: Handbuch der medizinischen Radiologie. Band I, Teil 2, Springer Verlag, Heidelberg, New York (1965), S. 224, Fig. 176.

Fig. V, 166 — Patent USP 2198479 vom 3. Nov. 1937 (filed), Irving Langmuir (GE): Image reproduction.

Fig. V, 167 — Donner, M.: John W. Coltman, PhD. Röntgen-Blätter 10 (1970) 445-446

Fig. V, 168 - 171 — Siemens Med. Archiv, Erlangen

Fig. V, 172 — Gebauer, A., J. Lissner, O. Schott: Das Röntgenfernsehen. Technische Grundlagen und klinisch-röntgenologische Anwendung. 2. Neubearb. und erweiterte Auflage, Georg Thieme Verlag, Stuttgart (1974) S. 48, Fig. 40

Fig. V, 173 - 174 — Siemens Med. Archiv, Erlangen

Fig. V, 175 — Bischoff, K., W. Gellinek: Geräte für die Anwendung ionisierender Strahlen. In: Vieten, H.: Physikalische Grundlagen und Technik, Teil 2, Springer Verlag, Heidelberg, New York (1965). Gesamtwerk Diethelm, L. O. Olsson, F. Strand, H. Vieten, A. Zuppinger: Handbuch der medizinischen Radiologie. Band I, Teil 2, Springer Verlag, Heidelberg, New York (1965), S. 233, Fig. 200.

Fig. V, 176 - 182 — Siemens Med. Archiv, Erlangen

Fig. V, 183 — Gebauer, A., J. Lissner, O. Schott: Das Röntgenfernsehen. Technische Grundlagen und klinisch-röntgenologische Anwendung. 2. Neubearb. und erweiterte Auflage, Georg Thieme Verlag, Stuttgart (1974) S. 41, Fig. 32

Fig. V, 184 — Siemens Med. Archiv, Erlangen

Fig. V, 185 — Deutsches Röntgenmuseum, Remscheid-Lennep

Fig. V, 186   Röntgentaschenbuch, Band II,
                     hrsg. von E. Sommer, Otto
                     Nemmich, Leipzig (1909)
Fig. V, 187 - 189   Siemens Med. Archiv, Erlangen
Fig. V, 190   Gocht, H.: Handbuch der
                     Röntgenlehre. 2. Auflage, Fer-
                     dinand Enke, Stuttgart (1903)
Fig. V, 191   Siemens Med. Archiv, Erlangen
Fig. V, 192   Albers-Schönberg, H.: Die
                     Röntgentechnik. 2. Auflage,
                     Lucas Gräfe & Sillem, Hamburg
                     (1910)
Fig. V, 193 - 196   Poppe, M.: Technik der Rönt-
                     gendiagnostik. Thieme Verlag,
                     (1961)
Fig. V, 197   Siemens Med. Archiv, Erlangen
Fig. V, 198 - 201   Poppe, M.: Technik der Rönt-
                     gendiagnostik. Thieme Verlag,
                     1961
Fig. V, 202 - 203   Med. Röntgentechnik, hrsg. von
                     W. Frommhold, H. Gajewski, D.
                     Schoen. Band I, Thieme Verlag,
                     (1979)
Fig. V, 204 - 210   Private source of the author

Epilogue

Fig. 1 - 2   Schumacher, P.H.: Die Rönt-
                     gendiagnostik in der Geburts-
                     hilfe. In: Holfelder, H. et al.
                     (Hrsg.): Ergebnisse der medizi-
                     nischen Strahlenforschung,
                     Band VI, Georg Thieme Verlag,
                     (1933) S. 253, Fig. 17 und
                     S. 251, Fig. 13
Fig. 3   Eig. Archiv
Fig. 4 - 5   Günther, R.W., M. Thelen
                     (Hrsg.): Interventionelle Ra-
                     diologie, Georg Thieme Verlag,
                     Stuttgart (1988) S. 46, Fig. 2a-c;
                     S. 47, Fig. 3a und b
Fig. 6   Radiology 156 (1986) 849
Fig. 7   Radiology 159 (1986) 285

Chronological Index

Years before 1895 can be found in chapter I, in the table on page 16 and in chapter V on pages 335, 336, 358, 458 and 459.

Pages in **bold** type contain illustrations.

Years: Pages:

1895: 4, 5, 6, 7, 8, **9**, **10**, 14, 15, 19, 20, 22, 37, 39, 51, 213, **282**, 336, 338, **339**, 359, **473**, 477

1896: 8, **9**, 10, **11**, 17, 18, 20, 25, 26, 27, 28, 29, **31**, 33, 34, 39, 40, **67**, 68, 69, 74, 76, 84, 116, **122**, 131, 163, **236**, 239, 281, 293, 294, 322, 335, 338, **339**, **340**, 357, **358**, **360**, 362, 366, **377**, 379, 383, 404, **405**, 408, 409, 411, 428, 442, 462, 463, 464, **471**, **472**, 477, 478

1897: 11, 14, 20, 29, **30**, **31**, 34, 40, 67, 68, 69, 70, 73, 74, 76, 80, 81, 131, 164, **339**, **346**, **360**, 364, 376, **399**, 405, **406**, 408, **440**, 442, 462, 464, 465

1898: 20, 29, **31**, 32, 40, 68, 69, 74, 78, 82, 84, 131, 132, **158**, 163, 164, 173, 253, 261, 341, 357, 383, 459, 460, 462, 463, 464

1899: **30**, 32, 34, 67, 69, 70, 72, 73, 74, 77, 78, 82, **122**, **361**, 400, **401**, 464, 478

1900: 5, 19, 20, 31, 37, **50**, 55, 70, 71, 74, 76, **171**, 173, 176, 472, **474**, 478

1901: 6, 14, **26**, 32, 34, 37, **50**, **67**, 68, 69, 70, 72, 73, 74, 76, 77, 80, 81, 84, 115, 132, 164, 167, 173, **357**, **361**, **373**, 386

1902: 6, 26, 68, 70, 72, 73, 74, 76, 164, **266**, 383, 386, **400**, 404, **405**, 412

1903: 32, 68, 69, 70, 72, 74, 75, **76**, 77, 78, 80, 83, 132, 164, 165, 261, 338, **362**, 383, 398, **399**, 461, 462, **471**, 478

1904: 32, 47, **48**, 68, 73, 77, 132, 133, 164, 173, **213**, 341, 364, 373, 404, 405

1905: 6, 14, 20, 29, **31**, **40**, 42, 49, 70, 72, 74, 76, 78, 99, **122**, 158, 281, 343, 364, 385, **386**, 398, **400**, 405, 406, 464, **471**

1906: **28**, **32**, **44**, 49, 51, 70, 73, 74, 77, 78, 79, 81, 82, 83, 84, 125, 133, **165**, 341, **363**, 386, 398, 404, 409, **410**

1907: **34**, **70**, 73, 74, 78, 79, 81, 82, 364, 374, 386, 397, 415, **416**, 464, **465**, 468

1908: 44, 72, 73, 75, 78, 82, 83, 116, 133, 136, 166, 167, 341, **360**, 364, 374, **399**, 400, **401**, **402**, **413**, 425, 429, **430**, 431, 459, 462, **471**

1909: **68**, **69**, 70, 73, 74, 77, 79, 81, **157**, **158**, 166, 248, 342, **374**, **386**, 408, **441**, **459**, 460, **461**, **462**, 464

1910: 20, **32**, 37, **39**, **40**, 73, 74, 76, 78, 79, 81, 84, **103**, 115, **122**, 123, 133, 138, 157, 158, 166, 167, 173, 213, 346, **362**, 364, **385**, 409, **410**, 425, 430, **431**

1911: 8, 74, 82, 83, 84, 85, 133, 138, 139, 143, 166, **343**, 374, 404, 429, **430**, 433, **460**, **461**

1912: 6, 8, 11, 12, 14, 36, 77, 78, 79, 81, 82, 83, 84, 115, 142, **262**, 343, 358, 362, 364, 373, 374, 382, **383**, **402**

1913: 11, 20, 32, 73, 77, 78, **79**, **80**, 81, 82, 83, 84, 85, **98**, **99**, 134, 138, **341**, 342, 343, 354, 363, 373, 374, 376, 380, 386, **387**, 441, 462, 464, **473**, 474

1914: 26, 77, 78, 79, **80**, 81, 82, 84, 85, 134, 167, 265, 342, 343, 347, 374, 383, **430**, **440**, 460, 461, 464

1915: 6, 18, 19, 37, 47, **49**, 77, 82, **122**, 123, 139, 262, 265, **267**, **268**, 346, 364, **365**, **380**, **388**, 446

1916: 20, 80, 84, **134**, **135**, **136**, 170, 262, 294, 364, **367**, 374, 384

1917: 37, **59**, 82, 84, 281, **282**, **344**, 374

1918: 82, 85, **122**, 123, **151**, **294**, 295, **344**, 367, **380**, **440**, 464, 473

1919: 6, 19, 79, 84, 157, **262**, **282**, 302, 304, **344**, 345, 367, **377**, 380, **426**, **444**, 461, 462

20s: 136, 176, 177, 182, 200, 300, 367, 464, 481

1920: 19, 78, 81, 82, 83, 84, 134, **347**, 367, **370**, **373**, **377**, **416**, 464, 473, **482**

1921: **31**, 47, **71**, 73, 77, 78, 79, 80, 81, 82, **84**, 85, 87, 88, 123, 135, **137**, 138, 158, **169**, 262, 265, **266**, **267**, 295, 302, 342, 402, **403**

1922: **32**, **75**, **76**, **77**, **78**, 84, 85, 87, 135, **136**, **137**, 170, **217**, 262, 265, 266, 295, 358, **359**, 382, 415, **417**

1923: **6**, 19, **122**, 138, 158, 161, 170, 176, 178, 213, 236, **237**, **345**, 367, 392, 465

1924: 29, 33, 84, 86, 87, 88, 159, 170, 176, **237**, 367, 405, **406**

1925: 35, 55, 84, 138, 159, 293, 349, 409, 415, **416**, **471**, 472

1926: 84, 87, 88, 124, **171**, **295**, **296**, 358, 362, 367, 374, 380, 383, **384**, 385, 387, 388, 418, **419**, **471**

1927: 85, 86, 87, 89, 90, 99, 123, 124, 139, 166, 170, **171**, 176, **267**, 300, 345, 346, 367, 368, 369, 371, **373**, 388, **416**, 465, **471**

1928: **32**, **82**, **83**, 85, 88, **122**, 139, **159**, **164**, **165**, **166**, 170, 213, 215, 262, 367, **368**, 369, 374, 388, **389**, 473

1929: **28**, 37, **57**, 85, 86, 87, 88, **124**, 141, 169, 170, **172**, 177, 200, **201**, **213**, 214, 218, 237, 238, **267**, 303, 346, **347**, 358, 361, **363**, 400, **401**, 446, 465, 477

30s: 100, 139, 189, 442, 465

1930: 14, 84, 87, 90, 100, 102, 124, 138, 141, 170, 176, 178, 248, **267**, 357, 368, 388, **417**, 441, 464, 465

1931: **26**, 86, 87, 88, **100**, 124, **140**, 160, 170, 213, 214, 248, **267**, 293, 297, 298, 300, **346**, 354, 368, 380, 401, 403, 404

1932: 85, 86, 87, 88, 99, 100, 123, **133**, 139, 140, 143, 214, 248, 354, 368, 381, **403**, 441, 446, **459**

1933: 32, 85, 86, 100, 125, 138, 140, 178, **179**, 214, 216, 297, 345, 347, 369, 372, 375, **377**, **381**, 388, 389, 393, 465, **477**, **478**

1934: 33, 54, 85, 86, 88, 100, 140, 141, 181, 219, 266, 271, 275, 276, 302, 346, 347, **348**, 375, 389, **417**, **418**

1935: 58, 85, 86, 87, 100, 142, 208, 265, 266, **267**, 276, 302, 364, 369, 377, **378**, 389, **419**, 434

1936: **67**, 85, 86, 87, 88, 89, 139, 178, 201, 214, 216, 263, 265, 266, **267**, 380, **381**, **416**, 447

1937: 33, 34, 35, 85, **86**, 101, **102**, 123, 139, **140**, 141, 145, 147, 160, 185, 214, 219, 266, 300, 301, 348, 401, 415, **425**, **431**, 432, **443**, 450, 462

1938: **31**, 84, 86, 87, 101, 139, 171, 178, 179, 181, 214, **218**, **266**, 375, 390, **402**, **414**, **434**, 468, 479

1939: **32**, 86, 87, 88, 89, 142, 178, 201, 214, 293, 300, 432, 434, **443**, **482**

40s: 182, 183, 184, 189, 300, 301, 389

1940: 85, 86, 88, 157, 177, 178, 214, 301, 374, 390, **404**, 446, 464, 473

1941: **87**, 142, 146, 178, 179, 202, 214, **267**, **347**, 369, 390, 402, 442, 447

1942: **86**, 87, 142, 170, 216, 390, 466

1943: 12, 100, **124**, 142, 182, 219, 357, 390, 391, **407**

1944: 33, 87, 125, 369, **370**, 389, **391**

1945: 35, 36, 87, 89, **132**, **140**, **141**, 142, **147**, 148, 179, 216, 342, 349, 392, **471**, **473**

1946: 85, 143, 180, **202**, **294**, 297, 364, 391, **403**

1947: 6, **39**, 86, 87, 88, 123, 178, 179, 208, 214, 266, **267**, 298, **299**, 314, 354, 391, 444, 479

1948: 33, 85, 86, 87, 88, 182, 185, 219, 266, **267**, 300, 303, 390, 394, 443, **444**, 446

1949: 8, 85, 86, 87, 88, 89, 142, **166**, **179**, **180**, 182, 202, 219, 266, **267**, 268, **300**, **348**, 370, 371, 375, 381, **425**, **435**, 446, 450

50s: 88, 103, 104, 127, 129, 140, 147, 152, 182, 183, 185, **186**, 188, 189, 192, 203, 206, 207, 208, 220, 225, 297, 301, 303, 381, 432, 444, 448, 468, 477

1950: **32**, **40**, 86, 87, 88, 126, 139, 141, 143, 182, **183**, 184, 191, 216, 266, **267**, 300, 301, 354, 371, 375, 376, 381, **388**, 392, **423**, 425, 444, 446, 450, 468

1951: **83**, 86, 90, **101**, 103, 115, **181**, 182, 183, 185, 187, 204, 214, 215, 219, **238**, 266, 375, 430, **431**, 432, **434**, **443**, 446, 465

1952: 88, **159**, 160, 184, 185, 193, 204, 216, 239, 248, 249, 301, 348, 375, 432, **444**, 479

1953: 88, 89, 125, 129, 144, 160, 169, **184**, 187, 188, 202, 205, 214, **266**, 301, 348, 375, 418, 425, 443

1954: **40**, 88, 89, 104, 125, 147, 221, **239**, **240**, **241**, 349, **365**, 418, 425, **427**, 444, 462, 468

1955: 85, 88, 89, 90, 104, 127, 145, 147, **166**, 185, **240**, **300**, 301, **344**, 375, 376, **378**, **391**, 403, **408**, 409, 418, 446, 450, 451

1956: 88, 89, 105, 163, **187**, 201, 202, 204, **205**, **213**, 281, 349, 371, 375, 376, 378, 392, **411**, 425, **444**, 446, 447, 448, **449**, 451, 459, 463, 465

1957: 88, 102, 104, 105, 134, **158**, **168**, 172, 185, 281, **294**, 349, **376**, **402**, 447

1958: 90, 104, 144, 145, 185, **188**, 217, 299, 364, 372, 392, 393, 402, **420**, **441**, 446, 447, 449, 451, 479

1959: 88, 89, 108, 185, 220, **240**, 248, 251, **276**, **277**, **278**, 348, 349, 362, 363, **391**, 410, 425, **432**, **445**, 447, 449

60s: 88, 118, 127, 147, 172, 185, 188, 189, 190, 191, 192, 194, 205, 206, 220, 225, 226, 248, 257, 281, 297, 303, 367, 376, 389, 407, **408**, 409, 412, 422, 425, 443, 445, 447, 449, 450, 453, 477

1960: 89, 90, 101, 102, 105, 126, 158, 191, 216, 219, 248, 251, 253, 272, 275, **350**, 354, 379, **415**, 420, **422**, **425**, 448, **474**, **475**

1961: 88, 90, 144, 145, 146, 169, **298**, 352, 382, 413, 427, 432, 444, **445**, 446, 447, **450**, **463**, **464**, **467**, **468**

1962: 89, 105, 146, 159, 191, 208, 248, 253, 257, 270, 274, 349, 371, 375, 447, **448**, 449, 451, 464

1963: 14, **35**, 89, **103**, 108, 145, 171, 220, 241, 248, 257, 259, 281, **282**, 295, 319, **344**, 346, **403**, 418, 448

1964: 90, 169, 171, 189, **239**, 248, **249**, 253, 254, 257, 353, **424**, 431, 445, 447, 449, 466, **482**

1965: **104**, 105, **106**, 108, 146, **159**, **160**, **161**, 248, 249, 254, 257, **301**, 364, 367, 369, 374, 377, 397, 400, 408, 418, 420, 427, 432, 433, 445, 447, 450, 462, 465

1966: **32**, 104, 105, 108, 148, 189, 217, 227, 248, 253, 259, 354, 358, **378**, **412**, 433, 445, **448**, **450**, **472**

1967: 105, 106, 147, 172, **191**, 209, 256, 259, 379, **381**, 445, 446, 447, 481

1968: 148, 249, 250, 253, 380, 382, 392, **411**, **417**, 418, **419**, 423, 445, 446, 448, 451, 465, 466, 469

1969: 102, 127, 134, 139, 148, 209, 248, 249, 252, 257, 259, 284, 350, **351**, 371, 392, **426**, 445, 446

70s: 89, 119, 146, 147, 192, 193, 194, 205, 206, 209, 210, 221, 239, 263, 282, 284, 290, 303, 304, 314, 353, 354, 367, 376, 393, 409, 423, 425, 427, 433, 434, 445, 448, 453, 454, 479, 480

1970: 89, **101**, 106, 108, 141, **227**, 249, 253, 354, 372, 379, 383, 392, 393, 417, 418, 420, 425, 427, 434, 435, 445, 450, 451, 459, 463, 465, 468, 483, 484

1971: 163, 145, 193, 249, 305, **351**, 369, 372, 384, 390, 392, 393, **410**, **421**, 445, 451

1972: 88, 102, 171, 192, 251, 259, 281, **282**, **286**, **347**, 350, **370**, 379, 390, 411, 412, 421, 427, 433, 446, 449, 451, 454

1973: 89, 90, 103, 108, 109, 194, 263, **282**, 297, **298**, 350, 353, 369, 372, 375, 382, 390, 393, **407**, **409**, **414**, **418**, **424**, 433, **450**, 454

1974: 89, 108, 144, 151, 192, **242**, 257, **282**, **283**, 284, 293, 305, 338, 350, 369, 375, **378**, 390, 442, 446, 447, 450

1975: 106, **107**, 108, 127, 194, **282**, 285, 353, **421**, 434, **435**, **454**

1976: 108, 144, 146, 151, 172, **173**, **218**, **228**, 249, 257, 350, 392, **406**, **424**, 448, 451, 452, 469

1977: 89, 103, 106, 108, 109, 151, 249, 253, 286, **354**, 372, 379, 392, 407, 414, 423, **426**, 446, 480

1978: **107**, 151, 303, 349, **353**, **370**, 379, 393

1979: 22, 90, 127, 128, **213**, 229, **282**, 306, 314, 350, 351, 352, 392, 452, 466, 467, 469

80s: 129, 194, 201, 209, 210, 221, 242, 290, 302, 352, 369, 385, 407, 414, 423, 428, 435, 446, 452, 455

1980:   161, 228, 249, 256, 257, **379**, 415, 425, 431, 452

1981:   128, 193, 228, **229**, **232**, 252, 349, 351, 352, **411**, 446, **452**

1982:   274, **351**, 380, **452**, 454

1983:   90, 107, **232**, **282**, **283**, 468

1984:   90, **103**, **151**, **229**, 249, **253**, **254**, **255**, 257, 258, **372**, 382, 434, 452

1985:   **217**, **232**, **268**, 352, **433**, 434, 452, **472**, **482**

1986:   35, 89, 90, 109, 110, **232**, 286, 338, 342, 372, 379, 392, 452, 454

1987:   108, 110, 144, 152, 257, 285, 323, 353, **370**, 382, **413**, 426, **453**, 454, **480**

1988:   33, 110, 128, 274, 286, 354, 372, 379, **412**, **453**, 466, **482**

1989:   110, 123, **282**, 286, **353**, 392, 468

90s: 290, 424, 434, 436, 446

1990:   119, **158**, 286, 290, 352, 353, 372, 379, 384, 393, 423, 425, **453**, 459

1991:   379, 414, **418**, **422**, **428**, **433**, 448, 481

1992:   109, 194, 287, 414, 427, **430**, 435, **436**, 448, 453, 454, 455, 484

1993:   110, **266**, **371**, 413, 414, 423, 424, **429**, 436, 453, 455, **475**, **484**

1994:   402, **413**, **423**, 436

1995:   **282**, **286**, **473**

Index of Names

Pages in **bold** type contain illustrations.
The numbers in brackets refer to the pages on which the reference numbers are given.

Aakhus   197 (191), 199 (194)
Abbes   248
Abeatici   183
Abel   158
Abram   188
Abrams   196 (187, 191)
Abreu de   86, 267
Ackermann   465, 466
Africa   2
Agatston   292 (290)
Agnew   99
Ahmed   102
Aichinger   384, 392, 393
Äkerlund   60 (42), 137
Alavi   199 (194)
Albarran   166
Albers-Schönberg   **31**, 32, 40, 47,
    48, 49, 68, 69, 70, 72, 74, 75, 76,
    77, 117, 164, 167, 261, 338, 384,
    386, 400, 406, 419, 461, 462, 471,
    473, 478
Albrecht   379, 418
Albright   54, 57
Alexander   60 (46)
Alken   171
Allbutt   74
Allen   60 (40)
Almén   127, 189, 196 (191), 198
    (193), 246 (238)
Altaras   249
Alwens   213, 236, 237
Ambrose   282, 304, 305, 313 (305)
Amendola   198 (193)
Ameuille   214
Ammann   1, 6, 22, 25, 37, 115, 335,
    338, 357, 369, 372, 375, 379, 390,
    393, 397, 433, 440, 458, 477
Ampère   17
Amplatz   145, 191, 193, 214, 217,
    483
Amundsen   197 (191)
Anacker   89, 333 (319, 325)
Anderson   197 (192)
Angerstein   466
Aquapendente   3
Archer   16, 459
Ardran   88, 146
Aristotle   248

Ariyama   211 (207)
Arnsperger   73, 77
Arnulf   217
Arrhenius   24
Arvay   248, 257, 259
Arvidson   225
Asage   110
Asellius   248
Assmann   75, 76, 77, 78, 79, 80, 81,
    84, 87, 135, 261
Atlee   355 (354)
Aub   54
Aubourg   73
Averroes   2, 3
Axén   182, 219, 425
Axhausen   60 (46, 59)

Baader   87
Baccaglini   333 (319)
Bachem   122, 129 (123), 133
Bade   70, 122
Baensch   32, 100, 170
Baese   262, 265, 267
Baetjes   60 (51, 58)
Baisch   60 (48)
Balfanz   451
Balthazard   131
Baraldi   100
Barclay   143, 146, 181
Barden   86
Barke   237
Barnal   20
Barnes   107
Baron   333 (325)
Bartelink   262, 266, 267, 270
Barth   412
Barthélemy   67
Barthels   248
Bartholinus   248
Bartstra   134, 144
Battersby   60 (40)
Bauer   54, 341, 461, 464
Baum   189, 192, 197 (190), 210
Becher   122, 131
Beck   158
Becker, H   305
Becker, G.J.   198 (193), (205), 211,
    305, 306, 313 (307, 312), 428

Becker, J.   451
Béclère   31, 32, 67, 68, 70, 72, 74,
    80, 84, 360
Becquerel   16, 20
Behling   353
Behr   86
Behring von   37
Beitel   344
Beitzke   60 (52)
Bell   144
Bellman   197 (190), 217
Beltz   120, 248, 249, 252, 256, 257
Benedikt   68, 69, 74
Benoist   383
Berberich   122, 130 (123), 176,
    178, 236, 246 (239)
Berczeller   301
Berenroth   73
Berg   119, 140, 349, 415, **417**
Berger   352, 413, 432
Bergmans   433
Bergonié   67, 70, 73
Berk   162 (161)
Bernard   24
Bernardeau   43
Berner   86
Berninger   313 (309)
Best   102
Bethge   172
Bezold   18
Bichat   22
Biergel   61 (51)
Bierman   183, 185, 191, 193, 203,
    204, 207
Biermanns   371
Bilgutay   217
Billroth   115
Bingel   295, 297
Binz   **124**, 130 (124, 125), 170, 171
Birch-Hirschfeld   471
Bircher   40, 60 (54)
Birkenfeld   60 (47)
Bischoff   60 (41, 50), 105, 369, 370,
    371, 375, 390, 393, 394 (389), 397,
    408, 418, 420, 432, 437 (398), 448,
    447
Bjoerk   214, 246 (238)
Blakemore   196 (183)

Blangey 86
Blencke 60 (48, 50)
Blickman 216
Bliss 479
Bluehbaum 122, 130 (123), 170
Boblitt 196 (189), 211
Bocáge 262, 265, **266**, 267
Bodart 145
Boehm 60 (49)
Boehminghaus 170, 171
Boerema 216
Bohr 20
Boijsen 120, 169, 176, 196 (190),
    197 (191), 200, 211 (205, 207,
    208, 209)
Bois du-Reymond 23, 28
Boles 139
Bollinger 247 (241)
Bolt 215
Borcke 463, 465
Borden 61 (40)
Bordet 83, 84
Bormann 381
Borsig 336
Bosniak 171
Bosnjakovic-Buescher 44
Bouchard 67, 68, 69, 74, 81, 82
Bouglé 451
Bouslog 142
Bouwers 85, 218, 345, 346, **347**,
    372, 442
Boveri 6, 8, 19
Boyd 286
Boyer 158
Braasch **166**, 167
Bracewell 281
Bragg 11, 384
Brailsford 61 (59)
Brakel 162 (161)
Brandt 61 (50)
Brandt-Zawadski 198 (194)
Brassel 428
Brauer 81, 84
Braun 371, 392, 471
Brauner 133
Brauning 84, 86, 87
Breen 292 (290)
Brennecke 228, 229
Bresler 286
Breuer 5
Brezovich 107
Brismar 130 (127)
Brodén 145, 180
Brody 102, 452
Brofman 216
Broman 189, 300
Brombart 146
Bronkhorst 465
Bronner 238
Brooks 176, 237, 246 (239), 291
    (283)

Broussais 22
Brown 145, 355 (349), 479
Bruce 87
Brunke 375
Brunner 84, 252, 253
Bruschke 214, 217, 218
Bruwer 246 (239)
Buchtala 425
Bucky 366, 402, **403**
Buechner 196 (189), 242
Buecker 145
Buehlmeyer 433
Buergel 61 (51)
Buersch 198 (194), 225, 227, 228,
    229, 230
Buffard 217
Bulay du 303
Bull 303, 313 (305)
Buono del 65 (44, 59), 248, 249,
    257
Burckhardt 161 (157, 158), 471
Burghardt 84
Burhenne 161, 483
Burns 122, 130 (123)
Buschke 61 (47)
Butler 107
Buttenberg 104, 105
Bynum 198 (193)

Cabot 70
Cadman 148
Caffey 87
Caldas 181, 200, 219
Callear 459
Calvé 46
Cameron 122, 130 (123)
Camp 141, 142
Camp de la 73, 74, 77, 83
Campi 183
Campo del 216
Cannon 122, 131, **132**, 133
Carman 134, 135, 136, 138, 161
    (157)
Carrière 70, 73
Carrington 91
Carroll 459
Carter 86
Carus 22
Carvalho 85, 248
Casciarolus 16
Case 32
Casper 170
Castaneda-Zuniga 198 (193)
Castellanos 178, 181, 214, 216
Castro 332
Cauley 86
Celis 214
Chaillet 214, 219
Chamberlain 89
Chantraine 367, 368, 371, 388,
    389

Chaoul 81, 84, 85, 87, 267, 276,
    344, 345
Chapman 225
Charbonnel 246 (237)
Charlie 442
Charlton 342
Chaussé 262, 266, 267, 303
Chavez 178, 214
Chérigié 420, 451
Chiro di 303
Christen 365, 383
Christensen 442
Christie 143
Chuang 198 (193)
Church 87
Churchill 87
Ciba 102
Cignolini 85
Citoler 109
Clapesattle 442
Clark 87, 127, 333 (325)
Clausius 18, 19
Clodius 249, 253
Cocchi 61 (41, 47), 86
Codman 61 (58)
Cohn 74, 79, 166
Cohnheim 23, 24
Colapinto 198 (192, 193)
Colcher 101
Cole 133, 134, 138, 139, 143, **158**,
    343
Colley 17
Collins 29
Colombo 3
Coltman 88, 185, 443, **444**
Contiades 214
Coolidge 85, 117, 134, **342**, 343,
    346, 363, 376, 380, 417, 441
Cooper 86
Cooperberg 161
Cope 197 (191)
Copernicus 3
Cormack 281, 282, 283, 314
Corvisart 22
Costa da 81
Costello 291 (287)
Cournand 214
Cowl 28, 31, 69, 74, 82, 460
Crafoord 179
Crane 14
Creevy 211 (203)
Criegern von 72, 74, 76
Crohn 140
Croizier 87
Cronquist 300
Crookes 12, 16, 338, 341
Cross 442
Crow 333 (316)
Crummy 198 (194), 228, 247
    (242)
Crystal 90

Cullen 102
Cullinan 468
Cummings 144, 151
Cunningham 173
Curie 20
Curry 333 (328)
Curschmann 78
Cushing 293
Czepa 26

Daguerre 16, 458
Dahlin 61 (58)
Dahm 146
Dalgaard 435
Dalrymple 89
Dandy **294**, 295, 297
Danelius 61 (41)
Darcy 247 (243)
Darwin 23
Dauvillier 446
Davis 211 (209), 477
Davy 17, 361
Dawson 198 (192)
Decker 304
Dedic 88
Degenhardt 468
Deichgraeber 107
Delherm 85
Denecke 445
Depréz 8, 360
Desormaux 163
Dessauer 8, 10, 14, **35**, 68, 77, 237,
    367, 386, 429, 430, **342**, 345, 363,
    462
Deutsch 88
Deycke-Pascha 62 (44, 52)
Dichiro 191
Dieck 61 (46)
Diedrich 162 (159)
Diethelm 61 (46, 55, 52)
Dietlen 62 (40), 77, 78, 80, 81, 82,
    83, 84, 88, 166
Dietz 350, 355 (351)
Dihlmann 61 (59)
Djindjian 191, 303
Dobretsberger 105, 106
Dodd 146
Dodds 146
Dodge 225
Doering 367
Dohrmann 104
Dohrn 162 (159)
Dominguez 100
Donald 479
Donner 146
Donzelot 84
Doppman 197 (191)
Dorbecker 214
Dos Santos 177, 180, 200, **201**,
    202, 208, 238, 246 (237)
Doss 180

Dotter 185, 189, 190, 216, 217,
    482, 483
Doub 86
Douglas 144
Drault von 360
Ducket 420
Duenner 130 (123)
Duex 217
Dufay 16, 358
Dumoulin 247 (245)
Dumstrey 68, 464
Dunham 87
Dunnick 333 (329)
Dupuytren 22
Durham 85
Dushman 374
Dussik 479
Dutreix 107
Dutto 122

Eastman 16, **459**
Eberlein 31
Ebersberger 380
Ebertz 84
Edebohls 173
Eder 34
Edholm 211 (204), 272, 275
Edison 17, 68, 163, 293, 303, 304,
    463, 472
Edsman 211 (203)
Edward 214
Egan 102, 103, 109, 354, 412
Eggert 465
Ehrenfeld 141
Ehrlich 37
Einstein 12, 20
Eisler 26
Ekberg 145, 146
Elder 216
Elema 425
Eliasberg 87
Elischer von 133
Elke 172, 249, 257, 258
Ellinger 85
Elliot 214
Ellis 87
Elsaß 349
Elster 344
Encarnacion 212 (210)
Engel 77, 78, 79, 84, 86, 87
Engelmann 61 (47)
Engels 61 (48)
Engstroem 61 (55)
Eppinger 82
Erasistratos 1
Erasmus 3
Erdély 61 (50)
Erdheim 53, 58, 61 (52)
Erikson 138
Ernst 61 (40)
Ertzbischoff 166

Espaillat 100
Esser 86
Evans 61 (58), 203
Evens 484
Ewald 28, 61 (48)
Exner 25, 26
Eykman 132, 143

Fallopio 3
Fantus 157
Faraday 16, 17, 19, 358
Fariñas 179, 180, 202, **238**
Fassbender 420
Fauré 89, 359
Feddema 420, 451
Fedder 61 (58)
Federle 333 (330)
Fehr 418
Feil 63 (46)
Feindt 451
Felder 128
Feleus 451
Felson 89, 90
Fenner 444, 445, 348, 349
Ferris 199 (195), 215
Fick 6, 8
Fiegel 144
Figley 219
Fink 247 (243)
Finkenzeller 418
Finny 73
Finsterbusch 100
Fischedick 61 (59)
Fischer 6, 23, 40, 61 (41, 42, 52,
    54), 85, 86, 87, 111, 128, 138, 144
Fischgold 85, 303
Flaskamp 471
Fleischner 26, 87, 90
Fobbe 247 (245)
Foehre 355 (342)
Foeldi 249
Foerster 82
Fomin 88
Forestier 85, 176, 213, 236, 303
Fork 145
Forssell 19, **32**, 136, 182, 300
Forssmann 177, 178, **213**, 238
Foucault 359
Fraenkel 40, 61 (58, 52, 53), 77,
    78, 81, 170
Frain 266, 267
Franck 213, 236, 246 (239)
Frangenheim 61 (53, 58)
Frank 61 (53)
Franke, H. 8, 85, 88, 367, 368, 390,
    465
Franke, K. 369, **370**, 371, 384, 392,
    393, 394 (372)
Franklin 16, 358
Fraser 89
Fray 100

Frazer 142
Fredzell 182, 196 (188), 425, **426**, 434
Freeny 333 (325)
Freiberger 61 (59)
French 142
Freud 5
Freund 26, 34
Frey 195 (178)
Frieben 471
Friedel 350, 355 (351)
Friedl 32, 62 (52), 170
Friedman 90, 147
Friedmann 62 (46), 247 (241)
Friedrich 11, **12**, 15, 36, 62 (46), 106, 107, 108, 110
Frik 40, 85, 88, 119, 138, 145, 170, 349, 447
Frische 185, 216
Fritz 61 (55), 384
Fromme 62 (52)
Frommhold 159, 160, 161, 466, 467
Fuchs 248, 249, 257, 259, 358, 382, 451, 459, 465
Fuerstenau 343
Fugazzola 104
Fulmer 90

Gaensler 91
Gaiffe 385
Gajewski 105, 106, 348, 392, 418, 423, 451
Galanski 292 (287), 313 (307)
Galen 1
Galilei 3, 19
Gallet 253
Garcia-Calderon 138
Garrigou 70
Gaulard 17
Gay 16, 333 (329)
Gebauer 85, 227, 266, 267, 268, 276, 277, 278, 333 (315), 392, 442, 447, 454
Gebbert 67, 339, 340, 341, 361, 383, 387, 399, 400
Gebhardt 62 (42)
Geißler 16, 338
Gelfland 138
Gellinek 60 (41, 50), 369, 397, 408, 418, 420, 432
Genant 292 (289), 351
Genereuse 89
Genereux 89, 90
Georgi 107, 211 (208)
Gerhardt 73, 77, 81
Gerkema 355 (353)
Gerlach 19, 20
Gerneth 437 (427, 434)
Gershon-Cohen 101, 102, 104, 109, 140, 142, 148

Gerteis 248, 259
Geschickter 62 (58)
Ghiselin 219
Gianturco 138, 483
Gibbs 19
Gidlund 182, 186, 187, 189, 196 (190), 425
Gilbert 16
Gilchrist 144
Gill 16
Gilman-Frost 472
Gindl 424
Ginzburg 140
Glaessner 82
Glancy 197 (192)
Glasser 25, 362
Glocker 15, 465
Gmeinwieser 292 (287)
Gmelin 198 (193)
Gocht **31**, 32, 68, 69, 70, 72, 77, 116, 261, 342, 459, 460, 461, 462, 463, 464, 366
Godart 248
Godlee 293
Goei 145
Goergeny-Goettche 87
Goeringer 435
Goerke 10, 27, 415, 431
Goethlin 198 (193), 211 (209)
Goetze 85, 167, **344**, 345
Golden 141, 142, 147
Goldstein 17, 249, 253
Gollman 185
Goodman 215
Goodspeed 12, 359
Gordon 216
Gough 90
Gould 89, 105, 301, 351
Goyanes 100
Goynes 354
Graf 437 (434)
Graham 130 (123), **158**
Grainger 90, 130 (124)
Grangérard 83
Grashey 31, **40**, 41, 42, 43, 62 (40, 41, 43, 46, 51, 59), 237, 409, 410, 419, 461, 462
Grassmann 436
Graux 86
Gray 358
Greenspan 198 (194)
Gregg 216, 217
Greineder 85, 87, 276
Greitz 189, 300
Greulich 41, 42
Gribbe 225
Griesbach 86
Grigg 364, 367, 374, 377, 400, 462, 465
Groedel 70, 71, 74, 75, 77, 79, 82, **83**, 84, 88, 430

Groh 450
Grolla 350, 351
Gros **103**, 104, 105, 107, 354
Gross 100
Grossmann 33, 85, 262, 265, 266, 267, 270, 358, 362, 364, 367, 373, 374, 382, 383, 434
Gruber 62 (47, 48)
Gruentzig **482**, 483
Grunmach 28, 67, 68, 167
Gruwez 248, 253
Gudden 451
Guenther 122, 133, 483
Guericke von 16
Guetgemann 250
Guglielmo di 185, 216
Guilleminot 69, 74, 82
Guleke 62 (40)
Gunning 18
Gutman 145
Guttadauro 185, 216
Gutzeit 371
Guy 195 (181)

Haas 107
Haasch 64 (50)
Haber 212 (209)
Haberrecker 350
Hach 247 (245)
Hackenbroch 62 (48)
Hacker 313 (305, 309)
Hackl 358, 361
Haendle 448, 450
Haenisch 32, 40, 62 (58), 77, 81, 138, 167
Haer van der 142, 143
Hagen 198 (193)
Hahn 62 (44, 46, 50, 52)
Haight 216
Halske 131, 336, 357, 358, 360, 362, 363, 364, 400
Halsted 99, 295
Hamilton 143
Hamman-Rich 87
Hammer 82
Hanafee 209, 211 (205)
Hann 63 (58)
Hanson 62 (46, 50)
Hantschmann 87
Harras 460, 462
Hart 62 (51)
Hartl 352
Hartmann 465
Harvey 1, 3
Haschek 25, 26, 87, 116, 122, 213, 333 (322), 236
Haslauer 449
Haslhofer 53, 62 (55)
Hasse 239, 240
Hasselwander 40, 44, 62 (41, 42), 77, 82, 85

Hatfield   162 (161)
Haubitz   313 (310)
Haubrich   85, 88
Haudek   26, 133
Hauksbee   16
Häuptli   62 (47)
Haus   468
Haut   198 (193)
Hawes   80
Hawkins   33, 130 (123)
Hearst   293, 303
Heberer   242, 246 (238)
Hecht   238
Heckmann   85, 434
Hedvall   87
Heijne   447
Heinecke   73
Heintzen   120, 194, 225, 226, 227, 228, 229, 302
Heisig   86
Heitzman   89, 90
Heiwinkel   85
Heller   446
Hellner   62 (51)
Helmholtz von   4, 10, 14, 17, 19, 23, 293
Helmstrom   216
Helmsworth   184
Hemmeter   131, 133
Henderson   142
Hendriks   103
Henline   201
Hennig   8, 137
Henshaw   33
Herfarth   62 (50, 55)
Herlinger   138
Hermann   6
Herophilos   1
Herrnheiser   86, 89
Herrschaft   449
Herschel   16
Hertz   6, 10, 13, 17, 19
Herxheimer   88
Hesse   145, 471
Hessel   198 (193), 211 (205)
Hettler   196 (190), 241, 433
Heuck   39, 62 (41, 52, 54, 55)
Heuer   294
Heuser   130 (123)
Heuss   106
Heyden   102
Hicken   102
Hickey   62 (41,44)
Hilal   303
Hilbertz   198 (194)
Hilpert   137
Hiltz   102
Hinck   197 (191)
Hippocrates   248
Hirsch   122, 176, 178, 236, 237
Hirschmann   355 (342)

Hittorf   16, 338, 339
Hitzenberger   26, 88
Hochenegg   26
Hochsinger   73, 78
Hodges   219, 392
Hoeffken   38, 98, 105, 106, 108, 109
Hoehne   227, 230, 288
Hoevels   211 (209)
Hofbauer   82
Hoff van 't   23, 24
Hoffa   40, 49, 62 (59)
Hoffman   74, 219
Hoffmann   62 (43, 48)
Hofmann   394 (378), 446, 451, 452
Holfelder   86, 471
Holm   86
Holmes   479
Holmstroem   425, 426
Holz   17
Holzknecht 26, 32, 40, 68, 69, 70, 72, 73, 74, 76, 77, 78, 80, 81, 82, 84, 119, 132, 133, 134, 139, 294, 404
Holzmann   88
Hom   451
Hooke   16
Hoppe   130 (125)
Horbaschek   448
Hornykiewytsch   95, 171
Hounsfield   281, 282, 283, 284, 303, 304, 305, 313 (306, 309), 314, 435
Howry   479
Hoxter   379, 414
Hoyes   216
Hruby   414, 424, 435, 436, 453, 455
Hryntschak   124, 170
Huard   162 (158)
Huber   27
Hueppe   107
Huepscher   146
Hufeland   24
Huizinga   86
Hurler   62 (48)
Husten   87

Ichikawa   145, 179, 333 (325)
Iimuma   291 (286)
Illeys   164, 173
Immelmann   31, 40, 41, 49, 69, 70, 74, 398, 399
Ingleby   101
Israel   62 (40)

Jacobi   130 (123)
Jacobsen   74, 78
Jacobsson   196 (190), 248, 251, 253
Jaeger   247 (245)
Jaffe   62 (52, 53, 54, 58), 63 (57)

Jaksch von   72, 73
Jamin   82
Janker   86, 88, 195 (181), 196 (187), 239, 240, 241, 247 (238), 425, 431, 432, 442, 444, 446, 451
Janowitz   333 (322)
Janssen   145
Jarre   144
Jaspers   20
Jastrowitz   27
Jefferson   216, 217
Jennings   359
Jirout   304
Joachim   349
Joachimsthal   28, 40
Joensson   178, 180, 181, 182, 214, 216
Joergensen   435
Joetten   107, 454
Joffé   19, 27
Johansson   62 (44, 51), 248, 251, 253
Johnen   110
Jones   146
Joseph   164, 165, 171
Jossifow
Jowsey   63 (52, 55)
Judkins   189, 191, 199 (194), 219, 217
Juengling   40, 63 (52, 55), 295
Junghanns   65 (46, 49)
Jungherr   63 (46)
Jutras   159, 197 (192), 420, 447, 449

Kabakian   144
Kaeser   446
Kaestle   74, 133
Kahlbaum   68
Kahlstorf   88
Kaick van   123, 253
Kaindl   248, 251
Kaiser   25, 26, 63 (40, 59)
Kaiser-Petersen   87
Kalender   281, 286, 291 (287), 292 (290), 313 (312)
Kamiya   198 (193)
Kamnitz   78
Kantor   142
Kantrowitz   197 (191)
Kappert   247 (241)
Karacson   35
Karger   27
Kassay   87
Kastert   61 (52)
Katayama   130 (128)
Katsch   344
Kattentidt   86
Kaude   451
Kauf   88
Kaufman   137, 138

Kawai 145
Kaye 346
Kazerner 313 (305)
Kazner 304
Keiling 105
Keith 214
Keller 446
Kelley 107
Kelvin **11**
Kemp 146
Kerley 90
Keyes 452
Kiefer 107
Kieffer 266, 267, 270, 434
Kienboeck 26, **40**, 53, 63 (46, 48,
    52, 55, 58, 59), 68, 69, 73, 78, 81,
    83, 138, 164, 460
Killoran 61 (59)
Kingston 102
Kinmonth 248, 249, 251
Kirch 88
Kirchner 63 (46, 50)
Kirklin 144
Kisch 63 (51)
Klason 88
Klayer 63 (52)
Klebs 23
Kleiber 137, 162 (159)
Kleinschmidt 99
Klingelfuss 383, 386
Klinkhamer 146
Klippel 63 (46)
Klose 164
Knese 63 (50)
Knipping 11, 36
Knothe 138
Koch 15, 37, 100, 115, 364, 386,
    389
Koehler, A. 31, 33, 35, **39**, 41, 42,
    45, 63 (41, 43, 44, 46, 48, 49, 50,
    51, 52, 58, 59), 70, 74, 75, 77, 79,
    81, 82, 166, 167, 248, 392, 420,
    462, 464
Koehler, R. 420
Koehler, K. 392
Koelliker von 4, 6, 10, **11**, 38
Koelsch 87
Koenig 27, 63 (51, 52), 163, 167,
    478
Koester 313 (307)
Kohlrausch 16, 18
Kolischer 164
Koslowski 448
Koster 228
Kotoulas 435
Kovats 89
Kraemer 420
Krahmann 110
Krampla 414, 424, 436, 453, 455
Kranberg 392, 393
Kranzfelder 68

Kratochvil 104
Kraus 133
Krause 73, 77, 79, 80, 81, 84
Krayenbuehl 303
Kremer 85
Kress 416
Krestel 379, 423
Kricheff 313 (307)
Krohmer 196 (185), 392
Kruger 452
Krupp 335, 336
Kubat 89
Kucher 345
Kuebler 104
Kuechler 110, 371
Kuehl 446
Kuehne 63 (46)
Kuehnel 372, 379
Kuemmel 40, 164
Kuenne 437 (421)
Kuentscher 41, 63 (41, 50)
Kuenzler 223 (216)
Kugler 301
Kuhlman 139
Kuhn 14, 107, 451
Kummer 63 (50)
Kumpan 333 (326)
Kundt 10, 15, 17, 18, 19
Kunlin 241
Kuntke 349
Kunz 124, 437 (434)

Labusch 104
Lacroix 266, 267
Laënnec 22
Lamas 200
Lambert 339
Lambertz 63 (41)
Lame 354
Lang 63 (46), 197 (190)
Lange 63 (44, 51, 59), 228
Langecker 130 (125, 126), 162
    (160), 246 (238)
Langenbuch 115
Langer 65 (47), 247 (243)
Langmuir 343, 344, 443
Lanyi 103, 109, 110
Laplace 22
Larrey 22
Laruelle 297
Lasser 364, **365**, 366, 374, 384
Laszig 313 (308)
Laub 247 (245)
Laue von 11, **12**, 36
Laufer 146
Laurell 138, 143
Lauterbur **480**
Lavoisier 22
Leborgne 100, 101, 109
Lecher 25
Lederer 211 (205)

Ledin 107
Ledley 284
Ledoux-Lebard 138
Lee 333 (314)
Leeuwenhoek 4
Legg 46
Lehman 196 (185), 216, 217
Lehmann 63 (51), 452
Leistner 367, 368, 369, 388
Leiter 163
Leitner 87
Lemp 364
Lenard 6, **13**, 14, 17, 338
Lenk 26, 87, 88, 108
Leonard 134, 173
Leppin 471
Léri 63 (47)
Leusch 379
Leuteritz 370
Levine 146
Levy 28, 67, 68, 355 (342), 462,
    463, 464, 472
Levy-Dorn **28**, 33, 68, 69, 70, 72,
    73, 74, 76, 82, 117, 404, 405
Lewis 85
Lexer 63 (50, 51, 59
Lichtenberg 16, 358
Lichtenberg von 122, 123, 124,
    165, **166**, 170, 171, 238
Lichtenstein 63 (57)
Lichtheim 84
Lichtlen 217, 218
Lichtwitz 171
Liebel-Flarsheim 422
Liebenow 376
Liebig von 23
Lilienfeld, A. von 43
Lilienfeld, E.J. 343
Lillehei 217
Lind 182, 219, 425
Lindblom 300
Lindemann 63 (45), 131, 340
Lindenthal 26, 116, 122, 213, 236
Lindgren 196 (185), 300, 301
Lindhardt 435
Lindner 144
Linke 451
Lissner 447, 451
Lister 115
Liucci de 3
Livstone 333 (325)
Lochtkemper 87
Locke 22
Lockwood 100
Lodge 87
Lodwick 63 (58)
Loeffler 63 (50), 86
Loefstedt 89
Loehr 119, 163, 172, 173
Loewenhardt 173
Lohmann 420, 451

Loichinger 139
Loman 178
Longscope 87
Looser 53, 59, 64 (47, 52, 53, 58)
Lorentz 15, 17, 18, 20, 281
Lorenz, A. 40, 64 (48)
Lorenz, H. 446
Lorenz, R. 64 (46)
Lorey 61 (52), 77, 79, 81, 84, 85
Losada 162 (158)
Ludwig 19, 23, 120, 213, 218
Luening 249, 257
Luessenhoop 197 (191)
Luisada 85
Lunderquist 198 (193), 209
Lutz 437 (433), 450
Lynah 85
Lyon 161 (157)
Lysholm 88, 298, **299**, 300, 409

Maatz 64 (50)
Mach 20
Mackie 141
Maddox 16, 459
Magendie 24
Maglinte 149
Mahieu 145
Malan 253, 254
Mallinckrodt 102, 125
Malmros 87
Malpighi 4
Maluf 163
Mann 246 (238)
March 384
Marchal 247 (245)
Margulis 144, 481
Marmolya 313 (307)
Marragliano 67, 80
Marshak 144, 147, 148
Marstaller 13
Martin 87
Martinez 334 (331)
Mascagni 248
Massabni 144
Massiot 266, 267, 420, 434
Mathiaschitz 436
Matthes 79
Maurer 25
Maxwell 17, 19
Mayer 23, 26, 64 (46), 262, 265, 297
Mayo 353
McAfee 196 (189), 201
McIntyre 68, 74, 163, 164
McLaughlin 87
McLoud 90, 91
McMaster 158, 468
Meaney 198 (194)
Meany 247 (242)
Medlar 87
Meige 253

Meiler 370, 371, 392, 434, 446
Meinertz 453
Melchior 64 (43)
Mellin 172, 173
Mendelssohn 27
Menees 162 (159)
Merwedel 64 (40, 51)
Metzner 68, 464
Meyer 133
Meyers 145, 333 (326), 459
Meyerson 178
Michaelis 64 (52)
Milkman 64 (52)
Miller 84, 107, 141, **151**, 152, 217
Milne 349
Milroy 253
Mintzer 333 (316)
Mirizzi 162 (158)
Mirvis 333 (319)
Mistretta 194, 227, 228, 302
Mobin-Uddin 197 (191)
Moeller 64 (46)
Moll 41
Moniz 123, 176, 177, 178, 181, 189, 200, 201, 214, 215, **300**
Montag 334 (332)
Montanari 213
Moon 446
Moore 201, 270, 303
Morales 85
Morel 418
Moreton 144
Morgan 85, 87, 88, 392, 446
Mori 286
Morin 198 (193)
Morino 205, 211 (204)
Moritz 74, 75, 76, 82, 83
Morkel 380
Morrow 214
Morse 336
Morson 144
Morton 115, 236
Mosely 445
Moser 132
Mosser 413
Mueller 4, 23, 64 (45, 47), 84, 89, 158, 341, 342, 344, 368, 371, 376, 390
Mueller-Lissner 145
Muhm 333 (316)
Muijderman 353
Muller 471, 472
Mundinger 313 (309)
Mundinus 3
Munk 81, 82
Muntean 64 (46), 104
Mutscheller 473
Myrden 102

Nachnani 197 (192)
Naegeli 64 (41)

Naidich 291 (287)
Napel 292 (287), 333 (327)
Nau 64 (46)
Naulleu 214
Nell 446
Nelson 142, 210 (201)
Neuhauss 27
Neuland 87
Neumann 16, 87
Neussner von 25
Newell 89
Newton 19, 303
Ney 291 (287)
Nielsen 338, 342
Niemann 368, 389
Niepce 16, 458
Nievelstein 105
Nishimura 199 (195)
Nissen 230
Nitatori 199 (194)
Nitze 163
Nobel 14
Noddack 349
Noix 89, 447
Nolan 148
Nonne 64 (52), 253
Nordenstroem 111, 196 (189), 217, 219, 425, 426
Noschis 86
Nudelman 227, 228
Nunez 214
Nusbaum 193
Nuvoli 178, 216
Nylander 145, 146
Nylin 88

O'Loughlin 208
O'Neil 453
Oedman 183, 185, 186, 205, 211 (204)
Oefner 219
Oehlecker 167
Oersted 17, 358
Oestmann 38, 67
Oetiker 374
Ohlsson 217
Ohm 17
Okazaki 198 (193)
Olin 196 (189, 190, 191), 211 (208)
Ollendorf 61 (47)
Olsson 169, 189, 202
Onnasch 229
Oosterkamp 447, 449
Oppenheimer 140
Orrin 246 (236)
Orth op den 145, 146
Orton 70, 76, 84
Osborne 130 (123), 170, 238
Osgood 471
Ostrum 107

Ostwald 24
Osypka 227
Otte 161 (157)
Otten 70, 73, 81
Ottens 145
Oudin 67
Oudkerk 1, 6, 22, 25, 37, 115, 149,
    261, 286, 335, 338, 357, 397, 440,
    458, 477
Ovitt 228

Paasche 387
Paatero 267, 268, 269
Paessler 239, 240
Paget 57, 73, 99
Pallardy 162 (158)
Palmaz 212 (209)
Palmer 130 (128)
Palmieri 83
Palugyay 26
Pancoast ·87
Pansdorf 138, 139, 140
Pape 85
Paré 89
Parker 484
Parschwitz 105
Pasche 374
Pasteur 22, 37
Paulin 197 (190), 217
Pavlov 24
Pecquet 248
Peirce 184
Peister 144
Pel 157
Pels-Leusden 64 (47)
Peltier 64 (41, 50)
Pendergrass 87, 170, 354
Penn 103, 483
Penning 303
Pereiras 214, 216
Perrin 89
Perthes 46, 64 (45)
Pervin 17
Pesquera 141, 142, 148
Peters 314, 247 (238, 242, 245),
    333 (327)
Petrucelli 161 (157)
Pettenkofer von 37
Pezieras 219
Pfahler 64 (58), 70, 72, 73, 74, 78
Pfaundler 64 (41)
Pfeiffer 78
Pfeiler 445, 451
Pfitzner 44, 51, 64 (42)
Pfluecker 16, 17
Phelps 292 (289)
Picard 16, 248, 253, 256, 257, 259
Picker 407
Piepgras 427
Piers 215
Pilarczyck 227

Pirquet 87
Plaats van der 105, 263, 420
Plakler 133
Planck 18, 19, 20
Planté 16, 359, 361
Ploke 446
Pochaczevsky 145
Pochhammer 64 (51)
Poech 26
Poeschl 64 (41, 44, 46, 47)
Pohl 262, 266, 267, 346, 418, 419,
    422
Poland 64 (42)
Policard 87
Polster 452
Pommer 55, 64 (50, 51, 52, 53)
Pond 215
Ponette 146
Ponsdomenec 214
Poppe 467
Porstmann 483
Porta della 16
Portes 262, 266, 267
Posniak 333 (320)
Potts 303
Preiser 64 (50, 59)
Prellwitz 338
Pressler 349
Prévôt 119, 145, 171
Pribram 130 (123)
Price 107
Pringot 145, 146
Prioton 190
Prokop 292 (287)
Proudfit 214
Psenner 64 (46)
Pugh 87
Puglionisi 253, 254
Pugno-Vanoni 369, 389
Pupin 68, 463
Putti 64 (46, 49)
Pyle 41, 42

Quarna 88

Racine 178, 216
Rackwitz 411
Radner 179, 180, 182, **183**, 185,
    202, 216, 300
Radon 281, 282, 283
Radt 177
Radtke 229
Raeth 124, 171, 214, 238
Raininko 198 (192)
Ramsey 195 (181)
Ranges 214
Ranke von 65 (42)
Rappaport 183, 185, 195 (191),
    204, 208
Raps 8, 16
Rath 452

Ratschow 238, 240
Rau 242
Rautenberg 167
Reboul 178, 216
Recklinghausen von 23, 53
Redeker 86, 87
Redlich 65 (54)
Redman 211 (209)
Regener 344
Rehn 115
Reich 65 (52), 161 (157)
Reichardt 212 (209), 363
Reiffenstuhl 259
Reimann 100, 369, 389
Reinbold 334 (332)
Reindell 88
Reinhardt 65 (46), 104
Reiniger 67, 339, 340, 341, 361,
    383, 387, 399, 400, 437 (429)
Reiser 20
Remy-Jardin 291 (287)
Rendich 138
Rentsch 65 (50)
Rethmeier 219
Reuleaux 335
Reuter 211 (207)
Revesz 445
Reynolds 65 (40)
Rhoads 141
Ribbing 65 (41, 45, 50)
Rice 147
Richards 214
Richardson 344
Richter 107, 303
Ricker 87
Ricketts 191
Ricklin 65 (44, 59)
Riechert 304
Riedel 65 (44, 46)
Rieder 31, 32, 68, 69, 70, 72, 73,
    74, 77, 78, 79, 80, 81, 84, 119, 132,
    133, 139, 462
Rienzo di 85
Ries 102
Righi 468
Rigler 89, 138, 196 (188), 211
    (203, 204)
Rimkus 279
Ringel 163
Ritman 227
Rivas 333 (314)
Robb 178, 181, 201, 214, 218, 227,
    286
Robinson 144, 162 (159), 198
    (193)
Rodeck 172
Rodriguez-Alvarez 196 (190)
Roeck 349
Roedel 106

Roentgen   6, 7, 8, 9, 10, 11, 13, 17, 25, 27, 29, 30, 39, 336, 338, 339, 340, 397, 404, 458, 463, 472
Roesch   209, 211 (208), 483
Roessle   65 (41, 54), 87
Rogers   87
Rohrer   88
Rokitansky   23
Rolleston   74
Rollins   68, 400, 401
Romberg von   82
Rond d'Alembert   22
Rønne   338, 342
Ronnen von   105, 148
Roo de   248
Roos   333 (317)
Rose   446
Rosen   198 (193)
Rosenbusch   1, 6, 22, 25, 37, 115, 152, 261, 293, 335, 338, 357, 397, 440, 458, 477
Rosenfeld   67, 74
Roseno   130 (123), 170
Rosenstein   169
Rosenthal   32, 65 (44), 69, 70, 74, 77, 132, 133, 462
Rossbach   131
Rossmann   107, 445
Roth   216, 421, 427
Rotky   72, 73
Rous   158
Rousthöi   178, 179, 214, 216
Rouviere   248
Roux   65 (50),131
Rowland   17, 29
Rowntree   158, 170
Roy   197 (192)
Rubens   20
Rubin   292 (287)
Rudbeck   248
Ruegsegger   292 (289)
Ruehmkorff   17, 357, 358, 359
Ruettimann   65 (44, 59), 248, 249, 257
Ruijs   119, 157, 162 (160)
Rumpel   65 (58), 131
Rumpf   67
Rusznyak   248
Rutherford   20, 292 (289)
Rutishauser   226
Rzewuski   355 (339)

Sabat   85
Sabiston   217
Sacks   198 (193)
Saebel   392
Salomon   **98**, 99, 354
Sanchez-Perez   182
Sanitas   401
Sansone   333 (319)
Sante   84

Sapeika   127, 130 (123)
Sauerbruch   82, 84, 115
Saupe   87
Sawada   198 (193)
Schad   214, 216
Schaffert   468
Schall   67, 339, 340, 341, 361, 383, 387, 399, 400
Scharmann   **480**
Schatzki   137, 142, 148
Schechter   303
Scheele   16
Schelling   22
Schenz   379, 414
Schermuly   90
Schertel   469
Scheuermann   65 (49, 50)
Schieffer   83
Schilling   62 (52)
Schinz   **32**, 62 (52), 65 (41, 43, 46, 48, 51, 54, 58, 59), 82, 83, 85, 86, 159, 165, 166, 169, 170
Schjerning   68
Schlatter   44, 65 (46)
Schleussner   **30**, 462
Schlossman   196 (190)
Schlotheim   65 (50)
Schmid   41
Schmidt   62 (52, 54, 55), 164, 471
Schmiedel   246 (238)
Schmitmann   369, 372, 375, 384, 390, 393, 396 (370), 433
Schmorl   65 (46, 49, 52, 57)
Schneider   17, 107
Schober   447
Schobinger   211 (204)
Schoenander   299, 300, 425
Schoenlein   24
Schoop   242, 247 (241)
Schorr   418
Schott   16, 105, 444, 447
Schreiber   143
Schrijvers   446
Schristenson   198 (192)
Schroeder   34, 79
Schroedinger   13
Schrott   130 (128)
Schuele   132
Schueller   26, 57, 65 (46), **294**, 297
Schuerch   65 (58)
Schuettmann   33
Schulz   387
Schulze   16
Schumacher   65 (41)
Schuster   423, 451
Schut   447, 449
Schwarz   26, 74, 83, 84, 139
Schwarzmann   379
Schwarzschild   219
Schwedel   88
Schwesig   418

Schwierz   446
Seabold   100, 354
Sehrwald   122, 162 (157)
Seidel   371, 376
Seldinger   69, **184**, 190, 202, 205, 214, 238, 241, 246 (239), 301
Sellink   119, 131, 144
Semmelweis   115
Servelle   248
Seyferth   247 (242), 452
Seyss   104
Shay   142
Shdanov   248
Shepard   293
Shields   376
Shimidzu   178, 185
Shinebourne   214
Shirakabe   145
Shirey   185
Sicard   85, 130 (124), 176, 213, 236, 303
Sick   41
Sidot   16
Siedentopf   447
Siegel   146
Siegelman   333 (317)
Siegert   65 (48)
Siemens   17, 131, 335, 336, 357, 358, 360, 362, 363, 364,400, 403, 429
Sigrist   103
Sigstedt   198 (192)
Silbermann   349, 350, 356 (344)
Siman   65 (51), 89
Simonyi   13
Simpson   115
Sinis   435
Sjoegren   196 (188), 425, 478
Skrabacz   286
Sloman   216, 217
Sluka   79
Smathers   110
Smith   198 (193)
Snell   141
Snellman   145
Snijder   215
Snook   364, 374
Sommer   262, 402, 437 (401), 459, 462
Sommerfeld   11, 12, 14, 15, 17, 20
Sones   185, 188, 190, 196 (187), 214, 217, 218
Sonesson   65 (46)
Sosman   303
Sovak   130 (128), 246 (238)
Speck   119, 121, 130 (123, 128), 246 (238)
Speiser   65 (48)
Spiegler   88, 107, 473
Spieß   78
Spranger   65 (47)

Stanford 107
Stangl 87
Staples 333 (319)
Staub 80
Stauffer 89, 446, 451
Staunig 384
Stechow 69
Steele 102
Stegmann 132
Steinberg 178, 181, 201, 214, 218
Steiner 369, 396 (370), 449, 454
Steinthal 99
Stender 38, 67, 89, 90
Stenvers 278, 297, **298**
Sterzel 100, 389
Steurer 65 (46)
Steven 65 (55)
Stevens 191
Stevenson 144, 266, 267, 447
Stewart 85, 100, 219
Stieda 44, 65 (59)
Stierlin 81, 135
Stieve 265, 280 (273), 417, 451
Stoeckl 26
Stoehr 6
Stokes 16
Stoll 363
Stolper 65 (44, 52)
Stomach 122
Stoney 17
Stormorken 198 (192)
Straubel 463
Strickler 101
Strijk 257
Strnad 418
Stroeer 65 (48)
Struempell 84
Stuermer 464
Stuertz 79, 84
Stumpf 85
Sturm 227, 446
Stutz 85, 87
Sudeck 50, 55
Swart 119, 333 (323, 329)
Swick 124, 125, 170, **171**, 172, 177,
    238
Swieringa 219
Swinton 357
Sylla 86

Tabar 103
Taenzer 246 (238, 242)
Tailland 270
Takahashi 198 (194), 266, 267,
    301
Takaro 198 (194), 211 (207)
Talbot 16, 458, 459
Taussig 214
Taveras 303
Templeton 216
Teschendorf 89, 141

Tesla 17, 357, 364, 360
Teubern von 84
Teubner 108, 473
Teves 444
Thibaut 304
Thiemann 66 (46)
Thienpont 303
Thijssen 302
Thoeni 144
Thompson 142
Thomson 12, 14, 17, 20, 67, 69, 74,
    76, 219, 261, 346, 357, 446
Thorner 27
Thurn 88, 247 (242)
Thurnher 25
Tichy 372
Tillander 185, 204, 205, 207
Titow 66 (52)
Tjernberg 248, 257
Toelle 379
Toendury 66 (46)
Toennis 304
Toepler 17
Tollman 102
Tomich 127
Toplar 357
Torricelli 16
Trapnell 90
Traube 24
Trenkle 343
Tricomi 333 (319)
Trout 107
Tschurlovits 35
Tsuzuki 217
Tuffier 70, 73, 81, 164
Twining 303

Uehlinger 65 (58), 66 (47, 51, 52,
    57, 58), 87
Ulrici 87
Ungar 214
Ungelenk 346, 356 (348)
Unschel 216
Unsoeld 313 (308)
Urra 147, 148
Uson 211 (203)

Valentino 427
Vallebona 85, 137, 262, 266, 267,
    268, 270
Valmaggiore 333 (319)
Vaquez 83, 84
Velpeau 99
Verse 418
Vesalius 1, 3
Viamonte 191, 197 (190), 257
Viehweger 241, 242
Vieten 85, 263, 265, 266, 267, **268**
Vijverberg 451
Villard 341
Vinci da 1, 330, 458

Virchow 4, 6, 23, 24, 27
Vlassenroot 219
Vock 286, 291 (287)
Voelcker 122, 129 (123), 165, **166**,
    167
Vogel 99, 100, 230, 354
Vogelsang 304
Vogl 79
Volhard 84
Volkmann 170
Vollmar 247 (241)
Volta 16, 358
Voorhoeve 66 (47)

Wachsmann 266, 268, 348
Wachter 88
Wackenheim 66 (50), 303
Wagner 107, 210 (201), 359
Waite 367, 377, 380, 402, 403, 441
Wall 333 (319)
Wallace 192, 483
Wallingford 125, 246 (238)
Wallmann 447
Walsh 70
Walsham 70, 73, 84
Walter 31, 86, 358, 362, 383, 384,
    385, 386
Walther 31
Warburg 10, 17, 18
Warenbourg 86
Warren 100, 354
Wassermann 68
Watanabe 355 (353, 354)
Watson 73, 266, 267, 268, 357
Watt 335
Weaver 107
Webb 333 (320)
Weber 25, 85, 138, 143, 144, 246
    (238)
Wedgewood 16
Wedgwood 458
Wegele 131
Wegelius 86
Wegener 292 (289)
Wehnelt 343, 344, 361, 365, 383
Weibel 90
Weigel 418
Weinberger 70, 72, 74, 76, 84
Weiss 26, 66 (48, 59)
Weissleder 107, 248, 249
Weld 130 (123)
Welin 144, 151, 152
Wellauer 427
Wells 88
Weltz 85, 147
Wende 304
Wentz 108
Wentzlik 239, 240
Wenz 247 (241)
Werf van der 230
Werner 104, 105

Wertheim Salomonson **32**, 33
Weskamp 106, 107, 108
Westinghouse 387, 392
Weyers 66 (48, 59)
Whittaker 161 (157)
Wholey 197 (191)
Wickbom 300, 447
Widal 22, 37
Widenmann 451
Wiechel 209
Wieda 86
Wiede **372**
Wiesner 77, 462
Wiewiorowski 86
Wilbert 66 (50)
Wilcke 16, 358
Wiljasalo 248, 257
Williams 32, **67**, 68, 69, 70, 73, 74, 80, 81, 82, 84, 132
Wilms 41
Wimberger 66 (41, 52, 53)
Winau 20
Winkelmann 463

Winthrop 102, 125
Wirsz, E. 436
Wirsz, N. 436
Wirth 248
Wiscomb 227
Woeke 451
Woelfflin 18
Wohlgemut 27
Wohlleben 195 (178)
Wolf 130 (128)
Wolfe 105, 469
Wolff 10, 66 (50)
Wollenberg 66 (44, 59)
Wolvekamp 152
Wood 225, 227, 303, 346
Wright 198 (193)
Wulff 173
Wurm 87
Wylick van 18

Yasargil 303
Young 276

Zadek 73
Zanetti 88
Zdansky 26, 85, 86, 88
Zehbe 84
Zehnder 8, 13, 17
Zeiss 17
Zeitler 120, 197 (190), 236, 246 (238), 247 (241, 242, 243, 244)
Zeitz 104
Zeyss 368
Ziedses des Plantes 85, 262, 263, 265, **266**, 267, 270, 271, 275, 293, 299, 302, 303, 333 (315)
Ziegler 130 (123)
Zimmer 40
ZimmermannG447
Zindel 170
Ziplack 239, 240
Ziskin 445
Zondek 477
Zseboek 89
Zuppinger 66 (50)
Zwerling 142

Index

A

Abdomen 322–324
Abdominal trauma
–, blunt 329f
Abdominal wall 326
Accumulator 359
Actinogram 167
Adrenal glands 328f
Advertisement 30
Akinometer 383
Allergic reactions 250
American X-ray Journal 29
Amipaque 127
Anaesthesia 217, 427
–, local 238
–, Urografin 217
–, Vasurise 217
Anatomy 250–252
Aneurysm 210
–, aortic 320
Angiocardiogram
–, biplanar 227
–, digital subtraction
– –, first 228
–, monitoring 425
Angiocardiography 88, 182, 218f,
   352, 429–434, 452
–, biplane
– –, special procedures room 433
–, digital 225–235
– –, functional 229–233
– –, HICOR 433
–, grid-controlled double
   focus 382
–, selective 178
Angiocardiometry 225
Angiogram
–, hepatic 204
Angiography 119, 184, 188f, 263,
   350–353, 402, 422, 427f
–, abdominal 200
–, automatic tabletop transport 242
–, balloon occlusion 207
–, biplane 426
–, cardiac 192
–, carotid 301
–, cerebral 176, 182, 193, 410

–, coronary 179, 192f, 217, 220
–, CT 287, 324
–, digital subtraction (DSA) 193f,
   205, 210, 215, 221, 242–245, 370,
   452
–, DYNAVISION 428
–, evolution of 176–199
–, exposure in 430
–, future of 194f
–, general 425–427
–, indications and methods 206f
–, interventional 193
– –, abdominal 209f
–, magnification 194, 207
–, MR 245
–, non-invasive 245f
– –, abdominal 210
–, peripheral 427
–, renal 202, 328
–, rotational
– –, DYNAVISION 429
– –, POLYTRON 429
–, selective 182, 184, 206f, 214
– –, abdominal 203–206
– –, coronary 185, 221
– –, pulmonary 215
–, serial 240
–, sliding table top 240
–, (with) spiral CT 288
–, superselective 207f, 352
–, table 240
–, three-phase technique 242
Angioplasty 210, 352f
Angiopneumography 214
–, Diodrast 214
–, Uroselectan 214
ANGIOTRON 228
Anode
–, CALOREX 350
–, composite 349
–, cooling by rotating 346f
–, dual-angle 349
–, lifespan of 350
–, molybdenum 349, 354, 412
–, radial cracking 350
–, rhenium 349
– –, tungsten alloy 350
–, rotating 218, 350

–, RTM 350
–, stress-relieved 351
–, tube
– –, rotating 389
– –, principal of 347
–, tungsten 349
Anorectal area 145
Anticathode
–, aluminium 338
–, platinum 338f
–, tantalum 341f
–, tungsten 341f
–, water-cooled 342
Aorta 74–77, 84
Aortogram 181
Aortography 200, 214
–, lumbar 177, 201–203, 206, 239
–, percutaneous translum-
   bar 200–202
–, supravalvular 185
Archives of Clinical Skiagraphy 29
Arterial calcification 239
Arterial tree 192f
Arteries 178–180, 184–186
–, catheterization of 179
–, coronary 178, 185, 215–222,
   290
– –, left 222
–, hand 245
–, thoracic 178
Arteriography 193
–, carotids 300
–, extra- and intracranial
   vessels 301
–, extremity 177
–, legs 237
–, percutaneous transfemoral 301
–, three-phase technique 241
–, upper leg 241
Arteriosclerosis 189
Arteriovenous shunt 192
Artery
–, brachial
– –, passage of catheter from 203
Asbestos 318

B

Back projection technique 283
Balloon pump
–, intra-aortic 191
Barium
–, particles 143
–, platincyanide 463
–, sulphate 133, 138
Battery
–, lead storage 359
Bearing
–, ball 353
–, helical fluid 353
–, liquid spiral 353
Benoist-Walter (BW) unit 383
Benzoic acid 125
Berlin 26–29
Berliner Klinische Wochen-
    schrift 27
Berlin Medical Society 27
Bilbao tube 148
Biochemistry 483
Biopsy 243, 263, 413
Bismuth
–, bicarbonate 133
–, meal 133
–, nitrate 133
Bladder
–, radiographic examination
    of 173
BLITZ 342, 386
Blood flow
–, cerebrovascular 310
–, hemodynamics of 239
Blurring 270
Board of Radiology 33
Bone
–, circulation disorders 55
–, density 290
–, dysplasia 57f
– –, fibrous 57
–, formation
– –, genetic disorders 52
–, generalized diseases 52–57
–, hormonal diseases 52
–, lymphogranulomatosis 52
–, microradiography 55–57
–, mineral content 289
–, transformation
– –, genetic disorders 52
–, tumour 58f, 331
Brake 397
Brightness 446f
British expeditionary corps 40
British Medical Journal 28
Bronchial asthma 79
Bronchial pneumonia 78
Bronchiectases 317
Bronchography 85
Brown tumour 54
Bubbly-barium method 145f

Bucky table 218

C

Cable
–, connector
– –, high-voltage 381
–, high-tension 403
–, high-voltage 380f, 389
Calcification 289f
–, intracranial 313
–, micro 354
Camera
–, 16-mm 220
–, 70-mm 448, 451
–, 70-mm film 241
–, 70-mm rollfilm 418
–, 70/100-mm 420
–, 100-mm 424
–, cine 418
–, laser 469
–, obscura 458
–, Odelka 219
Cancer
–, breast 98
–, curable 99
Carbon fiber table top 194
Carcinoma
–, bronchial
– –, central 87
– –, esophageal 324
–, gastric 145
–, hilus 81
–, lobar lung 81
Cardiac parameters 88
Cardiology 425, 429–434, 479
C-arm 243f, 378, 422f, 429, 448
–, ARCOSCOP 100 OP 411
–, BINO 425
–, first 410
–, mobile 411
– –, (with) digital imaging 453
Cassette 460
Cassette changer 181f, 186f, 206,
    218f, 240, 425, 429
–, (for) cerebral angiography 182
–, large-format serial 194
–, (for) radiographs of the
    heart 430
Cassette drum 239
Catheter 177, 185f, 206, 217, 425,
    428
–, 4 F 193
–, 4 and 5 F 242
–, balloon 185, 208, 482
– –, -tipped 193
–, closed-end 190
–, Cournand 178, 183
–, Ducor 191
–, end-hole 186
–, flow-directed 193
–, high-flow 192f

–, hook-tail 190
–, J-shaped 190
–, lumbar aortogram 186
–, Oedman-radiopaque 190
–, PE 190
–, pigtail 190
–, polyethylene 184
–, radiopaque polythene 205
–, Radner 180
–, side-hole 186
–, steerable 204
–, techniques 190f
–, thrombogenicity 190, 192
–, ureteral by retrograde
    injection 165
Catheterization
–, percutaneous 184
–, transfemoral route 193
–, transhepatic 193
Cathode
–, grid-controlled 348
–, rays 13f
Cava filter 191
Cavography 200, 208
–, Seldinger technique 208
Central bronchi 77
Ceramic 352
Chest
–, anatomy in various
    projections 72
–, changer 413
– –, THORAMAT 414
–, CT examination 316
–, fluoroscopy 68
–, paediatric unit
– –, THORAKOMAT 423
–, radiograph 71, 446
–, specific diseases 73
–, tumours 81
Cholangiography
–, intraoperative 160
Cholecystography
–, intravenous 159
–, oral 159, 161
Cholecystoses 160
Chronic idiopathic
    steatorrhea 141
Chylous effusion 256
Cineangiocardiography
–, biplane 187f
Cineangiography 215
Cine application 370
Cinedensitometry 225
Cinefluorography 187, 192
CINEMATIC 454
Cinematographic
    visualization 222
Cinematography 220, 348, 431
Cineradiographic unit 181
Cineradiography 194
Cinetomography 263

Circuitry
–, closed-loop   370
Classification of peripheral
   lymphedema   253
Closing light   373f
Coating
–, photosensitive
– –, doubling   462f
Coelioscopy   167
Colitis   138
Collimation   106, 400–402, 406,
   430, 440
–, Albers-Schoenberg   400
–, automatic   402
–, electronic   402
–, system
– –, Groedel   401
– –, principle function of   402
Collimator   397f, 408, 423
–, multileaf   401, 404
–, ROTAX universal   400f
Colon   132
–, cleansing of   144
–, examination   138f
– –, double contrast   144
–, irritable   138
–, tumour of   324
Comité de Coordination des
   Industries Radiologiques
   (COCIR)   382
Complications
–, abdominal angiography   201
–, (from) angiographic procedures   189
–, angiography   238
–, digital subtraction angiography   242
–, lumbar aortography   202
–, radiography   177
–, retrograde injection   166
–, selective abdominal angiography   206
–, vascular   192f
Compound scanning   479
Compression   106, 397f, 400, 406,
   410, 412
–, Albers-Schoenberg   400
–, patent   400
–, tube   136
Computed tomography see CT
Computer aided surgery
   (CAS)   290
Computer science   483
Contour   272
Contrast   466, 481
–, double   352
Contrast medium   100, 102, 176f,
   183, 189, 200, 236–238, 287, 434,
   450, 483
–, Abrodil   178
–, air   122

–, barium sulphate   122
–, bismuth nitrate   122
–, calcium sulphate
   (gypsum)   122
–, development of   121–130
–, Diodon   178
–, Diodrast   178, 180, 183
–, Halogens (iodide)   122
–, Hypaque   183
–, indicator   226
–, infusion   151
–, intravenous administration
   of   307
–, iodinated oily   249
–, lead acetate   122
–, Lipiodol   213, 236
–, low-osmolality   127f
–, Mercuric sulphide   122
–, Miokon   183
–, non-ionic   127f
– –, water-soluble   238
–, oral   167
–, organ-specific   128f
–, pathology-specific   128f
–, Perabrodil   178, 238
–, pharmacokinetics of   159
–, Renografin   183
–, silver   122
–, Skiodan   178
–, sodium iodide/bromide   122
–, strontium (bromide)   122
–, thorium dioxide   122
–, thorium (nitrate)   122
–, Thorotrast   177–179, 216, 300
–, Urografin   183, 217, 238
–, Urokon   183
–, Uroselectan   177, 213
–, water-soluble
– –, intravenous   171
– –, iodine   249
Contrast range   466
Contrast reaction   127
Control console   363, 370f
Control triode
–, high-voltage   370
Corona   381
Coronary   213–225
Cost-benefit   228
Costs   484f
Counterweight   397
Coupling   397
CT   194, 210, 263f, 304f, 313, 317,
   352f, 427, 435, 474, 478
–, 3D display   287f
–, 3D reconstruction   308f
–, ACTA   284
–, angiography   287, 324
–, chest examination   316
–, cine   286
–, conventional system
– –, continuously rotating   285

–, cost-effectiveness   290
–, -diskography   332
–, distortion   290
–, dual-energy techniques   290
–, first generation   284
–, fourth generation   285
–, high-resolution   307
–, -myelography   311, 332
–, performance characteristics
   of   286
–, principle of   282–284
–, quantitative (QCT)   290, 332
–, quantitative assessment of tissue
   properties   289
–, quantitative information   289
–, scan time   284
–, second generation   284
–, single photon emission
   (SPECT)   194
–, SOMATOM PLUS   372
–, spiral   286–288, 312, 353
– –, angiography with   288
– –, volume scans with   286-288
–, technical develop-
   ment   281–292
–, third generation   285
–, ultrafast   322, 354
–, value   284
–, volume scanner   285
–, Xenon-enhanced   309f
Current
–, reverse   359, 373f
Cushing's disease   54
Cystocopy   163
Cystographic evaluating   173
Cytostatics   264

D
Daniell cell   358
Dark room   467
–, lamp   461
–, table   461
Daylight
–, processor   468
–, system   468
DCI   228
Defecation studies   145
Defects
–, congenital   84
Deficiency pattern   142
Densitogram   225f
Densitometry   225f
Density   272, 284, 290
–, measurement   289
–, optical   392
–, tiny nodular   90
Dental medicine   268, 278
Dentistry   374, 378
Detector
–, double   393

Deutsche Roentgengesellschaft
  see German Roentgen Society
Developer 459
–, bath 461
Development 466
–, process 460
– –, controlled by sight 466
Diagnosis
–, intraoral 278
Diaphragm 82
–, Bucky 402
–, internal 400f
–, slit 269
–, vibrating Bucky patent 403
Diatrizoic acid 126
Differential diagnosis 253
DIGIMATIC 454
Digital luminescence radio-
  graphy 407, 409
Digital subtraction angiography
  (DSA) 193f, 205, 210, 215, 221,
  242–245, 370, 452
–, automatic control
– –, DIGIMATIC 452
–, intraarterial 244
–, intravenous 242f
–, stepwise 243
–, system 453
Digital videography 194
DIGITRON 228
Dilatation 193, 482
DIN/IEC 336/1981 349
Direct-sign-method 134
Disease
–, joint 481
Dislocation 331
Displacement current (roentgen
  current) 15–18
DIVAS 228
Documentation
–, 35-cm roll film 192
–, Amplatz' see-through
  changer 192
–, AOT changer 192
–, catheter 186–188
–, Diodrast 180
–, Franklin changer 192
–, injectors 191
–, radiographic 177, 206
–, rubber catheter 180
Dominant 392
Doppler Echography 479
Dose
–, considered permissible
– –, development 473
–, distribution within body 273
–, genetic effect 472
–, highest permissible 472
–, maximum permissible 472
–, Mutscheller 472
–, physical effect 472

–, rate 274, 388, 390, 423
–, reduction 110, 402, 451
– –, after new technical develop-
  ments since 1960 474
–, regulation 472
–, tolerance 472
Dosimetry 34f
Double contrast 133
Double focus principle 345
Drainage 243
Drift compensation 392
DSA see Digital subtraction angio-
  graphy
Dual-energy subtraction 228
Duodenal bulb 137
Duplex-doppler 194

E
EBT see Electron beam tomography
ECG 450
–, recording 433
–, triggered 186, 191, 215, 290
Education requirements 483
Efficiency coefficient 270
Ejection fraction 229
Electric shock 403
Electron beam scanner 285f
Electron beam tomography
  (EBT) 289f, 354
Electron gun 353
Electronic harmonizing 172
Electronic subtraction 220
Electrostatic inductor
  machine 357
Embolization 193, 210, 243, 427
Encephalography 295
Engineering 483
Enteroclysis 141
Equalizer
–, line-voltage
– –, PUGNO-VANONI 369
Ergonomic 417
–, situation 397
Esophageal
–, disorders 143
–, examination 143
Evoker 459
Examination
–, room 406
–, table
– –, development of 405–408
–, time 287, 434
– –, reduction 428
Exposure
–, angle 270f
–, avoiding 404
–, control
– –, automatic (AEC) 274,
  390–393, 412f, 454, 466
– – –, (for) tomography 392f
– –, system 391

–, fields
– –, irregular 401
–, forearm 378
–, hand 405
–, high energy 351
–, system 274
–, table 387
–, thoracic
– –, typical 472
–, time 219, 263, 352, 362, 368f,
  371, 385–393, 404f, 413, 432, 451
– –, patent 388
– –, reduction 134
Extremities 250f
Eye sensitivity 447

F
Fan beam 283–285
–, scanner 285
Filament 343
–, circuit 363
–, tungsten 364
Film 218, 459
–, 100-mm cut- 451f
–, blurring 466
–, camera 187
–, celluloid 464
–, changer 186, 192, 215, 239
– –, Amplatz' see through 192
– –, AOT 192, 242, 392
– –, cut- 241
– – –, AOT 241, 245, 427
– – –, PUCK 425, 427
– –, Elema roll- 187, 192
– –, Franklin 192
– –, long 192
– –, PUCK 193f, 241f, 352, 392,
  427
– –, roll- 182, 239
–, cine
– –, 35-mm
– – –, ARRIFLEX 433
– –, first German 444
–, density 391
–, double 367
–, format 465
–, magazine 407
–, processing machine
– –, electronically controlled 467
–, processor
– –, automatic 466f
– –, directly connected 407
– –, (for) mass fluorography
  films 467
– –, rack 466
–, production 466
–, roll-
– –, 25-mm 442
– –, 70-mm
– – –, ODELKA 442
–, screen system 263

–, shelf-life 464
–, single-coated 412
Filter 397
–, combination 110
–, Mo/Rh 413
Fistula
–, arteriovenous 210
Fistulography 86
Fixation 466
Flocculation 139f
–, (of) barium 147
Flow dynamics 210
Flow rate 184, 186
Fluidograph 105
Fluidography 106
Fluorography
–, chest 414
–, heart
– –, ODELKA 443
–, lungs
– –, ODELKA 443
–, unit built into a bus 415
Fluoroscopy 84f, 116, 182, 184f,
    204f, 213, 239, 347, 349, 351f, 370,
    393, 400f, 404, 406, 411, 415, 417,
    423, 425, 428, 432, 440–457, 482f
–, automation 453f
–, chest 68
–, edge enhancement 448
– –, TRANSICON 448
–, hand 404f
–, image
– –, HICOR 433
–, military X-ray unit 440
–, pulsed 425, 434, 454
–, recumbent patient 441
–, room 380
–, scene
– –, electronic storage 450
–, transition time 349
–, TV 451
Focal spot 108, 351f, 354
–, large 350
–, optical 344
–, size 342, 446
–, small 350, 428
–, spring 263
Focus
–, fine 352
Foreign body 261
Foreign object 265
Fourier reconstruction 283
Fracture 50f, 331
–, vertebral 312

G
Galactography 102–105
Gallbladder
–, (and) biliary tract 157–162
–, disease
– –, acalculous 160

Gap filling 434, 454
Gastrointestinal tract 323f
Generator 357–396
–, 2-pulse 106
–, 100-kW 371
–, (for) angiography
– –, PANDOROS OPTIMAT-
    IC 375
–, costs 369
–, DC 371
–, DC voltage 369
–, electrostatic 357f
–, GIGANTOS 368, 374
–, HELIODENT 378
–, HELIODOR 367
–, HELIOPAN R 373
–, HELIPHOS 369
–, high-frequency 369–371, 379,
    382, 414
– –, MOBIL XR 372
–, KODIAPHOS 353, 371, 390
–, large 369
–, MEDIO D 369, 374
–, MEGANOS 404
–, microprocessor-controlled 371
–, MONOPHOS 407
–, OPTIMATIC 369f, 372, 390,
    433
–, PANDOROS OPTIMATIC 369f
–, patient benefits 369
–, POLYDOROS 371, 392
–, POLYPHOS 354, 367, 379
–, quality 368
–, RENODOR 378f
–, secondary controlled
– –, PANDOROS 382
–, single-pulse 369
–, single-tank 263, 351, 376–380
– –, high-frequency
– – –, POLYPHOS 413
– – –, POLYPHOS B 411
– –, NANOPHOS 379
– –, POLYPHOS 351
– –, SIREPHOS 411
–, six-pulse 388f
–, small 369f
–, STABILIPAN 375
–, STATUS X 378, 423
–, three-phase 106, 368f, 371, 388
–, TITANOS 388
–, TRIDOROS 389
–, TRIDOROS 4 371
–, TRIDOROS OPTIMATIC 384
–, TUTO HELIPHOS 381
–, TUTOMAT 369
–, two-pulse 369
–, universal 366
–, x-ray 357, 364
– –, high-frequency 372
– –, three-phase 368
– – –, six-pulse 365

Geometric blurring 466
Geometric unsharpness 368
Geometry 397
Geriatrics 287
German Roentgen Society 29,
    31
Glass 352
Goetze-focus 345
Graphite 350
Grid 106, 397, 402f
–, Bucky 402
–, initial drive 403
–, mammography 108
–, moving 403
–, Potter-Bucky 100
–, technique 108
Guide-wire 180, 190, 192f, 242,
    425, 428
–, flexible 204
–, teflon-coated 192
–, torque control 193
Gynaecology 477f

H
Haematoma
–, intracranial 264
Halogens 157
Hardness 367
–, measurement 382–385
Head injury 306
Heart 74–77, 213–235, 321f
–, congenital disease 214
– –, Uroselectan 214
–, (and) large vessels 82–84, 88
–, positional anomalies 84
–, valvular diseases
– –, acquired 83
–, volume
– –, VOLUMAT 434
Heat storage capacity 349, 351f
Hemorrhage
–, acute cerebral 305
Hepatobiliary tract 324–326
Hexabrix 127
HICOR 228
High-frequency AC 364
High-kilovoltage tech-
    nique 370–372
High-voltage divider 384f
Hip dislocation 261
Hounsfield unit (HU) 284
Hydronephrosis 166
Hyperostosis generalisata 47
Hypotonic agent 146
Hysterosalpingography 478

I
ICRP 60 472
IDEAL apparatus 362, 364, 374
IDONTOMAT 379
IGNITRON 372

Ileum loops
–, examination via retrograde
    colon filling   139
Image
–, blurring   271
–, contrast   271
–, digital   413, 440–457
–, digitally acquired   469
–, display
– –, flicker-free   425
–, fusion   428
–, generation   271f
–, intensifier   88f, 118, 185, 187,
    192, 194, 204, 244, 411, 420, 426,
    442–446
– –, 14-inch   446
– –, 30-cm   451
– –, 40-cm   422
– –, 57-cm   446
– –, caesium iodide   451
– –, electron-optical design
    443
– – –, CINELIX   445
– –, image   440–457
– –, in the 1960s and 1970s   445f
– –, in the 1980s and 1990s   446
– –, large diameter   244
– –, mirror optics   445
– –, ODELKA   414, 427, 443
– –, optical   220, 432
– –, optical output   411
– –, patent   443
– –, radiography   448
– –, SIRECON   450
– –, SIRECON Duplex   445
– –, (in) surgery   448f
– –, surgical environment   448
– –, -TV system   201, 226
– –, unit BV   20
– – –, for surgical fluoros-
        copy   449
– – –, u-shaped
– – –, CARDOSCOP U   433
–, laten
– –, generation of   466
–, monitor
– –, digital   434
– –, flicker-free   434
–, processing
– –, quantitative   263
–, quality   283, 285, 393, 397–400,
    440, 451f, 454
– –, subjective   465–469
–, recording   119
–, sharpness   271
–, storage
– –, electronic
– – –, TONOTRON   447
–, time-parameter   232
–, transmission   271
–, unsharpness   271

Imaging
–, digital   110, 393
– –, 40-cm   426
–, magnetic resonance   208, 210
–, millisecond-range   290
–, planographic   265
–, system
– –, digital   422
–, vascular   287, 425–427
Induction
–, coil   358
–, electromagnetic   358
Inductor   358f, 362, 404
–, design   359
–, Ruhmkorff   357f
–, schematic   359
–, spark   363
–, voltaic   358
Industrial film   102
Infertility
–, female   478
Inflammatory diseases   51f
Inguinal region   251
Injection   177, 236, 239, 434
–, intravenous   228, 287
Injector   180, 186, 202, 206
–, Cordis   191
–, electrically powered   191
–, gas powered   191
–, Gidlund   186f, 191
–, high pressure   217
–, Viamont-Hobbs   191
Insulation
–, high-voltage   367f
Intensity   385
Intensive care unit (ICU)   379
Interference effect   271
International Commission on Ra-
    diation Units and Measurements
    (ICRU)   270, 274
Interrupter   360–363
–, Depréz   360
–, electrolytic   359
–, mercury   360f
–, mercury petroleum
– –, cross-section of   361
–, platinum   360
–, REKORD   360, 363
–, rotary mercury   359
–, Wagner hammer   359
–, Wehnelt electrolytic   361–363
Interventional procedures   263
Inverter technology   372
Ionization chamber   390–392
IONTOMAT   370, 391–393
IONTOMAT 7   392
IONTOMAT P   392f
Isodense method
–, (for) breast examination   105
Isotope   303

K
KENOTRON   374
Kerley
–, A and B lines, 1951   90
Kidney   327f
–, cavernous tuberculosis   166
–, solitary   166
Kinetic blurring   466
Kryptoradiometer   383
Kryptoskop   383, 411, 448
–, monitoring   425
kV   365
–, meter
– –, non-invasive   385
–, selection of   370
–, technique   139, 367, 381
–, value   370
– –, patent   367
Kymograph   146
Kymography   85, 172

L
Laminagraphy   263
Larynx   132
Laxative abuse   151
Layer
–, emulsion   466
–, half-value   383
–, protective   466
Lead acetate   131
Léri's melorheostosis   47
Lesion
–, traumatic   205
Level   271
Levocardiogram   227
Light box
–, adjustable shutters   465
Light distributor   444
Light localizer   402
Line
–, focus   344f
–, high-voltage   380–382
– –, open   380
Lipiodol   129
Lithotripsy   423, 483
LOADIX   353
Log-Electronics   104f
Loop control circuit
–, closed   367, 390
Loop control system
–, closed   392
Looser zones   58
Low-dose system   106
Low-radiation technique   106
Ludwig, Anna-Bertha   19
Luer lock   186
Lung   316
–, density   289
–, emphysema   79
–, field   72
– –, density changes   72

–, interstitial processes   90
–, pattern analysis to diffuse ~ disease   89
–, structural analyses   89–91
–, syphilitic   79
–, tumours
– –, benign   87
Lungenspitzenblende
–, Groedel   400
Lymphadenopathy   320
Lymphangiopathy
–, central   254f
Lymphatic cysts   255
Lymphatic system   254
–, retroperitoneal   327
–, tumour of   256
Lymphatic vessels
–, anatomy   248
–, diseases   252–256
Lymphedema   248, 252f
–, acquired primary   252
–, peripheral
– –, classification of   253
–, post-traumatic   252
–, primary   253f
–, secondary   252–254
Lymph node
–, disease   256f
– –, malignant   257–259
–, enlarged   77
–, metastases   258f
Lymphographic technique   249
Lymphoma
–, primary malignant   257f

M

Magnetic resonance imaging see
  MRI
Magnification   352, 446
Malformation   210
Mammogram
–, craniocaudal view   100
–, lateral-oblique   100
Mammograph   98
–, requirement for techniques   101
Mammography   98–114, 469, 479
–, automatic exposure control   106
–, scattered radiation   106
–, system
– –, MAMMOMAT   3000   413
–, technical developments   105f
mAs
–, meter   388
–, product   106, 365, 385, 388
–, relay   389f
–, selection of   370
–, value   370
– –, patent   367

Mastectomy   99
Mastopathy   100
Maximum intensity projection
  (MIP)   288
Measurement
–, quantitative   483
Mechanical stability   274
Mediastinal masses   320
Mediastinum   78, 319f
Medical science before   1895   22–24
Medullar osteopathies   55
Method
–, direct   218
–, indirect   218
Methylcellulose   138
Microcalcification   100f, 109
Microfocal spot   352
Microfocus magnification technique   108–110
–, magnification mammography   108
Microprocessor technology   379
Military   379
–, medicine   40
Milliampere setting   365
MIMER   299, 410
MOBIL XR   379
Modulation transfer function
  (MTF)   445
Molybdenum   109
–, anode   103
– –, tube   104
–, filter   104
Monitor
–, SIMOMED   448
Motion blurring   345, 352
Moulage sign   142
Movement   266f
–, circular   266
–, multi-dimensional   266
–, one-dimensional   266
–, plane-parallel   266
–, pluridirectional   271
–, undirectional (linear)   271
MR angiography   194
MRI   194, 264, 312, 480–484
Multidirectional view   352
Multiplanar reconstruction
  (MPR)   288
Multiscope   244
Musculoskeletal system
  330–332
Mutation
–, genetic   472
–, spontaneous   472
Myelography   302
Myocardial perfusion   229f

N

NANOMOBIL   379

National Council on Radiation
  Protection and Measurements   274
Needle aspiration   104
Nephrolithiasis   166
Nephroptosis   167
Neuroradiology   263, 350, 427f, 481

O

Object plane   270
Obstetrics   477f
Odelka camera   219
Oesophageal motility   146
Operating room   411, 448
–, TV   449
Orthodiagraph   76, 404f
–, vertical by Kienboeck   460
Orthodiagraphy   75,82
Orthodontic   268
Orthopaedics   404
Orthopantomography   278, 478
Osmolality   189, 238
–, contrast media
– –, ionic   193
– –, non-ionic   193
Osteitis deformans (Paget's
  disease)   57f
Osteoarticular diseases   59
Osteochondronecroses   46f
Osteodensitometry   332
Osteodystrophia fibrosa generalisata cystica Recklinghausen   53
Osteogenesis imperfecta   47
Osteomalacia   52
Osteoporosis   54, 289f
Overload warning   353f
OZONEX principle   381

P

Paediatrics   287, 423–425, 479
Palpation   420
Pancreas   205, 209, 325f
Pancreatitis
–, acute   326
–, chronic   326
Panoramic view   378
Pantomography   268, 279
Parenchyma   105
Patient positioning   397–439
Pelvis   330
Pencil beam   283f
Perceptibility   271
Percutaneous techniques   194
Percutaneous transluminal angioplasty (PTA)   189, 243, 482
Perfusion   289
–, tissue   290
Pericardial effusion   84
Peritoneal cavity   326
Peritoneogram   145

Perivision 244
PET *see* Positron Emission Tomography
Pharmacoangiography 183, 189, 191, 208f
Pharmacology 483
Pharyngeal swallowing mechanism
–, cinematographic studies on 143
Phenoltetrachlorophthalein 158
Phlebography 238
–, abdominal 208f
Phlebolymphedema
–, combined 253
Photoacoustic effect 15
Photofluorography 194
–, 100-mm 192
Photosensitivity 459
Phototimer 106–108, 392
Physical prolegomena of the discovery of X-rays
–, electricity and magnetism 16f
–, evacuation 16
–, fluorescence examination 16
–, manufacture of discharge tubes 16
–, photography 16
Physics 483
Pixel 282
Placenta 478
Planigraph 266
Planigraphy 263, 270
Plate
–, double-coated 463
–, dry
– –, double-coated 464
– –, photographic 459
–, gelatin
– –, silver-bromide 459
–, glass
– –, coating 459
–, selenium 468
Pleura 318f
–, diseases 81f
–, effusion 73,81
–, punctures 86
Pneumocephalography
–, MIMER 427
Pneumoconioses 80
Pneumoencephalogram 264
Pneumoencephalography 263, 297
Pneumomycoses 86
Pneumoradiography 169
Pneumothorax 319
–, diagnostic 86
Polycystography 167
Polyester 466
POLYMATIC 454
Polytome 266
Portal circulation 193

Portal system 183
Portography
–, transhepatic 208
Position
–, lock-in 397
–, Trendelenburg 397
Positron Emission Tomography (PET) 194, 484
Presse 25
Primary hyperparathyroidism 54
Projection
–, beam
– –, multidirectional 426
–, caudocranial 221
–, craniocaudal 221
–, frontal 221
–, lateral 221
–, multiplanar 243
–, oblique 420
–, orthogonal 425
Protection
–, electrical 397
–, electric shock 403f, 415
–, mechanical 397
–, radiation 404, 415
–, standards 35
Pseudoaneurysm 192
PUGNO-VANONI 389
Pulmonary
–, circulation 178
–, diseases 86–87
– –, disseminated 87
–, infections
– –, opportunistic 317
–, lesions
– –, echinococcal 73
–, masses
– –, benign 81
–, metastases 81
– –, small 316f
–, opacities 72
–, parenchyma 78f
–, tuberculosis 74,79
Pulsed exposure 220
Puncture 186
–, intercostal 216
–, needle 190
–, percutaneous 177
–, suprasternal 216
–, transhepatic 160
–, transsternal 216
Pyelography 172
–, intravenous 169–173
–, retrograde 167

Q
Quality
–, assurance 274
–, control 34f
Quantification 243

R
Radiation 188
–, biological effects 471
–, biology 34f
–, burn 404, 471
–, characteristic 104
–, cooling
– –, high-temperature 346
–, dose 181, 412, 468, 485
– –, quality of 368f
–, effects
– –, deterministic 471
– –, stochastic 471
–, exposure 103, 220, 272–274, 278f, 287, 354, 412f, 420, 424, 434, 454, 469, 478f, 484
– –, development 472–475
– –, reduction 102f, 393, 409, 430
– –, risk and benefit 471–475
–, extrafocal 342
–, hardness 340f
– –, technical parameters 387
–, hardness measurement
– –, Benoist 384
– –, Benoist-Walter 384
– –, half-value layer (Christen) 384
– –, sparking distance 384
– –, Walter 384
– –, wavelength 384
– –, Wehnelt 384
–, hard technique 348f, 389
–, high-temperature cooling 348
–, hygiene 393
–, intensity
– –, distribution 339f
–, output 368
–, patient exposure 369, 371
–, protection 34f, 345f, 397, 400, 404, 411, 414, 483
–, protective housing 398
–, scattered 269, 271, 398, 402f
–, soft 367, 387–389
–, spectrum 384
–, standard hand 386
Radiocarousel 219
Radiograph
–, chest 423, 446
– –, paediatric 423
–, dental 479
–, (as) evidence 29
–, foot 408
–, hand 408
–, medical
– –, first 25f
–, panoramic 378
–, postevacuation 138
–, skull 339, 408
–, stereoscopic
– –, chest 413
– –, heart 413

–, surgical specimen   99
–, table   406
–, viewing   462
Radiographic technique   387
Radiography   347, 350, 400
–, 70-mm roll-film   451
–, body section   270
–, chest   371, 413–415, 474
–, cine   443
– –, digital   452
– –, (with) image intensifier   450f
– –, pulsed   431
–, dental   478
–, digital   453
– –, luminescence   393, 414
– – –, system   110
– –, (with) X-ray image intensi-
    fier   452
–, electron   468
–, expansion of observa-
    tions   77–84
–, Fuji computed   194
–, further expansions
    1920–1950   84–88
–, hand   404f
–, image intensifier   448
–, indirect   451
–, intraoperative   423
–, luminescence
– –, digital   453
–, skeletal   408–410
– –, ORBIX   409
–, skull
– –, perdiagraph after
        Grashey   409f
–, spot film   392f
–, stereo   428
–, Thorax   314–322
– –, after   1950   88–91
– –, early years   67–70
– –, further expansions
        1920–1950   84–88
–, transition time   349
Radiology
–, birth in Vienna   26
–, board of   33
–, cardiovascular   180
–, digital   435f, 453
–, forensic   479
–, interventional   119, 189, 481
–, paediatric   451
–, pioneering age   25–36
–, quality control in   202
–, small intestinal   142
Radiolucency
–, decreased   78
–, increased   78
Radioscopy   70, 134
Radiosurgery
–, GAMMAKNIFE   428
Radiotherapy   34, 263

Radiotomy   270
Radner technique   190f
Rectification
–, Graetz   367
–, high-voltage   373f
–, six-pulse   368
Rectifier   364, 387
–, high-vacuum   374f
–, high-voltage   364
– –, mechanical cross-arm   373
–, rotating   373f
–, selenium   375f
– –, semiconductor   375
–, semiconductor   376
–, silicion   376
–, spark gap   373f
Regeneration
–, mica   341
–, osmotic   341
–, palladium   341
Regional enteritis   140
Regurgitation fraction   229
Rehfuss tube   148
Remote-control equipment   146
Renal stones   163f
Reporting
–, soft copy   455
–, system   454
–, workstation
– –, SIREP   454
Resolution   274f, 448
–, contrast   263
–, spatial   263
Respiration   82
Retroperitoneal organ   205
Retroperitoneography   263
Retroperitoneum   251, 326
Retropneumoperitoneum   169
Revolution per minute   351
Rheumatic diseases   52
Rhodium   109
Roentgen
–, apparatus for single-pulse
    operations   363
–, Association   29
–, cinematography   133
–, Episkop   402
–, examination
– –, prophylactic   101
–, film   464f
– –, sensitivity   465
–, instrumentarium   362
– –, single-pulse   386
–, Kugel   345, 369, 377
–, photography   458–470
– –, early years   459–462
– –, history   458f
–, plate in advertisement   459
–, Society   29
–, Vereinigung see Roentgen
    Association

Roentgen, W. C.
–, (in) Apeldoorn   18
–, doctorial thesis   18
–, (in) Giessen   19
–, (in) Lennep   18
–, letter by   340
–, Nobel Prize   14
–, scientific activities   15
–, scientific integrity   14
–, (in) Utrecht   18
–, (in) Zürich   18
Roll-film changer   182
–, Elema   187
Rotation   349
Rubber   381

S
Scan time   285
Scattered radiation   106
Screen
–, blurring   466
–, densitometry   225
–, fluorescent   440–442
– –, KRYPTOSKOP   440f
–, input
– –, caesium iodide   446
–, intensifying   69, 102, 465
– –, blue-fluorescent lanthanum
        oxybromide   468
– –, green-fluorescent gadolinium
        oxysulphide   468
– –, rare earths   468
– –, red fluorescent yttrium
        oxysulphide   468
–, rare earths   275, 414, 452
–, split   227
Screening   103
–, mammographic   103
Section
–, coronal   307
–, interval   270f
–, thickness   270
Segmentation
–, temporal   232
Selective studies   182
Selectivity   270
Senograph   104
Sensitivity
–, improvement   473
Serialography   389, 410, 417, 451
Serial roentgenography   133
Sharpness   466
Shock-waves
–, extracorporeal   423
Shunt
–, arteriovenous   192
–, portocaval   209
SIENET system   435
Silver salt   463
Single Photon Emission Computed
    Tomography (SPECT)   194

Skeletal abnormalities
–, congenital
– –, genetically determined
     47–50
Skeletal ossification   41–47
Skeleton   39–66
–, syphilitic infection   52
Skiameter   383
Skull
–, bony   294–297
–, special views   298
–, unit   410
Slice
–, transverse axial   263
Small bowel   139
–, series   142
Sodium-iodide solution   170
Soft tissue   59f
Sonography   479
–, duplex   245
–, real-time   479
Spalding's sign   478
Spark
–, gap   363, 373
– –, measurement   383
–, machine
– –, single-   363
Spatial frequency   446
Spatial resolution   210
Spectroscopy   481
Spinal
–, cord   311
–, trauma   311
Spine   331f
Spiral   263
Spirometric control   290
Spleen   325
Splenoportography   208
Spot film   350, 421
–, device   415–422
– –, Berg   417
–, (with) fluorescent screen   444
–, (with) image intensifier
     449–452
Spot-filming   370
Staging   328
Stand   397–439
–, 3D   408
–, chest
– –, paediatric
– – –, THORACOMAT   424
– –, with a 57 cm image intensi-
     fier   413
–, cinematography
– –, Janker   431
–, development   405–408
–, floor to ceiling   408
–, Immelmann's
– –, (with) collimation
     system   399
–, Lysholm's   410

–, (with) overtable tube   420
–, (of) skull and extremities   410
–, small   399
–, stationary   408
–, surgical C-arm   411
–, VERTIX B   411
–, wooden   398
–, (with) wooden clamps   398
–, (for) x-ray tubes   398–400
Stenosis   193, 210
Stent
–, metallic expandable   209
Stereo   352
Stereolaminagraphy   263
Stereoradioscopy   351f
Stereoscopic method   261
Stereoscopic radiographic
     images   49
Stereoscopy   262
Stereotactic
–, localization   110
–, principle   111
–, surgery   309
Stereotaxy   428
Stomach   131–133
–, tumour of   324
Stone's technique   190f
Stratigraphy   263, 270
Structure
–, superimposed   265
Subtraction   302, 450
–, photographic   218f
Sudeck's bone atrophy   50
Superimposition   275
SUPERORTHICON   446f
Superselective technique   191
–, steering devices   191
Surface   273
–, dose   272f
–, rendering (SSD)   288
Symptom-complex-method   134
System   397–439
–, ATLAS   409
–, low-dose   412
–, movement   397
– –, image receptor   398
– –, one-dimensional
– – –, curved   398
– – –, linear   398
– – –, rotational   398
– –, patient positioning   398
– –, tabletop   398
– –, three-dimensional   398
– –, two-dimensional   398
– –, x-ray tube   398
–, skeletal diagnostics   404–410
Systemic osteoscleroses   55

T
Table   397–439
–, Bucky   407

–, BUCKYMAT
– –, magazine technique and film
     processor   407
–, catheterization
– –, KOORDINAT   425
–, Gilmer   410
–, KLINOSKOP
– –, Kress   416
–, (for) radiographs   406
–, tilting   415–423
– –, FLUOREX
– – –, (with) image intensi-
     fier   443
– –, Kress   416
– –, OMNISKOP   418f
– –, (with) overtable tube
     418–422
– –, POLYSTAR universal   422
– –, principle   418
– –, (with) PUCK film chang-
     er   421
– –, (with) remote control   420
– –, (with) tube under table
     top   415–418
– –, UROSKOP B   423
–, tomography
– –, POLYTOME   434
–, top
– –, carbon-fibre   408
– –, floating   408
– –, lock-in   408
– –, plastic   408
–, (for) urological examina-
     tions   422
Technical factors   67–72, 100f,
     105, 117f, 132, 143f, 164
–, exposure technique improve-
     ments   68f
–, mammographic examina-
     tion   102
Teichmann's mixture   236
TELEPANTOSKOP   381
Teleradiography   75
Teleroentgenography   82
Television system *see* TV-system
Temporomandibular joint   278
Tesla instrumentarium   358
Therapy planning   264
Thoracic
–, duct   251f
–, wall   322
Thorax   67–97, 314–322
Three-phase circuit   364
Thrombogenicity   190, 192
Thrombosis   327
Thymus
–, tumour of the   320
Timer   387–389
–, electronic   389
–, photo
Tomogram   104, 263, 410

–, automatic exposure
    control 434
–, curved 269
Tomograph
–, transverse 263
–, whole body 285
Tomography 262f, 270, 350, 370,
    392, 420
–, 3-phase 366
–, abdomen 278f
–, attachments 266
–, chest 276f
–, conventional 265–280, 434f
–, heart 277
–, indication 275f
–, large vessels 277
–, linear 407
– –, UNIVERSAL PLANI-
    GRAPH 434
–, mediastinum 277
–, multiple 270
–, nomenclature 270–272
–, panoramic 269
–, skeletal system 277f
–, system 434
–, table
– –, POLYTOME 434
–, transverse
– –, axial 266, 435
– –, conventional 264
– –, principle of 435
–, universal 435
Tomosynthesis 279
Total body dose 103
Toxic osteopathies 55
Trachea 78
Training requirements 483
Transducer 479
Transformer 364–366, 387
–, AC 374
–, high-frequency 357, 372
–, high-voltage 364, 372
–, single-phase 366
–, Tesla 357
–, windings ratio-control 365
Traumatology 287, 331, 479
Tri-odobenzoic acids 126
Tube
–, bifocal 109
–, current 388
– –, setting 367
–, exchange 399
–, grid-controlled 389
– –, PANTIX 443
–, high-vacuum 342–345
–, holder 362
–, ion 341, 386
– –, water-cooled 373
–, medium-hard
– –, technical parameters 387
–, operation

– –, multiple 366
–, overload 367
–, rectifier
– –, high-voltage 366
–, stand 373
–, voltage 367, 389
– –, measurement for 356
– –, measuring system 390
– –, setting 367
Tuberculosis 415
Tuberculous diseases 51
Tuberculous spondylitis 51f
Tumour 73f, 166
–, (of) bone 331
–, Brown 54
–, (of) chest 81
–, (of) colon 324
–, dental
–, diagnosis 427
–, (of) lymphatic system 256
–, mediastinal 73
–, metastases in the lungs 73
–, oral 278
–, sella turcica 262
–, (of) stomach 324
–, (of) Thymus 320
Tungsten 385
TV 204, 446–448
–, -camera 444, 448
–, -monitor 192
–, operating room 449
–, -system 185, 220
– –, high-resolution 448

U
Ulcera
–, artificial 133
Ulcerative gastritis 138
Ultrasonography 194, 210, 264,
    478
–, duplex-Doppler 208
Ultrasound 303, 479
–, real-time 161
U- or C-arm equipment 193f
Urografin 129
Urography
–, infusion 172f
–, intravenous 263
–, rapid sequence 172
Urokon 125
Urology 422f
Uroselectan 124

V
Valve
–, control 375
–, high-vacuum 364
–, SIMPLEX 367f
–, switching 375
Varices
–, esophageal 209

–, gastric 209
Varicography 238
–, Uroselectan 238
Vascular processes 320f
Vasoconstrictor 208
Vasography 238
Vein 178, 183, 208
–, portal 208
Vena cava inferior
–, anomalies of the 327
Venography 183, 200
–, abdominal 208f
–, portal system 208f
–, splenoportal 183
Venous system 254
Ventricular volumes 227
Ventriculogram 295
Ventriculography 297
Vertebral canal 302f
Vertigraphy 270
Vessels
–, abdominal 200–212
–, peripheral 194, 236–247
–, pulmonary 215
Videodensitometer 227
Videodensitometry 225–227
Videometry 226f
VIDOMATIC 454
Vision
–, three-dimensional 261
Visual characteristics 447
Voltage
–, measurement
– –, non-invasive 384
–, peak 367
–, peak high- 386f
Volume scan 263
Volumetry 225f
Voxel 282

W
Wall motion 229
Walter unit 383
Wash-in phase 290
Wash-out phase 290
Water bag 263
Wave shape 371, 386f
Whipple's disease 147
World Health Organization
    (WHO) 274, 279, 379, 412

X
Xenon 290
–, -enhanced CT 309f
–, stable 289
Xeroradiogram 469
Xeroradiography 105, 412, 469
–, principle 468
X-ray 11
–, biologic effects 33
–, examination

– –, military environment
      411–413
– –, room   362
– –, traumatology   411–413
–, film
– –, double-coated
– – –, microcut   463
–, frequency   475
–, generator   364
– –, three-phase, six-pulse   365
–, METALIX   345
–, plate   462
–, room   405
– –, diagnostic   380
–, shoe store   406
–, system for children
– –, INFANTOSKOP   423
–, tomography   85
X-ray tube   108, 118f, 218,
      338–356, 363
–, 50 kW   379
–, BIANGULIX   349f

–, bimetallic   109
–, (and) breast cancer   354
–, CALOREX   351
–, cooling   343
–, DOFOK   345
–, double focus   345
–, DURALIX   353
–, grid-controlled   382
–, high-vacuum   363
–, Hittorf   339
–, holder
– –, self-centring   399
–, hot cathode   365
–, housing assembly
– –, oil-filled   348
– –, PANTIX P20   348
–, ion   338f
–, lifespan   350
–, Lilienfeld   343
–, mammography   354
–, MAMMUT   342
–, MAMMUT-MEDIA   368, 388

–, MAXIMUS ROTALIX
      ceramic   353
–, MEDIA   345
–, OPTILIX   350, 352
–, output   371
–, PANTIX   347f, 352
–, protective housing   362
–, regeneration   341
–, ROTALIX   347
–, rotating   346
– –, anode   348
–, stand   398–400
–, stereo   261
–, STEREOLIX   352
–, Super ROTALIX   349
–, Super-ROTALIX ceramic   352
–, thermal loading   352
–, TUTO   345f, 380

Z
Zonography   423